Medicine and Clinical Engineering

BERTIL JACOBSON

Karolinska Institute, Stockholm, Sweden

JOHN G. WEBSTER

University of Wisconsin, Madison

Prentice-Hall, Inc., Englewood Cliffs, New Jersey 07632

Library of Congress Cataloging in Publication Data

JACOBSON, BERTIL.
  Medicine and clinical engineering.

  Translation of Medicin och teknik.
  Includes bibliographies and index.
  1. Medicine. 2. Biomedical engineering. I. Webster, John G.,   (date) joint author. II. Title.
[DNLM: 1. Diagnosis. 2. Therapeutics. WB141 J17m]
RC48.J313 1977   616   76-13842
ISBN 0-13-572966-1

10 9 8 7 6 5

Printed in the United States of America

PRENTICE-HALL INTERNATIONAL, INC., *London*
PRENTICE-HALL OF AUSTRALIA PTY. LIMITED, *Sydney*
PRENTICE-HALL OF CANADA, LTD., *Toronto*
PRENTICE-HALL OF INDIA PRIVATE LIMITED, *New Delhi*
PRENTICE-HALL OF JAPAN, INC., *Tokyo*
PRENTICE-HALL OF SOUTHEAST ASIA PTE. LTD., *Singapore*

Contents

PREFACE TO .THE SWEDISH EDITION   xi

PREFACE TO THE AMERICAN EDITION   xiii

1   MEDICAL TERMINOLOGY   1

GENERAL MEDICAL TERMINOLOGY   2

Tissue Terminology   11
    The Cell   *12*
    Tissue Types   *15*
    Body Fluids   *26*
Pathological Terminology   27

TERMINOLOGY OF ORGANS   *35*

Terminology of General Anatomy   *35*
    Parts of the Human Body   *35*
Locomotive System   *42*
    Skeletal System   *42*
    Muscular System   *47*
Metabolic Apparatus   *51*
    Digestive System   *51*
    Respiratory System   *56*
    Circulatory System   *58*
    Excretory System   *67*
Reproductive System   *69*
Skin   *72*
Regulatory Systems   *74*
    Endocrine System   *74*
    Nervous System   *77*
    Regulatory Functions   *88*
Sensory Organs   *96*

2   PHYSICAL DIAGNOSIS   **102**

MEDICAL HISTORY   *105*

PHYSICAL EXAMINATION   *109*

    Inspection   *114*
    Smell   *121*
    Palpation   *122*
    Percussion   *124*
    Auscultation   *127*
    Pressure Measurement   *132*
    Temperature Measurement   *136*
    Reflexes   *138*

CLINICAL DEATH   *140*

3   CARDIOPULMONARY PHYSIOLOGY   **142**

RESPIRATION   *145*
    Lung Function Tests   *146*

CIRCULATION *160*

Hemodynamics *160*
Cardiac Catheterization *161*
Phonocardiography *167*
Blood Pressure Measurement *170*
Blood Flow Determination *174*
Fluid and Tissue Compartments of the Body *184*
Electrocardiography *188*
Measurement Considerations for Electrocardiography *202*
Recording and Transmission of ECG *209*
Computer Analysis of ECG *214*
Cardiac Defibrillation *217*
Pacemaker Therapy *219*

PHYSICAL WORK CAPACITY *227*

4 CLINICAL NEUROPHYSIOLOGY *230*

THE CENTRAL NERVOUS SYSTEM—EEG *232*

Recording Techniques *234*
Wave Types *236*
Provocation of EEG *240*
Clinical Use of EEG *241*
Automatic Signal Analysis of EEG *246*

PERIPHERAL NERVES AND MUSCLES *251*

Electromyography *253*
Conduction Velocities in Motor Nerves *256*
Electroneurography *258*

NEUROPHYSIOLOGICAL MEASUREMENT TECHNIQUES *260*

5 CLINICAL CHEMISTRY AND HEMATOLOGY *267*

MEDICAL DIAGNOSIS WITH CHEMICAL TESTS *270*

Blood *270*
Blood Plasma and Blood Serum *271*
Blood Cells and Blood Diseases *285*
Bleeding Diseases and Blood Clotting *291*

Urine   *293*
    Renal Function   *293*
    Composition of the Urine   *295*
Gastric and Intestinal Juice and Feces   *299*
Cerebrospinal Fluid   *301*

METHODS OF CHEMICAL ANALYSIS   *302*

    Methods of Optical Analysis   *302*
    Methods of Electrochemical Analysis   *307*
    Chromatography   *310*
Automated Analytical Methods   *312*
Automatic Data Processing in Clinical Chemistry   *315*

RADIONUCLIDE METHODS   *318*

6   CLINICAL MICROBIOLOGY AND IMMUNOLOGY   *321*

CLINICAL MICROBIOLOGY   *323*

Microbiological Culture Techniques   *329*
Sterilization and Disinfection   *335*
    Sterilization   *336*
    Disinfection   *338*
Hospital Hygiene   *340*

IMMUNOLOGY   *343*

Antigens and Antibodies   *346*
Immunological Diseases   *350*
Serology   *354*
Technical Aspects of Microbiological Diagnosis   *357*

7   BLOOD AND TRANSPLANTATION   *359*

BLOOD   *360*

Blood-Group Serology   *361*
Blood Transfusions   *369*

TRANSPLANTATION   *372*

Tissue Typing   *374*
Tissue Storage and Preservation   *375*

8   **DIAGNOSTIC RADIOLOGY**   *377*

X-RAY DIAGNOSIS   *377*

Radiography and Fluoroscopy   *378*
Contrast   *380*
X-ray Examination of the Organs   *383*
X-ray Techniques   *399*
The X-ray Object   *399*
X-ray Generators   *402*
Image Detection   *410*
Information Content of Radiographs   *416*
Data Analysis in Diagnostic Radiology   *437*
Quantitative Radiological Measurements   *439*

VISUALIZATION OF ORGANS CONTAINING RADIONUCLIDES   *449*

PHOTOGRAPHY   *453*

VISUALIZATION WITH NONIONIZING RADIATION   *454*

Thermography   *454*
Physical Basis   *455*
Medical Applications of Thermography   *457*
Thermographic Measurement technique   *460*
Ultrasonics   *463*
Physical Principles   *463*
Medical Applications of Ultrasonics   *467*
Technical Aspects of Ultrasonic Diagnosis   *472*

9   **INTERNAL MEDICINE AND GENERAL PRINCIPLES OF TREATMENT**   *479*

General Treatment Principles   *485*
Forms of Treatment   *485*
Pharmacology   *488*
Examples of Treatment for Internal Medical Diseases   *494*

10   SURGERY   500

PRINCIPLES OF SURGICAL TREATMENT   *501*

Antisepsis   *502*
Anesthesia   *505*
　　Regional Anesthesia   *505*
　　General Anesthesia   *508*
Surgical Techniques   *518*
　　Incisional Methods and Similar Procedures   *519*
　　Suturing   *523*
　　Transplantation Techniques   *525*
　　Implantation of Prostheses   *527*
　　Dressing Techniques   *529*

EXAMPLES OF TREATMENT OF SURGICAL DISEASES   *530*

11   INTENSIVE CARE   538

RESPIRATION   *540*
　　Artificial Ventilation and Free Airway   *540*
　　Ventilators   *545*
　　Hyperbaric Treatment with Oxygen   *551*

CIRCULATION   *554*

Cardiac Arrest   *554*
Shock   *557*
Myocardial Infarction   *560*
Extracorporeal Circulation and Assisted Circulation   *562*
　　Heart-Lung Machines   *563*
　　Apparatus for Assisting the Circulation   *568*
　　Artificial Hearts   *569*

INTERNAL ENVIRONMENT AND NUTRITION   *570*

Nutrition   *570*
Fluid Balance   *572*
Electrolyte Balance   *573*
Acid-Base Balance   *574*

DIALYSIS   *577*

　　Hemodialysis   *579*
　　Peritoneal Dialysis   *580*

TECHNICAL ASPECTS OF INTENSIVE CARE *582*

Parameters in Intensive Monitoring *582*
 Respiration *583*
 Blood Circulation *583*
 Level of Consciousness *587*
 Temperature Measurement *587*
Automatic Data Analysis in the Intensive Care Unit *587*
 Automatically Controlled Administration of Drugs *588*

12 OBSTETRICS *591*

Pregnancy *593*
Delivery *599*
 Obstetric Anesthesia *603*
 Obstetric Complications *604*
 Surgical Techniques in Obstetrics *607*
Technical Aspects of Obstetric Diagnosis *610*

13 RADIOTHERAPY AND PHYSICAL THERAPY *615*

RADIOTHERAPY *616*

Radiobiology *619*
Radiophysics *624*
 Treatment Planning *624*
 Dose Measurement *629*

PHYSICAL THERAPY *631*

14 HOSPITAL INFORMATION SYSTEMS *635*

The Medical Record *637*
 Content of the Medical Record *637*
 Design of the Medical Record *640*
Planning of Medical Care *642*
Computer Diagnosis *643*

APPENDIX *645*

INDEX *649*

Preface
to the Swedish Edition

This book presents an introduction to medical diagnosis and therapy. The contents explain how the physician works and the problems that face him. There is an emphasis on the technical aspects of medicine. Medical terminology is introduced throughout the book so that the language of the doctor is readily understood.

The book is intended for medical engineers and other workers in the medical field who are concerned with clinical medicine, including radiophysicists, scientists, physiotherapists, pharmacists, and administrators. The engineering sections may be of interest both to the physician and the surgeon.

The material is arranged to give the reader a picture of what actually happens in the various departments and laboratories of a hospital, rather than according to a logical classification of material. Thus, sections on physiology are found in several of the chapters. The dominant theme is the care of the patient.

The questions inserted in the text serve two purposes; to test knowledge and to present examples. Programmed learning has been somewhat modified to help check the reader's knowledge and to provide further information on typical cases.

The author has found this system more instructive than a strictly programmed presentation. Because these questions contain many new facts, they are also of interest to the reader who does not read the text primarily to answer them.

The preparation of this book has only been made possible by the assistance of many colleagues. Each chapter has been scrutinized by at least two specialists, and the author is indebted to them for their constructive criticism and suggestions. Several hundred students have also made their contributions to improved clarity.

Sylvi Morén typed numerous drafts and the manuscripts of the two editions and read the proofs. Most of the illustrations are ink drawings by Elsa Holmgren made from the author's sketches. He has enjoyed excellent cooperation with them both.

BERTIL JACOBSON

Stockholm, 1975

Preface
to the American Edition

Most of this American edition of the book closely follows the original. This is because medicine in Europe and the United States is practiced according to very similar principles. However, there are subtle differences. These have prompted certain changes, deletions, and additions. Since our aim was to present a book of general application, we felt it necessary in some parts to describe more than one principle, followed by a clear statement of the application areas. The alterations have also resulted in the addition or revision of a few figures. Some of the questions have also been rewritten in the hope of increasing their pedagogic value.

In the Swedish edition, the internationally accepted SI units have been used throughout. In this American edition, we have often retained old units according to current usage and have added SI units in brackets. A conversion table is given in the Appendix.

A preliminary American version of this book was class-tested in a course at the University of Wisconsin-Madison, and in this connection, various chapters were read by specialists. The authors are grateful for the numerous corrections and improvements which resulted. Particular thanks are due to Myrna Larson who rewrote a number of paragraphs in Chapter 7 on blood transfusion problems. Many students also made their contributions.

Again, Sylvi Morén typed, and corrected the manuscripts and read the proofs, and Elsa Holmgren drew new figures and relettered all the previous figures. Their help is greatly appreciated.

The authors welcome suggestions for improvement in concept, emphasis, and clarity.

BERTIL JACOBSON
Department of Medical Engineering,
Karolinska Institute,
S-104 01 Stockholm 60, Sweden

JOHN G. WEBSTER
Department of Electrical and
Computer Engineering,
University of Wisconsin
Madison, Wisconsin 53706

| chapter 1 | # Medical Terminology |

A common language is essential for meaningful communication. To be able to best cooperate with the physician it is important for supporting personnel to possess a knowledge of medical terminology.

The physician's language is often regarded as unnecessarily obscure. So far as the actual terms are concerned, however, the difficulties largely disappear once a knowledge has been acquired of the word-stems, prefixes and suffixes. The medical terms are simply constructed, and unlike the words in engineering specialities, they have the advantage of being international. With a working knowledge of a foreign language a medical text can therefore be read, as long as the internationally accepted medical words, derived from the Greek and Latin, are familiar.

For anyone concerned with the field of medicine and medical research some acquaintanceship with medical terminology is therefore essential. This does not mean, however, that one should prefer the less commonly known expression. In fact, it is important to avoid this where possible until an adequate knowledge of the nuances and the appropriate use of the words has been acquired. To be able to speak a language, one needs more than just to understand it.

To provide an introduction to medical nomenclature, some fundamental concepts in anatomy, physiology and pathology are described in the main body of this chapter. A background of these basic sciences is important for an understanding of all other branches of medicine. The principles applied in investigations in clinical engineering are to a large extent linked with the anatomy and physiology of the organs, and the names of the methods used with these organs are usually derived from their anatomical and physiological terms. Before dealing with the special terminology of the organ systems, certain general principles of the structure of medical language will be outlined.

GENERAL MEDICAL TERMINOLOGY

Medical words and terms are constructed from word-stems, prefixes and suffixes. Use is commonly made of words borrowed from Greek and Latin, a reflection of the fact that so many fundamental discoveries in anatomy and pathology were made during times when these were the languages of the learned. The terms for the organs and organic systems thus provide a structural basis for medical language.

From the nouns are derived the adjectives and adverbs. For instance, a principle division of the windpipe is known as the **bronchus**, which has the adjective **bronchial** and the adverb **bronchially** (Fig. 1.1). Bronchial cancer is a malignant tumor of the windpipe. Bronchial respiratory sounds occur in the

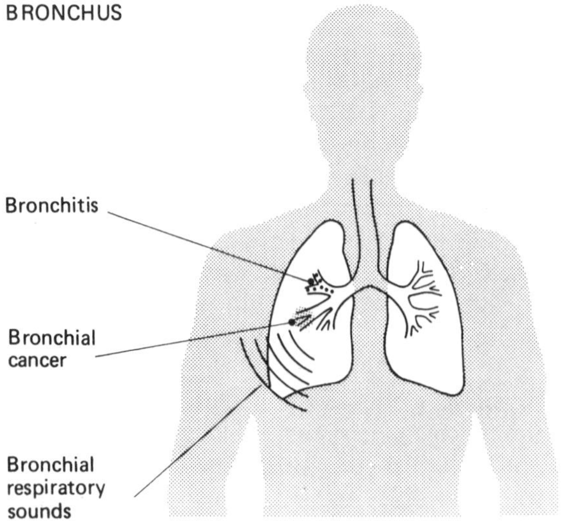

BRONCHUS

Bronchitis

Bronchial cancer

Bronchial respiratory sounds

Figure 1.1 Example of the structure of medical language.

windpipe and can be heard with the aid of a stethoscope by the physician performing a lung examination.

Word-stems are often modified. For example, the word for mouth is **os**, but in the genitive **oris** and in the plural **ora**. A medicine to be administered by mouth is said to be taken **per os** (per, through) or, in the adverbial form, **perorally**, and in the adjectival form by the **peroral** route. In the same way, **abdominal** is the adjective for **abdomen**, **thoracic** for **thorax** (the chest) and **rectal** for **rectum**.

As is evident from the above examples, many originally Greek or Latin nouns and their derivatives are now anglicized in their spelling and endings.

Many words are formed by using prefixes. A medicine injected into a vein is said to be given **intravenously** (intra, in). Certain vaccines are injected into the skin so that a blister forms; they are given **intracutaneously (cutis**, the skin). Other vaccines and many drugs must be given **subcutaneously** or in the **subcutis** (sub, under).

In compound words the endings have greater weight than the prefixes. A chicken hawk is a hawk that hunts chickens, not a chicken that hunts hawks. **Hematuria** is the term for a pathological change in the urine when it contains blood (**hemat-** denotes blood and **-uria** urine); it does not describe the condition when the substances normally excreted in the urine collect in the blood. When this occurs—that is, when the kidneys are unable to eliminate the body's waste products from the blood—the state is known as **uremia** (the ending **-emia** denotes blood).

Many endings are known from general usage. For example, **-logy** denotes a subject and **-logist** a specialist dealing with this subject, biology—biologist. The prefix **oto-** denotes ear so that **otology** is the branch of medicine dealing with ear diseases and an otologist is an ear specialist. The ending **-itis** denotes inflammation, as in **bronchitis**. Inflammation of the ear is known as **otitis**. The word for nose is **rhino** (cf, rhinoceros) so the common cold is called **rhinitis**. The cavity at the upper end of the windpipe is the **larynx**, and inflammation at this site is known as **laryngitis**. The ending **-spasm** denotes cramp; in the larynx this is known as **laryngospasm**, and in the bronchus, as occurs in asthma, **bronchospasm**. The physician's language is thus simply and logically constructed.

The text is followed by a compilation of important facts presented as questions, and further informative material is often presented as brief case histories. Cover the page below each question and try to answer it. When the following square is exposed, the answer to the question will be found on the right. If you did not answer the question correctly refer back to the text.

Question		*Answer*
1.1	Medical terminology contains many words borrowed from .... and	
1.2	One such foreign word is "os" (genitive, oris), which means	Greek Latin

1.3	A sedative must be taken "per os," that is	mouth
1.4	Adjectives are often formed with the ending ...., and adverbs with	by mouth
1.5	A sedative may be taken .... (adverb form) or by the .... (adjectival form) route.	-al -ally
1.6	A physician examines a patient with abdominal pains "per rectum," that is by exploring the .... with a finger.	perorally peroral
1.7	The physician in the previous question performed a .... examination.	rectum
1.8	A gynecologist performs a vaginal examination on a female patient by feeling in the	rectal
1.9	Iron deficiency can be remedied by administering iron ...., that is, by injection into a vein.	vagina
1.10	The ending -itis denotes	intravenously
1.11	Hematuria is a pathological change of the	inflammation
1.12	Uremia is a state in which the waste products of the body accumulate in the	urine
1.13	A person with bronchial inflammation has	blood
1.14	A person with otitis has inflammation of the	bronchitis
1.15	In rhinitis there is secretion from the	ear
1.16	A person with an inflammation of the upper part of the windpipe has	nose
1.17	An oto|rhino|laryngologist is a physician specializing in the	laryngitis
1.18	The study of ear, nose and throat disease is known as	diseases of the ear, nose and throat
		otorhinolaryngology

Some common prefixes

Many of the prefixes used in medical language are also in general use. The following examples show that the original meaning of the prefix has often undergone modification or has been broadened.

a(n)-	without, not	anemia—deficiencies in blood
		anesthesia—lack of feeling
		anesthesiology—the study of methods of anesthesia
		anoxia—deficiency of oxygen
anti-	against	antibacterial—acting against bacteria
		antibiotic—a substance produced synthetically or by certain organisms.and capable of damaging others, especially bacteria
		antispasmodic—relieving spasms or preventing them
bi-	double-, two	bifocal lens—eyeglass lens with two areas of different powers (focal lengths)
		bipolar—having two poles
di-	double, two	dichotomy—cut into two
dys-	bad, mis-, disorder, faulty	dysfunction—disorder of function
		dyspepsia—digestive disorder
		dystrophy—faulty nutrition and growth
end(o)-	within, inward	endogenous—produced within the organism
		endocrine glands—glands secreting into blood
		endoscope—instrument for examining the inside of body cavities
extra-	outside	extraperitoneal—outside the peritoneal membrane
		extrasystole—premature heart beat
hemi-	half, unilateral	hemianopia—defective vision in one half of the visual field
		hemiparesis—slight paralysis affecting one side of the body
hyper-	abnormally high, excessive	hyperemia—excess of blood in a part
		hyperopia—farsightedness
		hypertension—abnormally high blood pressure
		hypertrophy—increased volume due to enlargement of cells or tissue

hyp(o)-	abnormally low, deficient	hypothermia—greatly decreased body temperature
		hypotension—abnormally low blood pressure
		hypotrophy—underdevelopment
		hypoxia—oxygen deficiency in tissues
inter-	between	intercellular—between the cells
		intercostal—between the ribs
		intermittent—occurring at intervals
		interstitial—in spaces in tissue or structure
		intervertebral—between the vertebrae
intra-	within	intra-arterial—within an artery
		intracellular—within the cell
		intracranial—within the cranium
		intramuscular—within the muscle
		intrauterine—within the uterus
		intravascular—within a blood vessel
macr(o)-	large	macrocyte—an abnormally large red blood cell
		macroscopic—visible to the unaided eye
mega-	large	megacolon—excessive dilation of the colon
micro-	small	microcyte—an abnormally small red blood cell
para-	several meanings, including beside, faulty	parallel
		paralysis
		parasite—individual or species nourishing itself at the expense of organisms of another species
		paratyphoid fever—a disease resembling typhoid fever
path(o)-	disease, morbid	pathology—the study of diseases
		pathogenic—producing disease
per-	through	per rectum—through the rectum
		peroral—through the mouth
		perforation—hole through a part
		permeable—porous, not impassable
peri-	around	pericardium—the sac enclosing the heart
		peripheral—remote from the midpoint
		perioral—around the mouth
		periosteum—the membrane covering bones
		peritoneum—membrane lining walls of abdominal and pelvic cavities and covering the viscera

poly-	many	polyarthritis—inflammation of several joints at once
		polysaccharide—macromolecular compound consisting of several monosaccharides
retro-	behind, backward	retrograde—going backwards
		retroperitoneal—located behind the peritoneal membrane
		retrosternal—located behind the sternum
sub-	under	subacute—somewhat acute; between acute and chronic
		subclinical—without clinical manifestations
toxi-, toxo-	poisonous	toxicity—state of being poisonous
		toxicology—the study of poisons and poisoning
		toxicosis—poisoning
		toxin—poison produced by living organisms

1.19	A patient with anuria .... (does, does not) secrete urine.	
1.20	An antirheumatic agent is used .... rheumatism.	does not
1.21	Poison that is produced by bacteria is known as a toxin; a substance counteracting a toxin is called an	against
1.22	Kinesis means movement; a patient with dyskinesia has	antitoxin
1.23	An endoscope is an instrument for examining	difficulty in moving
1.24	In extrauterine pregnancy the fetus develops .... the uterus, for example, in the oviduct or the abdominal cavity.	a body cavity
1.25	A patient with hemiparesis has slight paralysis of one .... of the body.	outside

1.26	An abnormally high blood pressure is known as .... -tension, and abnormally low, as	half
1.27	Intervertebral discs are located .... the vertebral bodies.	hyper- hypotension
1.28	An intrauterine pregnancy is .... (normal, abnormal), since the fetus develops .... the uterus.	between
1.29	The prefix macro- means ...., and mega- means	normal within
1.30	Microtia is a congenital deformity in which the pinna of the ear is too	large large
1.31	The prefix para- has several meanings, including	small
1.32	Pathophysiology is the physiology of the vital functions in	beside, faulty
1.33	Many medicines must be taken .... (through the mouth).	disease
1.34	Inflammation of joints is known as arthritis, inflammation around a joint as	perorally
1.35	A patient with polyneuritis has inflammation of .... nerves.	periarthritis
1.36	The kidneys are located retroperitoneally, that is .... the peritoneal membrane.	several
1.37	The hard membrane covering the brain is known as the dura, the intervening space (under the dura) the .... space.	behind
1.38	The study of poisons and poisoning is known as	subdural
		toxicology

Some common suffixes

Suffixes are formed from nouns, adjectives or verbs. Just as with the prefixes, some suffixes are used also in everyday language.

-algia	pain	myalgia—muscle pain
		neuralgia—nerve pain
-esthesia	feeling	hyperesthesia—abnormally increased sensitivity (to touch)
		hypoesthesia—abnormally diminished sensitivity (to touch)
		paresthesia—abnormal sensation; pins and needles
-gen,	origination	hematogenous—deriving from the blood
-genesis		neurogenic—deriving from the nervous system
-opia,	vision	hemianopia—defective vision in one-half of the visual field
-opsia		hyperopia—farsightedness
-path,	disease	myopathy—disease of the muscles
-pathy		neuropathy—disease of the nerves
		psychopathy—disease of the mind
-plegia	paralysis	hemiplegia—unilateral paralysis
		paraplegia—paralysis of symmetrical muscles, e.g., of both legs
		quadraplegia—paralysis of all four extremities
-scope	viewing	microscope
		endoscope—an instrument for examining inside body cavities
-trophy	nourishment, development	atrophy—wasting
		hypertrophy—increase in volume due to enlargement of existing tissues

1.39	Some .... (neuropathies), cause .... (neuralgia).	
1.40	Some neuropathies cause hyperesthesia, ...	nerve diseases nerve pain
1.41	Malignant tumors can spread hematogenously, that is	increased sensitivity to touch

1.42	A patient with myopia is near-..........	through the blood
1.43	In quadriplegia all four extremities are..........	sighted
1.44	With a proctoscope the rectum can be	paralyzed
1.45	A hypertrophied organ is	viewed
		enlarged

General terminology of diseases

A disease can produce physical—**somatic**—or mental—**psychic**—symptoms. A **psychosomatic** disease has mental causes but produces bodily symptoms.

Symptoms vary in **duration** from a brief moment to years. They can **progress**, remain unchanged **(stationary)** or subside **(regress)**.

The cause, or **genesis**, of a disease may be known or unknown. Diseases vary in their frequency of occurrence in a population. The frequency, or **morbidity**, is usually indicated by the number of cases per thousand (or per million) of the population per year. The frequency of death from a particular disease, the **mortality** (mors, death), is usually expressed as the number of deaths per thousand (or per million) of the population per year. A disease leading to death is **lethal**—fatal.

1.46	A psychosomatic disease has mental causes but produces .... symptoms.	
1.47	Most diseases probably have at least a contributing mental cause, although they usually are considered to be of physical origin. It is difficult to know how to characterize a broken leg of an alcoholic. His alcohol problems are very likely of .... (mental) origin but his broken leg of .... (physical) origin even if the accident occurs because of intoxication.	physical
1.48	A disease can be progressive, i.e. .... or regressive, i.e.	psychic somatic
1.49	Genesis of a disease refers to its .... and the ending -gen means	getting worse getting better
1.50	The morbidity for the common cold is about .... and the mortality about	cause causing or producing

1.51	A lethal disease is	1,000 (or million), i.e. nearly everyone gets it 0 (almost no one dies from it)
		fatal

TISSUE TERMINOLOGY

The human body is composed of cells. After fertilization of the ovum, this divides repeatedly, and at first a group of similar cells appears. Later on, however, cells differing in size, appearance and function develop. Groups of similar cells are referred to as **tissue**. Tissue has a structure that gives it a certain consistency and color but no particular shape.

Different tissues make up the **organs** of the body, which, however, have a specific shape and position in the body. The organs contain both tissue that furnishes some mechanical strength, and specialized tissue that gives a particular function. The liver, for example, consists of connective tissue and gland tissue, in which a vital part of the body's metabolism occurs. Similarly, the lungs contain a tissue that enables gaseous exchange between the blood and air to occur. Such tissue that is specific for the organ is known as **parenchyma**—e.g., liver parenchyma, lung parenchyma and kidney parenchyma. The organs also contain other tissues, such as nerve, muscle, connective tissue, etc.

A number of organs can function in **coordination** as a system. For example, the heart, arteries, capillaries and veins together constitute the circulatory system.

1.52	A group of cells of the same type is called	
1.53	The organs of the body are composed of various	tissue
1.54	The parenchyma is the tissue that is . . . . for a particular organ.	tissues
1.55	A tissue . . . . (has, does not have) a given shape.	specific
1.56	A number of organs in the body that function in a coordinated manner form a	does not have

1.57	The tissue that is specific for a particular organ is known as	system
		parenchyma

The Cell

A cell consists of a core, the **nucleus**, and a cell body, the **cytoplasm**, surrounded by a **cell membrane**. The nucleus contains the carriers of the biological units of heredity, the **genes**. These consist of chromatin granules, which coalesce during cell division to form **chromosomes** (Fig. 1.2). The genes are coded by the

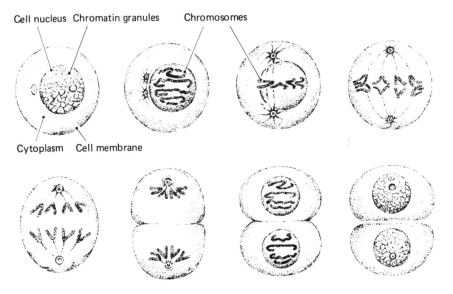

Cell nucleus   Chromatin granules   Chromosomes

Cytoplasm   Cell membrane

Figure 1.2 During cell division the chromatin granules in the cell nucleus gather into clumps and chromosomes are formed. These divide into identical halves, producing daughter cells, where the chromosomes again dissociate into chromatin granules.

structural arrangement of nucleic acids—the most important substance in the cell nuclei.

The cells differ in size. The smallest ones in the body are about 5 μm across and the largest, the ova, are 250 μm. An erythrocyte (red blood cell) is 7.5 μm.

About 75 percent of a cell is water, while the greater part of the solid constituents are proteins. Cells also contain fats, carbohydrates and inorganic salts. The proteins consist almost entirely of enzymes, which control the chemical processes in the cell.

Cells display certain characteristics of life: metabolism, motility, irritability and a capacity for reproduction.

Cell metabolism occurs through the uptake of nutrients and oxygen from the surrounding fluid. The substances taken up are broken down and converted into substances, many of which have a chemical composition specific for the individual. The nutrients are also burned by means of the oxygen taken up, thereby providing the energy required for the cell metabolism. The waste products then formed and the carbon dioxide produced during cell respiration are excreted into the fluid surrounding the cell.

Motility differs greatly according to the type of cell. In all cells the fine granules move in the cytoplasm. Many cells have also specific forms of motility: white blood cells move like amoebas in their search for foreign organisms, and muscle cells have the power of contraction. Cells that cover many of the mucous membranes of the body are furnished with hairs—**cilia**—which have the power of movement. The cilia on the surface of these cells cause a film of liquid on the mucosa to move by means of periodic undulating wavy movements, which are synchronized for closely spaced cells.

The **irritability** also differs widely from one type of cell to another. Nerve and muscle tissues show the greatest irritability. It is characteristic that if some part of a cell in these tissues is subjected to a stimulus that exceeds a threshold, this stimulus spreads to the entire cell. The stimulus may be chemical, electrical, optical, thermal or mechanical.

Cells **reproduce** by division. For many tissues, such as bone marrow and lymphatic tissue, the rate of cell division is high; on the other hand, there is no cell division after birth for nerve cells.

cyt(o)-, **-cyte**	cell	cytology—the scientific study of cells cytoplasm—cell body erythrocyte—red blood cell leukocyte—white blood cell

1.58	Nucleus means . . . . and cytoplasm	
1.59	The biological units of heredity, the . . . . , are coded through the . . . . arrangement of the nucleic acids present in the cell nucleus.	cell core cell body
1.60	Cells vary widely in size according to their type, ranging from . . . . to	genes structural

1.61	About .... percent of a cell is water.	5 μm 250 μm
1.62	The solid constituents of cells consist mainly of ....; there are also small amounts of ...., ... and	75
1.63	Cells display four characteristics of life, namely ...., ..., ... and	proteins fats carbohydrates salts
1.64	Cell metabolism occurs: through the .... of nutrients and oxygen from the surrounding fluid; through the partial .... of the substances taken up (to obtain energy); through the .... of the substances taken up (into those required by the individual); and through the .... of waste substances and carbon dioxide (into the surrounding fluid).	metabolism motility irritability reproduction
1.65	Some cells have a pronounced motility; for example, ... move like amoebas.	uptake combustion conversion excretion
1.66	Some cells that cover many of the mucous membranes of the body are provided with ...., which, by undulating movements, can move a film of fluid on the surface of the membrane.	white blood cells
1.67	The tissues having the greatest irritability are .... and .... tissues.	cilia
1.68	The stimulus may be ...., ..., ..., ... or .... in type.	nerve muscle
1.69	In bone marrow and lymph tissue the rate of cell division is .... (high, low).	chemical electrical optical thermal mechanical
1.70	Cell division does not occur after birth in .... tissue.	high
		nerve

Tissue Types

There are five different types of tissue: epithelial, connective, muscle, nerve and fluid tissue.

Epithelial tissues

All surfaces of the body, both external and internal, are covered by epithelial tissue. It follows that there are different types of epithelial tissue, which differ greatly in their function and appearance (Fig. 1.3). The epithelial tissue of the skin not only protects the body against infections, but among other things, regulates the body temperature by evaporation of liquid. The thin epithelial cells of the blood capillaries enable an exchange of oxygen, carbon dioxide and many other inorganic and organic substances to take place between tissues and blood. The

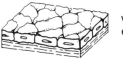
Vascular epithelium

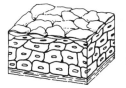
Dermal epithelium

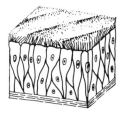
Ciliated epithelium

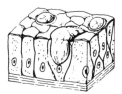
Glandular epithelium

Figure 1.3 Epithelial tissues of various kinds cover the body surfaces.

mucous membrane of the intestines takes up nutrients from the food; together with the epithelial cells of the large glands, namely, the liver and the pancreas, it also secretes juices necessary for digestion. The cells having the specific function of secreting these fluids are known as **glandular epithelium**.

There are two kinds of glands. **Exocrine** glands secrete to a free surface—for example, salivary glands to the mouth, the glands of the gastric and intestinal mucous membranes, and the liver and the pancreas, to the gastrointestinal tract; the prostate gland to the urethra; and the sweat and sebaceous glands to the skin. **Endocrine** glands have no secretory ducts, and their products, **hormones**, enter the blood. The endocrine glands are part of the endocrine organ system, which regulates the function of many other organs in the body.

Other epithelial cells are converted to **sensory epithelium**, and they constitute the most important functional parts of the sensory organs. Sensory stimuli are received by the cells of the sensory epithelium and the stimulus is transduced into a form suitable for processing by the nervous system.

1.71	The tissue covering the surface of the body is known as . . . . tissue.	
1.72	Epithelial tissue covers both . . . . and . . . . surfaces of the body.	epithelial
1.73	By means of epithelial tissue an . . . . of organic and inorganic substances takes place between tissues and blood.	internal external
1.74	Epithelial tissue that produces secretion is known as	exchange
1.75	Glands that secrete to free surfaces are known as . . . . glands.	glandular epithelium
1.76	Glands producing secretion that enters the blood circulation are known as . . . . glands.	exocrine
1.77	In the sensory organs certain epithelial cells are converted into . . . . , which transduces sensory stimuli into a form suitable for processing by the nervous system.	endocrine
		sensory epithelium

Connective tissue

The body's mechanical stability and strength are provided by the connective tissue: **fibrous tissue, adipose tissue, cartilage** and **bone**. A characteristic of connective tissue is that the actual cells make up only a small part of the volume of these tissues (except for the adipose cells, which are filled with fat); the greater part consists of intercellular substances, which give this tissue its mechanical properties (Fig. 1.4). The intercellular substance contains **collagen** fibers, which

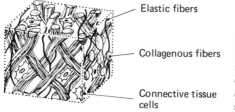

Elastic fibers

Collagenous fibers

Connective tissue cells

Figure 1.4 In connective tissue, collagenous fibers provide tensile strength and elastic fibers provide elasticity. The connective tissue cells are interspersed in the intercellular space.

have great tensile strength, and **elastic** fibers, which have great elasticity like rubber. Both consist of proteins. The mechanical properties of the connective tissue depend on the relative number of these fibers. The least elastic are the tendons, which consist mainly of collagenous connective tissue fibers.

In addition to the collagenous and elastic fibers there are other intercellular substances. Thus, bone contains bone mineral, an inorganic salt of calcium and phosphorus (hydroxyapatite). Just as reinforcing iron rods give greater strength to the cement in concrete, so the collagenous fibers reinforce the bone.

lip(o)-	fat, adipose	lipids—fat and fat-like substance lipoma—a fatty tumor lipemia—abnormally elevated fat content of the blood
oste(o)-	bone, skeleton	osteology—the scientific study of the skeleton osteogenetic—deriving from the skeleton osteogenic—forming bone osteoporosis—reduced bone mass, resulting in lack of strength

---

1.78   The mechanical stability and strength of the body are provided by the connective tissues: . . . . tissue, ... tissue, ... and . . . .

1.79	A common feature of connective tissues is that they are held together by two types of fibers, namely, ... and	fibrous adipose cartilage bone
1.80	The collagenous and elastic fibers constitute an important part of the . . . . substance of the connective tissues.	collagenous elastic
1.81	The collagenous fibers have a high	intercellular
1.82	The elastic fibers have high	tensile strength
1.83	Besides collagen fibers the intercellular substance of bone contains	elasticity
1.84	Bone mineral consists of an inorganic compound containing . . . . and	bone mineral
1.85	Osteosarcoma is a malignant tumor of	calcium phosphorus
1.86	A person has had a swelling on the back for a number of years. The swelling can be displaced relative to the skin. The physician says it is a lipoma, that is to say, a benign tumor consisting of	the skeleton (bone)
		fat

Muscular tissue

There are in the body three types of muscle. The first type is **smooth muscle**, which is not under voluntary control. The second type is skeletal muscle or **striated muscle**, which is under voluntary control. The third type is **heart muscle**, which is similar to skeletal muscle in that it is striated, but is different in that it is not under voluntary control. A common feature of all three types of muscle is that the cells have the power of active contraction.

Smooth muscle consists of cells of varying lengths. The cells are spindle-shaped fibers, about 0.1 mm long. Such smooth muscle is found in, for example, the gastrointestinal tract, the bronchi, the uterus, the urinary bladder and the iris. The contraction of smooth muscle is often modified by the brain via the autonomic nervous system (page 87).

In striated muscle each muscle is composed of a large number of **muscle fibers**, 1–40 mm long and 0.01–0.1 mm in diameter. Each fiber consists of a muscle cell.

which has transverse lighter and darker parts; hence the term "striated". The power from the muscle fibers is transmitted via connective tissue fibers to tendons, which are usually attached to skeletal bones.

Fatigue in a muscle is due partly to consumption of the nutrients, which provide energy for contraction, and partly to accumulation of the products of contraction, such as pyruvic and lactic acids. Fatigue occurs not only in the actual muscle but also in the motor nerve cells and in conduction paths between nerve and muscle. The nervous system is affected by fatigue more rapidly than the muscle itself.

Muscular contraction requires energy, which is derived from the liberation of chemically bound energy, mainly from adenosine triphosphate (ATP), which is converted to the lower energy form: adenosine diphosphate (ADP). ADP is normally reconverted to ATP by an **aerobic** (oxygen-demanding) process. Here, glucose is oxidized, yielding carbon dioxide, water and chemical energy. When high muscular performance is required, ADP can also be reconverted to ATP by an **anaerobic** process (non-oxygen-demanding), which occurs when the demand on the muscle exceeds the available amount of oxygen. The balance between the various energy-rich compounds in the muscle is then disturbed, and the oxygen consumption is elevated a fairly long time after the muscular work has ceased in order to correct the **oxygen deficit**.

my(o)-	muscle	myoglobin—a red protein in muscle myoma—a tumor consisting of muscle cells myocarditis—inflammation of the heart muscle

1.87	There are three kinds of muscle in the body, ..., ... and	
1.88	The .... muscle can be contracted voluntarily.	smooth muscle striated muscle heart muscle
1.89	The .... muscle and .... muscle cannot be contracted voluntarily.	striated
1.90	In the gastrointestinal tract, bronchi, uterus, urinary bladder and iris there is .... muscle.	smooth heart
1.91	Smooth muscle fibers are about .... long.	smooth
1.92	Muscle fibers in striated skeletal muscle are .... in length and .... in diameter.	0.1 mm

1.93	Contraction of muscle requires energy. This is obtained first by oxidation of .... (substance), which then supplies energy to the muscle cells via the reaction: ATP⇌ADP.	1–40 mm 0.01–0.1 mm
1.94	This process is normally aerobic, that is to say, it	glucose
1.95	For high energy output, energy can be developed for a short period through a process not requiring oxygen, that is an .... process.	demands oxygen
1.96	There is then a temporary .... in the muscle.	anaerobic
1.97	A myoma is a benign tumor that is often located in the uterus and consists of	oxygen deficit
1.98	The root "*cardi*(o)" denotes heart. The heart muscle is therefore called the .... -cardium.	muscle cells
		myo

Nerve tissue

Nerve tissue is constructed from **nerve cells** and **glial cells**. The glial tissue has a supporting function and is also considered to participate in the metabolism of the nerve cells.

The functional unit of the nervous system is the nerve cell or the **neuron**.

Each nerve cell body has several short processes, or **dendrites**, and a long nerve fiber, an **axon**, which can have many branches (Fig. 1.5).

The neurons form an extremely complex network, which connects all parts of the body. While the size of the central body of the nerve cell is the same as that of the other cells of the body (10–$100\,\mu$m), the axon can be a meter in length. For example, the axons of the foot muscle originate in the lower part of the spinal cord, where the associated nerve cells are located.

Information is transmitted through an axon by means of short impulses of constant amplitude, in accordance with the "all-or-nothing law" (cf, the monostable flip-flop of engineering). When the stimulation threshold is exceeded, a nerve impulse is generated and conducted along the axon at a speed dependent on its diameter. For axons of 20 and $0.5\,\mu$m the velocity is about 100 and 0.5 m/s, respectively. The duration of the impulse is about 1 ms. The information is coded through the rate of conducted impulses—a process known as pulse frequency

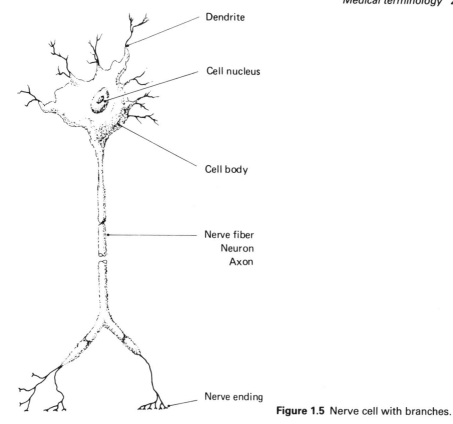

Dendrite

Cell nucleus

Cell body

Nerve fiber
Neuron
Axon

Nerve ending

Figure 1.5 Nerve cell with branches.

modulation. This nervous activity, which is of a biochemical nature, is accompanied by electrical phenomena which can be picked up and recorded (see also Chapter 4).

A connection between two excitable cells, in the form of a contact surface between a neuron and another cell (a neuron, a muscle cell, a sensory cell, etc) is called a **synapse**. In the nervous system there are thus a large number of synapses between each neuron and the cell bodies of other neurons, the dendrites of neurons, and branched end-fibers of the axons (Fig. 1.6). In the synapse a nerve impulse can be transmitted, blocked, changed from a simple to a repetitive pulse or integrated with impulses from other nerve cells. This leads to complex impulse patterns in subsequent cells, depending on the function of the synapse.

In the synapse the information is carried by a chemical substance called a **neurotransmitter**, which diffuses across the gap. The nerve cells synthesize the neurotransmitters, of which two types are known: **acetylcholine** and **norepinephrine** (noradrenalin). The two types of nerves that contain them are different and are called cholinergic and adrenergic, respectively.

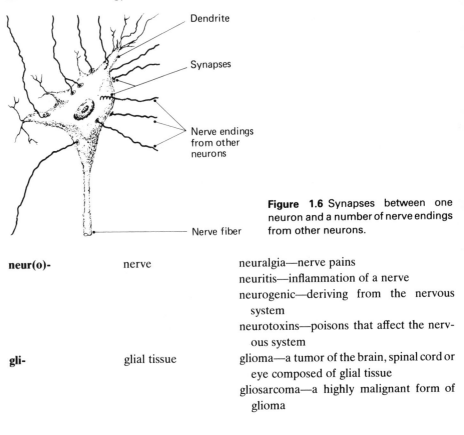

Figure 1.6 Synapses between one neuron and a number of nerve endings from other neurons.

neur(o)-	nerve	neuralgia—nerve pains neuritis—inflammation of a nerve neurogenic—deriving from the nervous system neurotoxins—poisons that affect the nervous system
gli-	glial tissue	glioma—a tumor of the brain, spinal cord or eye composed of glial tissue gliosarcoma—a highly malignant form of glioma

1.99	The brain tissue consists of .... cells and .... cells.	
1.100	The functional unit of the nervous system is the	nerve glial
1.101	A dendrite is a .... (short, long) process from a neuron.	neuron (nerve cell)
1.102	The long process from a neuron is called an	short
1.103	The body of the nerve cell measures between .... and	axon
1.104	The axon can be .... long.	10 μm 100 μm

1.105	Connections between nerve cells are called	1 m
1.106	The structure in which nerve impulses can be conducted, blocked, altered or integrated is known as a	synapses
1.107	The "all-or-nothing law" means that an impulse is spread throughout the axon if the neuron receives a stimulus exceeding the	synapse
1.108	The velocity of conduction in thick neurons is .... m/s and in thin neurons .... m/s.	threshold
1.109	In the nervous system the information is coded by means of .... modulation.	100 0.5
1.110	The scientific study of the physiology of the nervous system is known as	pulse frequency
1.111	Gliosarcoma is a highly malignant form of tumor known as a glioma, which is formed from glial tissue, one of the .... of the body.	neurophysiology
		nerve tissues

Liquid tissue

The liquid tissues of the body are the blood and lymph. Blood consists of **plasma** and **blood cells**. Plasma contains proteins, inorganic salts, varying amounts of nutrients, products of metabolism and hormones.

There are three kinds of formed elements in the blood, see Fig. 1.7. The red cells—the **erythrocytes**—of which there are about 4.5 million per μl, are

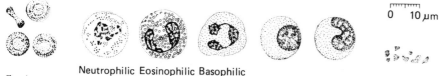

0   10 μm

Erythrocytes   Neutrophilic   Eosinophilic   Basophilic   Lymphocyte   Monocyte   Thrombocytes
            granulocyte   granulocyte   granulocyte

Figure 1.7 Various types of blood cells. The granulocytes are designated according to their reaction to stains.

biconcave discs with a diameter of about 7.5 μm. They contain the protein **hemoglobin**, which transports oxygen and carbon dioxide. The white cells—**leukocytes**—number about 5000 per μl, and measure 6–20 μm in diameter. They are concerned with, among other things, the body's defenses against infections and foreign substances. There are several types of leukocytes: eosinophilic, basophilic and neutrophilic granulocytes, lymphocytes and monocytes.

The blood platelets, or **thrombocytes**, number about 300,000 per μl, are of irregular shape and measure 1–3 μm. They are necessary for the clotting of the blood.

The lymph consists of lymphatic liquid and white blood cells. The lymph enters the other tissues by filtration of blood plasma through the capillary walls. The lymph is returned to the blood stream via the lymph ducts.

hem(o)- **hemato-**	blood	hemangioma—blood-vessel tumor (page 33) hemodynamics—study of the movement of the blood hemoglobin—protein in blood cells hematogenic—derived from the blood
-emia	blood	uremia—poisoning by urine, caused by nitrogen-containing constituents of the urine remaining in the blood
lymph-	lymph(atic) (oid)	lymphadenitis—inflammation of lymph nodes lymphangioma—benign tumor consisting of dilated lymph ducts lymphangitis—inflammation of lymph ducts lymphatic capillaries—minute vessels for lymph

1.112	The liquid tissues of the body are . . . . and	
1.113	The blood consists of . . . . (liquid) and	blood lymph

1.114	There are three groups of formed elements in the blood: ...., ... and	plasma blood cells
1.115	The erythrocytes contain the blood protein ...., which transports oxygen and carbon dioxide.	erythrocytes (red) leukocytes (white) thrombocytes (platelets)
1.116	The number of erythrocytes in normal blood is about ...., and they have a diameter of	hemoglobin
1.117	Eosinophilic, neutrophilic and basophilic granulocytes, lymphocytes and monocytes are the .... of the blood.	4.5 million/μl 7.5 μm
1.118	The leukocytes number about	white blood cells (leukocytes)
1.119	The formed elements participating in the coagulation of the blood are known as	5,000/μl
1.120	The lymph consists of .... and	thrombocytes (platelets)
1.121	Hematology is the scientific study of .... and its diseases.	lymphatic liquid leukocytes (white blood cells)
1.122	A person has had a hemangioma on his forehead since birth; this is a .... -vessel tumor.	the blood (e.g., the blood forming organs)
1.123	Hematuria is a condition in which the urine contains	blood-
1.124	Hemorrhoids are nodular dilations of .... around the orifice of the rectum.	blood
1.125	Hyperkalemia is a condition in which the .... contains excess potassium ions.	blood vessels (veins)
1.126	The condition in which the blood contains an abnormally small amount of potassium is called	blood
1.127	The presence of urinary constituents in the blood is known as	hypokalemia

1.128	Hyperglycemia is a condition in which the .... contains too .... (much, little) glucose (blood sugar).	uremia
1.129	A patient with diabetes took too large a dose of insulin; the blood sugar concentration has consequently fallen too low, resulting in coma because of .... (Greek term).	blood much
1.130	A patient has neglected a wound on his leg and infection has occurred, leading to lymphangitis and lymphadenitis—that is, spread of infection to lymph .... and lymph	hypoglycemia
		ducts nodes

Body Fluids

The body water accounts for about two thirds of the body weight of a lean person of normal health. About two thirds of this body water is distributed among about 10^{12} cells and comprises the **intracellular** fluid. The remaining third constitutes the **extracellular** fluid. The greater part of this is located in the space between the cells—the **interstitial** fluid. Part of the extracellular fluid is also located in the blood plasma, part in the gastrointestinal tract and part in the cerebrospinal fluid (the liquid surrounding the brain and filling its cavities).

There is a continuous circulation of water between the various fluid compartments of the body (Fig. 1.8). The chemical composition of the fluids in these

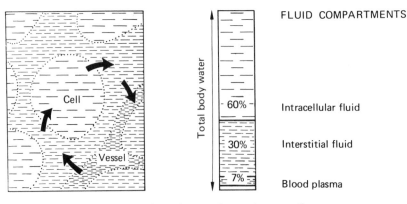

Figure 1.8 There is a constant interchange of water between the different fluid compartments of the body.

compartments varies with the location, however, because of the varying permeability of the cell membrane and capillary walls.

Disturbances in the fluid compartments of the body occur in many pathological conditions. During intensive care, after accidents, or surgical operations, or in other critical conditions, it is of vital importance to maintain the correct **fluid balance** in the body (see also Chapter 11).

1.131	Two thirds of the body water consists of .... fluid, and one third of	
1.132	Blood plasma, the fluid portion of the blood, is part of the .... fluid.	intracellular extracellular
1.133	Because of a stomach infection a child has not taken food or drink for 2 days, and he is dehydrated. The skin is dry and wrinkled and the cheeks hollow, due mainly to the reduction in volume of the interstitial fluid. By intravenous infusion of liquids the child's condition can be improved immediately, since in this way the body's .... is restored.	extracellular
		fluid balance

PATHOLOGICAL TERMINOLOGY

Pathology is the scientific study of the alterations in the body caused by disease. Pathological processes can lead to changes in the tissues—**tissue degeneration**. This can take many forms. In **lipidosis**, fat is deposited in the cells (e.g., fatty degeneration of the liver, in which fat is deposited in the liver parenchyma). In **fibrosis**, conversion to connective tissue takes place. If the tissues are at the same time hardened and possibly calcified, the condition is known as **sclerosis** (e.g., arteriosclerosis, in which the blood vessels are converted to connective tissue and calcium salts are deposited). Local death of tissues is called **necrosis**. If there is also decomposition, **gangrene** develops (e.g., gas gangrene).

These changes have several causes: poisoning (alcohol, bacterial toxins) and oxygen deficiency in lipidosis; infections, mechanical trauma, hormonal and unknown causes in fibrosis and sclerosis; impaired blood supply, bacterial toxins, heat and cold in necrosis.

Tissue degeneration can lead to destruction of the organ; or it can cease when the cause is removed, and **regeneration** of the affected cells and tissues can follow.

-osis	pathological condition	necrosis—tissue death fibrosis—conversion to fibrous tissue sclerosis—conversion to fibrous tissue, especially when the tissue hardens and is possibly calcified lipidosis—deposit of fat in cells

1.134	A patient suffering from chronic alcoholism dies from a mild infectious disease, due to, among other things, impairment of liver function resulting from lipidosis—that is to say, ... in the liver parenchyma.	
1.135	Arteriosclerosis is a disease that occurs mainly in elderly people, and results in . . . . of the vessel walls.	deposition of fat
1.136	Necrosis is . . . . , gangrene is necrosis accompanied by	calcification
1.137	Conversion of tissues or organs to nonfunctioning tissue is known as	tissue death decomposition
1.138	Reconstruction of tissue through the formation of new cells is known as	degeneration
		regeneration

Circulatory disorder

Many pathological conditions are due to disorders of the blood circulation. Irradiation with ultraviolet light, infection and many other conditions result in reddening of the skin—**hyperemia**. This is due to an increase in the blood flow through the superficial tissue layers, owing to dilation of the fine arteries. In obstruction of flow, **stasis** occurs, and the tissues contain an increased amount of blood that is not saturated with oxygen. The tissue then takes on a bluish hue and is said to be **cyanotic** (blue coloration, **cyanosis**). When there is an abnormal increase in the interstitial tissue fluid, swelling or **edema** results.

A particular form of circulatory disorder is **pulmonary edema** in which fluid from the blood plasma (serous fluid) passes into the alveolar sacs. This may be due to a number of pathological conditions; the cause is often heart failure, resulting in too high a pressure in the pulmonary vein (see Chapter 9, page 497).

Lowering of the blood supply by a reduction of the flow in an artery causes a local deficiency of blood, **ischemia**. A general deficiency of the quantity of hemoglobin in the blood is known as **anemia**. Another word for bleeding is **hemorrhage**—e.g. cerebral hemorrhage (*cerebrum*, brain). A local collection of blood in the tissues is called a **hematoma**. When the blood coagulates in the vessels a clot, or **thrombus**, forms.

The clot can become detached and be carried by the blood stream to another site where it may obstruct a vessel—**embolus**. If the clot is so large that the affected part of the tissue dies this affected part is called an **infarct**.

Emboli can also arise in other ways. If air enters the vascular system—for example, through a hole in a vein, where the blood pressure is negative—an air embolus appears. In the case of major bone fractures, fat droplets can detach from the bone marrow and produce fat emboli.

1.139	Hyperemia is the presence of a local excess of	
1.140	Obstruction of blood flow is known as	blood
1.141	To become "blue with cold" is, in medical language, to become . . . .; in other words, ... occurs.	stasis
1.142	A person awakens one morning with "swollen eyes"—that is to say, eyelid	cyanotic cyanosis
1.143	A patient has been troubled for some time by fatigue and giddiness, and has fainted on several occasions. The patient, who is very pale, may have a reduced quantity of hemoglobin, i.e.	edema
1.144	A deficient local blood supply is known as isch-	anemia
1.145	A boy is punched in the eye and a "black eye" results; that is, the boy is said to have developed a	emia
1.146	An elderly patient has cerebral hemorrhage—that is, ...	hematoma
1.147	After a major abdominal operation blood coagulates in a vein in the lower leg; venous . . . . has developed.	bleeding in the brain

1.148	When the clot is detached and carried away in the blood stream to and through the heart an .... arises, and sudden death may follow due to blocking of the pulmonary artery.	thrombosis (blood clot formation)
1.149	In an automobile accident a person receives multiple fractures of the legs, and fat droplets in the bone marrow are detached and carried in the blood stream through the heart and to the lung capillaries where they lodge. The patient cannot get his breath due to impaired oxygenation of the blood. The patient is said to have developed	embolus
1.150	In an injury to the neck, air enters the veins and is carried by the blood to the lungs, where due to the high surface tension between air and blood, the air bubbles block the finer blood capillaries. An .... is formed.	fat emboli
		air embolus

Inflammation and infection

Inflammation is a state of irritation of a tissue. The irritation is often due to **infection**—that is, to the entry of bacteria or virus into the body. Inflammation can, however, also arise in other ways—for example, due to the effect of chemical substances or irradiation. The term "inflammation" thus denotes a condition of the tissue; "infection" denotes an abnormal presence of microorganisms.

An inflammation provides four early signs of disease. Hyperemia produces **reddening** of the skin and increased tissue **warmth**; **swelling** and **pain** also occur early.

Many changes in tissues and organs are due to infections. An infection near a body cavity can result in an inflammatory discharge of fluid in it—**exudate**. In body cavities, stones—**concretions**—can also form; for example, renal concretions (nephrolithiasis—kidney stone) and bile-duct concretions (cholelithiasis—gallstone). If tissue decomposes, there may be an accumulation of **pus**—an **abscess**. If the abscess is not drained, but the infection spreads to the blood stream, **bacteremia** occurs. This can result in hematogenous spread to other organs. If this bacteremia is severe, there may be fever and the condition is then called **sepsis**. A further stage in the pathological process is reached when clumps of bacteria circulate in the blood—this is known as **pyemia**, or pus in the blood. Toxins excreted by the bacteria in the blood can produce blood poisoning, or **toxemia**.

-itis	inflammation	otitis—inflammation of the ear
		hepatitis—inflammation of the liver
		nephritis—inflammation of the kidneys
-lith	stone	nephrolithiasis—kidney stone
lithiasis		cholelithiasis—gallstone

1.151	If a tissue is irritated by microorganisms, chemical substances, etc, it is in a state of	
1.152	The abnormal presence of disease-producing microorganisms in the body is known as	inflammation
1.153	Early signs of inflammation are ...., ..., ... and	infection
1.154	A patient with a lung disease has exudate in the pleural cavity—that is, a .... into it.	reddening warmth swelling pain
1.155	After repeated urinary tract infection which ascended into the kidneys, a patient has concretions in these; that is	discharge of fluid
1.156	When there is decomposition of tissues with the accumulation of pus, an .... has formed.	kidney stones (nephrolithiasis)
1.157	An abscess is filled with	abscess
1.158	Bacteremia, sepsis and pyemia are conditions with an ascending degree of severity, in which .... circulate in the	pus
1.159	Toxemia is	bacteria blood

1.160	After an illegal abortion, performed with nonsterile instruments, the woman develops an infection of the uterus. The infection spreads to the blood stream and . . . . results. High fever and chills develop and the patient is admitted to hospital with a diagnosis of . . . . The patient dies after a day or so from pus in the blood, or . . . . At autopsy, purulent foci are found in several organs due to . . . . (via the blood circulation) spread of the bacteria. The organs also show the effect of bacterial toxins due to the . . . . (blood poisoning) that developed.	blood poisoning
		bacteremia sepsis pyemia hematogenous toxemia

Tumor diseases

A tumor—**neoplasm**—is an uncontrolled growth of cells that serve no useful purpose. Tumors displace and destroy surrounding normal tissue. Toxic products are also produced, which have a general detrimental effect on the body.

Tumors may be **benign** or **malignant**. An untreated malignant tumor kills the patient wherever it grows in the body, even if it is in a hand or a foot. A benign tumor can lead to death only if it happens to obstruct a vital organ, such as the brain.

Tumors originate in any of the normal tissues of the body and are designated accordingly; for example, myoma—muscle tumor. The more the various tumor cells differ from the cells of the original tissue, the more malignant the tumor generally is. Such a tumor is, however, more sensitive to radiation than a tumor composed of cells that more closely resemble the various cells in the tissue giving rise to the tumor.

A malignant tumor **infiltrates** the surrounding tissue and the tumor cells grow in between the normal cells. Therefore, it is difficult to be sure that all the tumor cells have been removed. A benign tumor has borders that are well defined. It grows like a bladder then gradually **expands**, displacing the normal tissue. In a malignant tumor, there is a high rate of cell division which can be seen under the microscope, whereas in a benign tumor none of the cells can be seen to divide.

A malignant tumor extends in various ways: by **infiltrative** growth, by spread of tumor cells **via** the **blood** vessels and **lymph** ducts (see emboli, page 29), and by **implantation**—that is, by dissemination of daughter tumors in body cavities such as the abdomen. Spread by implantation can also occur during a surgical operation if tumor cells are transferred to healthy tissue in the operative field.

The tissue from which dissemination has occurred is known as the **primary tumor**; secondary tumors are daughter tumors or **metastases**, which have originated from the primary tumor.

-oma	tumor in general	fibroma—connective tissue tumor (benign) lipoma—fat tumor (benign)
-angioma	tumor from vascular tissue	hemangioma—blood-vessel tumor (benign) lymphangioma—lymph-duct tumor (benign)
-carcinoma	malignant tumor from epithelial tissue	adenocarcinoma—malignant tumor from glandular tissue
-sarcoma	malignant tumor from connective tissue	osteosarcoma—malignant tumor in bone lymphosarcoma—malignant tumor originating from lymphoid tissue
glioma	tumor originating from glial cells in nerve tissue	

1.161	Neoplasm is another word for	
1.162	A tumor that infiltrates is said to be .... and one that does not is said to be	tumor
1.163	Tumors can originate from any of the body's normal	malignant benign
1.164	A malignant tumor displays .... growth.	tissues
1.165	A benign tumor displays .... growth.	infiltrative
1.166	Microscopic examination of malignant tumors discloses a high rate of	expansive
1.167	A malignant tumor spreads in three ways, by .... growth, by spread of tumor cells via .... and .... or by .... (dissemination of daughter tumors in a body cavity or in the area of an operation).	cell division

1.168	A female patient is operated on for a nodule in a breast, which microscopic examination shows to be a fibroma—that is, a tumor originating from .... tissue.	infiltrative blood vessels lymph ducts implantation
1.169	During surgery on the patient in the previous question no metastases were found because the tumor was a .... one.	connective
1.170	An osteosarcoma originates from .... tissue.	benign
1.171	A patient was troubled for a year by alternating constipation and diarrhea, with bloody stools and hemorrhoids. Examination disclosed a tumor in the colon, an adenocarcinoma, which was removed surgically. At the operation .... (daughter tumors) were found, since there had been spreading from the tumor, which was a .... one.	bone
		metastases malignant

Trauma

An injury produced by external force is called a **trauma**; the science of the associated diseases is known as **traumatology**. An external blow can cause a **wound** (cut), **perforation** (hole), **rupture** (break), **contusion** (bruise), **dislocation** (displacement of bones in a joint) or **fracture** (break in a bone).

1.172	A motorcyclist has an accident and his head hits the ground. The physician finds five problem areas. The motorcyclist suffers from skull	
1.173	He has cuts, ..., on the right hand.	trauma
1.174	Rupture, ..., of the right Achilles tendon occurred.	wounds
1.175	There was .... of the left shoulder-joint.	breaking
1.176	There was also a fracture, ..., of the lower leg.	dislocation

1.177	At many places on the body there were contusions, or	break
		bruises

TERMINOLOGY OF ORGANS

A knowledge of the structure of the living body and its function is essential for an understanding of all aspects of medicine. The science of the structure of the body is known as **anatomy**, and that of its function, **physiology**.

Anatomy is divided according to different bases. **Gross anatomy** is the study of the structure of the organs as seen by the naked eye on dissection. The shape, size, components and appearance are described. **Topographical anatomy** deals with the position of the organs in relation to each other, for example, as they are seen in sections through the body in different planes. **Microscopic anatomy** or **histology** is the study of the minute structure of the organs by means of various kinds of microscopy (light, phase contrast, polarization, interference, electron and x-ray microscopy). One special field of histology is **cytology**, in which the structure, function and development of the cells are studied.

For practical reasons, gross anatomy is described and systematized in somewhat different ways by different medical specialists; one speaks, for example, of surgical, pathological and radiological anatomy.

Physiology can also be divided into different bases. In its general sense the term **physiology** relates to the normal function of the organs of the body. The vital functions of the cells are studied in **cell physiology**. The pathological functions of organs are treated in **pathophysiology**. In addition, a division into various sub-areas dealing with different organs can be made; in **circulatory physiology** the blood circulation is studied, in **respiratory physiology** the breathing and in **renal physiology** the excretory organs.

TERMINOLOGY OF GENERAL ANATOMY

Parts Of The Human Body

The body is divided into the head, neck, trunk and extremities (Fig. 1.9). The head consists of the **face** and **skull** (cranium). The head is connected to the trunk by the **neck**. The trunk consists of the **thorax, abdomen** and **pelvis**. These three parts form a cavity in which the **viscera** are located. This cavity is divided into two parts by a hemispherical muscle, the **diaphragm**; the upper part contains the organs of the chest, and the lower part the abdominal organs.

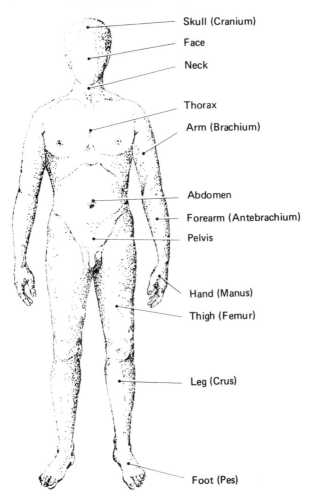

Skull (Cranium)

Face

Neck

Thorax

Arm (Brachium)

Abdomen

Forearm (Antebrachium)

Pelvis

Hand (Manus)

Thigh (Femur)

Leg (Crus)

Foot (Pes)

Figure 1.9 Parts of the human body. The Latin terms in parentheses are frequently used to form adjectives.

The upper extremities consist of the **arm** (brachium), the **forearm** (antebrachium) and **hand** (manus). The hand consists of the **wrist** (carpus), the **mid-hand** (metacarpus) and the **fingers** (digits).

The lower extremities consist of the **thigh** (femur), the **lower leg** (crus) and the **foot** (pes). The foot consists of the **ankle** (tarsus), **mid-foot** (metatarsus), and the **toes** (digits).

1.178	The head is composed of the . . . . and the . . . .

1.179	Other major divisions of the body are . . . ., ... and	face skull (cranium)
1.180	The trunk consists of the . . . ., ... and	neck trunk extremities
1.181	The trunk contains the	thorax abdomen pelvis
1.182	The cavity of the trunk is divided into two parts by a hemispherical muscle, the	viscera
1.183	The upper extremities consist of the . . . ., ... and	diaphragm
1.184	The lower extremities consist of the . . . ., ... and	arms forearms hands
		thighs legs feet

Terms for indicating location

Certain fundamental terms are used to indicate position unambiguously in the body; some of these are shown in Fig. 1.10. The body is divided by three planes at right angles to each other: the **sagittal**, **frontal** and **transverse plane**. A synonym for the frontal plane is the **coronal plane**. The transverse plane through the navel is known as the **umbilical plane** (from umbilicus, navel). A synonym for the transverse plane is the **horizontal plane**.

The sagittal plane, coinciding with the midline of the body, is known as the **median plane**. This divides the body into a right and a left half (**dexter**, right, and **sinister**, left). In each half of the body, **lateral** means towards the side of the body, and **medial** towards the midline. **Bilateral** means on both sides. Two other terms in common use are **proximal** and **distal**. Proximal means nearer to the body or to some other point constituting the center of the part of the body in question, and distal, analogously, away from the body, or any other central part.

The terms indicating direction perpendicular to the frontal plane are **ventral**, meaning towards the belly surface and **dorsal**, towards the back.

In the case of man, the term **anterior** is often used synonymously with ventral, and **posterior** for dorsal; for four-footed animals, anterior means towards the

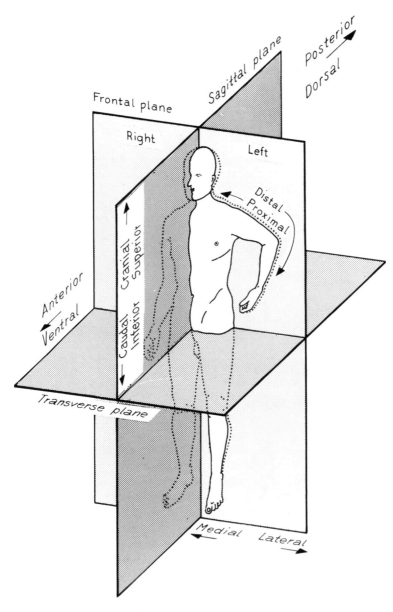

Figure 1.10 Terms for indicating direction.

head and posterior towards the tail. The terms indicating direction perpendicular
to the transverse plane are **cranial**, towards the head, and **caudal**, towards the tail;
superior (upper) and **inferior** (lower) have the same meanings.

Locations inside and outside the dividing wall of the body cavity are indicated by the words **internal** and **external**; proximity to the body surfaces is often indicated simply by **superficial**, and positions remote from the body surface by **deep**.

1.185	A plane through the tip of the nose, back of the neck and navel is known as the .... or	
1.186	The line formed by the intersection of the median plane and the body surface is known as the **median line**. The ventral median line is on the body's .... side, and the dorsal on the	sagittal median plane
1.187	The Latin for right is .... and for left	belly back
1.188	The clavicle (collar bone) lies on the .... side of the trunk, and the scapula (shoulder blade) on its .... side.	dexter sinister
1.189	A point closer to the median plane is located medially, and a point further to the side, ...	ventral dorsal
1.190	The clavicle lies .... to the shoulder.	laterally
1.191	The shoulder is located .... to the clavicle.	medial
1.192	An injury on both sides is	lateral
1.193	Posterior, in the context of man, means a position on the back of the body, and is therefore synonymous with	bilateral
1.194	Anterior, in the context of man, means a position on the belly side, and is therefore synonymous with	dorsal
1.195	The direction towards the head is denoted as	ventral
1.196	The direction towards the tail is denoted as	cranial

1.197	The blood flowing towards the heart from different parts of the body collects in two arteries, namely, the **superior** and **inferior vena cava**. The blood flowing into the superior vena cava comes from the . . . . (upper, lower) part of the body.	caudal
1.198	The venous blood from the lower part of the body collects in the	upper
1.199	The **carotid artery** in the neck is divided into an inner and an outer branch. The blood flow to the brain is carried mainly by the inner branch, that is the . . . . carotid artery.	inferior vena cava
1.200	The arterial blood to the face is carried by the	internal
		external carotid artery

Terms of movements of the extremities

The various types of joints (plane, ball-and-socket, hinge, rotational, ellipsoidal and saddle-shaped joints) enable the body to execute a large range of useful movements. In **flexion** (bending) and **extension** (straightening) the angle between the two bones is respectively diminished and increased. In **dorsiflexion** of the hand (or foot) it is moved so that the angle between the back of the hand (or foot) and the forearm (lower leg) is reduced. In **palmar flexion** of the hand (**palma manus**—palm of the hand) the angle between the palm and the forearm is reduced. The corresponding movement for the foot, downward bending of the

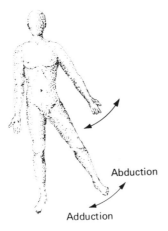

Abduction

Adduction

Figure 1.11 Terms for indicating movements of the extremities towards and away from the median plane.

sole of the foot, is known as **plantar flexion (planta pedis**—sole of the foot). Flexion of the hand towards the side of the thumb (towards the radius) is **radial deviation**, also towards the side of the little finger (towards the ulna), **ulnar deviation** (see page 44).

Abduction—adduction denote movement of the extremity away from and towards the median plane, respectively (Fig. 1.11). In abduction of the fingers, they are moved away from, and in adduction towards, the middle finger.

Rotation can occur in, for example, the ball-and-socket joints in the shoulders and hips.

Rotational movements of the forearms are denoted by **pronation** and **supination** (Fig. 1.12).

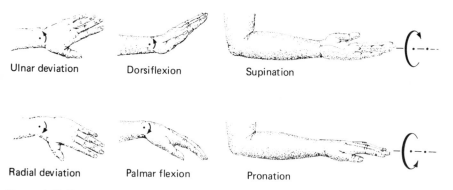

Ulnar deviation   Dorsiflexion   Supination

Radial deviation   Palmar flexion   Pronation

Figure 1.12 Terms for indicating bending and rotating movements of the hand and arm.

1.201	When jumping astride a horse in the gymnasium the legs are	
1.202	When one is riding and gripping the saddle firmly the legs are	abducted
1.203	When diving, the feet should be held in .... (dorsiflexion, plantar flexion).	adducted
1.204	If a person falls forward and saves himself with his hands (the palms on the ground) these are in the ....-flexed position.	plantar flexion

1.205	In the resulting fracture of the radius, there may be a misalignment, with dorsiflexion of the distal part of the fracture. During reduction (setting in the right position) the hand should be strongly . . . .- flexed. (Reduction also requires other movements.)	dorsi-
1.206	Screws usually have a right-hand thread. This is because a greater muscular power can be exerted in supination than in pronation (and because most people are right-handed). When a right-handed person removes a screw he performs a movement of	palmar-
1.207	When a left-handed person tightens a screw he performs a movement of	pronation
1.208	When one looks at the palm of one's own hand, the rotation is called	pronation
		supination

LOCOMOTIVE SYSTEM

Skeletal System

The main purpose of the skeleton is to give the body mechanical stability, to protect delicate organs, and to serve as an anchorage for the muscles, thus making body movements possible through lever action. The skeleton also serves as a reservoir for calcium and phosphorus, and contains the bone marrow, the most important bloodforming organ.

Structure and function of the skeletal bones

Bone can be **compact** or **cancellous**—spongy (Fig. 1.13). The trabeculae (the thin bony structure) in cancellous bone are arranged parallel to the line of action of the forces, so as to provide maximum strength with a minimum of weight, just as in a mechanical framework. In some cancellous bones, the spaces between the trabeculae contain **red bone** (hemopoietic) **marrow** in which blood cells are formed—the red cells, most of the white cells, and the platelets. The cavity of the long bones is filled with **yellow bone marrow**, a fatty tissue. As described above, bone is composed of a compound of calcium and phosphorus, hydroxyapatite, and connective tissue, the fibers of which are oriented so that they reinforce the bone and thus strengthen it. The hydroxyapatite also acts as an **ion exchanger**, the

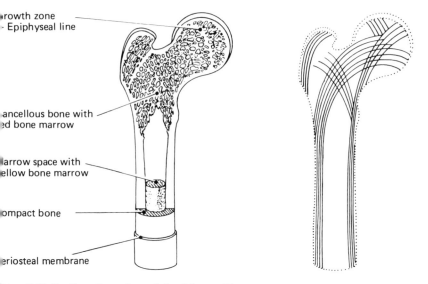

rowth zone
- Epiphyseal line

ancellous bone with
ed bone marrow

arrow space with
ellow bone marrow

ompact bone

eriosteal membrane

jure 1.13 Section through a skeletal bone. The cancellous
ne is composed of trabeculae oriented in the direction of the
es of force.

skeleton thus serving as a reservoir for calcium and phosphorus. This maintains
the correct concentration of these ions in the blood, which is of vital importance
for the organism (Chapter 5).

Except for the cartilage-covered surfaces, the skeletal bones are completely
enclosed by a membrane, the **periosteum**, from which bone is formed in the
healing of fractures. When a bone grows normally, however, it does so from the
epiphyseal line (Fig. 1.13).

oste(o)-	bone, skeleton	see page 17

1.209	The main purpose of the skeleton is to provide . . . . for the body, afford . . . . for delicate organs and to serve as an anchorage for muscles in order to make . . . . possible.	
1.210	The skeleton also serves as a reservoir for . . . . and	stability protection body movements
1.211	There are two types of bone, ... and . . . . (spongy).	calcium phosphorus

1.212	Cancellous bone contains the .... bone marrow in which the .... are formed.	compact cancellous
1.213	In the case of a fracture, new bone is formed from the bone membrane: the .... During growth in length, bone forms from the	red blood cells
1.214	Osteoporosis is reduced mass of	periosteum epiphyseal line
1.215	An inflammatory process in the bone is known as	bone
		osteitis

The skeleton

The skeleton consists of some 200 bones (L. **os**, pl. **ossa**.) They are held together by **cartilage** or by bands of connective tissue, **ligaments**, in such a way that the individual bones can move with relation to one another to a limited degree (Fig. 1.14).

The skeleton of the head consists of the brain case and the facial bones. The head rests on the **spine** (vertebral column), which consists of seven **cervical**, twelve **thoracic** and five **lumbar vertebrae**. The lowest lumbar vertebra rests on the **sacrum**, which is formed by the fusion of five vertebrae. In man the "tail" vertebrae are usually fused into a single bone, the **coccyx**. Between the **vertebrae** are the **intervertebral discs**. A disc consists of a firm outer covering enclosing a gelatinous core. The discs allow the vertebral column to have a certain degree of mobility. Sometimes the covering ruptures and the gelatinous core is extruded; this is known as disc herniation.

The vertebral column has the form of a double S: the curves that are convex in the dorsal direction are known as **kyphoses** while the concave ones are **lordoses** (Fig. 1.15). A lateral curvature is known as a **scoliosis**.

From the twelve thoracic vertebrae extend twelve pairs of ribs (**costae**). The ten uppermost ones are attached to the **sternum** (breastbone) by costal cartilages, while the lower two end freely in the trunk wall. The **clavicle** (collar bone) articulates (joins) medially with the upper part of the sternum and laterally with the **scapula** (shoulder blade), which provides a ball-and-socket joint for the **humerus** (bone of the arm). The forearm consists of two bones: the **ulna** and the **radius**. The distal parts of these articulate with the proximal bones of the hand. When the hand is rotated about an axis parallel to the forearm, the radius also rotates, but not the ulna, which is connected to the humerus by a hinge joint.

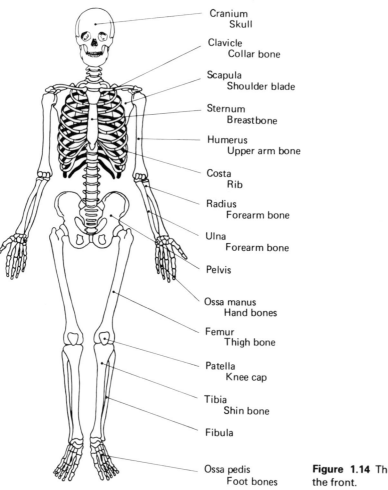

Cranium
  Skull

Clavicle
  Collar bone

Scapula
  Shoulder blade

Sternum
  Breastbone

Humerus
  Upper arm bone

Costa
  Rib

Radius
  Forearm bone

Ulna
  Forearm bone

Pelvis

Ossa manus
  Hand bones

Femur
  Thigh bone

Patella
  Knee cap

Tibia
  Shin bone

Fibula

Ossa pedis
  Foot bones

Figure 1.14 The skeleton seen from the front.

Attached to the sacrum is the **pelvis**. The pelvis articulates with the proximal part of the **femur** (thigh bone) in a ball-and-socket joint. The head and the shaft of the femur are connected by an angulated part known as the **femoral neck**; here **fractures** (bone breaks) often occur at advanced ages. The femur articulates with the **tibia** (shin bone). This and the **fibula** constitute the skeletal components of the lower leg.

Over the articular space between the femur and the tibia, and in contact with the femur, is the **patella** (knee cap). When the leg is extended, this transmits force from some of the thigh muscles to the tibia. The distal articular surfaces of the tibia and fibula articulate with one of the bones in the foot.

Friction in the joints is reduced by a smooth articular cartilage that covers the bone surfaces. These surfaces, together with the articular capsule attached to the

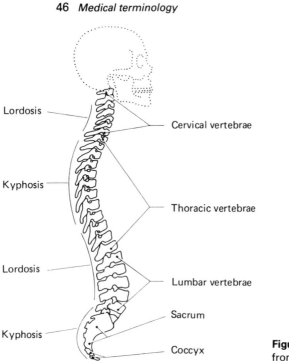

Lordosis

Kyphosis

Lordosis

Kyphosis

Cervical vertebrae

Thoracic vertebrae

Lumbar vertebrae

Sacrum

Coccyx

Figure 1.15 The vertebral column seen from the right side.

bones, form a closed cavity. The inner surface of the articular capsule is covered by a membrane that secretes a viscous lubricating fluid.

spine	belonging to the spinal region	spinal anesthesia—injection of an anesthetic into the spinal canal in the lumbar region
		spinal puncture—insertion of a puncture needle into the spinal canal to obtain a specimen of cerebrospinal fluid
sternal	belonging to the sternum	sternal line—an imaginary line along the border of the sternum
		sternal puncture—insertion of a puncture needle into the marrow space of the sternum to obtain a specimen of red bone marrow

1.216 The vertebral column consists of . . . . ,
. . . . and . . . . vertebrae.

1.217	The lowest lumbar vertebra rests on the first .... vertebra.	cervical thoracic lumbar
1.218	The lumbar spine forms a curve called a	sacral
1.219	The cervical spine forms a .... (lordosis, kyphosis).	lordosis (both start with l)
1.220	The sacrum forms a	lordosis
1.221	Scoliosis is a .... curvature of the spine.	kyphosis
1.222	The breastbone is known as the ....; pertaining to the breast bone, ...	lateral
1.223	The bones of the upper extremity are the scapula, ..., the humerus, ..., the ulna and radius, ..., and the bones of the hand.	sternum sternal
1.224	The bone of the forearm on the thumb side is known as the	shoulder blade arm bone forearm bones
1.225	The bones of the lower extremity are the femur, ..., patella, ..., tibia, ..., the .... and the bones of the foot.	radius
1.226	The patellar reflex is an involuntary contraction of the extensor muscles of the thigh when the tendon is struck below the	thigh bone knee cap shin bone fibula
		knee cap

Muscular System

The human body has some 300 skeletal muscles, which produce the voluntary body movements. The muscles are often arranged in pairs so as to act antagonistically. For example, on the anterior side of the arm are the muscles that flex the elbow-joint, and on the posterior side those that extend the joint (Fig. 1.16).

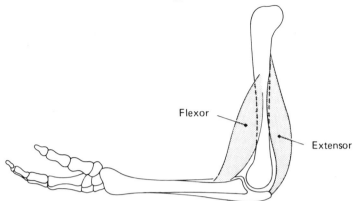

Figure 1.16 Skeletal muscles that work in opposition are known as antagonists.

A muscle that is exercised to a great extent increases in size; that is, it becomes **hypertrophied**; a muscle that is inactive becomes **atrophied**. Contraction of the muscles is regulated via nerves. If the nerve is damaged the muscle cannot be voluntarily contracted; that is to say, it is paralyzed. The muscle is still able to contract; for example, if it is electrically stimulated. Incomplete paralysis, or muscular weakness, is known as **paresis**.

Muscular contraction

There are two types of contraction, **isotonic** and **isometric**. In isotonic contraction, the muscle is shortened under constant load; in isometric contraction, the muscle contracts without shortening. The first stage in a muscular movement is usually an isometric contraction. This is followed by isotonic contraction.

The efficiency of a muscle is comparatively low. In an isotonic contraction, less than 20 percent of the energy is converted into mechanical work; the rest is converted into heat. In isometric contraction, no work is performed and all energy is converted into heat. Muscular contraction is the body's most important mechanism for generating heat; when we shiver with cold we involuntarily contract our muscles to increase the amount of heat generated.

Regulation of muscular contraction

To each skeletal muscle runs a **motor nerve**, which conducts impulses that cause contraction. The nerve consists of a large number of individual nerve fibers. Each fiber is divided into several branches and supplies a group of muscle fibers. Each group consists of a hundred or so muscle fibers. Such a group is known as a **motor unit**, because all the muscle fibers contract simultaneously when stimulating the nerve fiber.

Each contraction of a motor unit produces a constant force. The movement of a whole muscle is regulated by a change in the contraction frequency and by adding motor units as required.

Fine movements are obtained by means of a feedback signal which is transmitted from the muscle to the controlling unit in the central nervous system. The sensors in the muscles are the **muscle spindles** which contain their own muscle fibers (Fig. 1.17). The spindles are connected with the central nervous system via

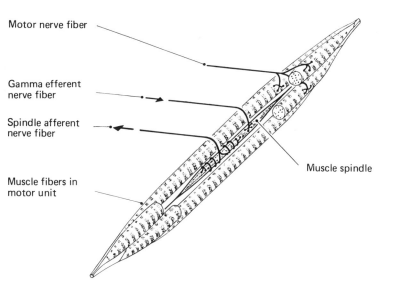

Motor nerve fiber

Gamma efferent nerve fiber

Spindle afferent nerve fiber

Muscle spindle

Muscle fibers in motor unit

Figure 1.17 The location and innervation of a muscle spindle in a motor unit.

nerve fibers (Fig. 1.18). **Efferent** gamma fibers (conducting **from** the central nervous system) adjust the spindle length to the required degree of contraction (cf, a "desired" value of a servo system), and **afferent** fibers (conducting **to** the central nervous system) conduct the error signal—that is, the difference between the "actual" and "desired" value.

There are also receptors for muscle control in the joints for transmitting to the central nervous system the rate of movement and the position of the joint. This **deep sensibility** is extremely well developed. It enables the extremities to be positioned with great precision without the aid of vision; for example, with the finger tip a person can touch any chosen part of his body, even when it is placed in an unusual position.

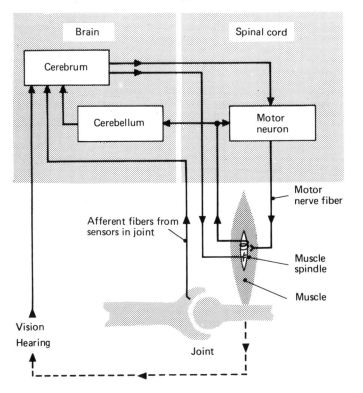

Figure 1.18 Simplified block diagram for the contraction of a muscle.

1.227	The muscles of a wrestler become . . . . and those of a sick person spending a long time in bed, ...	
1.228	Loss of muscular power is known as . . . . and muscular weakness as	hypertrophied atrophied
1.229	The bundle of muscle fibers in a muscle supplied by a single motor nerve fiber is called a	paralysis paresis
1.230	Each contraction of a motor unit has a constant	motor unit
1.231	The movement of a whole muscle is controlled by a change in . . . . and by adding	force

1.232	The setting of the "desired" value of contraction in a skeletal muscle and the measurement of the instantaneous "actual" value are effected by .... in the motor units.	contraction frequency motor units
1.233	From the muscle spindle an error signal (which is a function of the difference between the "actual" and the "desired" values for the contraction) is transmitted via an .... (conduction to the central nervous system) nerve fiber to higher nerve centers.	muscle spindles
1.234	To the muscle spindles and to the motor units run .... (conducting from the central nervous system) pathways.	afferent
1.235	The sensory system which controls the body movements and the relative positions of parts of the body, enabling us, for example, to eat a hot dog in complete darkness, without getting ketchup on our face, is known as	efferent
		deep sensibility

METABOLIC APPARATUS

For the vital processes energy is required, and this is obtained by metabolism. The food is disintegrated and absorbed by the **digestive system**, oxygen is taken up by the **respiratory system**, and these essential nutrients are carried via the **circulatory system** to the individual cells, where combustion takes place. The body can burn carbohydrates, fats and proteins. The products of combustion, which consist of carbon dioxide, water, urea and other nitrogenous substances, are carried via the circulatory system to the **excretory system**, where the nitrogenous substances and some of the water are separated from the blood and leave the body as urine. Carbon dioxide and some of the water are excreted by the respiratory system.

Digestive System

In the digestive system, the food is treated mechanically and chemically so that it can be absorbed. In the **mouth**, the food is chewed and mixed with saliva from the salivary glands, after which it passes through the **esophagus** and the **cardiac orifice** (the upper opening of the stomach) to the **stomach** (prefix **gastr-**). The stomach wall contains various kinds of glandular cells which secrete **hydrochloric acid**, **pepsin** (an enzyme that breaks down protein) and **mucus**. The cells are located in tubular glands in the gastric mucosa. There are about 50 million such glands in the stomach. When the food is mixed with gastric juice at the correct level of acidity, pH 1, the **pyloric orifice** (lower opening of the stomach) opens and the food passes through the **duodenum** where bile and pancreatic juice are added and the pH becomes slightly alkaline.

The bile is produced by the **liver** (prefix **hepat-**), the body's largest gland, and is led through the bile ducts to the **gallbladder** (prefix **cholecyst-**) where the bile is concentrated.

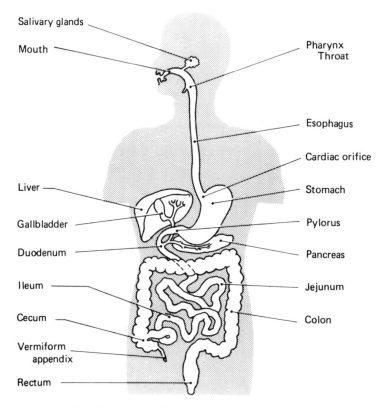

Salivary glands

Mouth

Pharynx
Throat

Esophagus

Cardiac orifice

Liver

Stomach

Gallbladder

Pylorus

Duodenum

Pancreas

Ileum

Jejunum

Cecum

Colon

Vermiform
appendix

Rectum

Figure 1.19 The digestive system.

The bile empties through the **common bile duct** (combined cystic and hepatic ducts) into the duodenum. The **pancreas** excretes the pancreatic juice and it empties directly into the aperture of the common duct, or through a short common excretory duct, into the duodenum.

The small intestine, which is about 5 m long, consists of the **duodenum**, the **jejunum** and the **ileum**. The gland cells in the mucous membrane of the small intestine secrete digestive enzymes. The absorption of the food takes place mainly in the small intestine.

Between the ileum and the **cecum**, which is the first part of the **colon**, there is the **ileocecal valve**, which prevents the reflux of the intestinal contents from the colon. The cecum has a wormlike part, the **appendix**, which is often the site of inflammation—a condition known as appendicitis.

The large intestine, which is about 1 m long, first runs cranially on the right side, the **ascending colon**, crosses the abdomen from the liver to the spleen, the **transverse colon**, and then runs caudally, the **descending colon**, after which it passes through an S-shaped curve, the **sigmoid colon**, into the **rectum**. In the colon, water is absorbed from the intestinal contents, which thus assume a solid consistency.

The small intestine and the greater part of the colon obtain their blood supply from vessels in the **mesentery**, which is anchored to the dorsal wall of the abdomen (Fig. 1.20). Because of the mesentery the intestines are highly mobile in the peritoneal cavity, a fact that is exploited in operations. The whole of the inner surface of the abdominal cavity and all the organs within it are covered by the **peritoneum**.

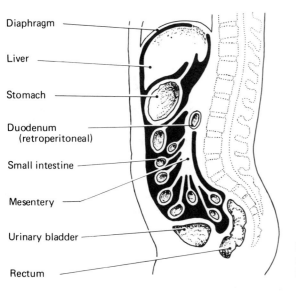

Diaphragm

Liver

Stomach

Duodenum
  (retroperitoneal)

Small intestine

Mesentery

Urinary bladder

Rectum

Figure 1.20 In the abdominal cavity (black in the figure) the stomach and intestines are highly mobile.

The digestive apparatus thus consists essentially of a long tube. The food is advanced by **peristaltic** movements, produced by automatic rhythmic contractions of the smooth muscles present throughout the wall of the digestive tract. Only at its upper end, the mouth, and the lower orifice, the **anus**, is there striated muscle, which makes possible voluntary activity.

gastr(o)-	stomach	gastritis—inflammation of the stomach
		gastroenteritis—inflammation of stomach and intestine
		gastroscope—instrument for examining the stomach
chol-	bile	cholangitis—inflammation of the bile ducts
		cholelithiasis—gallstones
cholecyst-	gallbladder	cholecystography—x-ray examination of the gallbladder
col-	colon	colitis—inflammation of the colon
		colostomy—creation of an artificial opening in the colon through the outer abdominal wall

1.236	The vital processes require energy, which is obtained through metabolism, whereby the body burns . . . ., ... and	
1.237	In the combustion process . . . . is consumed; it is taken up by the respiratory organs.	carbohydrates fats proteins
1.238	The combustion products consist of . . . ., ..., ... and other nitrogenous substances.	oxygen
1.239	The combustion products are excreted by the . . . . system and the . . . . system.	carbon dioxide water urea
1.240	A patient experiences difficulties when swallowing food. The physician refers the patient for x-ray examination of the . . . . (the tube connecting the throat and the stomach).	respiratory excretory
1.241	At the same time he has an examination of the stomach, during which the contrast media passes through the . . . . (upper opening of the stomach), and also through the . . . . (lower opening).	esophagus
1.242	A person with gastritis has inflammation of the	cardiac orifice pyloric orifice

1.243	A person with hepatitis has infection of the	stomach
1.244	Cholecystitis is inflammation of the gall-..........	liver
1.245	The ending -iasis denotes a pathological state; lith- means stone. The Latin term for gallstone is	bladder
1.246	Inflammation occurs when a body cavity, such as a gland or part of the gastrointestinal tract, is blocked. When a gallstone is located in the narrowest part of the gallbladder at the entry into the common duct, ... develops.	cholelithiasis
1.247	The excretory ducts of the pancreas often emerge together with the common duct. In such cases, a gallstone located in the orifice of the common duct can easily give rise to inflammation of the pancreas. This pathological condition, which is known as ...., often leads to death. A person with gallstones should therefore have the gallbladder, where the stones are formed, removed by an operation.	cholecystitis
1.248	A wound caused by a pathological process is known as an **ulcer**. A lesion in the stomach is known as a	pancreatitis
1.249	A lesion in the first part of the small intestine is known as a	gastric ulcer
1.250	The adjective of ulcer is ulcerative or ulcerous. A person with ulcerative colitis has an	duodenal ulcer
1.251	When the bile cannot pass through the common duct to the intestine, biliary stasis arises. Bile pigment then cannot be excreted through the liver but collects in the blood, and this gives a yellowish color to all the organs; the patient has jaundice. Jaundice can also be caused by infection of the liver, which is known as	inflammation of the large intestine with ulcerations
1.252	Cholecystitis that goes untreated may cause rupture of the gallbladder, with resulting spread of the infection to the peritoneal cavity; .... then develops.	hepatitis

| 1.253 | Inflammation of the wormlike part of the cecum is called . . . . | peritonitis (inflamma-tion of the peritoneal membrane) |
| | | appendicitis |

Respiratory System

The oxygen consumed in the combustion of food is absorbed through the lungs, and it is also through the lungs that the carbon dioxide formed is eliminated. Ventilation consists of **inspiration** (breathing in) and **expiration** (breathing out).

The air passes from the nose to the **pharynx**, then via the **larynx** and **trachea** (windpipe) to the two **bronchi**, where it is distributed to the left and right **lungs**. The bronchi are kept distended by cartilage rings. In the lungs, the air stream is distributed throughout the bronchial tree via **bronchioles**—air tubes less than 1 mm in diameter with no cartilage—to the **alveoli**, where gas exchange takes place. The alveoli number some $3 \cdot 10^8$, with a total area of $70 \, \text{m}^2$. The lungs consist mainly of these alveoli.

The lungs have the shape of rounded cones. The **apex** of the lung is uppermost and the **base** is towards the diaphragm. The right lung has three lobes and the left

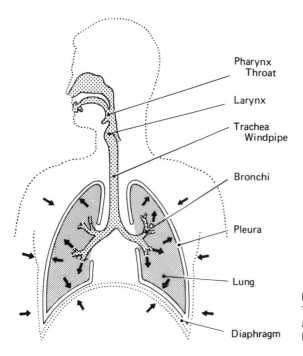

Pharynx
Throat

Larynx

Trachea
Windpipe

Bronchi

Pleura

Lung

Diaphragm

Figure 1.21 The respiratory organs. The pleural cavity is normally empty and the lungs are thus kept distended by the air pressure.

one two. The **lobes** are well defined by deep fissures, which facilitate surgical removal of a complete lobe in the case of pathological changes. Infection in the lung may be either localized in one or more of the lobes (**lobar pneumonia**), or in patches around the bronchial tree (**bronchopneumonia**).

Between the lungs, and passing in the median plane, there is a thick wall—the **mediastinum**—which encloses the **heart**, the **esophagus** and the **trachea** (windpipe).

On each side of the mediastinum are the lungs, located in a cavity that is bounded by the chest and the diaphragm. The cavity and the lungs are lined with a smooth membrane—the **pleura**, forming a sac, the **pleural cavity**. This cavity normally contains no air, and the lungs are thus kept distended by the negative pressure in the pleural cavity (Fig. 1.21).

The larynx contains two bands of mucous membrane—the **vocal cords**. These can be stretched, and they are then set vibrating by the passage of air. The sound so generated is modified and amplified by acoustic resonators formed by the cavities in the throat and mouth and by the nasal cavities. Speech sounds are formed by movements of the tongue, lips and soft palate, which vary the properties of the resonators.

laryng(o)-	larynx	laryngitis—inflammation of the larynx
		laryngoscopy—examination of the larynx with a mirror
		laryngospasm—spasm of the vocal cords, preventing air from passing
bronch(o)-	bronchi	bronchitis—inflammation of the bronchi
		bronchoscope—instrument for inspecting the larger airways
		bronchospasm—spasm of the bronchi
pleur-	pleura	pleural exudate—accumulation of fluid in the pleural cavity
		pleural puncture—puncture of the pleural cavity
		pleurisy—inflammation of the pleura
pneumo-	air, lung	pneumonia—inflammation of the lung
		pneumothorax—accumulation of air in the pleural cavity

1.254	In inflammation of the larynx, the vocal cords swell, causing hoarseness. Temporary hoarseness can thus be a sign of	

1.255	Laryngitis is often combined with inflammation of the throat, called	laryngitis
1.256	Infection easily spreads down to the trachea, resulting in . . . . , and on to the bronchi, causing	pharyngitis
1.257	Asthma is recurrent respiratory distress due to, among other things, spasm in the smooth muscles of the bronchial walls; this is known as	tracheitis bronchitis
1.258	There are two kinds of pneumonia. These are . . . . and	bronchospasm
1.259	In pneumonia, the . . . . are filled with an inflammatory exudate, which interferes with gaseous exchange.	lobar pneumonia bronchopneumonia
1.260	Between the lungs, in the median plane, is a thick wall, the . . . . , which encloses the . . . . , ... and the	alveoli
1.261	If a perforation appears in the thoracic wall (e.g., in an accident or during an operation in the thoracic cavity) or the lung, the . . . . fills with air; and the whole lung collapses; this is known as . . . . -thorax.	mediastinum heart esophagus trachea
1.262	In an operation in the thoracic cavity when the pleura is opened, collapse of the lung must be prevented by applying a . . . . (positive, negative) pressure via a tube connected to the trachea.	pleural cavity pneumo
		positive

Circulatory System

For the transport of oxygen, carbon dioxide, numerous chemical compounds and the blood cells, there are two systems: the blood-vascular system and the lymphatic system.

The **heart** pumps the blood through the **pulmonary** (lesser) **circulation** to the lungs, and through the **systemic circulation** to the other organs of the body (Fig. 1.22).

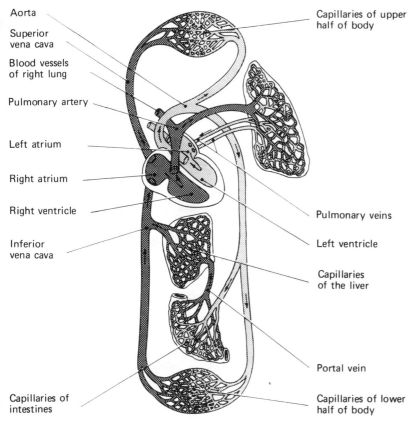

Aorta

Superior
vena cava

Blood vessels
of right lung

Pulmonary artery

Left atrium

Right atrium

Right ventricle

Inferior
vena cava

Capillaries of
intestines

Capillaries of upper
half of body

Pulmonary veins

Left ventricle

Capillaries
of the liver

Portal vein

Capillaries of lower
half of body

Figure 1.22 The circulatory system. (Redrawn from T. Petrén, Anatomi, AB Nordiska Bokhandelns Förlag, Stockholm, 1962, by permission.)

In the pulmonary circulation, the **venous** (non-oxygenated) blood flows from the **right ventricle**, through the **pulmonary artery**, to the lungs, where it is oxygenated and gives off carbon dioxide. The **arterial** (oxygenated) blood flows through the pulmonary veins to the **left atrium**. It then flows to the **left ventricle** and is pumped through the **aorta** and its branches, the **arteries** (Fig. 1.23), out into the body. Through the **arterioles** (small arteries) the blood is distributed to the capillaries in the tissues, where it gives up its oxygen and chemical compounds and takes up carbon dioxide and products of combustion.

The blood returns to the heart along different routes in different parts of the body (Fig. 1.24). It usually passes from the venous side of the capillaries directly via the venous system to either the **superior vena cava** or the **inferior vena cava**, both of which empty into the **right atrium**.

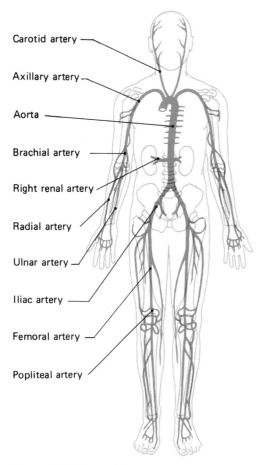

Carotid artery

Axillary artery

Aorta

Brachial artery

Right renal artery

Radial artery

Ulnar artery

Iliac artery

Femoral artery

Popliteal artery

Figure 1.23 The arterial system.

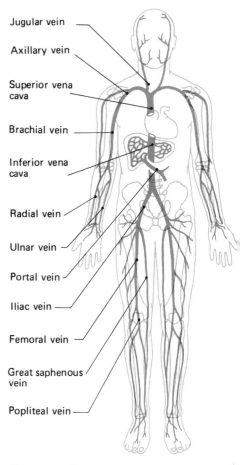

Jugular vein

Axillary vein

Superior vena cava

Brachial vein

Inferior vena cava

Radial vein

Ulnar vein

Portal vein

Iliac vein

Femoral vein

Great saphenous vein

Popliteal vein

Figure 1.24 The venous system.

In other cases the return is more complex. For example, the blood from the capillary network in the intestines, stomach and spleen flows back via the **portal vein** to the liver, where it is again distributed in a capillary network. Then it is collected by the **hepatic vein**, which feeds into the inferior vena cava. By means of this **portal circulation**, the liver is able to directly convert substances absorbed in the intestines—for example, glucose, which is stored in the liver as glycogen (animal starch). Detoxification of many substances also takes place in the liver. The liver receives oxygenated blood via the **hepatic artery**.

Arteries and veins (and also nerves) are named after the organ they supply or one near their route. For example, the artery of the arm is known as the **brachial artery**. It divides into two branches, one passing along the radius, the **radial artery**, and the other along the ulna, the **ulnar artery** (Fig. 1.25). The largest artery of the

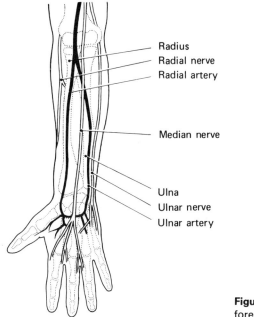

Radius
Radial nerve
Radial artery

Median nerve

Ulna
Ulnar nerve
Ulnar artery

Figure 1.25 Arteries and nerves of the forearm.

femur is the **femoral artery**, in which pulsations can be felt in the groin of the supine body. The names of the major arteries and veins are given in Figs. 1.23 and 1.24.

The heart is supplied by two small but highly important arteries, the **coronary arteries**. They branch from the aorta just above the heart. If they are occluded by coronary thrombosis, myocardial infarction follows.

Through the capillary walls a thin clear fluid exudes into the **interstitial space** between the cells (page 26). This tissue fluid, which is derived from the blood by ultrafiltration, contains no blood cells or macromolecular substances, such as proteins. The tissue fluid supplies the cells with vital nutrients and takes up waste products of metabolism and substances to be used in other parts of the body. The tissue fluid is returned mainly to the venous side of the capillaries, but some is taken up by **lymph capillaries**, which begin in the interstitial space. The tissue fluid, which at this stage is known as **lymph**, is conveyed in **lymph ducts** via **lymph nodes**, also incorrectly called lymph glands, through ducts of increasing diameter back to the blood stream. The largest duct, the **thoracic duct**, empties into the **left subclavian vein**, and another smaller lymph duct empties into the **right subclavian vein**.

cardi(o)-	heart (also in cardiac orifice of the stomach)	cardiogram—electrocardiogram cardiologist—heart specialist tachycardia—too high a pulse rate

cardi(o)-(*continued*)

bradycardia—too low a pulse rate
myocardium—heart muscle
myocarditis—inflammation of the heart muscle
pericardium—the sac enclosing the heart
pericarditis—inflammation of the pericardium
(but cardiospasm—spasm in the stomach's upper orifice, close to the heart)

arteri-   artery

arteriosclerosis—a disease that results in calcification of arteries
arteritis—inflammation of arteries

phleb(o)-   vein
also **ven(o)-**

phlebitis—inflammation of veins
phlebography—x-ray examination of veins (also venography)
phlebectasia—varicose (dilated) veins

vas(o)-   vessel

vascularization—development of new vessels
vasodilation—dilation of vessels
vasoconstriction—contraction of vessels
vasomotor—change of vessel diameter to modify the blood supply

lymph-   lymph

lymphangitis—inflammation of lymph ducts (see also page 24).

1.263	The circulatory system consists of two parts, the . . . . system, which contains blood, and the . . . . system.	
1.264	The blood-vascular system also consists of two parts, the . . . . and the	blood-vascular lymphatic
1.265	A vein is a vessel that conveys . . . . (venous blood, arterial blood, blood to the heart, blood from the heart).	pulmonary circulation systemic circulation
1.266	In the systemic circulation the arteries convey . . . . (arterial, venous) blood, and in the pulmonary circulation . . . . blood.	blood to the heart

1.267	From the left ...., blood passes via .... (type of vessels) out to the capillaries. There, a thin fluid exudes into the .... space, from which most of it is collected and carried to the heart via the .... (type of vessels).	arterial venous
1.268	Some interstitial fluid is also taken up by .... ducts and is conveyed as .... via .... to the left and right subclavian veins.	ventricle arteries interstitial veins
1.269	After an abdominal operation, when the patient must rest in bed for several days, the blood may clot in the veins of the lower leg; this condition is known as venous thrombosis. This presents a risk of an embolus for if such a blood clot becomes detached it is carried away in the blood stream. It passes through the venous system to the ...., on into the .... atrium and ventricle, and through the .... artery to the lungs.	lymph lymph lymph ducts
1.270	If the clot is large, the blood flow will be completely blocked and death will occur in a minute or so from a pulmonary .... It is thus important to diagnose .... (blood clot in the vein) as early as possible and to give an anticoagulant.	inferior vena cava right pulmonary
1.271	If the clot is small, it will pass through the pulmonary artery to a smaller lung artery. The part of the lung supplied by the artery then dies; that is, a pulmonary infarction occurs. The patient has pain in the chest, fever, and coughs up blood, but he may survive because the blood can pass through the rest of the .... circulation.	embolus venous thrombosis
1.272	Tissue death resulting from blockage of an artery is known as	pulmonary
1.273	Myocardial infarction can occur when a piece of calcified material from an arteriosclerotic area becomes detached from one of the .... that supply the heart muscle with blood, and blocks the lumen of the vessel. In myocardial infarction part of the .... (heart muscle) dies.	infarction

1.274	A few days after an infarction, a coating of coagulated blood forms on the heart chamber wall. If the clot is detached from the left ventricle, it is carried in the blood stream through the . . . . , and then blocks the blood flow in a peripheral	coronary arteries myocardium
1.275	The patient is said to have an arterial	aorta artery
1.276	Inflammation of the heart muscle is known as	embolus
1.277	Inflammation of the heart sac is known as	myocarditis
1.278	Blood flows to the liver in the hepatic . . . . and the	pericarditis
1.279	The pulsations in the femoral artery can best be felt in the	artery portal vein
1.280	The radial artery passes in the forearm on the side of the . . . . (little finger, thumb).	groin
1.281	Cardiovascular diseases are diseases of the . . . . and	thumb
1.282	Thrombophlebitis is inflammation of a . . . . , resulting in thrombosis.	heart vessels
1.283	Periarteritis is a disease in which there is inflammation and thickening of the . . . . walls.	vein
		arterial

Hemodynamics

From the hydrodynamics viewpoint the heart consists of two pumps connected in series to form a closed circulatory system (Fig. 1.26). An analogy can be drawn between the hydraulic quantities of the circulatory system and the electrical quantities of a circuit. The electromotive force corresponds to the blood pressure E_R and E_L, the current to the flow, I, and the electrical impedance to the hydraulic impedance Z_P and Z_S. The impedance has a real component, which is dependent on the blood's viscosity and the length and radius of the blood vessel. It also has an imaginary component, which is dependent both on the elasticity of the vessel wall

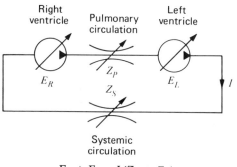

Right
ventricle   Pulmonary   Left
circulation ventricle

E_R Z_P E_L I

Z_S

Systemic
circulation

$$E_R + E_L = I(Z_P + Z_S)$$

Figure 1.26 The circulatory system consists of two pumps and two impedances in series.

(capacitive component) and on the mass of the blood, etc. (inductive component). A hydraulic analog to Ohm's Law can then be used to relate the above quantities.

The left ventricle is more powerful than the right. The blood pressure is therefore higher in the systemic circulation than in the pulmonary circulation, as is evident from Fig. 1.27, which shows the mean pressure. The greatest drop in pressure in the system occurs in the arterioles.

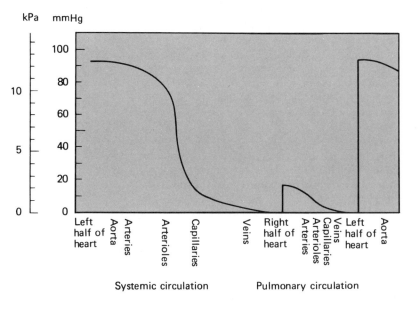

Figure 1.27 Mean blood pressure in the systemic and pulmonary circulation. Note the comparison between the two vertical scales. New SI units (see Appendix, page 646) are given in kilopascal and old units in mm Hg.

The rate of flow of the blood varies greatly. In the aorta it averages about 0.5 m/s and in the capillaries less than 1 mm/s. The contraction of the heart generates a pressure wave that travels in the arteries at a speed of about 5 m/s. Thus this surface wave (page 172) travels much faster than the average rate of flow.

When the heart of a healthy young person is functioning normally at rest, it is capable of performing useful work at a rate of about 1.5 W. During extreme effort this figure may be increased tenfold.

During the heart's working cycle the blood pressure varies periodically. The maximum pressure, the **systolic** pressure (**systole**: the heart's contraction phase) is normally about 120 mm Hg ($\approx$16 kPa), and the **diastolic pressure** (**diastole**: the heart's expansion phase) about 75 mm Hg ($\approx$10 kPa), Chapter 2. Too high blood pressure is known as **hypertension**, and too low **hypotension**.

1.284	The greatest drop in blood pressure occurs in the	
1.285	Symptoms of too high and too low blood pressure differ. In too low blood pressure, the blood flow to the brain is low. Oxygen deficiency leads to a feeling of exhaustion, cold sweat, visual blackouts, and sometimes fainting. To prevent this, a person troubled by these symptoms should increase the blood pressure in the brain by keeping the head at a .... level. A person who has frequent fainting attacks may be suffering either from anemia or from a shunting of blood away from the brain, resulting in cerebral .... (low blood pressure).	arterioles
1.286	High blood pressure rarely produces any symptoms until after it has caused complications. Occasionally it results in headache, dizziness and buzzing in the ears. The condition may be due to spasm in the vascular muscles or to arteriosclerosis. Either problem causes an increase in hydraulic impedance and blood pressure. To ensure adequate flow to the tissues, the circulatory centers in the brain send signals to the heart, causing it to pump harder. Arteriosclerosis can thus cause .... (too high blood pressure).	low hypotension
1.287	The maximum pressure during the heart's working cycle is known as the .... pressure.	hypertension

1.288	The lowest pressure is known as the .... pressure.	systolic
		diastolic

Excretory System

The body has several methods of eliminating the metabolic combustion products and the non-useful substances absorbed from the food. The lungs remove carbon dioxide and water, the sweat glands remove water and salts, and the liver, via the bile, removes certain waste products. There is also some excretion through the colon.

The greater part of the non-volatile waste products are, however, excreted through the kidneys (adj. **renal**, or in compound words, **nephr(o)-**). Nitrogenous breakdown products, formed in the combustion of proteins, are excreted only through the kidneys. If neither kidney is functioning, the nitrogenous substances (e.g. urea) accumulate in the body and **uremia** (urine poisoning of the blood) occurs.

The blood flows to the kidneys through the **renal artery**. In the kidneys the blood undergoes ultrafiltration (a passing of only the small molecules through filter pores) with formation of, at first, very dilute urine, which is then concentrated by reabsorption of water and other useful substances (Chapter 5). The urine collects in the **renal pelvis** (in compound words **pyel(o)-**) and is carried through the two **ureters** to the urinary bladder (in compound words **cyst(o)-**). During **micturition** (urinating) the urine leaves the body through the **urethra** (Figs. 1.28–1.30).

ren-	kidney	suprarenal—pertaining to the suprarenal glands (adrenal glands)
nephr(o)-	kidney	nephrogenic—originating in the kidneys
		nephrolithiasis—kidney stone
		nephrosis—degenerative kidney disease
		nephritis—renal inflammation
		hydronephrosis—distension of the renal pelvis by urine
pyel(o)-	renal pelvis	pyelitis—inflammation of the renal pelvis
		pyelography—x-ray examination of the renal pelvis
		pyelonephritis—simultaneous inflammation of the renal pelvis and the kidney
uretero-	ureter	ureterography—x-ray examination of the ureter(s)

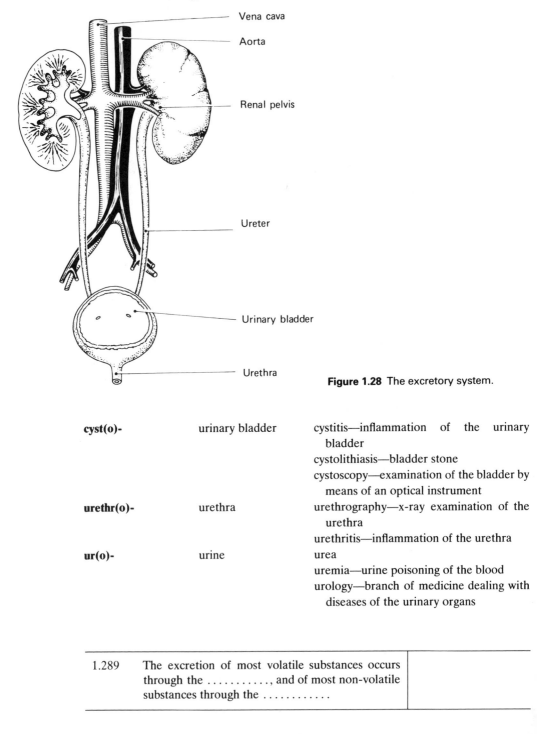

Figure 1.28 The excretory system.

cyst(o)-	urinary bladder	cystitis—inflammation of the urinary bladder
		cystolithiasis—bladder stone
		cystoscopy—examination of the bladder by means of an optical instrument
urethr(o)-	urethra	urethrography—x-ray examination of the urethra
		urethritis—inflammation of the urethra
ur(o)-	urine	urea
		uremia—urine poisoning of the blood
		urology—branch of medicine dealing with diseases of the urinary organs

| 1.289 | The excretion of most volatile substances occurs through the . . . ., and of most non-volatile substances through the . . . . | |

1.290	A patient has apparently recovered from a throat infection, but 2 weeks later has a relapse with blood in the urine, headache and reduced urine output. The condition is due to inflammation of the kidney(s), ..., caused by an immunologic response (Chapter 6).	lungs kidneys
1.291	A patient falls ill with fever, chills, the urge to urinate and back pains, which radiate downwards. The urine is found to contain many bacteria. The patient has inflammation of the renal pelvis or . . . . and infection of the bladder, ...	nephritis
1.292	One of the meanings of the ending -osis designates a degenerative disease; such a condition in the kidney is known as	pyelitis cystitis
1.293	In the case of ureteral obstruction—for example, by a kidney stone—there is distension of the renal pelvis by urine, a condition known as hydro-	nephrosis
1.294	Kidney stone is also known as	nephrosis
1.295	The tubes carrying the urine from the kidneys to the bladder are known as . . . ., and that carrying the urine from the bladder is the	nephrolithiasis
		ureters urethra

REPRODUCTIVE SYSTEM

The male genital organs are shown in Fig. 1.29. The two **testicles** (prefix **orchi-**) are located in the **scrotum**. Two duct systems collect the sperm at the **epididymis** and carry them through the **ductus deferens**, which run, one through each groin, into the abdominal cavity. The ductus deferens continue to the dorsal wall of the urinary bladder, where they have two protuberances, the **seminal vesicles**. They then emerge into the **urethra**, which is surrounded at this junction by the **prostate gland**. The seminal vesicles and the prostate gland produce two secretions which form the semen. This semen activates the **sperm** and makes them mobile. The anterior part of the **penis**, the **glans**, is surrounded by a loose fold of skin, the **prepuce** (foreskin).

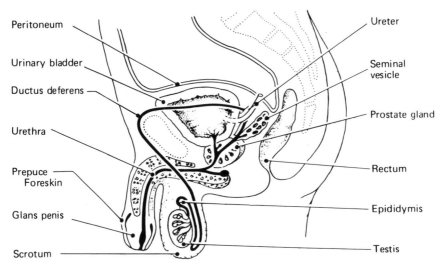

Figure 1.29 The male genital organs.

The female genital organs are shown in Fig. 1.30. In the **ovaries** (prefix **oophor-**) the ova, eggs, are generated. In **ovulation**, usually one is detached and spends a few days passing through the **fallopian tube** (oviduct, in compound words **salping-**) to the **uterus** (womb). Fertilization takes place in the fallopian tube, to which the sperm have swum through the uterus (Chapter 12). When the ovum

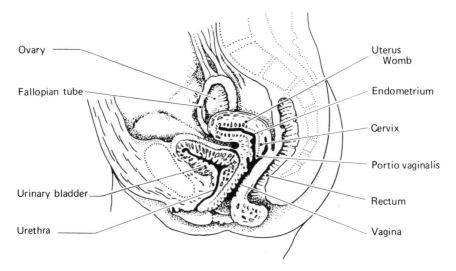

Figure 1.30 Sagittal section through the female pelvis.

70

reaches the uterus it becomes embedded in the **endometrium** (mucous membrane in the uterus). The **fetus** develops through repeated cell division. The fetus receives nourishment from the mother via the umbilical cord and the **placenta**, which is attached to the uterine wall. The lowermost part of the uterus is known as the **uterine cervix** (neck of the womb) and its protrusion into the **vagina** is known as the **portio vaginalis**.

A common term for both male and female sex glands is the **gonad**. For example, in exposure to ionizing radiation, we speak of the gonad dose; this is important in its genetic effect on the human race.

orchi-	testicle	orchidic—pertaining to the testes
		orchitis—inflammation of a testis
testo-	testicle	testosterone—male sex hormone
prostat-	prostate	prostatomegaly—hypertrophy of the prostate
		prostatitis—inflammation of the prostate
oophor-	ovary	oophoron—an ovary
		oophoritis—inflammation of an ovary
salping-	fallopian tube	salpingitis—inflammation of a fallopian tube
		salpingography—x-ray examination of a fallopian tube

1.296	Sterility in man may be due to epidemic parotitis (mumps) during adulthood, when infection of the testes can occur. As there is no successful treatment for this infection, it is advantageous for boys to have mumps before puberty; .... (infection of the testes) is then rare.	
1.297	Another possible cause of sterility in man is untreated gonorrhea, which can spread to the epididymis and cause an inflammation, called	orchitis
1.298	The prostate is also often attacked at the same time, resulting in	epididymitis
1.299	Inflammation of the fallopian tube can result in sterility through fusion of the mucous membrane during lengthy healing. Therefore, it is important to diagnose and treat .... (inflammation of a fallopian tube) as early as possible.	prostatitis

1.300	Salpingitis is often preceded by inflammation of the mucous membrane of the uterus, ...	salpingitis
1.301	The ovaries may also be involved, ...	endometritis
1.302	The womb is known as the . . . ., the neck of the womb as the . . . . and the protrusion into the vagina as the	oophoritis
1.303	The fetus is nourished through the	uterus cervix portio vaginalis
		placenta

SKIN

The skin has several functions. It protects the body, is part of the body's heat regulating system, is an excretory organ and is the origin of many sensations. The skin, **cutis**, consists of the outermost layer, the **epidermis**, and the inner layer, the **corium** or **dermis**; below this is the **subcutaneous tissue** (Fig. 1.31).

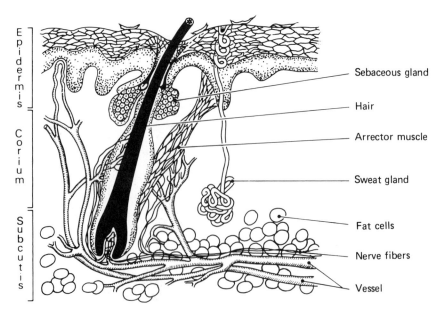

Figure 1.31 Section through the skin.

The epidermis consists of stratified squamous (platelike) epithelium, the surface of which is a horny layer. It has no blood vessels, but since it is usually thin it assumes a light reddish color from the vessels of the corium.

The corium is richly provided with blood vessels and nerves, which are connected to the sensory organs of the skin. The subcutaneous tissue is a loose tissue rich in fat cells.

Through its elastic structure and high fat content, the skin is able to withstand great mechanical stress. It affords comparatively effective protection against chemicals and is impermeable to most gases and substances dissolved in water. It also forms a barrier to bacteria.

The skin regulates the body temperature within narrow limits. Because of the fat layer in the subcutaneous tissue, the skin is a poor thermal conductor, and thus protects the body against heat losses. The sweat glands are the body's most important organ for heat dissipation.

The skin aids in the excretion of fluids, salts and, to a limited extent, urea. The **mammae**, or breasts, consist of glandular tissue, specialized for producing milk.

The somatic sensory system is located in the skin; it is sensitive to touch, pressure, pain, heat and cold.

derma-	skin	dermatology—a branch of medicine dealing with diseases of the skin
		dermatitis—inflammation of the skin
		dermatomycosis—skin disease due to microscopic fungi
cutan-	skin	subcutaneous—beneath the skin
		intracutaneous—in the skin
		percutaneous—through the skin

1.304	The skin protects the body against . . . . and . . . . action and against	
1.305	The skin protects the body from heat loss through the insulating property of the . . . . layer in the	mechanical chemical bacteria
1.306	Heat is given off by the skin by action of the	fat subcutaneous tissue
1.307	The main substances excreted through the skin are . . . . and	sweat glands
1.308	The skin contains sensory organs for the perception of . . . . , ... , ... , ... and	water salts

1.309	The breasts are known as the	touch pressure pain heat cold
1.310	Dermatosis is a	mammae
1.311	Tetanus vaccine is injected subcutaneously, that is, ...	skin disease
		beneath the skin

REGULATORY SYSTEMS

The regulatory systems of the body consist of the nervous system and the endocrine system. The nervous system governs the rapid events, such as muscle contractions and the secretion of most of the glands, while the endocrine system mainly regulates the slower, metabolic processes.

Endocrine System

The endocrine system acts by using hormones, which are carried through the circulatory system. The hormones are generated in the **endocrine glands** or the **glands of internal secretion** and are discharged directly from the gland cells into the blood or lymph.

The endocrine system is represented diagrammatically in Fig. 1.32. The system is controlled by nerve impulses from the autonomic nervous system and by chemical substances, including hormones secreted by other endocrine glands. The **pituitary** (hypophysis) is the principal endocrine gland and influences several other glands through the action of a large number of hormones. Nerve impulses from a part of the brain called the **hypothalamus** are conducted to the median eminence, where they release hormone releasing factors, which are carried down to the pituitary by the circulation. Thus the hypothalamus controls the pituitary.

The **thyroid gland** secretes, among other things, **thyroxin**, which increases the metabolism in the body. A deficiency of thyroid hormone leads to **hypothyroidism** or **myxedema**, which results in a low metabolic rate and mental retardation. An excess of the hormone results in **hyperthyroidism**. One of the results of this high metabolic rate is nervousness.

The **parathyroid glands** are located on the dorsal side of the thyroid. They regulate the body's calcium and phosphorus metabolism. If they are removed, the calcium level in the blood falls; this leads to muscle spasms, known as **tetanus**, which can be fatal.

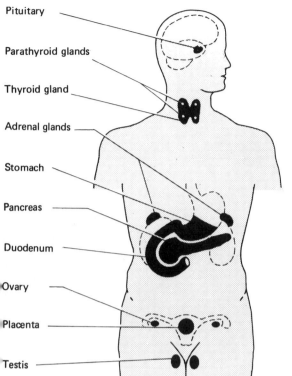

Pituitary

Parathyroid glands

Thyroid gland

Adrenal glands

Stomach

Pancreas

Duodenum

Ovary

Placenta

Testis

Figure 1.32 The most important organs of the endocrine system.

The **adrenal** (suprarenal) **glands** are divided into the **cortex** and **medulla**. The cortex is important to life, since it secretes a number of hormones—**corticoids**. These influence, for example, the metabolism of salts, the water-electrolyte balance, muscular activity and renal function. In the adrenal medulla epinephrine and norepinephrine form. One of their functions is to regulate blood pressure and flow.

The **pancreas** has an endocrine function. In the gland tissue, which secretes pancreatic juice, there are cells known as the **islets of Langerhans**; these secrete **insulin**, a hormone that regulates the metabolism of glucose. A deficiency of insulin results in increased glucose in the blood, a condition known as **diabetes**.

The mucous membrane of the **duodenum** generates a number of hormones as the acid contents of the stomach pass down into the intestine. These regulate the secretion and composition of the pancreatic juice, induce emptying of the gallbladder, and reduce stomach contractions and the production of hydrochloric acid. The lower part of the stomach also has an endocrine function.

The sex glands, the **gonads**, like the pancreas, have a dual function. Besides the sex cells, a number of sex hormones are generated (e.g., in the male, **testosterone**, and in the female, **estrogen** and **progesterone**). These hormones regulate the sex drive, pregnancy, and the development of secondary sex characteristics (the male and female features that develop at puberty).

The **placenta** generates a number of hormones that are of importance in pregnancy.

thyro-	thyroid	thyrogenic—deriving from the thyroid gland thyroidectomy—surgical removal of part of the thyroid gland thyrotropic—affecting the thyroid gland (e.g., from the pituitary)
supraren-	adrenal, suprarenal	suprarenal—(1) pertaining to the adrenals (2) located above the kidneys
cortico-	adrenal cortex	corticoids—adrenal cortical hormones corticotropic—affecting the adrenal cortex (e.g., from the pituitary)

1.312	The endocrine system regulates the body's .... (rapid, slow) functions.	
1.313	The principal endocrine gland, the ...., governs several other endocrine glands.	slow
1.314	The pituitary is controlled by the .... (part of brain).	pituitary
1.315	Too low an output of thyroid hormone is known as ....-thyroidism.	hypothalamus
1.316	A patient consults a physician for nervousness, thumping heart, loss of hair and finger tremor. The physician finds signs of excessive production of thyroid hormone, or .... (disease).	hypo-
1.317	Hyperparathyroidism is a disease in which there is excessive production of ...., which leads to disturbance of the calcium and phosphorus metabolism.	hyperthyroidism
1.318	A patient with suprarenal symptoms has signs of functional disorder of the	parathyroid hormone
1.319	Corticosteroids are hormones from the	adrenal glands

1.320	Diabetogenic factors are ones that favor the development of	adrenal cortex
1.321	A patient with diabetes has too low an output of .... (hormone) due to a disorder involving the .... (organ).	diabetes
		insulin pancreas

Nervous System

The nervous system coordinates the functions of the organs. This occurs by the action of external and internal **stimuli**, which result in **reflexes**—that is, the transmission of stimuli via nerve fibers and groups of neurons to muscles or glands which are caused to contract or secrete in an appropriate manner. The neurons and their branches, the nerve fibers, form an extremely complex network, which links up all parts of the body.

The nervous system consists of a central and a peripheral part. The **central nervous system** is made up of the **encephalon** (brain) and the **spinal cord**. The **peripheral nervous system** comprises all the nerves and groups of neurons outside the brain and spinal cord.

A group of neurons is known as a **ganglion** (pl. ganglia) or **nucleus**. They occur peripherally, for example, along the spinal cord associated with certain nerves, and in the brain in the form of **basal ganglia**. They are responsible for certain specialized and complex regulatory functions.

The basal ganglia together with the **cortical layer** of the brain, which is also rich in neurons, constitute the **gray matter** of the brain. The intervening **white substance** consists of conducting pathways, which are bundles of nerve fibers. In the spinal cord the distribution of the gray matter composed of neurons gives a characteristic H-shaped cross-section, which is surrounded by white matter comprising conducting pathways.

A peripheral nerve, such as those branching from the spinal cord, consists of bundles of nerve fibers. The nerves contain two types of pathways. The **afferent** ones conduct inwards and are called **sensory** pathways because they conduct impulses from the sensory organs of the skin, or from the deep sensibility of the muscles. The **efferent**, outward conducting pathways, are called **motor** pathways because they conduct impulses to the muscles and the various gland systems.

encephal-	brain	encephalitis—inflammation of the brain encephalography—x-ray examination of the brain

cerebr(o)-	brain, cerebrum	cerebral—pertaining to the brain
		cerebrospinal—pertaining to the cerebrum and the spinal cord
		cerebrospinal fluid—the fluid in the brain, and around the brain and spinal cord
cerebell-	cerebellum	cerebellar—pertaining to the cerebellum
spinal-	spinal cord	spinal nerve—nerve arising from the spinal cord
		spinal anesthesia—anesthesia of the lower half of the body by injection of an anesthetic into the spinal canal (not the spinal cord)

1.322	The nervous system governs the body's . . . . (rapid, slow) control functions.	
1.323	The nervous system coordinates organs by the action of external and internal . . . . , which produce	rapid
1.324	The nervous system consists of two parts, a . . . . and a . . . . part.	stimuli reflexes
1.325	The central nervous system includes the . . . . and the	central peripheral
1.326	A group of neurons is known as a	brain (encephalon) spinal cord
1.327	The gray matter of the brain consists mainly of	ganglion
1.328	The intervening white matter consists of	neurons
1.329	Basal ganglia in the brain are nuclei with special . . . . (purpose in the body).	bundles of nerve fibers (conducting path- ways)
1.330	In the spinal cord the neurons are arranged in an . . . . -shaped cross-section, which consists of . . . . matter.	regulatory functions

1.331	The outer parts of the cross-section of the spinal cord consist of .... matter, that is, ...	H gray
1.332	An afferent pathway conducts .... (inwards, outwards).	white conducting pathways
1.333	A pathway conducting outwards is said to be	inwards
1.334	A sensory pathway is	efferent
1.335	A motor pathway is	afferent
1.336	Softening (malacia) of the brain is known as	efferent
1.337	Encephalitis is	cerebromalacia
1.338	A boy dives in shallow water and breaks his neck. This severs the .... and leads to a paralysis (page 48) of all skeletal muscles below the neck.	inflammation of the brain
		spinal cord

Central nervous system

The brain, the **encephalon**, consists of three parts, namely, the **cerebrum**, **cerebellum** and the **brain stem**. The brain stem continues directly into the spinal cord. The number of neurons in the brain has been estimated at 1.2×10^{10}. Each neuron is connected by means of synapses with on an average 10,000 other neurons. In the brain stem, where all vital centers are located, the synapses number tens of thousands per neuron.

Cerebrum. The cerebrum consists of two well demarcated **hemispheres** separated by a deep fissure in the median plane. At the bottom of the fissure the hemispheres are connected by the corpus callosum. The hemispheres are divided into lobes: **frontal lobe**, **parietal lobe**, **occipital lobe**, and **temporal lobe** (Fig. 1.33). The outer layer of the brain, the cerebral cortex, contains numerous convolutions. Various areas are responsible for sight, hearing, touch, and control of the voluntary muscles of the body.

The cerebral cortex is also the center of intellectual functions (Fig. 1.34). The frontal lobes are essential for intelligence, constructive imagination and abstract thought. Here, large quantities of information can be temporarily stored and

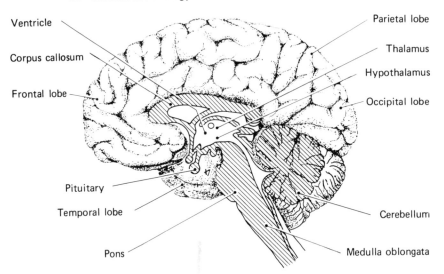

Ventricle

Corpus callosum

Frontal lobe

Pituitary

Temporal lobe

Pons

Parietal lobe

Thalamus

Hypothalamus

Occipital lobe

Cerebellum

Medulla oblongata

Figure 1.33 Median sagittal section through the brain.

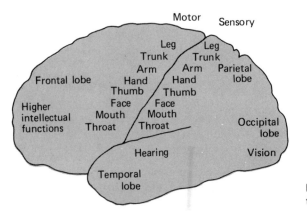

Motor Sensory

Leg Leg
Trunk Trunk
Arm Arm Parietal
Frontal lobe Hand Hand lobe
Thumb Thumb
Higher Face Face
intellectual Mouth Mouth
functions Throat Throat Occipital
lobe

Hearing Vision

Temporal
lobe

Figure 1.34 Sites of some centers in the cerebral cortex.

correlated, thus affording a basis for higher mental functions. In **lobotomy**, an operation that was formerly performed in cases of, among other things, severe anxiety that could not be cured by other means, all the conducting pathways to the anterior parts of the frontal lobes were severed. The patient's anxiety disappeared, but at the same time so did his higher mental functions; the patient could, however, perform low level tasks.

The posterior part of the frontal lobe is the center for the body's voluntary activity. Here, an important pathway originates, the **pyramidal tract**, through which nerve impulses are conducted to the muscles in the opposite half of the body—opposite because the pyramidal tracts from the respective hemispheres cross as they pass through the brain stem. Each pyramidal tract consists of about 250,000 nerve fibers. Each point in the **motor center** in the cerebral cortex corresponds to a certain body movement; such a movement can be elicited by electrically stimulating the brain surface.

In the anterior part of the parietal lobe lies the terminal station for the nerve pathways conducting sensation from the opposite half of the body. This **sensory center** contains counterparts of the various areas of the body in different locations of the cortex, similar to that of the adjacent motor cortex (Fig. 1.34).

The visual pathways terminate in the posterior part of the occipital lobe. If a metal splinter damages a certain part of this **visual center**, this produces a blind patch in the visual fields of both eyes, with a size and shape corresponding approximately to the extent of the damage to the cortex. The rest of the occipital lobes store visual memories, by means of which we interpret what we see. An injury to these parts of the occipital lobes can therefore lead to psychic blindness, a condition in which the person can see but cannot interpret what he sees.

On the upper side of the temporal lobe the acoustic pathways terminate. This is the location of the **hearing center**. Acoustic sensations are interpreted by means of acoustic memories stored elsewhere in the temporal lobes. In bilateral temporal lesions, word deafness can develop in which the patient, analogously with psychic blindness, cannot interpret the sounds he hears. For example, he is unable to distinguish between music and speech on the radio, since he cannot see who is producing the sound. The temporal lobes are also of importance for the storage process in the long term memory. In the case of damage to certain parts of these lobes, the patient is unable to remember recent events but can recall experiences that occurred prior to the damage.

1.339	The brain consists of three parts: ...., ... and	
1.340	A patient with brain damage has lost his hearing. The injury is probably located in the .... lobe.	cerebrum cerebellum brain stem
1.341	A soldier has been hit by grenade splinters and the physician has found a blind patch in the visual field of both eyes. There are splinters in the .... lobe.	temporal
1.342	A patient with a brain tumor has become paralyzed in the right leg. If the injury is located in the cerebral cortex, it is in the .... (anterior, posterior) .... (right, left) part of the .... lobe.	occipital

1.343	If the tumor is not located in the cortex, it is probably in the .... tract, which originates in the motor cortex.	posterior left frontal
1.344	The sensory cortical centers are located in the .... (anterior, posterior) part of the .... lobe.	pyramidal
		anterior parietal

Cerebellum. The cerebellum likewise consists of two hemispheres. They regulate the coordination of muscular movements elicited by the cerebrum—for example, the automatic relaxation of the flexor muscles when the extensors are activated. The cerebellum is also a balance center.

Brain stem. An important formation known as the brain stem extends from the region just below the cerebral cortex. It consists of the diencephalon, midbrain, the pons, and the medulla oblongata (which continues down into the spinal cord). A part of the diencephalon, the **thalamus**, is a relay station for sensory pathways to the cortical sensory center of the cerebrum.

In the lower part of the diencephalon, the **hypothalamus**, there are several vital centers for temperature regulation, metabolism and fluid regulation; they include the centers for appetite, thirst, sleep and drive (aggression, fear, rage, maternal feelings and sexual drive). The hypothalamus is important for subjective feelings and emotions.

The **medulla oblongata** contains centers for regulating the work performed by the heart, the vasomotor centers, which control blood distribution, and the respiratory center, which controls the ventilation of the lungs.

A knowledge of the location of the various centers in the brain is important for understanding the symptoms in various kinds of epilepsy (Chapter 4).

The brain contains a system of cavities, known as the **ventricles**, where the **cerebrospinal fluid** is generated. The fluid passes through a hole in the brain stem and surrounds both the brain and the spinal cord. These thus float in the fluid which helps to resist the stresses due to acceleration.

Spinal cord. The spinal cord is a downward continuation of the medulla oblongata. It extends to the level of the first or second lumbar vertebra. The spinal cord is protected by the spinal canal; this is formed by the vertebral arches, which are situated one above the other.

In the H-shaped gray matter of the spinal cord are located the neurons that control many reflexes, for example, the knee reflex and the bladder-emptying.

The brain and the spinal cord are covered by the **meninges**. Next to the brain is the **pia mater** (soft brain membrane), outside this the **arachnoid** (intermediate brain membrane), and outermost the **dura mater** (hard brain membrane). The cerebrospinal fluid is located between the pia mater and the arachnoid.

1.345	Examination of a patient with disturbed balance discloses signs of damage to the central nervous system, namely in the .... (cerebrum, cerebellum, brain stem, spinal cord).	
1.346	Centers for temperature regulation, metabolism, fluid regulation, appetite, thirst, sleep and sexual drive are located in the part of the brain stem called the	cerebellum
1.347	The vasomotor center, and the center that regulates ventilation are located in the	hypothalamus
1.348	In the .... there are centers for the knee reflex.	medulla oblongata
1.349	The fluid in the brain ventricles and surrounding the brain and spinal cord is known as the	spinal cord
1.350	A patient with meningitis has inflammation of the	cerebrospinal fluid
1.351	Inflammation of the brain, that is, ..., often follows meningitis.	meninges
		encephalitis

Peripheral nervous system

The peripheral nervous system consists of motor and sensory nerve fibers which are arranged in bundles to form nerve trunks, usually referred to as "nerves". These peripheral nerves branch and lead to all the organs of the body (Fig. 1.35). The motor nerve fibers control the muscles and glands, while the sensory fibers convey to the central nervous system information on the state of various parts of the body.

Twelve pairs of cranial nerves arise from the brain. The first pair conducts impulses from the organ of smell to the brain, the second pair, the **optic nerve**, runs from the eyes, the eighth, the **vestibulocochlear**, runs from the inner ear to the brain, and the tenth, the **vagus nerve**, connects the brain to the viscera.

From each side of the spinal cord emerge the **ventral roots**, which conduct motor impulses to the muscles, and the **dorsal roots**, which conduct sensory

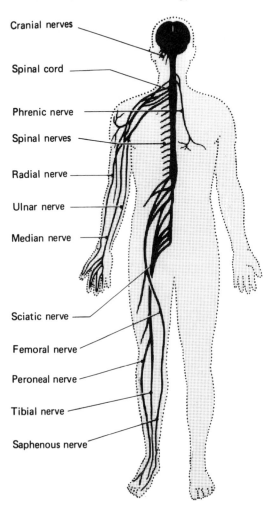

Cranial nerves

Spinal cord

Phrenic nerve

Spinal nerves

Radial nerve

Ulnar nerve

Median nerve

Sciatic nerve

Femoral nerve

Peroneal nerve

Tibial nerve

Saphenous nerve

Figure 1.35 The peripheral nervous system consists of all the nerves that leave the brain and spinal cord. The tenth cranial nerve, the vagus nerve, which runs to most of the organs in the trunk, is not included in the figure.

impulses to the central nervous system (Fig. 1.36). The motor pathways thus conduct outwards, and are described as **efferent**, and the sensory ones conduct inwards, **afferent**. Figure 1.37 shows the areas of the skin that are innervated by the various sensory spinal nerves. A knowledge of these areas is of importance in locating injuries to the spinal cord roots—for example, in disc herniation.

1.352	A peripheral nerve consists of bundles of	
1.353	The nerve fibers are of two types, ... and	nerve fibers

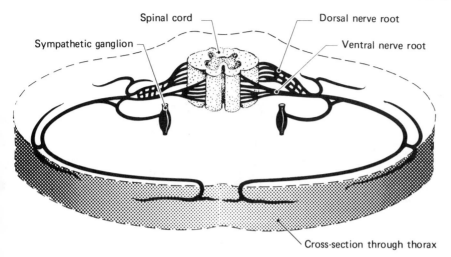

Spinal cord — Dorsal nerve root

Sympathetic ganglion — Ventral nerve root

Cross-section through thorax

Figure 1.36 Diagram showing the arrangement of the spinal nerves.

1.354	The motor nerve fibers control .... and	motor sensory
1.355	The sensory nerve fibers conduct impulses to the	muscles glands
1.356	The tenth cranial nerve, the ...., runs to the	central nervous system
1.357	The dorsal roots from the spinal cord conduct .... impulses.	vagus viscera
1.358	The ventral roots conduct .... impulses.	sensory
1.359	In disc herniation, a substance extruded from an intervertebral disc presses on the nerves that leave the spinal cord. If they press on the dorsal roots, which contain sensory fibers, the person feels pain. This is perceived in the corresponding area of the skin. If they press on the ventral roots, which contain motor fibers, ... results.	motor

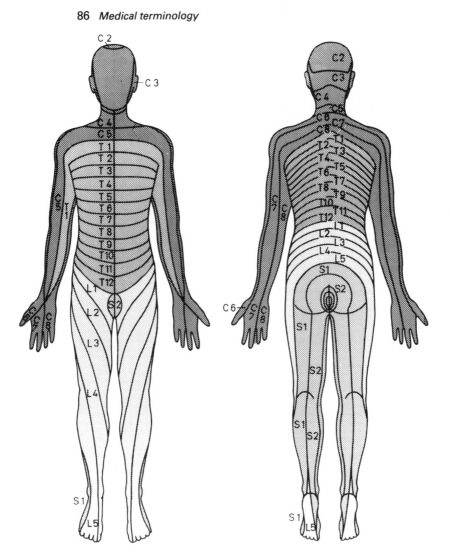

Figure 1.37 Areas of the skin that correspond to the various nerve roots (C, cervical; T, thoracic; L, lumbar; S, sacral).

1.360	A patient with disc herniation has pain that extends from outside the right knee over the front of the lower leg down to the foot. From Fig. 1.37 locate the vertebra where the hernia is located.	paresis (slight paralysis)
		L5 (fifth lumbar vertebra)

Autonomic nervous system. All the body functions that are not conscious or under the control of the will—for example, the circulation, digestion, excretion, gland function and smooth muscle activity—are regulated by the autonomic nervous system. This system is not anatomically well defined, however, but it does function as a unit.

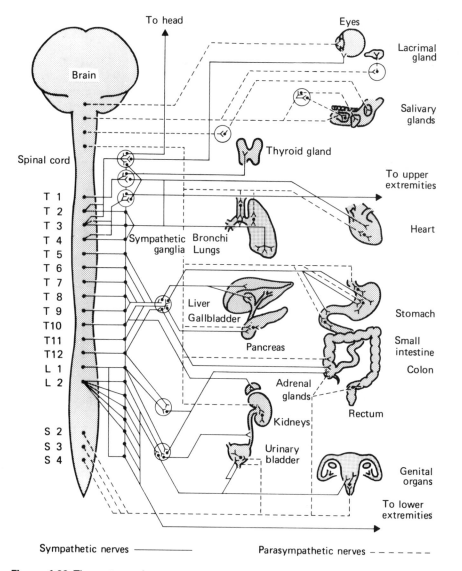

Figure 1.38 The autonomic nervous system consists of two functionally opposite systems, the sympathetic and the parasympathetic.

The autonomic nervous system consists of two purely motor systems working in opposition, the **sympathetic** and the **parasympathetic** systems. Nerve impulses conducted through one of the systems stimulate activity in an organ in one direction, and those conducted through the other system evoke the opposite effect. For example, the pupil of the eye is dilated by the sympathetic system and contracted by the parasympathetic. There is thus a state of equilibrium, or **homeostasis**, in the activity of the organ.

The sympathetic nervous system consists of, among other things, **sympathetic ganglia**, which are located along each side of the spinal column (Fig. 1.36). From here sympathetic fibers lead to the viscera, blood vessels and skin. When stimulated by the sympathetic system, the vessels contract, the heart rate increases, the peristaltic activity of the intestine is decreased, the uterus contracts, secretion by the sweat glands is stimulated, and secretion by the glands of the digestive organs is inhibited. The parasympathetic nerve fibers run in certain cranial nerves (e.g., the vagus nerve) and in certain spinal nerves (Fig. 1.38).

The antagonistic function of sympathetic and parasympathetic systems is evident also from their different modes of reaction to certain drugs.

1.361	The autonomic nervous system is a(n) .... (anatomic, functional) unit.	
1.362	The autonomic nervous system consists of the .... and the .... nervous systems.	functional
1.363	The sympathetic and parasympathetic nervous systems act	sympathetic parasympathetic
1.364	Through the coordinating action of the two systems, homeostasis develops, that is, ... in the activity of the organs.	in opposition (antagonistically)
		equilibrium

Regulatory Functions

There are literally thousands of regulatory functions in the body. Some of them are comparatively simple, and are then often known as reflexes; in other cases many reflexes work together in complex regulatory systems which include both endocrine and nervous functions.

Reflexes

A receptor must first be activated in order to excite a reflex. The stimulus is next conducted from the receptor, through nerve fibers in an afferent nerve, to the spinal cord or the brain. There the stimulus is transmitted to other neurons, causing the nerve fibers in an efferent nerve to excite a muscle or a gland, which then contracts or secretes. These reflexes regulate the vital functions. In diseases of the nervous system, disorders of the reflexes appear, and therefore it is often necessary to test the reflex function.

There are different types of reflexes and these can be classified in different ways. Many reflexes are congenital—**inborn reflexes** (e.g., the cough reflex occurs when the bronchi are stimulated). Others develop later in life and some are acquired through experience; the latter are known as **conditioned reflexes** (e.g., salivary secretion evoked by the smell of food). The reflexes can also be divided according to the number of neurons that are involved: we speak of monosynaptic and polysynaptic reflexes (**synapse**: site of contact between two neurons).

Most reflexes serve an obvious purpose; for example, blinking occurs when the cornea is touched—the **corneal reflex**; sneezing follows stimulation of the nasal mucosa—the **sneezing reflex**; the pupil contracts when light enters the eye—the **pupillary reflex**; the hand jerks back when it touches a hot object. In body movements—for example in working or jumping—a number of reflexes are involved; this is necessary for coordinated motion. Here, **tendon jerk reflexes** act—that is, if a muscle or its tendon is stretched, the muscle contracts.

The patellar reflex is an example of a tendon jerk reflex. When the patellar tendon is tapped it stretches, as do the extensors of the femur (Fig. 1.39). The

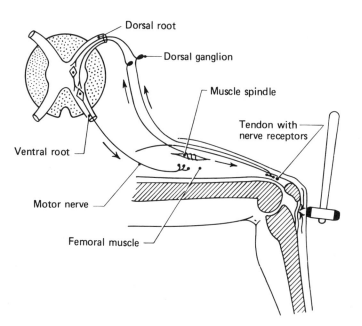

Figure 1.39 The nerve mechanism in the patellar reflex.

receptors in the muscle spindles and in the tendon are activated and impulses are transmitted in afferent pathways via a dorsal root into the spinal cord. There the signals, after passing through a single synapse, excite the motor neurons. These emit impulses through efferent nerve fibers in a ventral root to the extensors of the thigh muscle, which contract with a jerk.

1.365	A child suddenly runs into the road, which causes the driver of a car to immediately apply the brake. This is the result of a . . . . reflex.	
1.366	The rapid movement of the leg used in braking, and the jerk that occurs when the foot meets the brake pedal causes a sudden pull on the heel tendon and calf muscles, resulting in a . . . . reflex. (The combination of mechanical load from the pedal and the muscular contraction caused by the reflex can result in tearing of the calf muscle or Achilles tendon.)	conditioned
		tendon jerk

Example of compound regulatory functions

A knowledge of the vital regulatory functions in the body is of immediate practical importance in intensive care therapy (Chapter 11). For example, disturbances in the regulation of breathing and blood pressure are common, and rapid counter-measures are of vital importance.

Control of ventilation. The ventilation of the lungs is governed by the respiratory center which controls the inspired volume and breathing rate. The respiratory center, located in the medulla oblongata, receives information from the **chemoreceptors**, which sense the oxygen and carbon dioxide content of the blood and its pH (hydrogen ion concentration), and also from the stretch receptors in the lungs, which determine the extent to which they are filled. The chemoreceptors are located (1) at the bifurcation (branching) of the **common carotid artery**, (2) in the **aortic arch** (the semicircular part of the aorta next to the heart), and (3) in the actual respiratory center in the **medulla oblongata**. The nerve impulse frequency for the carotid artery chemoreceptors is shown in Fig. 1.40 as a function of the oxygen and carbon dioxide partial pressures, PO_2 and PCO_2.

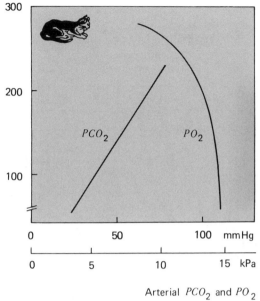

Number of nerve
impulses per second

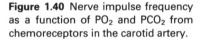

Arterial PCO_2 and PO_2

Figure 1.40 Nerve impulse frequency as a function of PO_2 and PCO_2 from chemoreceptors in the carotid artery.

Ventilation can also be voluntarily controlled—the breath can be held for a limited time. It is also governed by certain reflexes, for example, in coughing, sneezing, vomiting and yawning. Figure 1.41 shows a block diagram of the respiratory control system.

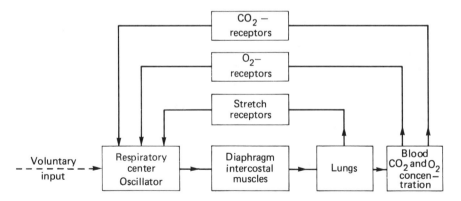

Figure 1.41 Block diagram showing respiratory control.

1.367	The respiratory center is located in the.	
1.368	Ventilation is governed by . . . .-receptors for the oxygen and carbon dioxide concentration and pH, and by . . . . receptors located in the lungs.	medulla oblongata
1.369	The chemoreceptors are located in the . . . ., ... and	chemo- stretch
		common carotid artery aortic arch medulla oblongata

Regulation of blood pressure. The blood pressure is kept at a relatively constant level by a complex regulatory mechanism (Fig. 1.42). There are, however, certain physiological variations—for example, the blood pressure elevates during effort,

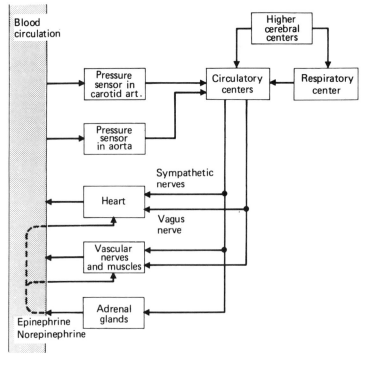

Figure 1.42 Block diagram for control of circulation.

after intake of food, and in emotional states, but falls during sleep. The mean blood pressure is adjusted to obtain optimal blood flow through the organs.

The blood pressure is sensed by **baroreceptors** in the arch of the aorta and in the carotid sinus (a widening of the carotid artery located where it branches into the **internal** and **external carotid arteries**). A change in blood pressure produces a change in the vessel wall tension; this is sensed by the baroreceptors, which change the impulse frequency of the nerves leading to the circulatory centers in the **medulla oblongata**.

From these centers the blood pressure is regulated by the heart (which varies its power output) and by the vessels (which vary their hydrodynamic impedance).

The activity of the heart is lowered by the **parasympathetic** nerve fibers of the **vagus nerve**, so that the blood pressure is lowered; the heart activity is stimulated via the **sympathetic** nerves, so that the blood pressure is raised. In addition, the heart is influenced indirectly by hormones from the adrenal glands, namely **epinephrine** and **norepinephrine**, which reach the heart through the blood stream.

There are also two opposing influences that affect the vessels. The lumen of the vessel is reduced by **vasoconstriction** (vascular contraction of the smooth muscle in the vessel wall), or it is increased by **vasodilation** (widening of the vessels). The vessel muscles are controlled directly via the autonomic nerve impulses from the vasomotor centers in the medulla oblongata, and indirectly by the adrenal hormones, which reach the vessels through the blood stream. Epinephrine and norepinephrine both increase the systolic pressure, but have differing effects on the heart and various parts of the vascular system.

1.370	The centers for regulation of blood pressure are located in the	
1.371	The blood pressure is controlled through .... (pressure sensors) located in the aortic arch and carotid sinus.	medulla oblongata
1.372	The blood pressure is regulated by actions of the .... and the .... (organs).	baroreceptors
1.373	The activity of the heart is lowered by the .... nerve fibers in the .... nerve, so that the blood pressure is lowered.	heart vessels
1.374	If the heart is stimulated by the ...., the blood pressure is raised.	parasympathetic vagus
1.375	The heart is also regulated by the endocrine system through epinephrine and norepinephrine, which come from the	sympathetic nerves

1.376	The hydrodynamic impedance in the vascular system is varied by .... and .... (narrowing and widening of the vessels).	adrenal glands
1.377	The muscles in the vessels are controlled directly via nerve impulses from vasomotor centers in the .... and, indirectly, by hormones from the	vasoconstriction vasodilation
1.378	Too high a blood pressure is known as	medulla oblongata adrenal glands
1.379	Too low a blood pressure is known as	hypertension
		hypotension

Temperature regulation. The body temperature in man remains within narrow limits, even when the environmental temperature undergoes great changes. Temperature stability is achieved through several mechanisms.

The body temperature is determined by the balance between heat generation and heat loss. Heat is generated by chemical combustion. Heat is given off by conduction, convection, irradiation and evaporation. The relative magnitudes of these factors are dependent on the external temperature, relative humidity, wind velocity, clothing and type of physical activity.

The body requires a complex regulatory system to maintain the temperature within $\pm 0.1°C$ ($\pm 0.2°F$) in spite of large differences in heat loss (Fig. 1.43). The sensors for the temperature regulating system are located in the skin (for sensing environmental temperature) and in the hypothalamus (for sensing body temperature). The hypothalamus contains the temperature regulation centers and the temperature reference sensor.

Several reflex centers in the central nervous system are involved in the control of temperature. A drop in the environmental temperature results in an error signal—the difference between the temperature reference and the body temperature. This error signal in the hypothalamus activates the autonomic nervous system so that the heat losses are reduced and the heat generating mechanisms are increased. The latter is accomplished by an increase in metabolism; for example, involuntary muscle activity is produced in the striated muscles—"we shiver with cold". If the external temperature rises, another part of the hypothalamus is activated, producing the opposite effect via the autonomic nervous system. There are increases in sweat gland secretion, peripheral blood flow in the skin and breathing rate, but decreases in muscle activity.

The normal **rectal temperature** (the body temperature measured in the anus) is 36.5–$37.5°C$ (97.7–$99.5°F$). If there is a slight rise in temperature to 37.5–$38°C$

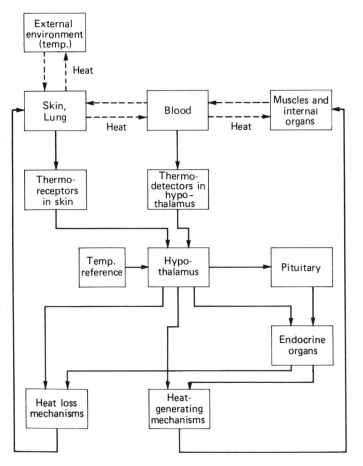

Figure 1.43 Block diagram for temperature regulation.

(99.5–100.4°F) the patient is said to be **subfebrile**, and if there is an increase to above 38°C (100.4°F) he is **febrile**.

1.380	The center for temperature regulation is located in the	
1.381	The temperature reference sensor lies in the	hypothalamus
1.382	Heat is generated by	hypothalamus
1.383	When we shiver with cold, ...	chemical combustion

1.384	Thermal conductivity, convection, radiation and evaporation are mechanisms for	heat is generated
1.385	A patient with a temperature of 37.9°C (100.2°F) is	loss of heat
		subfebrile

SENSORY ORGANS

The sensory organs serve as receptors of information from the environment. The information is carried by nerves to the brain, where sensory perception takes place. All the sensory organs have the power of **adaptation**; that is, adaptation of the organ's sensitivity to the level of stimulus. This occurs with a certain time constant and the process is similar to automatic volume control in a radio.

The somatic sensors react to touch, pressure, warmth, cold and pain, each with its own receptors. These receptors are small and sparsely distributed; thus it is possible to distinguish them separately. The **touch receptors** are most closely spaced on the fingertips, on the lips and the tip of the tongue. Sensitivity to touch is intensified by the hairs on the skin, which act as levers for the touch receptors. The sense of touch displays rapid adaptation. **Pressure receptors** are located deeper and adaptation is slower. They are also used to sense vibrations, which are most clearly perceived at about 200 Hz. The **warm and cold receptors** are most dense on the chest, abdomen and inner surfaces of the arms; and most sparse on the face and hands. Their adaptation is relatively slow. The **pain sensors** are free nerve endings. These serve to protect the body from mechanical damage, and there is little adaptation. A pain stimulus is generated in the skin and in some internal organs.

-esthesia	feeling	hyperesthesia—abnormally elevated sensitivity of the sense of feeling (see also page 9)

1.386	The sensory organs display an automatic gain control (similar to that in a radio), which is known as	
1.387	Lack of sensitivity to touch is known as	adaptation
		anesthesia

The olfactory organ is located in the mucous membrane in the upper part of the nasal cavity, where 10–20 million receptor cells cover an area of about 5 cm². The stimulus is generated by volatile substances, which are soluble in the thin film of liquid that covers the membrane. The sense of smell displays great adaptation. Its primary purpose is to serve as a protection against unsuitable inspired air and, together with the sense of taste, to identify unsuitable food. Both these senses also provoke by **reflex action** the secretion of saliva and gastric juices, which are important for the digestion of food. The **taste receptors** are located on the tip, border and base of the tongue, on the soft palate and certain parts of the throat. We are able to distinguish four basic tastes: sweet, sour, bitter and salt. The perception of taste is limited to dissolved substances or ones soluble in the saliva.

The visual sense responds to radiation in the wavelength range of 0.4–0.8 μm. The wall of the eye is composed of three layers. The outermost is known as the **sclera**. Its anterior part, the **cornea**, is transparent. The middle layer, the **choroid**, merges in the front with the **iris**, which contains a round hole, the **pupil**. The innermost layer is the **retina** (Fig. 1.44). The diameter of the pupil adapts to the light intensity by contracting annular and radial smooth muscles in the iris, which are controlled by the autonomic nervous system.

Incident light is refracted at the interfaces between the air, cornea, aqueous humor, lens and vitreous humor. **Accommodation**, the adaptive mechanism that enables us to focus on objects at different distances, is regulated by means of the smooth muscles, which modify the shape of the lens.

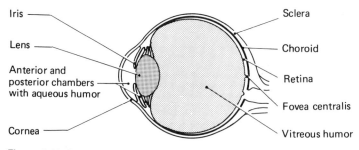

Iris —
Lens —
Anterior and posterior chambers with aqueous humor —
Cornea —

Sclera
Choroid
Retina
Fovea centralis
Vitreous humor

Figure 1.44 Structure of the eye.

The retina contains optical receptors, called **cones** and **rods**, which are linked to the optic nerve. The human eye contains some 3 million cones and about 60 million rods, whose signals converge to about 400,000 nerve fibers in the optic nerve. In the **fovea centralis**, where the central part of our gaze is projected, there are only cones. The fovea has a relatively low light sensitivity but high color sensitivity. The cones of the fovea number about 34,000, and have a diameter of 1–3 μm. There are many optic nerve fibers carrying information from the fovea, so high visual acuity (resolution) is possible there. At the periphery of the retina there are few cones, compared with the number of rods. The rods have a high sensitivity to light but no color sensitivity and are used in weak light—that is, for seeing in the dark. The rods and cones are connected to the optic nerve by a highly complex network, where complicated image preprocessing takes place.

Color vision uses three types of cones, with maximum sensitivity for blue, green and red light; thus, the eye performs a spectrum analysis of the image.

One means of regulating the sensitivity of the retina, known as **dark and light adaptation**, is a photochemical process using a pigment, **rhodopsin**. This pigment is broken down by light, which reduces the sensitivity. In the dark, the pigment is slowly restored and the sensitivity increases, a process that takes about 20 minutes. The ratio of maximum to minimum light sensitivity, including the changes due to the pupil area, is about 10^6.

ophthalm(o)-	eye	ophthalmology—study of the eye and its diseases
-opia	vision	myopia—near-sightedness (see also page
-opsia		9)

1.388	The wall of the eye is composed of three layers: (1) the . . . . , which in the front has a transparent part, the . . . . , (2) the . . . . , which is fused anteriorly with the . . . . , and (3) the	
1.389	The adaptation of the eye for seeing at different distances is known as	sclera cornea choroid iris retina
1.390	The eye's sensitivity to light is regulated by adjustment of the . . . . and by adaptation, which relies on a . . . . process.	accommodation
1.391	Inflammation of the iris is known as	iris photochemical
1.392	Inflammation of the retina is known as	iritis
1.393	The prefix meaning eye is	retinitis
1.394	A far-sighted person has	ophthalm(o)-
		hyperopia

The sense of hearing responds to acoustic signals over a frequency range of about 20 to 20,000 Hz (in young persons). The sound is received by the **external ear** and transmitted by the external acoustic meatus (ear canal) to the ear drum, through the **middle ear** by means of the ossicles (the malleus, the incus and the stapes) to the **inner ear** (Fig. 1.45).

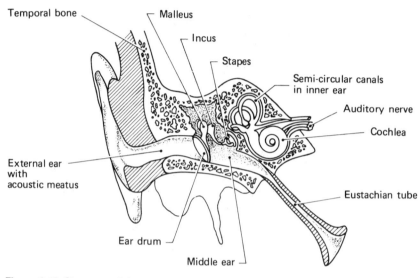

Figure 1.45 Structure of the ear.

The movement of the stapes is transmitted by the oval window to the labyrinth, which is filled with fluid. The fluid conducts the sound to the **cochlea**, where the receptors are located which convert the acoustic signal to nerve impulses. Different frequencies cause wave resonances to occur at different locations along the cochlea, and frequency discrimination occurs by stimulation of receptors in different positions in the cochlea.

The middle ear communicates with the pharynx via the **eustachian tube**, thus keeping the mean pressure in the middle ear at atmospheric pressure. The passage is normally closed but it opens when swallowing or yawning.

The tympanic membrane, or ear drum, is critically damped by the auditory ossicles; this is of importance in perceiving sounds with rapidly varying pitches. Two muscles issuing from the bony wall of the middle ear are attached to the ossicles. One goes to the malleus (when it contracts, the ear drum is stretched), and the other to the stapes (when it contracts, the conduction of sound by the stapes to the inner ear is reduced). These muscles are thus responsible for reflex control of hearing sensitivity.

The range of greatest sensitivity, namely 1–5 kHz, is determined primarily by the resonant frequencies of the various parts of the ear. For example, the resonant frequency for the external acoustic meatus is about 3 kHz, and for the middle ear 1 kHz, both strongly damped and therefore broad-band (low value of Q in engineering terms).

Since the middle ear contains air and the inner ear liquid, the acoustic impedance is different. (The acoustic impedance is defined as the ratio between the pressure perturbation and the particle velocity caused by the sound, and is measured in acoustic ohms.) The ossicular chain of the middle ear functions as an acoustic impedance transformer consisting of pistons and levers, with a lever ratio of about 1 : 10. This reduces the acoustic impedance of the fluid-filled cochlea by a factor of about 100, thereby improving the efficiency of the sound transmission from the air.

The sense of balance is located in the inner ear, and controls the body's static and dynamic equilibrium.

Three semicircular canals are used for sensing rotational movements. They are oriented in three mutually perpendicular planes and contain a fluid. Since the fluid has inertia, it flows with respect to the canals when the head is rotated. Sensory hair cells, which project into the fluid, are bent and generate signals that control the body's dynamic equilibrium. Another part of the balance system senses and controls the static equilibrium of the body.

-acusia	hearing	hypoacusia—diminished acuteness of hearing
ot(o)-	ear	otologist—ear specialist

1.395	The ear is sensitive over the frequency range ...., and the maximum sensitivity lies in the range	
1.396	The auditory ossicles serve as an acoustic .... for the conversion of impedance between the .... and the	20–20,000 Hz 1–5 kHz
1.397	Sound vibrations are transmitted from the tympanic membrane via the auditory ossicles to the oval window, where the loosely attached stapes serves as a piston. In calcification of the tissues, **sclerosis**, the mobility of the stapes is reduced causing a hearing loss, which may be a sign of	transformer external meatus cochlea
1.398	Inflammation of the ear is known as	otosclerosis
		otitis

REFERENCES

Fox, T. A. *Manual of Orthopaedic Surgery.* Chicago (American Orthopaedic Association) 1966. 183 pages.

Ganong, W. F. *Review of Medical Physiology.* Los Altos (Lange) 1975. 587 pages.

King, B. G. and Showers, M. J. *Human Anatomy and Physiology.* Philadelphia (W. B. Saunders) 1969. 432 pages.

Lewin, R. *Hormones: Chemical Communicators.* Garden City (Anchor) 1973. 113 pages

Preece, W. E. (Ed.): *Human Health and Diseases.* Sections listed in Propaedia, pp. 217–241, Encyclopaedia Britannica, Chicago (Encyclopaedia Britannica) 1974.

Rothenberg, R. E. *The New American Medical Dictionary and Health Manual.* New York (Signet) 1968. 496 pages.

Smith, G. L. and Davis, P. E. *Quick Medical Terminology.* New York (Wiley) 1972. 248 pages.

chapter 2

Physical
Diagnosis

A correct diagnosis is usually a prerequisite for effective treatment. The diagnosis is determined by examining the results of a number of
techniques. First a **medical history** is taken, in which the patient is questioned on
various aspects of his disease. A **physical examination** is then performed by
utilizing a series of simple methods. From an evaluation of the findings appropriate chemical and bacteriological laboratory tests are carried out and the patient
is referred to special laboratories and departments for diagnostic x-ray and other
examinations.

The results are entered in the patient's **medical record** (Fig. 2.1). This serves as
a basis for the **diagnosis**, the **choice of treatment** and the **prognosis**—that is, an
appraisal of the most likely outcome of the disease and treatment.

If the resulting picture does not point conclusively to a particular disease, but
there are several alternatives, further examinations must be made; that is, a
differential diagnosis must be performed. For example, jaundice may be due to
hepatitis, gallstones or a tumor, and examinations must be carried out to

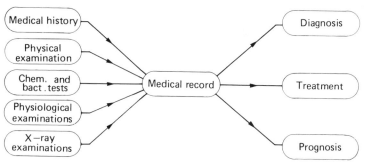

Figure 2.1 The results of clinical examinations are entered in the medical record; from these data the type of the patient's disease can be established, a suitable method of treatment chosen and the outcome of the disease determined.

determine which of these diseases is responsible. The need for differential diagnosis often arises.

The **physical diagnosis** includes the medical history and the physical examination, in which certain simple methods are used. The basis for these simple methods is treated in this chapter, while some of the next chapters are concerned with other, technically more advanced, examination procedures which have been developed from the simpler techniques. Here, a description is given of what can be seen directly by external **inspection**, and what can be examined with relatively simple optical instruments, while Chapter 8 deals with the methods of x-ray diagnosis. The physician's **smell** is of diagnostic significance only in exceptional cases, because the procedure of chemical analysis (Chapter 5) provides thorough quantitative measurements of the patient's metabolism. Two other simple methods are **palpation**—feeling the patient's body with the hands and fingers—and **percussion**, that is, listening to the sounds and feeling the vibrations emitted by organs when striking the surface of the body over the respective organs. These methods may be supplemented with ultrasonic examination (Chapter 8). Another simple technique is **auscultation**, that is, listening to the sounds generated in the patient's organs; the use of electronic methods such as phonocardiography is described in Chapter 3. The **measurement of blood pressure** is one of the most common clinical examinations and can be performed by a simple indirect method; for direct pressure measurement advanced techniques are often required (Chapter 3). **Temperature measurement** with a simple mercury thermometer is of fundamental medical importance; the procedure may be supplemented by the technically complicated method of thermography (Chapter 8). In testing the body's many **reflexes** the central nervous system can be examined with simple aids; examples of a number of electronic methods relying on advanced measurement techniques are given in Chapter 4. All the simpler methods are extensively used, whereas the more advanced procedures require special equipment and competent personnel, and for this reason are generally performed only at larger hospitals.

Question		*Answer*
2.1	One prerequisite for the proper choice of patient treatment is usually a correct	
2.2	The first step towards making a diagnosis is to take the medical	diagnosis
2.3	A physical examination is then made in which the patient is examined by using certain	history
2.4	The medical history and results of the physical examination and other technically more advanced examinations are entered in the medical	simple methods
2.5	The medical record provides a basis for the . . . ., the choice of . . . . and the	record
2.6	The medical history and the physical examination are known collectively as the	diagnosis treatment prognosis
2.7	Many diagnostically important findings can be made on the basis of an external . . . ., that is, by looking at the patient.	physical diagnosis
2.8	Feeling the patient's body with the hands and fingers is called	inspection
2.9	In an examination of patients with abdominal disorders the physician feels in the rectum with one finger; this is called	palpation
2.10	Two simple, fundamentally different, acoustic methods are used in the physical examination. In one, the physician listens to the sounds generated by the patient's organs; this is called	palpation per rectum

2.11	The other acoustic method is to listen to the sounds emitted by the organs after striking the surface of the body over the organs; this is known as	auscultation
2.12	In percussion one relies on .... as well as hearing.	percussion
2.13	Inspection, palpation, percussion, auscultation, blood pressure and temperature measurement and observation of reflexes are among the techniques used in the	feeling
2.14	Headache has many causes. Exhaustive examinations are therefore often needed in the required	physical examination
		differential diagnosis

MEDICAL HISTORY

The number and the type of questions that the patient is asked varies greatly, depending on his reason for consulting the physician. Therefore, some of the following questions may be omitted. For the purpose of **identification** the name, age, occupation and address are noted. Questions are then asked about hereditary factors (**heredity**: transmission of characteristics from parents or ancestors to offspring), the state of health of parents and siblings, causes of death and the occurrence of any diseases in the other members of the family. As far as possible, **earlier** illnesses are distinguished from the patient's **present** illness. When the history is taken, the patient's own words are recorded in order to avoid a tentative diagnosis that may subsequently prove to be incorrect.

Symptoms and signs of disease are of the following kinds:

- **subjective** symptoms, which only the patient can observe; for example, headache
- **objective** signs, which others can also observe, such as a skin eruption
- **general** symptoms, which do not indicate a diagnosis; for example, fever
- **specific** symptoms, also known as **pathognomonic** symptoms, which point directly to a specific disease, for example, the eruption in shingles

When a medical history is taken the patient is therefore questioned on the location, duration, development and nature of the symptoms of the current disease and their possible relation to different body positions and functions (physical and mental effort, meals, etc). The recording of the medical history is thus an essential preparation for the physical diagnostic examination; only with a correctly recorded medical history can the appropriate examinations be chosen.

The importance of questioning of the patient is also evident from the fact that about one half of all tentative diagnoses made on the basis of a medical history are confirmed by later examinations.

2.15	The state of health of the patient's family and their causes of death are recorded in the medical history under the heading	
2.16	An indication of illness that only the patient can observe is called a	heredity
2.17	A symptom or sign that others can observe is called an	subjective symptom
2.18	A symptom or sign that by itself does not determine a diagnosis is called a	objective sign
2.19	A symptom that points directly to a certain disease is called a pathognomonic or	general symptom
2.20	Which of the four types of symptoms or signs does a patient have who is suffering from diarrhea?	specific symptom
2.21	Which of the four types of symptoms or signs does a patient have who is troubled by nausea?	objective sign and general symptom
2.22	Which of the four types of symptoms or signs does a patient have who consults a physician for poor long distance vision, but good short distance vision?	subjective symptom and general symptom
		subjective symptom and specific or pathognomonic symptom

Location of pain

Pain is a common symptom of disease. It is a subjective feeling of discomfort that helps to protect the body from injury and, in case of injury, induces the body to rest. Among the various kinds of pain are a dull pain, a sharp pain, a stabbing pain, a throbbing ache and a dull ache. The patient's description of pain can be of diagnostic value. Of still greater importance are the pain's location, radiation and whether the pain is intermittent or constant.

Not all organs are sensitive to pain. The brain, for example, is insensitive. Organs controlled by the autonomic nervous system are also insensitive to localized stimuli. It is therefore possible to cut and perform surgery on heart muscle, stomach, bowel, liver and kidneys without the patient feeling it. Traction on the mesentery, however, induces a very unpleasant sensation (Fig. 1.20), since diffuse stimulation can be felt.

Despite this insensitivity to direct contact, pathological conditions in the viscera produce pain. Pain sensation is often located in another part of the body than the affected organ. For example, the pain experienced in **angina pectoris** (caused by deficient oxygenation of the heart muscle due to arteriosclerosis in the coronary artery) is located not only in the chest over the heart region but also in the left shoulder, and radiates along the arm to the little finger (Fig. 2.2). Pain due

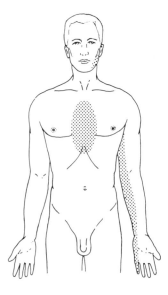

Figure 2.2 Site of pain in angina pectoris.

to gallstones is felt in the right shoulder and shoulder blade (Fig. 2.3). The location of pain in renal calculus is often so typical that a diagnosis can be made solely on the patient's description of the site and change in position of the pain. It moves from the hip to the inside of the leg, over the whole of its length, and finally to the groin and scrotum (Fig. 2.4). Pain felt in a place other than the affected organ is known as **referred pain**, and pain in or over a diseased organ is known as **local pain**. The mechanism in referred pain may be described as "cross talk" (engineering term) of nerve impulses between sensory nerves that lead to the spinal cord through the same dorsal roots.

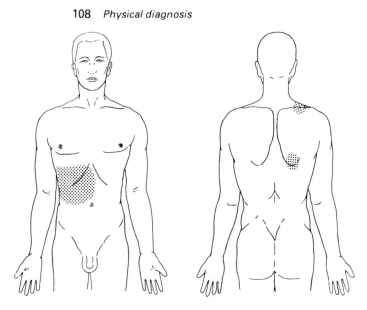

Figure 2.3 Site of pain with gallstones.

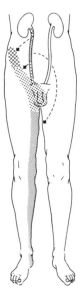

Figure 2.4 Migration of pain with kidney stones as the stone passes through the ureter. (Redrawn from R. H. Major & Mahlon H. Delp, Physical Diagnosis, Philadelphia, Pa, W. B. Saunders Company, 1962, by permission.)

2.23	Pathological processes in the viscera often produce pain elsewhere in the body than in the vicinity of the affected organ; this phenomenon is called	

2.24	Pain near a pathological process is known as	referred pain
2.25	In the case of diminished blood supply to the heart muscle a pain, called angina pectoris, arises not only in the chest region but also in the	local pain
2.26	Referred pain in an attack of gallstones is located in the	left shoulder and left arm on side of little finger
2.27	In an attack of renal calculus the pain shifts characteristically from the .... to the .... and the	right shoulder and shoulder blade
2.28	The mechanism in referred pain may be described as "cross talk" of nerve impulses between sensory nerves that lead to the spinal cord through the same	hip inside of the leg groin and scrotum
		dorsal roots

PHYSICAL EXAMINATION

The physical examination is performed in a definite sequence according to anatomical regions. A few of the many possible components follow:

General condition. Weight, height, physical build, coloration, temperature, breathing rate, skin eruptions, mental condition; for example, the patient's emotional attitude to his illness.

Mouth. Inspection of the teeth, tongue, the back of the throat and tonsils; poorly repaired teeth that may give trouble are looked for; as are mucosal changes, such as inflammation, patches and accumulation of pus, which are signs of infection. The swallowing reflexes are elicited; any irregularity may be indicative of an organic nervous disorder.

Thyroid gland. Palpation of size and consistency; enlargement of the thyroid may be indicative of a metabolic disorder.

Superficial lymph nodes. Palpation of the neck, axillae, groin, etc; enlarged lymph nodes may point to infection or a tumor.

Lungs. Percussion and auscultation; signs of infection, asthma, tumor diseases and senile changes are looked for.

Heart. Determination of the heart rate and rhythm; the heart rhythm may be regular or irregular. Palpation of the position of the apex of the heart and the strength of the pulsations; percussion of the heart borders; enlargement of the heart may be a sign of a pathological condition, often a valvular defect. Auscultation: tones generated when the valves close or when the blood is forced through the valve orifices are useful in appraising valve function.

Abdomen. Inspection; a search is made for, among other things, scars from previous operations. Palpation of the liver, spleen, kidneys, urinary bladder; enlargement of these organs is a sign of disease, as also is tenderness on palpation. Percussion; accumulation of gas in the intestines produces a characteristic percussion tone, which may be a sign of intestinal obstruction or impaired bowel function. An accumulation of fluid in the abdominal cavity may also be detected by percussion.

Rectum (per rectum). Palpation; a search is made for hemorrhoids, tumors and enlargement of the prostate.

Reflexes. Reflexes can be produced by tapping certain tendons and muscles with a reflex hammer or by touching the skin at certain places; an abnormal reflex may be a sign of an organic nervous disease.

Surface anatomy

In the physical examination a number of special terms are used to indicate the position of pathological changes. On the chest the ribs are used to indicate levels. The first rib cannot be palpated, the second one can be felt below the collar bone; the ribs are then counted in the caudal direction. The spaces between the ribs are known as the **intercostal spaces** and they are numbered with reference to the overlying rib; the second intercostal space is thus the one palpated caudal to the second rib.

For indicating positions on the circumference of the thorax a number of lines are used that run parallel to the axis of the body (Fig. 2.5): the **median line** in the middle, the **sternal line** at the border of the sternum, the **parasternal line**, the **midclavicular** line from the midpoint of the clavicle (also known as the **mammillary** line because it passes through the nipples) the **anterior axillary**, **midaxillary** and **posterior axillary lines** and the **scapular line**.

On the body there are a number of easily identifiable landmarks consisting of **depressions** or fossae: the **supraclavicular fossa**, the **infraclavicular fossa**, the epigastric fossa, usually abbreviated to the **epigastrium** (pit of the stomach), and the **iliac fossa**; the last three are observable only on persons of slender build.

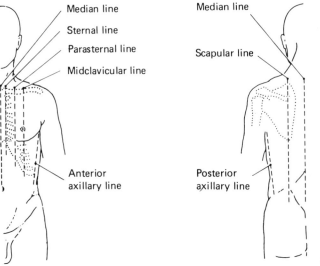

Median line
Sternal line
Parasternal line
Midclavicular line

Anterior
axillary line

Median line

Scapular line

Posterior
axillary line

Figure 2.5 Reference lines used in specifying positions on the chest.

Other readily identifiable formations are the **costal arch**, the **iliac crest**, which ends ventrally in a process, the **anterior superior iliac spine**, the **spine of the scapula** and **angle of the scapula** (Fig. 2.6).

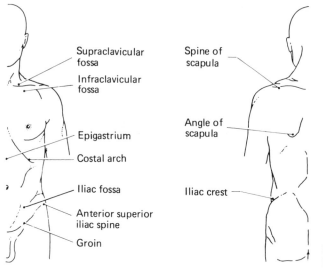

Supraclavicular
fossa
Infraclavicular
fossa

Epigastrium
Costal arch

Iliac fossa
Anterior superior
iliac spine
Groin

Spine of
scapula

Angle of
scapula

Iliac crest

Figure 2.6 Some commonly used landmarks on the trunk.

It is also important to know the position of the viscera in relation to the above landmarks (Fig. 2.7). The following should be observed: the lower border of the liver reaches only one centimeter lower than the costal arch in the right

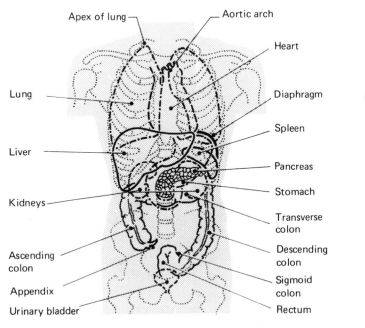

Figure 2.7 Position of the viscera in relation to the skeleton.

midclavicular line, the spleen lies in the upper quadrant left of the abdominal cavity protected by the costal arch, the diaphragm reaches approximately to the level of the fifth intercostal space, and the apex of the heart is on a level with the fifth intercostal space.

2.29	The spaces between the ribs are called . . . . and are counted . . . . (cranial, caudal) to the respective rib.	
2.30	On the ventral side of the body five lines are used for indicating position; reckoned from the middle these are: the . . . . , ... , ... , ... and	intercostal spaces caudal
2.31	On the dorsal side of the body three lines are used, namely the . . . . , ... and	median line sternal line parasternal line midclavicular line anterior axillary line

2.32	Fossae are	median line scapular line posterior axillary line
2.33	The supraclavicular fossa and the infraclavicular fossa are two depressions located cranial and caudal to the	depressions
2.34	The epigastrium is the	clavicle (collar bone)
2.35	An important landmark is the costal arch; this is the arch formed by the	pit of the stomach
2.36	The iliac crest means	lower ribs
2.37	The spina scapulae is the	prominence of the hip bone
2.38	The scapular angle is the	upper border of the shoulder blade
2.39	The anterior superior iliac spine is the tip in which the .... terminates.	lower tip of the shoulder blade
2.40	A person has appendicitis. From Figs. 1.19, 2.7 and 2.6, try to locate the place in the abdomen where the pain is most intense.	iliac crest
2.41	A patient with gastric ulcer complains of pain and tenderness in the	right iliac fossa (right lower quadrant)
2.42	The liver is normally palpated .... cm below the right costal arch in the midclavicular line.	epigastrium
2.43	As a complication after an attack of gallstones, a patient has acute inflammation of the pancreas; there will be tenderness in the	one
2.44	A man has received a deep knife stab in the left parasternal line of the fourth intercostal space. The man will .... (survive, not survive) because the knife has entered the	epigastrium

2.45	A child fell from a window and ruptured his spleen, causing bleeding in the abdominal cavity. The spleen was therefore removed immediately. To reach the spleen the surgeon had to make an abdominal incision parallel to the .... (left, right) .... (arch formed by the ribs).	not survive heart
2.46	A 70-year-old woman fell on her left side and fractured the neck of the femur. Since the femoral neck was compressed, the left leg was then shorter. To record the shortening a measurement is made with a measuring tape from the ankle to the process of the crest of the hip bone, the	left costal arch
		anterior superior iliac spine

Inspection

A simple visual observation of the patient is an important diagnostic aid, for many diseases can be diagnosed on this basis alone.

Mental state. In connection with the recording of the medical history and the physical examination the physician can often obtain an impression of the patient's **mental state** by observing his facial expression, pattern of movements, and response to questions.

Such an inspection may be sufficient for diagnosing certain disorders of hormonal origin that affect the mental state. Patients with toxic goiter (hyperthyroidism or thyrotoxicosis), which is due to excessive production of thyroid hormone, are nervous, have difficulty sitting still, and may have tremor. They give an impression of intellectual activity, and often display a personal charm. These observations, plus other signs such as the appearance of protruding eyeballs (exophthalmos), provide the basis for diagnosis even before beginning the physical examination of the patient. The opposite state to this disease, myxedema or hypothyroidism, which is due to an inadequate output of thyroid hormone, has observable signs which are almost as useful in diagnosis.

Of major importance for diagnosis and treatment is the patient's attitude to his illness: the patient may **simulate** symptoms—for example, malingering in the armed services; or for insurance compensation he may **exaggerate** or **feign**. In applying for insurance policies he may **conceal** symptoms.

Body posture and malformations. The posture can give valuable clues. The patient described in question 2.46, was probably admitted to the hospital lying on her back with the left foot characteristically rotated outwards and the leg shortened, signs that are practically unmistakable in fracture of the femoral neck. A patient with a perforated gastric ulcer lies still with the abdomen distended because of irritation of the peritoneal membrane, while a patient with kidney stones wanders around in agitation. The fact that a patient suspected of having appendicitis is unable to straighten his right leg at the hip supports the diagnosis and indicates the site of the appendix. The sign is due to inflammatory irritation of a muscle that runs in the dorsal wall of the abdominal cavity from the spine to the femur.

Color changes. The presence of **exanthem** (skin eruption) and **enanthem** (eruption on the mucous membrane) is of obvious diagnostic value. Its appearance, distribution on the body and time of onset in relation to other symptoms should be recorded.

The color of the lips is also an indication of the level of the oxygenation of the blood: poor oxygenation (due to impaired circulation or respiration) results in blue lips—lip cyanosis. If a patient has blue lips plus other findings, such as pulsations in the neck, it is possible merely by inspection to determine that the patient has heart trouble, and sometimes even to determine where in the heart the lesion is located.

2.47	In far advanced stages of a number of diseases, such as heart conditions, chronic inflammation of the kidneys, high blood pressure and brain tumors, a characteristic type of ventilation is sometimes found. The breathing is interrupted for 15 seconds or so, slowly increases to full amplitude, and then diminishes again. This phenomenon, known as Cheyne-Stokes breathing, is due to damage to the respiratory center in the medulla oblongata. The center does not react adequately to a change in the carbon dioxide content of the blood and results in an intermittent oscillation (as in a poorly adjusted servo-system). A diagnosis of brain damage can be made solely by .... (Cheyne-Stokes breathing implies a poor but not necessarily hopeless prognosis).	
2.48	In measles, enanthem consisting of small bluish patches develops on the oral mucosa. The enanthem, which occurs only in measles, appears and disappears before the exanthem develops. Thus, from a simple inspection the physician can reach the right diagnosis, since enanthem is a ...., or a ...., (alternative term) sign.	inspection

2.49	In order not to risk losing his license, a professional pilot denies to the physician that physical effort produces pain in the chest which radiates in the left shoulder and arm (angina pectoris). From his observation of the patient while noting the history the physician suspects that the patient is .... and refers him to a specialist for a more thorough heart examination.	specific pathognomonic
2.50	A man that has been hit by a car and suffered a fracture of the lower leg, which healed after 4 months, states that he cannot return to work because he still has pain in the ankle. At a physical and an x-ray examination the physicians can find no explanation of the patient's symptoms apart from slightly reduced mobility. It is therefore probable that the patient is .... the symptoms.	concealing symptoms
2.51	In an infantry unit the day before a march, 250 men report sick—25 percent of the unit. The duty medical officer finds a wide variety of symptoms among the men that have reported sick, but no signs of an epidemic infection. As the unit has only recently been recruited from young healthy persons it is statistically highly likely that most of the men that have reported sick are .... It is probable that a few of the men that have reported sick really are ill. The physician is thus presented with a difficult diagnostic problem of quickly identifying the men that require closer examination. Since the time available is about 1 minute per man, only the simple form of .... can be used.	exaggerating
		feigning physical examination

Endoscopy

To permit inspection of body cavities not visible to the naked eye, a tubular optical instrument known as an **endoscope** is used. Depending on its specific use this varies greatly in form, size and optical principle. It may be a straight tube with no other optical system than an external electric bulb, or a complex flexible instrument with 50 or so optical components (Fig. 2.8). Many instruments are equipped with small forceps for taking samples of tissues—**biopsy** specimens—for microscopic examination in cases of suspected tumor. The endoscope is designed for easy sterilization.

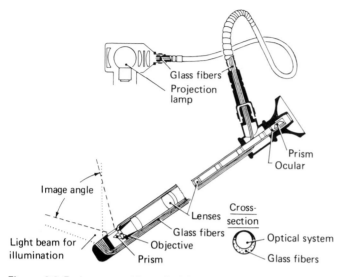

Figure 2.8 Endoscope with optical lens system for transmitting the image and light fiber optics system for illumination. (Redrawn from pamphlet by Richard Wolf GmbH, Knittlingen, W. Germany, by permission.)

Most of the body's cavities can be inspected either through existing orifices in the body or through passages created with a sharp instrument so that the endoscope can be inserted. The body cavity is filled with air or isotonic saline so as to keep the walls distended and to improve the optical transmission.

Illumination. The quality of the image seen in the endoscope is dependent not only on the properties of the optical system but also on the illuminating system. In earlier instruments a miniature lamp was used as the light source. The lamp was fixed to the internal part of the endoscope or to a tube which was inserted in the endoscope, as in certain bronchoscopes and rectoscopes. These miniature lamps had several disadvantages: the intensity of illumination was low because of the small dimensions; the lamp had a short life because of the high filament temperature required for maximum intensity.

In modern endoscopes fiber optics are often used instead to transmit light from an external light source with low loss. The fiber optics utilize special fibers consisting of two transparent materials, an internal core with a high refractive index and an external shell with a low refractive index. A light beam incident on one end is then transmitted to the other end by total reflection. Many fibers are combined to form a tube or a flexible cable, or are molded into the walls of the endoscope (Fig. 2.8). Fiber optics have good transmitting properties so the system yields a high enough intensity of illumination to take color pictures.

Table 2.1   Some types of endoscopes

Type	Range of use	Example of diagnostic problem or operation
bronchoscope	trachea larger airways	tumors foreign bodies infections aspiration of mucus
cardioscope	heart cavities	valvular defects septal defect—that is, a hole between right and left atria
cystoscope	urinary bladder	tumors inflammation stones catheterization of ureters to obtain separate specimens, and for x-ray examination of each kidney
esophagoscope	esophagus	bleeding from veins tumors
gastroscope	stomach	gastritis gastric ulcer tumors
laparoscope	abdominal cavity	tumors
laryngoscope	larynx	inflammation tumors
mediastinoscope	mediastinum	insertion of pacemaker electrodes on the outside of the heart
ophthalmoscope	eye fundus	state of vessels in high blood pressure retinal detachment inflammation tumors
otoscope	tympanic membrane	infections perforation of ear drum pressure conditions in the middle ear
proctoscope	rectum	hemorrhoids tumors minor operations
sigmoidoscope	rectum and distal part of colon	side pockets of the bowel (diverticulosis) bowel lesions tumors
thoracoscope	pleural cavity	tumors air in the pleural cavity

Optics.   The optical system of the simplest endoscopes consists of a positive **lens** located in the external part of the endoscope, as in the case of an otoscope. With such an arrangement, however, the ray geometry gives a small field of view. For this reason in other instruments, such as gastroscopes and cytoscopes, a telescope system is added, which is located in the internal part of the endoscope; this provides a wider field of view and a considerably better image quality.

In many examinations it is desirable to have a flexible endoscope. Some gastroscopes have been designed with highly complex optical lens and prism systems where part of the instrument has been made somewhat flexible. The introduction of **fiber optics** has enabled the design of endoscopes that are flexible over their whole length (Fig. 2.9). Here, coherent—that is, ordered—bundles of fiber optics are used which enable the image to be transmitted by a number of image elements equal to the number of fibers. With a fiber diameter of 30 μm about 10^5 image elements per square centimeter are obtained; this usually gives an acceptable image quality. The coherent fiber optics system is produced by winding a continuous fiber in a groove on a drum. The fibers are cemented together at one place on the periphery of the drum and then cut transversely at this one place. In this way a flexible bundle is obtained in which the two ends of a particular fiber are located in corresponding positions in the two cut surfaces.

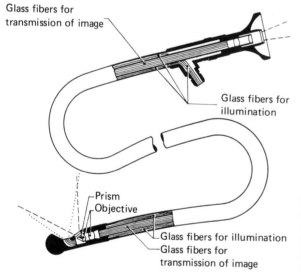

Glass fibers for transmission of image

Glass fibers for illumination

Prism
Objective
Glass fibers for illumination
Glass fibers for transmission of image

Figure 2.9 Endoscope with light fiber optics system for image transmission and illumination. (Redrawn from pamphlet by Richard Wolf GmbH, Knittlingen, W. Germany, by permission.)

Endoscopic pictures can be recorded with color film or by television and videotape recorders; but the resulting endoscope is heavier and somewhat less maneuverable.

| 2.52 | Most of the body cavities can be inspected by inserting an .... | |

2.53	To keep the walls distended the body cavities can be filled with .... or	endoscope
2.54	Many endoscopes are furnished with small forceps for obtaining tissue samples, ..., where a tumor is suspected.	air isotonic saline
2.55	A patient complains of pain in one ear. While inspecting the ear drum with an .... the physician finds infection with an accumulation of pus in the middle ear.	biopsy specimens
2.56	A patient at the dentist aspirated a piece of a broken drill. At a thoracic disease clinic the fragment was removed with the aid of a	otoscope
2.57	A patient had observed blood-tinged urine for some days. Examination of the bladder with a .... disclosed a bleeding polyp, which was immediately removed.	bronchoscope
2.58	A patient had long been troubled by increasing loss of appetite, lack of energy and loss of weight. As an x-ray examination of the stomach aroused suspicion of a tumor, an inspection of the stomach was made with a ...., and a biopsy of a suspected tumor tissue was performed.	cystoscope
2.59	The biopsy specimen was sent to a pathologist for microscopic examination, and the suspicion of a tumor was confirmed. To find whether the tumor had spread into the abdominal cavity the physician used a ...., which he inserted by puncturing the abdominal wall.	gastroscope
2.60	In a patient complaining of headache, the physician found reduced physical work capacity, pounding of the heart and high blood pressure. The patient was referred to an ophthalmologist for an examination of the blood vessels in the eye fundus, which may be done with an	laparoscope
2.61	A patient with hemorrhoids consults a physician who examines the patient with a	ophthalmoscope

2.62	A patient consults a physician for bowel trouble, with alternate constipation and diarrhea and blood in the stools. To examine the bowel a .... is inserted. Part of the mucous membrane is thickened and ulcerated, and a .... is taken with a biopsy instrument.	proctoscope
2.63	For illuminating body cavities in endoscopy it is advantageous to use a .... for transmitting light from an external light source.	sigmoidoscope tissue specimen
2.64	Fiber optics can also be used for transmitting endoscopic images, and then a fiber optics system that is .... must be used.	fiber optics system
2.65	One advantage of endoscopy using a fiber optics system for transmitting images is that the instrument is	coherent
		flexible

Smell

Even one not versed in medicine can recognize the smell from a person that is under the influence of **alcohol**. Another odor of medical interest is that of **acetone** which forms in the body in diabetes or starvation. Acetone is formed when fat is burned; it is carried by the blood to the lungs and expired. The use of the sense of smell in diagnosis is mainly of historical interest because today chemical analysis (Chapter 5) enables detailed examinations of the metabolism to be carried out.

2.66	A physician is called to see a patient who during the past month has been troubled by increasing thirst and urine output, weakness and nausea. As the patient smells of acetone, the physician immediately suspects .... (diagnosis) and has the patient conveyed to the hospital by ambulance for treatment.	

2.67	A two-year-old child has not been eating his food for two days due to an acute cold and fever. The physician smells acetone, but no immediate examination is made for this sign since this may be due to the patient's	diabetes
		starvation

Palpation

The sense of touch is an important diagnostic aid. By means of palpation it is possible to determine the shape, size, surface structure and mobility of many organs. Signs of infection, tumors and other signs of disease are looked for. The abdomen is particularly accessible to palpation, since on the ventral side it is not protected by the skeleton; palpation is the most important method in the physical examination of the abdomen.

Palpation of the superficial lymph nodes is especially important. Pathological processes easily spread to these via the lymph ducts, and an enlarged lymph node may be a sign of infection or a tumor. In the case of an infection the lymph nodes are tender and may be displaced in relation to the skin and underlying tissues; an enlarged node that is not tender and firmly attached to the skin or underlying tissues is usually a sign of a tumor.

By the sense of touch it is possible to estimate the temperature of the patient and to feel the state of the skin in other respects. A dehydrated patient has a skin that can easily be raised in folds; in a patient with excessive fluid the skin is edematous (swollen).

The pulse can be palpated at several places on the body, but most easily over the radial artery on the palmar side of the wrist, against the most distal part of the radius. The following factors are assessed:

Pulse rate. Normally 70 beats a minute; a slow pulse is known as **bradycardia** and a rapid pulse rate as **tachycardia**.

Pulse rhythm. The rhythm is normally regular. However, there is some acceleration on breathing in and retardation on breathing out which is called respiratory arrhythmia.

Pulse pressure. The difference between the diastolic and systolic pressure.

Pulse type. The duration of the systolic pulse peak (abrupt or prolonged).

2.68	In a physical examination of the abdomen it is found that an organ is palpated 7 cm below the costal arch in the right mid-clavicular line. The patient thus has an/a .... (enlarged, normal-sized, reduced) .... (organ).	
2.69	A patient is admitted, feeling ill, with slightly raised temperature and abdominal pain that has moved from the epigastrium to the right iliac fossa. Palpation discloses tenderness and muscular defense—local contraction of the abdominal muscles over an inflammatory focus in the abdominal cavity—over the iliac fossa. From Figs. 1.19, 2.6 and 2.7, make a diagnosis.	enlarged liver
2.70	The child in question 2.45, with ruptured spleen and bleeding into the abdominal cavity, is admitted to the hospital; the examining physician immediately feels the patient's pulse and finds that the pulse pressure is .... (strong, weak) because of the loss of blood.	appendicitis
2.71	The heart tries to compensate for a loss of blood and the consequent drop in blood pressure by increasing the heart rate. The child described in the previous question thus had .... -cardia on admission to the hospital.	weak
2.72	The child's history, with the description of the fall from the window and the state of shock, prompts an immediate examination of the abdomen. The physician finds that it is distended and decides on an immediate operation solely on the basis of the findings from .... (method of examination).	tachy
2.73	A youth involved in an accident on his motorcycle received abrasions on the left lower leg. He did not clean and disinfect the wound and an infection developed. He was admitted to hospital with an oozing wound and fever. Palpation of the left groin disclosed a lymph node that was .... (enlarged, not enlarged), ... (tender, not tender) and .... (mobile, fixed) in relation to the skin and underlying tissue.	palpation

2.74	A woman notices a swelling in the right breast. On examination the physician finds that the patient probably has mammary carcinoma, since in the right axilla several lymph nodes can be felt which are . . . . (enlarged, of normal size, reduced), ... (tender, not tender) and . . . . (mobile, attached) to the skin and underlying tissue.	enlarged tender mobile
2.75	An operation was performed on the patient described in the previous question, but it is not known whether all the tumor tissue was removed. Therefore the . . . . (outcome of the disease) was uncertain.	enlarged not tender attached
		prognosis

Percussion

Percussion is performed by a right-handed physician by placing the fingers of the left hand somewhat spread on the patient's body and tapping the middle phalange of the left middle finger with the bent right index finger (Fig. 2.10). The blow sets the organ vibrating. Of particular importance are the resonators formed by organs containing air or gas, such as the lungs, stomach and bowels. The vibrations, which are rapidly damped, can be heard by the examiner and felt by the hand resting on the body.

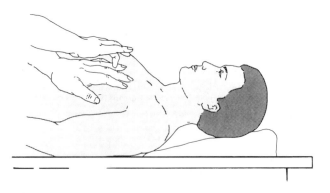

Figure 2.10 Tapping position in percussion.

The qualities of the resulting sound can be readily explained on a physical basis. The **pitch**, that is the frequency, is dependent on the size of the resonator. The **quality of the note**, that is, the harmonic content, is also dependent on the mechanical properties of the resonator. The decrease in the amplitude of the vibrations with time, the **damping**, is dependent on the sound absorption by the tissues (the Q value of the resonator (engineering term)). The **intensity**, or the amplitude of the vibration, is dependent on a number of factors, including the acoustic coupling between the percussing finger and the resonator and between the resonator and the ear of the examiner, on the reflection of sound by the various anatomic structures, and on the damping within the resonator. It is not necessary to understand a physical explanation of the method in order to find it valuable. With experience, the physician learns to recognize various conditions by listening and feeling with his hand.

Over the greater part of the normal thoracic cavity, percussion produces a note of moderate intensity with many harmonics. Over the lower left quadrant, on the ventral side a more powerful sound with fewer harmonics is obtained—a so-called tympanitic note. This is due to resonance in the stomach, which always contains some air. On the right side over the liver and directly over the heart a short, well damped, dull percussion note is obtained (Fig. 2.11).

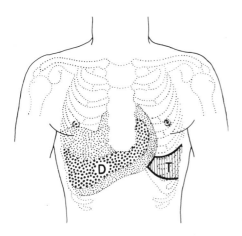

Figure 2.11 Normal percussion boundaries. Over the stomach a tympanitic note is obtained, T, because of the contained air, and over the liver and heart a damped note, D, because of the absence of air.

By means of percussion the boundaries of certain organs can be located. For example, the method is used for assessing the size and position of the heart, and the borders and mobility of the lungs during breathing. In the case of pathological alterations of the lungs—for example, in pneumonia, infarction and tumors—there is damping over the region of the pathological process. There is also large damping where there is an accumulation of fluid in the pleural cavity, as in **hydrothorax** (water in the pleural cavity) and **hemothorax** (blood in the pleural cavity). In **pneumothorax** (air in the pleural cavity) a tympanitic note is heard.

Attempts have been made to render percussion more objective by recording the sounds with a microphone, storage on an endless magnetic tape loop and analysis of the frequency spectra. The method has been tested experimentally for demonstrating fragility of bone due to a reduction in the bone mineral content (osteoporosis). The value of the percussion method lies in its simplicity, however, rather than in the application of advanced measurement techniques; for quite different methods, and in particular radiological examinations, yield more exhaustive diagnostic information.

2.76	In percussion, tissues, especially those containing gas or air, are set in mechanical	
2.77	The mechanical vibrations in the tissues are produced by the examiner by . . . . with a finger.	vibration
2.78	The tapping sets up vibrations in the . . . ., which are located in the underlying tissues.	tapping
2.79	Over the stomach a . . . . note is obtained because it always contains air.	resonators
2.80	Over the liver and the heart a . . . . percussion note is obtained because these organs do not contain air and are therefore poor resonators.	tympanitic
2.81	The man described in question 2.44 was unlucky that the knife entered the heart region. If it had entered the right side he might have survived. It is true that there would have been severe bleeding from the damaged lung, but if air had flowed into the pleural cavity the lung would have collapsed and the bleeding would have diminished. If on admission to the hospital a percussion examination had been performed on the upper right side of the chest with the patient in the seated position a . . . . percussion note would have been obtained because of the . . . . -thorax (air in the pleural cavity) that appeared when air entered the pleural space.	damped

2.82	Over the lower part of the lung a . . . . percussion note would have been obtained because of the . . . . -thorax (blood in the pleural cavity) which occurred due to the hemorrhage.	tympanitic pneumo
2.83	The diagnostic procedure in which the examining physician uses both hearing and tactile senses is known as	damped hemo
		percussion

Auscultation

In auscultation the physician listens to the sounds generated in the organs. For practical reasons a **stethoscope** is usually employed for the acoustic coupling between the patient and the examining physician, although direct application of the ear gives better transmission of the sound. The stethoscope may consist of a straight wooden tube with flared contact surfaces at each end. European physicians prefer such an instrument for listening to the sounds of the fetal heart (fetal stethoscope). In the United States metal binaural fetal stethoscopes are preferred.

The ordinary stethoscope consists of a chest piece; this is connected by a rubber tube to two bent metal tubes that are pressed against the physician's external acoustic meatuses by spring tension. The chest piece has two alternative sound channels, which can be selected by a valve: a small open bell about 2 cm in diameter intended for low tones (some heart murmurs), and a larger and shallower bell with a diaphragm intended for sounds with a higher pitch (most heart murmurs and breath sounds).

Because of the poor acoustic impedance matching, the frequency response of an ordinary stethoscope is not ideal (Fig. 2.12). Stethoscopes furnished with an electronic microphone and with transistorized amplifiers have a better frequency response but they have not been adopted for general use.

Auscultation of the lungs. When listening over the lung field of a normal person, a sound is heard like the wind through the trees, the dominant frequency of which lies in the range 100–200 Hz; this is known as a **vesicular sound** or "**vesicular breathing**". Over the sternum in a position corresponding to the esophagus and the larger bronchi, the sound has a higher frequency, 800–2000 Hz, **bronchial sound**. The distribution of these sounds over the chest changes in the case of pathological processes. With fluid in the lung, for example, in pneumonia, the sound generated in the bronchi is better conducted to the thoracic wall. In other conditions the sound is weaker or abolished—for example, in pneumothorax. This is partly due to reduced ventilation in the lung and partly to poor sound

Sound transmission, dB

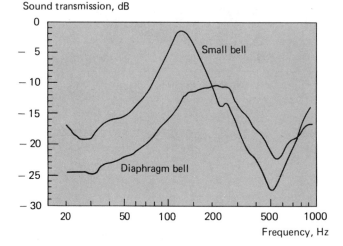

Figure 2.12 Frequency response for sound transmission of an ordinary stethoscope. (By permission of D. E. Winer, F. Siegel, R. J. Kuchlewski and C. A. Caceres.)

transmission through the air mass. Various forms of secondary sounds arise in certain pathological conditions of the lungs—for example, the wheeze heard in asthma.

Auscultation of the heart. This is an important method of examination. By means of the simple stethoscope it is possible in most cases to determine the nature of an organic heart defect. In order to understand the principles, a brief description of the valve system of the heart and the various pressures in the circulatory system are given.

The heart beat occurs in two time phases: first the two atria contract—**atrial systole**—over a period of about 0.1 s, and the ventricles then fill to their greatest extent. The ventricles then contract simultaneously—**ventricular systole**—for about 0.3 s, and the blood is forced from the right ventricle into the pulmonary artery and from the left ventricle into the aorta. During **ventricular diastole**, lasting about 0.4 s, the ventricles fill again.

Flow in the wrong direction—**regurgitation**—is prevented by a valve system between the atrium and the ventricle of each half of the heart and between the ventricles and the respective arteries. The atrio-ventricular valves consist of cusps or leaflets, three on the right side and two on the left, which during ventricular systole are pressed together and prevent return flow. So that the cusps are not forced through the valves there are attached to their margins a number of fibers which are anchored to the papillary muscles arising from the walls of the ventricles (Fig. 2.13).

The right system is called the **tricuspid valve** and the left system the **mitral valve**. The valve system between the right ventricle and the pulmonary artery is called the **pulmonary valve**, and that between the left ventricle and the aorta the **aortic valve**. Each consists of three semilunar structures (Fig. 2.14).

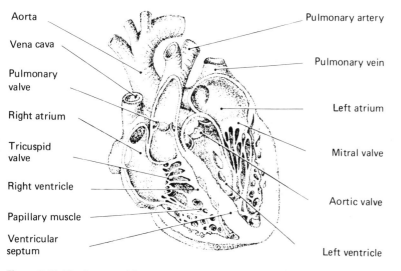

Aorta

Vena cava

Pulmonary valve

Right atrium

Tricuspid valve

Right ventricle

Papillary muscle

Ventricular septum

Pulmonary artery

Pulmonary vein

Left atrium

Mitral valve

Aortic valve

Left ventricle

Figure 2.13 The heart cavities, valve systems and related vessels.

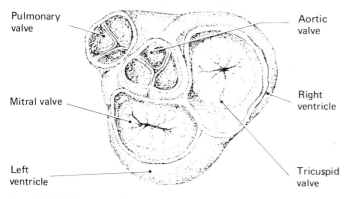

Pulmonary valve

Mitral valve

Left ventricle

Aortic valve

Right ventricle

Tricuspid valve

Figure 2.14 The valve system of the heart, seen from above. The atria and the vessels leaving the ventricles are omitted.

The pressure in the left ventricle and aorta, the ventricular volume and a number of other parameters are shown (Fig. 2.15). During diastole the ventricles fill to more than two thirds their volume, and during atrial systole more blood is added. At the beginning of ventricular systole the tricuspid and mitral valves close and the pressure in the ventricles increases. When the pressure exceeds the pulmonary and aortic pressure the respective valves open and blood is ejected. The valves close at the beginning of diastole when the pulmonary artery and aortic pressure exceed the ventricular pressures.

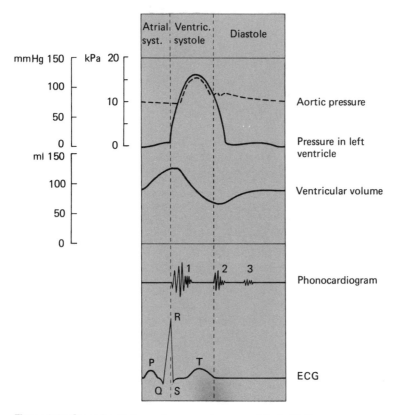

Figure 2.15 Some hemodynamic parameters associated with the cardiac cycle.

When the heart is beating, mechanical vibrations are generated which can be heard during auscultation or recorded electronically by, for example, phonocardiography (page 167). The first heart sound is a somewhat drawn out "lub" with a peak intensity in the frequency range 25–50 Hz; it is generated when the mitral and tricuspid valves close and vibrations are set up in the walls of the ventricles. The second heart sound is a shorter "dup", with a slightly higher frequency, the peak intensity occurring at 50–100 Hz; it is generated when the aortic and pulmonary valves close.

The flexibility and form of the four valves are normally such that during the cardiac cycle they open wide enough for the blood to flow and then close tightly. The normal function can be disturbed by two pathological alterations. In **stenosis**—that is, constriction due to scar formation and shrinking—the valve does not open sufficiently. In **insufficiency**—incomplete closure for the same reason—the blood regurgitates during phases when the valve should be tight. Such anatomical defects cause turbulence in the blood flow and this produces

murmurs; a laminar blood flow is quiet. The origin of the murmurs can be determined by noting the time of occurrence during the cardiac cycle and observing the distribution over the chest.

The time when the murmurs occur is determined by observing whether they are **systolic** or **diastolic**, that is, whether they occur during ventricular systole or diastole. From a knowledge of the openings of the valves during the cardiac cycle the following relationships are derived:

Valves	Pathological change	Time of murmur
Aortic or pulmonary valves	stenosis	systolic
	insufficiency	diastolic
Mitral or tricuspid valves	stenosis	diastolic
	insufficiency	systolic

The maximum sounds for the murmurs in auscultation do not lie over the respective valve systems on the chest (Fig. 2.16). This is because the sound from the valves is conducted out to the surface of the chest in certain preferential directions.

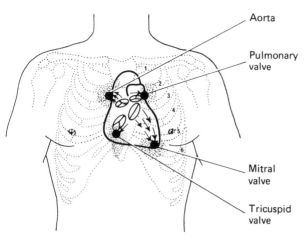

Aorta

Pulmonary valve

Mitral valve

Tricuspid valve

Figure 2.16 The location of the sound maxima in auscultation of the heart valve system does not coincide with their projection on the chest. Redrawn from R. H. Major & Mahlon H. Delp, Physical Diagnosis, Philadelphia, Pa, W. B. Saunders Company, 1962, by permission.)

2.84	Mitral insufficiency results in regurgitation to the left atrium, generating a .... (systolic, diastolic) murmur.

2.85	The murmur in mitral insufficiency is best heard in the .... intercostal space to the .... (right, left) of the sternum. (Use Fig. 2.16.)	systolic
2.86	When does the murmur in mitral insufficiency occur in relation to the first and second heart sounds? (Use Fig. 2.15.)	fifth left
2.87	In mitral stenosis a .... (systolic, diastolic) murmur is heard because of turbulence that arises when the blood flows into the	between the first and second heart sounds (and also at the same time as these)
2.88	In aortic insufficiency a .... (systolic, diastolic) murmur is heard.	diastolic left ventricle
2.89	The murmur in mitral stenosis has two components corresponding to two maxima in the rate of blood flow. From a knowledge of the function of atrial systole, determine the time for the second sound peak in relation to ventricular systole.	diastolic
2.90	A patient had rheumatic fever as a child. There is permanent damage to the heart valves due to the disease. During auscultation both systolic and diastolic murmurs are heard, with peaks over the apex of the heart. The patient has .... and	just before the systole; "presystolic murmur"
2.91	In a patient with syphilis that has gone untreated, the disease has damaged the heart. A soft blowing diastolic murmur is heard in the second intercostal space to the right of the sternum. The patient has .... (Use Fig. 2.16.)	mitral insufficiency mitral stenosis
		aortic insufficiency

Pressure Measurement

For normal body function the pressure in various organs should lie within certain limits. For example, the intracranial pressure should not exceed about 30 mm Hg ($\approx$4 kPa); an increase in the pressure after a skull injury or brain operation is a development that can lead rapidly to death; when the intracranial pressure approaches the systolic pressure the circulation of blood in the brain ceases and the patient dies. Likewise, the normal pressure in the bowels, gallbladder and urinary bladder should not be exceeded if function is to remain unimpaired. The pressure in the eyeball should also lie between certain values; both an increase and a decrease are signs of serious pathological conditions. The same applies to the pressure in the circulatory system.

In a **direct measurement of pressure**, a cannula is inserted into a body cavity and connected to a manometer. This often consists of a simple glass capillary tube or a plastic tube. The pressure can be measured by means of a ruler or scale. The method requires no complicated equipment and the accuracy is good enough for static measurements. For the registration of pressure on a recording instrument—for example, in order to be able to examine rapid fluctuations in pressure—electrical pressure transducers are used (page 171).

In some cases a direct puncture of the organ cavity is impractical (for example, in blood-pressure measurements) or harmful (for example, in the measurement of intra-ocular pressure). Use is then made of **indirect pressure measurements**. It is then necessary for the cavity to have a soft wall which can be subjected to a varying external pressure, and to be able to observe when the wall yields. For measuring blood pressure in physical diagnosis an indirect procedure is always used.

Blood-pressure measurement. The measurement of blood pressure is an important examination, since any changes in it—hypertension and hypotension—usually indicate conditions that call for medical treatment. A cuff

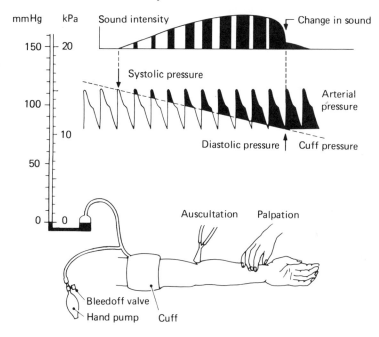

Figure 2.17 Principle for indirect measurement of blood pressure. (Middle and lower half of figure redrawn from Robert F. Rushmer, Cardiovascular Dynamics, Philadelphia, Pa, W. B. Saunders Company, 1970, by permission.)

consisting of a flat rubber bag with an inelastic external collar is placed round the arm and inflated to a pressure above the systolic blood pressure (Fig. 2.17). The pressure, which is observed on a manometer, is then steadily lowered, and it is noted when the pulse first passes the cuff. This can be done by feeling the pulse in the radial artery, or with a stethoscope just distal to the cuff listening to the tapping sound generated by turbulence in the flow as the blood is forced past the cuff. The pressure noted is equal to the systolic blood pressure.

As the cuff pressure is lowered further, the tapping sounds are gradually prolonged until a longer murmuring sound is heard, after which the sound changes and becomes weaker. The diastolic pressure is noted as the cuff pressure when the sound changes, not when it disappears (Fig. 2.18).

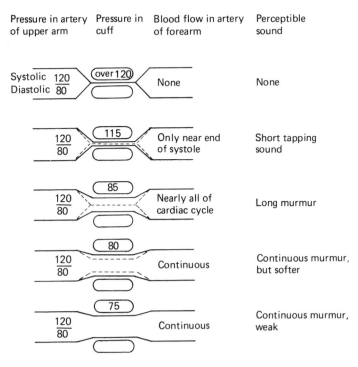

Pressure in artery of upper arm	Pressure in cuff	Blood flow in artery of forearm	Perceptible sound
Systolic 120 Diastolic 80	over 120	None	None
120 80	115	Only near end of systole	Short tapping sound
120 80	85	Nearly all of cardiac cycle	Long murmur
120 80	80	Continuous	Continuous murmur, but softer
120 80	75	Continuous	Continuous murmur, weak

Figure 2.18 Pressure conditions, blood flow and auscultatory sounds in indirect measurement of blood pressure. (To convert from mm Hg (shown) to kPa (SI units), multiply by 0.133 or see scales in Fig. 2.17.)

It is preferable to measure blood pressure with the patient in the supine position to eliminate the hydrostatic error due to a difference in level between the site of measurement and the heart. In addition, the slight physical effort caused by sitting or standing may cause a blood pressure increase that results in an erroneously high value.

Differences in the blood pressure in different extremities are a sign of obstruction in the arterial system. In the case of such obstruction—for example, constriction of the aorta—the pressure is higher in the arteries branching before than after the obstruction.

The systolic blood pressure is normally 120–140 mm Hg ($\approx$16–19 kPa) and the diastolic 60–90 mm Hg ($\approx$8–12 kPa). The two values are written with the systolic value first and a slash between, for example, 120/80, ($\approx$16/11 kPa). During effort and under stress the blood pressure is raised, and during sleep it is lowered. Pathological alterations in the blood pressure can have many causes; most of the functional blocks that are involved in blood pressure regulation (Fig. 1.42) can cause disturbances which result in hyper- or hypotension.

2.92	In physical diagnosis . . . . (direct, indirect) pressure measurements are mostly used.	
2.93	In indirect measurement of the pressure in a soft-walled cavity an external pressure is applied to the cavity and it is observed when the wall	indirect
2.94	In indirect measurement of blood pressure, the compression of the vessel is observed either by . . . ., when only the systolic blood pressure can be determined, or by . . . ., when both systolic and diastolic pressures can be measured.	yields (is compressed)
2.95	A patient consults a physician for headache, giddiness and buzzing in the ears. The blood pressure is found to be 180/110 ($\approx$24/15 kPa). Diagnosis:	palpation auscultation
2.96	During a physical examination the patient's blood pressure is found to be 95/60 ($\approx$13/8 kPa). Diagnosis:	hypertension (high blood pressure)
2.97	Examination of a child in the supine position shows the blood pressure in the arms to be 120/80 ($\approx$16/11 kPa) and in the legs 90/60 ($\approx$12/8 kPa). The patient therefore has a . . . . of the aorta (congenital malformation that can be treated by surgical removal).	hypotension (low blood pressure)

2.98	In measurement of the blood pressure by auscultation it is found in a patient that the systolic pressure is 120 ($\approx$16 kPa) but no change in the sound is heard until the pressure in the cuff is extremely low. From Fig. 2.15 make a diagnosis:	constriction
2.99	In auscultation over the aortic valves in the patient in the previous question a .... murmur is heard.	aortic insufficiency
		diastolic

Temperature Measurement

The measurement of body temperature is of great importance in diagnosis and treatment. The temperature is usually measured with a mercury thermometer of the "maximum" type: the capillary tube has a constriction that prevents the mercury column from running back during cooling. An electrical instrument using a thermistor as the transducer is used for continuous recording of temperature, especially in intensive care (Chapter 11).

The body temperature is measured in the rectum, axilla or mouth. Measurement in the rectum, which has disadvantages from the hygienic aspect, gives more accurate values, since the rectal temperature is less dependent on air temperature. However, most temperature measurements are made in the mouth for simplicity. The oral temperature is about 0.5°C (0.9°F) lower than the rectal temperature.

Many diseases give a characteristic temperature curve which is of diagnostic significance. A classical example is malaria (Fig. 2.19), where the intermittent

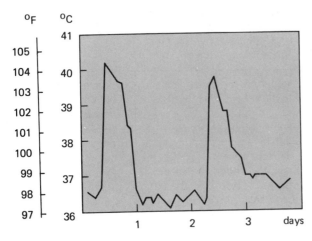

Figure 2.19 Temperature curve in a form of malaria.

fever peaks are produced by the developmental stages of the malaria parasites. Untreated lobar pneumonia (question 1.258) gives a temperature curve similar to that shown in Fig. 2.20, but such fully developed curves are rarely seen today

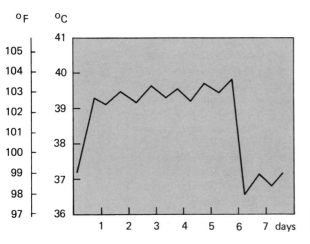
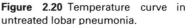

Figure 2.20 Temperature curve in untreated lobar pneumonia.

because antibiotic therapy is given so that the temperature falls before the seventh day. In measles (morbilli), one temperature peak occurs when the mucosal eruption appears, and a second when the skin eruption develops, Fig. 2.21. (See also question 2.48.)

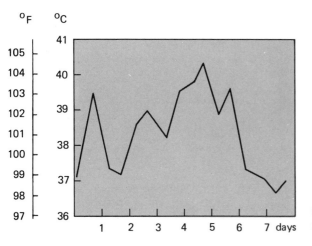

Figure 2.21 Temperature curve in measles.

2.100	Many infectious diseases begin with a sudden chill. The skin is pale, dry and cyanotic, due to the reduced peripheral circulation, and the patient shivers—that is, there is involuntary activity in the striated muscles. This raises the body temperature because of the increased .... (see Fig. 1.43).	
2.101	When the body temperature rises after a while so that the patient has fever, the skin becomes warm, moist and red (increased peripheral circulation). This state increases the .... so that the body temperature is adjusted to a suitable level.	heat generation
2.102	A patient that has undergone a major abdominal operation has a high temperature for the first few days after the operation. Fever-causing substances are emitted during the healing process by the tissues around the large surgical wound. When the physician sees the high temperature he takes .... (immediate, no) measures.	heat emission
2.103	Six days later, after the temperature has been normal for a couple of days, there is a slight rise in temperature, to 38°C (100°F). This is an unexpected change in the patient's condition and prompts an immediate examination. The physician finds a tender area in one of the calves due to venous thrombosis. This is a dangerous state because the blood clot may come free, be carried in the blood stream to the heart, pass through it and result in .... embolus. (See questions 1.269–1.271.)	no
2.104	Treatment to prevent blood coagulation is immediately introduced—an important, often life-saving measure, which is taken because of the physician's observations of the patient's	pulmonary
		temperature curve

Reflexes

In diseases of the nervous system, reflex disturbances may occur, which motivate testing of the reflex functions. For example, tests are made of the deep tendon reflexes, corneal reflex and pupillary reflex (page 89).

As an example of one of the many reflexes tested the patellar reflex will be described. By striking the patellar tendon with a reflex hammer, tension is set up in this tendon and also in the extensor muscle of the femur (Fig. 1.39). The receptors in the muscle spindles and in the tendon are then activated and impulses are conducted in afferent pathways to a dorsal root in the spinal cord. Here, a connection occurs in synapses to a motor neuron, which emits impulses through the efferent nerve fibers in a ventral root to the extensors of the thigh muscles, which contract.

If the reflex arc is broken—for example, as a result of an injury to a nerve or the spinal cord (Fig. 2.22 right)—the reflex cannot be elicited, that is, the reflex is **absent**. The reflex response may also be increased in relation to the normal—**increased** reflex. This is due to an injury to the nerve pathways from certain centers in the brain, which normally inhibit the reflex (Fig. 2.22 left). Such injuries occur in certain organic nervous diseases.

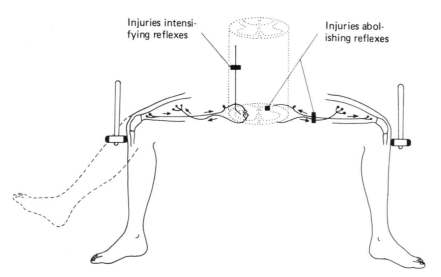

Injuries intensi-
fying reflexes

Injuries abol-
ishing reflexes

Figure 2.22 Reflexes can be strengthened or weakened depending on the location of an injury to the nervous system. (Redrawn from R. H. Major & Mahlon H. Delp, Physical Diagnosis, Philadelphia, Pa, W. B. Saunders Company, 1962, by permission.)

An examination of the nervous system comprises much more than a test of certain reflexes. Thus, all the sensory organs are checked: smell, vision, hearing, taste and touch. Neurological diagnosis is among the most advanced specialities in modern medicine. It is based on a detailed knowledge of the nerve pathways of the brain and spinal cord and the many centers of the brain. Such diagnostic knowledge is important in, for example, the location of a brain tumor.

2.105	The pupils of the eyes normally contract when light falls on one of the eyes, or when the eyes are focused on a near object (accommodation reflex). In syphilis a sign occurs in the central nervous system that is not found in other diseases: the pupil does not react to light but it does to accommodation. An examination of the pupillary reflex is therefore important, since it is possible to exploit a .... symptom.	
2.106	A patient in his thirties has for several years been troubled periodically by double vision and recently also by shaking and loss of power in the legs. The examining physician diagnoses multiple sclerosis, MS, a disease that is due to local lesions in the conducting pathways of the central nervous system. The physician finds .... (decreased, increased) reflexes in the legs.	specific or pathognomonic
2.107	A man aged 40 has been an alcoholic for a number of years. In the last year he has been troubled by pins and needles and a crawling sensation in the hands and feet, pain in the arms and legs, and paralysis in the distal parts of the extremities. The physician diagnoses polyneuritis—inflammation of several peripheral nerves due to a toxic effect—on the basis of a neurological examination in which .... (decreased, increased) reflexes in the extremities have been demonstrated.	increased
		decreased

CLINICAL DEATH

There is usually no doubt when death has occurred. When breathing and cardiac activity cease the cells receive no oxygen and the products of metabolism cannot be removed: the cells gradually die. Most sensitive to oxygen deficiency are the nerve cells of the brain, which at normal body temperature are irreparably damaged after a few minutes. The viscera can be deprived of oxygen for about 20 minutes. The cells of the skin are the least sensitive, probably because they can take up oxygen directly from the air.

In diagnosing that **death** has occurred, breathing and cardiac activity and the pupillary and corneal reflexes are observed. If none of these vital functions can be demonstrated, the patient is dead. Further evidence is found in the appearance, after an hour or so, of blue discoloration of the skin, **hypostatic spots**, caused by the falling of the blood to the lowest parts of the body under gravity. (This enables the forensic specialist to determine the position of the body after death and any subsequent changes in position.) Some hours after death **rigor mortis**, rigidity of the skeletal muscles, sets in. This is due to contraction of the muscles and ceases after a day or so.

The use of the above criteria of clinical death have changed with the introduction of technological aids. Breathing and circulation can be maintained by intensive care so that oxygen is supplied to the cells, which can thus survive. However, the vital centers in the brain may have irreversibly ceased to function, and for this reason the term "**cerebral death**" has been introduced. There is a difference in opinion as to whether the conventional concept of death, namely the arrest of the circulation and ventilation, or the concept of cerebral death should be used.

REFERENCES

DEGOWIN, E. L. and DEGOWIN, R. L. *Bedside Diagnostic Examination*. New York (Macmillan) 1976. 952 pages.

DELP, M. H. and MANNING, R. T. *Major's Physical Diagnosis*. 8 Ed. Philadelphia (Saunders) 1975. 356 pages.

KRUPP, M. A., SWEET, N. J., JAWETZ, E., BIGLIERI, E. G. and ROE, R. L. *Physician's Handbook*. Los Altos (Lange) 1976. 754 pages.

MORGAN, W. L., JR. and ENGEL, G. L. *The Clinical Approach to the Patient*. Philadelphia (Saunders) 1969. 314 pages.

PRIOR, J. A. and SILBERSTEIN, J. S. *Physical Diagnosis: The History and Examination of the Patient*. St. Louis (Mosby) 1973. 470 pages.

chapter 3

Cardiopulmonary Physiology

Many of the methods of clinical examination are performed by specialists, using specialized equipment. For such examinations the patient is referred to appropriate laboratories within the hospital. Measurements are made to determine such things as respiratory function, circulatory function and the body's work capacity.

The purpose of respiration is to supply the body's cells with oxygen and to eliminate the carbon dioxide. In the broad sense, respiration involves several mechanisms (Fig. 3.1). In external respiration, pumping movements of the thoracic wall and the mediastinum result in **ventilation**—gas exchange between the environment and the alveoli. Gas exchange or **diffusion** between the air and the blood occurs in the alveoli, which are surrounded by capillaries of the pulmonary circulation. The cardiovascular system provides **circulation**, by pumping the oxygenated blood out into the capillary network of the systemic circulation. There, internal respiration occurs by a gaseous exchange between the blood and the cells—**cell respiration**.

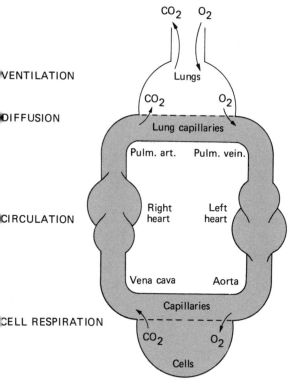

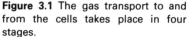

Figure 3.1 The gas transport to and from the cells takes place in four stages.

Functional disturbances may arise in any of the component processes of ventilation, diffusion, circulation or cell respiration. A general disturbance of the internal respiration in the cells is rare. One example is cyanide poisoning, in which the respiratory enzymes in the cells are blocked, a situation leading in a few minutes to arrest of cell respiration and death through internal suffocation.

Circulatory disorders are the most common pathological state, and their investigation accounts for a large portion of the laboratory work in hospitals. In order to determine the condition of the cardiovascular system, hemodynamic examinations are performed; these include measurement of blood pressure, blood flow and blood volume. A record of the electrical activity of the heart indicates the state of the heart muscle.

Respiratory measurements for examining the ventilation and diffusion processes include determinations of inspired volume, airway resistance, oxygen and carbon dioxide concentrations of the expired air and the blood, and pH of the blood.

The various physiological processes interact. For example, ventilation is affected not only by pathological processes in the respiratory organs, but also by changes in other organs. Shortness of breath that is not due to physical effort may be due to reduced ventilation, impaired diffusion in the lungs, circulatory disorders due to heart failure, or increased metabolism, which results in higher oxygen consumption. Some pathological conditions are difficult to detect and require a number of supplementary examinations.

Question		*Answer*
3.1	Transport of oxygen and carbon dioxide to and from the body's cells occurs in four stages, namely, ... , ... , ... and	
3.2	When we use the term "ventilation", we mean the . . . . (external, internal) respiration, which takes place in the	ventilation diffusion circulation cell respiration
3.3	Breathing is driven by an air pump, which consists of the thoracic wall and the diaphragm. It produces . . . .—gas exchange between the environment and the	external lungs
3.4	Gaseous exchange, or . . . . , is possible because the alveoli are surrounded by the . . . . network of the pulmonary circulation.	ventilation alveoli
3.5	The most common pathological conditions are those affecting the	diffusion capillary
3.6	The cardiovascular system is examined by . . . . examinations and by recording the heart's . . . . activity.	circulatory organs
3.7	Respiration is examined by determining inspired . . . . and airway . . . . ; the concentrations of . . . . and . . . . in the expired air; and by measuring the . . . . of the blood.	hemodynamic electrical
		volumes resistance oxygen carbon dioxide pH

RESPIRATION

Ventilation occurs by changing the volume of the thoracic cavity. This is accomplished by lowering the diaphragm, and by outward and upward rotation of the costal arches, which articulate with the vertebral column.

The ventilation, $\dot{V}$, measured in liters per minute, is also known as the minute ventilation. It is defined as the product of the volume of gas expired per breath, the tidal volume, V_T, and the breathing rate, f; thus, $\dot{V} = fV_T$. A portion of the tidal volume does not reach the alveoli, since it remains in the airways at the end of inspiration. To obtain the minute volume of the alveolar ventilation, $\dot{V}_A$, the tidal volume must be diminished by the volume, V_D, of this dead space; that is:

$$\dot{V}_A = f(V_T - V_D)$$

For a desired alveolar ventilation, the ventilation must therefore be somewhat larger; a reduction in tidal volume cannot be compensated for by a proportional increase in the breathing rate. This has practical implications in artificial ventilation, especially if the dead space is increased by connecting the airways to an anesthesia unit or ventilator. In artificial ventilation we seek a large tidal volume.

The diffusion of oxygen and carbon dioxide between the alveolar air and the individual blood cells in the capillaries takes place in less than one second. In pulmonary edema, when plasma leaks from the capillaries into the alveoli, there is an acute (short term) reduction in diffusion. Chronic (long term) reduction in the diffusion capacity occurs with permanent anatomic alterations in the lungs, such as thickening of the alveolar membrane caused by corrosive gases and liquids. In both cases cyanosis may occur if the diffusion resistance is so great as to reduce oxygenation of the blood.

3.8	Ventilation is expressed in .... (units).	
3.9	Ventilation is defined as the product of the .... and the	liters per minute
3.10	The alveolar ventilation is less than the ventilation because of the .... located in the airways.	tidal volume breathing rate
3.11	If f is the breathing rate, V_T the tidal volume and V_D the dead space, the alveolar ventilation $\dot{V}_A =$	dead space
3.12	In order to maintain adequate ventilation it is therefore more important to have a large .... than a high	$f(V_T - V_D)$

3.13	Even when adequate ventilation can be maintained, oxygenation of the blood is low if the . . . . is reduced.	tidal volume breathing rate
3.14	If the diffusion resistance increases, ... (bluish coloration of the mucous membranes and skin) occurs even though the ventilation may be adequate.	diffusion
3.15	Increased diffusion resistance occurs in . . . . edema, when the alveoli are filled with	cyanosis
3.16	In a patient with "interstitial lung fibrosis" the membranes separating the capillary blood from the alveolar air are greatly thickened. Oxygenation of the blood is low because of impaired	pulmonary serous fluid (page 28)
3.17	A mother finds her baby lifeless and cyanotic, with his face covered by a plastic bib. The cause of death is obstructed	diffusion
3.18	Ten days after a major abdominal operation a large pulmonary embolus develops—that is, a blood clot has become detached from the deep veins of the lower leg, has been carried in the blood stream up through the heart and has occluded the pulmonary artery. The patient died immediately from arrested	ventilation
3.19	A worker in a silver-plating factory happens to inhale hydrogen cyanide and dies within a few minutes from suffocation caused by blocking of the . . . . in spite of adequate pulmonary ventilation.	circulation
		cell respiration

Lung Function Tests

Ventilatory volumes

The lungs have a capacity of 5 to 6 liters, 1–1.5 liters of which remain even after maximum expiration—**residual volume** (Fig. 3.2). At rest the **tidal volume** is 0.5 liters. After normal inspiration a further 2–3 liters can be inspired—**inspiratory**

Volume
liters

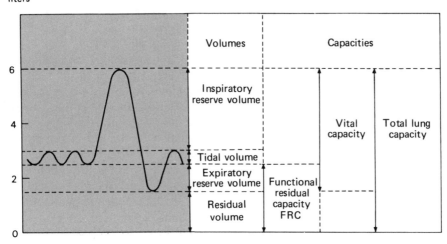

Figure 3.2 Static lung volumes.

reserve volume, and after normal expiration a further 1 liter or so can be expired, **expiratory reserve volume**.

The total enclosed volume at maximum inspiration is the **total lung capacity**. The difference between total lung capacity and residual volume is the **vital capacity**. The **functional residual capacity**, *FRC*, is the residual volume after normal expiration.

These volumes can be determined by **static spirometry** (spiros, breath), with the exception of the residual volume, the functional residual capacity and the total lung capacity. The patient breathes into a spirometer, which records gas volumes (Fig. 3.3).

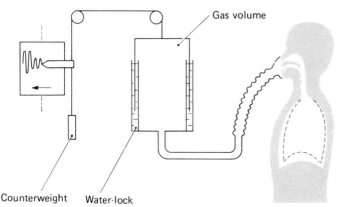

Figure 3.3 Spirometer for determining the relative lung volumes.

The lung function is often determined by measuring the **maximum voluntary ventilation**, MVV. The patient performs maximum inspiration and expiration into a spirometer for a 10 second period and then the ventilation is calculated in liters per minute. The test is easy to perform and of great practical value.

The absolute value of the lung volumes must be determined by an indirect method, such as the **indicator dilution method**. After normal expiration, the airways are connected to a balloon containing a known volume of a gas. A gas such as helium is chosen because it does not diffuse rapidly into the blood. During breathing, the gas mixes with the air in the lung, and after equilibrium has been established, the helium concentration is determined. By knowing the balloon volume and the resultant helium dilution, the total volume of the balloon and FRC can be calculated. The accuracy of the method is limited, especially in pathological conditions where some parts of the lungs are less well ventilated than others.

Absolute lung volumes can also be determined by a **body plethysmograph**. This consists of a closed airtight chamber in which the patient is placed (Fig. 3.4).

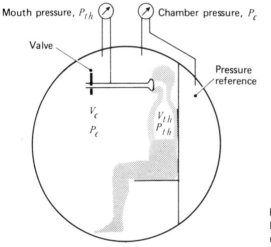

Mouth pressure, P_{th} Chamber pressure, P_c

Valve

Pressure reference

V_c
P_c

V_{th}
P_{th}

Figure 3.4 Determination of absolute lung volumes with a body plethysmograph.

The method is based on the application of Boyle's law to the gas volume in the lungs and to the gas volume in the chamber. Boyle's law can be expressed by the equations, $PV = \text{const}$ and $P/V = -(dP/dV)$.

The patient breathes the air enclosed in the plethysmograph through a mouthpiece. At the end of a normal expiration (lung volume, V_{th}) a valve in the mouthpiece is closed. The patient then performs respiratory movements and generates positive and negative pressures in his lungs through compression and expansion of the air. The pressure difference, dP_{th}, is measured with a pressure transducer connected to the mouthpiece. During the inspiratory movements the thorax volume increases, which expands the air in the lungs. This expansion can be determined by measuring the increase in pressure, dP_c, in the air enclosed in the plethysmograph, V_c. It can be shown that

$$V_{th} = -(dP_c/dP_{th})\,V_c$$

This method for determining lung volumes by plethysmography is rapid, reliable and comfortable for the patient.

3.20	The difference in volume between maximum inspiration and expiration is known as the	
3.21	The lung volume at maximum inspiration is the	vital capacity
3.22	The lung volume after normal expiration is the	total lung capacity
3.23	For a person in normal health with a vital capacity of 4 liters, the tidal volume at rest is about	functional residual capacity (*FRC*)
3.24	The sum of the inspiratory reserve volume, the tidal volume and the expiratory reserve volume is known as the	0.5 liter
3.25	These three lung volumes can be measured by static	vital capacity
3.26	The functional residual capacity can be measured with a gas, which is used as an .... The respiratory tract is connected to an apparatus of known .... with a gas, such as ...., which does not diffuse into the blood. The lung volume is obtained by determining the .... of the gas.	spirometry
3.27	The functional residual capacity can also be determined with a ...., which is essentially an .... chamber, which encloses the patient. The calculation is based on .... law.	indicator volume helium dilution
3.28	A drop in pressure in the body plethysmograph occurs during .... (inspiratory, expiratory) movements; this is caused by .... of the air enclosed in the lungs.	body plethysmograph airtight Boyle's
		expiratory compression

Respiratory work

During ventilation the body performs work. The work is required to overcome the **airway resistance** and the elastic forces in the lungs and chest; these forces are described by the term **compliance** (flexibility). When the respiratory work cannot be increased above a certain level, the rate of oxygen uptake is limited, thus limiting the body's physical work output. In severe pathological conditions the respiratory work must sometimes be taken over by a ventilator (page 545).

Airway resistance. When air flows from the mouth to the alveoli, it causes a pressure difference, which overcomes frictional losses in the airways. In analogy with Ohm's law, the flow resistance, R, of a gas through a tube system is related to the pressure difference, ΔP, and the flow, $\dot{V}$, as follows:

$$R = \Delta P / \dot{V}$$

The pressure is measured in centimeters of water, Pa, and the flow in liters per second; thus, units of airway resistance are cm $H_2O \cdot$ s/liter (SI units, Pa $\cdot$ s/liter).

For laminar flow of a gas or liquid, the flow resistance, R, is directly proportional to the viscosity, η, and the length, l, of the tube, and inversely proportional to the fourth power of the radius, r. Thus,

$$R = 8\eta l / \pi r^4$$

The radius is thus critically important in determining the flow resistance. The body utilizes this fact for regulating the flow, for example, to ensure an equal distribution of air and of blood into different portions of the lungs. If the cross-sectional area of an airway is reduced by a pathological process, it can cause major functional disturbances. One example of this is the increased flow resistance in asthma, due to the contraction of the smooth muscles in the walls of the bronchioles, the swelling of the mucous membranes of the bronchioles and the accumulation of mucus.

Dynamic spirometry is used to gain an impression of the airways' flow resistance. After maximum inspiration, the patient exhales as rapidly as possible, and the spirometer records the change in volume with time. Special instruments, **pneumotachographs** or **pneumotachometers**, are also often used for this purpose; these are often based on the principle that air flowing through a flow resistance causes a pressure drop that is a function of the velocity. A low forced expiratory volume during the first second, $FEV_{1.0}$, may be due to a low vital capacity; therefore a percentage, $FEV\%$, is used. If the vital capacity is normal, a low $FEV_{1.0}$ indicates an increased resistance to respiratory movements, which may be located either in the airways, the lung tissues or the chest wall. Normally, $FEV_{1.0}$ is 3 liters/s and $FEV\%$ is 70. Typical values in asthma during attack-free periods are 1.5 liters/s and 35; during attacks the values are still lower. The method is easy to use and is valuable in screening—that is, the rapid elimination of normal persons, saving more sophisticated and time-consuming tests for patients who require more thorough examination.

An exact measurement of air-flow resistance can be performed with a **body plethysmograph** (Fig. 3.5). The arrangement is the same as that used in the determination of the total lung capacity, and Boyle's law is also used. Two separate measurements are made. First, as in lung volume determinations, the mouthpiece valve is closed. The change in pressure in the chamber, dP_{c1}, is

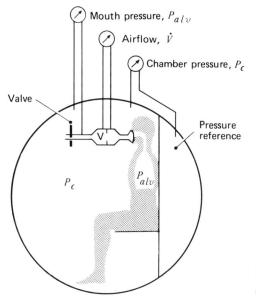

Mouth pressure, P_{alv}

Airflow, $\dot{V}$

Chamber pressure, P_c

Valve

Pressure reference

P_c

P_{alv}

Figure 3.5 Determination of airway resistance with a body plethysmograph.

determined as a function of the change in alveolar pressure, dP_{alv}; this quantity is equal to the mouth pressure when no air is flowing through the airways. Second, with the valve open, the change in pressure in the chamber, dP_{c2}, is measured as a function of the change in flow, $d\dot{V}$, when panting through the mouthpiece. The airway resistance is

$$R = (dP_{c2}/d\dot{V})(dP_{alv}/dP_{c1})$$

The airway resistance varies with lung inflation. The method is comfortable for the patient, sensitive, rapid and gives reliable values, which are independent of the mechanical resistance in the chest wall and the lung tissues.

Compliance. Surface tension within the lungs normally tends to collapse the lungs, whereas the elasticity of the thorax tends to expand it. In respiratory equilibrium, the forces balance each other; in order to disturb this balance, muscular work is required. The elasticity of the lung tissues and the thorax is described by the term **compliance**, C, which is defined as the change in volume, dV, per unit change in the alveolar pressure, dP_{alv}. Thus

$$C = dV/dP_{alv}$$

The compliance is determined by recording changes in lung volume as a function of the pressure in the pleural cavity. This is performed during slow breathing, when the frictional loss is negligible. The pleural pressure is equal to the pressure in the esophagus. It is measured with a balloon connected by a catheter to a pressure-recording instrument and inserted in the esophagus. The compliance is normally 0.2 liters/cm H_2O (SI units, 2 ml/Pa).

3.29	The flow resistance is defined as the ratio of .... to	
3.30	For laminar flow of a gas or liquid, the relationship between the flow resistance, R, the viscosity, η, the length, l, and the radius, r, of the tube is given by the formula	pressure difference flow
3.31	The flow resistance in a tube then depends mainly on the area of its cross-section. The body utilizes this relationship to regulate the .... of blood and air to the lungs.	$R = 8\eta l/\pi r^4$
3.32	In asthma, one factor which increases the airway resistance is the contraction of smooth .... in the	flow
3.33	In dynamic spirometry the change in volume per .... is measured during as rapid an .... as possible.	muscle bronchioles
3.34	During dynamic spirometry, if the vital capacity is normal, too slow expiration may be due to increased resistance in ...., ... or	unit time expiration
3.35	A reliable method for measuring airway resistance is	airways lung tissue chest wall

3.36	Determination of the resistance by plethysmography is a .... (sensitive, insensitive) method, yielding .... (reliable, unreliable) values, which are .... (dependent on, independent of) the resistance of the lung tissues and chest wall.	body plethysmography
3.37	The elasticity of the lung tissues and the chest wall is known as .... and is defined as the ratio of the change in lung .... to the change in alveolar pressure.	sensitive reliable independent of
		compliance volume

Blood gases

A measure of the total net effect of respiration and circulation can be obtained by determining the concentration of oxygen and carbon dioxide in the blood.

Oxygen is normally taken up by the lungs in the following way. The inspired air is humidified with water vapor to give a partial pressure (tension) of about 50 mm Hg (6.7 kPa). The oxygen tension in the inspired air in the airways is then 21 percent of (760–50) or 150 mm Hg (20.0 kPa). (At standard pressure the oxygen tension in air is 160 mm Hg (21.3 kPa).)

The oxygen diffuses from the alveoli into the pulmonary capillaries and is replaced by carbon dioxide, $PCO_2 = 40$ mm Hg (5.3 kPa), from the pulmonary capillaries. This lowers the oxygen tension in the alveolar air to about 110 mm Hg (14.7 kPa). During the short passage of the capillary blood in the lung alveoli (0.75 s at rest and 0.3 s during strenuous exercise), both carbon dioxide and oxygen attain diffusion equilibrium. Due to the mixing of some venous blood, the oxygen tension in the arterial blood is about 100 mm Hg (13.3 kPa).

At a given oxygen tension in the blood, the hemoglobin has a certain level of oxygen saturation—a certain percentage of the hemoglobin is bound to oxygen. At an oxygen tension of 100 mm Hg (13.3 kPa) in the arterial blood, the saturation level is close to 100 percent. In mixed venous blood before oxygenation in the lungs, where the oxygen tension is about 40 mm Hg (5.3 kPa), the oxygen saturation is about 70 percent (Fig. 3.6). One gram of hemoglobin binds 1.34 ml of oxygen; thus,

$$\text{oxygen content} = \text{oxygen saturation} \times \text{Hb concentration} \times 1.34$$

	(ml/100 ml)	(percent)	(g/100 ml)
SI units	(ml/l)	(percent)	(g/l)

Percentage oxygen saturation

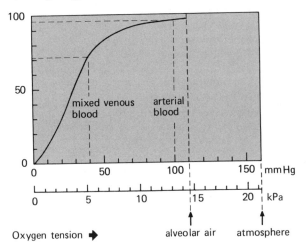

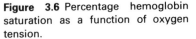

Oxygen tension ➡   alveolar air   atmosphere

Figure 3.6 Percentage hemoglobin saturation as a function of oxygen tension.

A small part of the oxygen transport is normally due to oxygen physically dissolved in the plasma. If the oxygen tension is increased, the amount dissolved also increases; when pure oxygen is breathed at a pressure of 3 atm (300 kPa), the entire oxygen requirement of the cells can be transported without relying on the hemoglobin. This fact is exploited in some forms of intensive care (page 551).

The body tends to keep the carbon dioxide tension in the arterial blood constant at about 40 mm Hg (5.3 kPa). One reason for this is that the carbon dioxide tension affects the blood's pH, which must be maintained within narrow limits. The respiratory center in the medulla oblongata regulates the tension by adjusting the ventilation.

Carbon dioxide diffuses through the capillary and alveolar walls more easily than oxygen, which is the limiting factor in gas exchange. Thus, the carbon dioxide tension in the alveolar air is about 40 mm Hg (5.3 kPa). Since the alveolar ventilation is inversely proportional to the carbon dioxide tension in the arterial blood, the alveolar ventilation can be determined indirectly by blood gas analysis.

Blood gas analyses. The oxygen tension in the blood can be measured by polarography. A Clark PO_2 electrode consists of a platinum electrode which is at a 0.7 V negative potential with respect to a silver–silver chloride reference electrode (Fig. 3.7). The two metal electrodes are surrounded by a phosphate buffer with a constant pH of 7, saturated with potassium chloride. The solution is separated from the sample—in this case, blood—by a thin polyethylene membrane, which is permeable to oxygen. Oxygen diffuses through the membrane, with equilibrium attained within 10–20 s. The measured oxygen is reduced at the platinum electrode, yielding an electric current proportional to the oxygen tension. The platinum electrode is usually small, with a diameter of about 0.01 mm. The current depends on the design; a typical value is $10^{-8}–10^{-11}$ A per mm Hg (0.13 kPa) of oxygen tension.

The carbon dioxide tension can be measured with a Severinghaus electrode (Fig. 3.8). This consists of a glass electrode for measuring pH (see below),

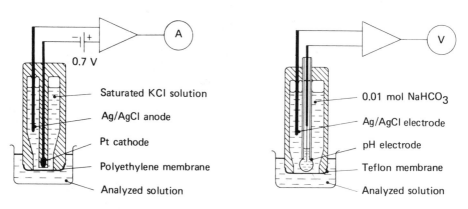

Figure 3.7 Polarographic determination of the oxygen tension, PO_2, with a Clark electrode.

Figure 3.8 Severinghaus electrode system for determining the carbon dioxide tension.

surrounded by a solution of sodium bicarbonate. A Teflon membrane, which is permeable to carbon dioxide, separates the solution from the sample. The carbon dioxide tension is related to pH as follows: $\log (PCO_2) = K + pH$, where PCO_2 is the carbon dioxide tension and K is a constant. A typical internal resistance for a PCO_2 electrode is $5 \cdot 10^8$ ohm. A change of 1 mm Hg (0.13 kPa) of the carbon dioxide tension at 40 mm Hg (5.3 kPa) corresponds to 0.01 pH unit, or 0.6 mV. Both the oxygen and the carbon dioxide electrodes are sensitive to temperature, thus, thermostatic control is essential.

3.38	The oxygen tension in air at standard pressure is ...., in normal arterial blood is .... and in mixed venous blood is about	
3.39	A certain oxygen tension results in a certain level of .... of the blood.	160 mm Hg (21.3 kPa) 100 mm Hg (13.3 kPa) 40 mm Hg (5.3 kPa)

3.40	Oxygen saturation means the percentage of .... bound with oxygen.	oxygen saturation
3.41	In arterial blood the oxygen saturation is normally .... and in mixed venous blood it is about	hemoglobin (Hb)
3.42	The oxygen content (ml/100 ml) of arterial blood is equal to the product of .... (each gram of Hb binds 1.34 ml oxygen).	100 percent 70 percent
3.43	Through the respiratory center in the medulla oblongata the .... is regulated so that the normal carbon dioxide tension in the arterial blood is constant at about	oxygen saturation, Hb concentration and 1.34
3.44	Carbon dioxide diffuses .... (more, less) easily than oxygen through the capillary and alveolar walls.	ventilation 40 mm Hg (5.3 kPa)
3.45	As a result the carbon dioxide tension of the arterial blood is equal to the tension in	more
3.46	The carbon dioxide tension in arterial blood is inversely proportional to the alveolar ...., a fact that is utilized in determining this quantity.	alveolar air
3.47	The oxygen tension in the blood can be determined with a .... (proper name) electrode, which is based on a .... principle.	ventilation
3.48	A Clark electrode consists of a .... electrode which is made 0.7 V negative with respect to a reference electrode.	Clark polarographic
3.49	At the platinum electrode the oxygen is reduced, which generates an electric .... proportional to the	platinum
3.50	A PCO_2 electrode consists of a .... electrode for measuring ...., surrounded by a solution of	current oxygen tension

3.51	As the PCO_2 varies, the . . . . of the sodium bicarbonate changes according to a . . . . function. The instrument for measuring the . . . . of the pH electrode can be graduated directly in PCO_2.	glass pH sodium bicarbonate
		pH logarithmic potential

Blood pH

The hydrogen ion concentration of the blood is affected by the respiration (due to the carbon dioxide tension), and by the metabolism (due to the formation of non-volatile acids). The pH of the blood is normally 7.40 and that of the arterial blood can range from 7.35 to 7.45. When the value is below this range, **acidosis** occurs, and when the value is higher, **alkalosis**. The limits compatible with life are 6.8–7.8. According to the Henderson-Hasselbalch equation, the acidity of the blood can be calculated from the bicarbonate ion concentration $[HCO_3^-]$ and the concentration of dissolved carbonic acid $[H_2CO_3]$:

$$pH = pK + \log \frac{[HCO_3^-]}{[H_2CO_3]}$$

where pK is a constant that is dependent on the first dissociation constant of the carbonic acid, and has the value 6.1 in blood plasma. Since the concentration of carbon dioxide is equal to the product of the carbon dioxide tension and the solubility constant of carbon dioxide, 0.03 (in SI units, 0.23), we have

$$pH = 6.1 + \log \frac{[HCO_3^-]}{0.03 \, PCO_2}$$

Normally the ratio $[HCO_3^-]/[H_2CO_3] = 20:1$. This can increase or decrease either because of a change in the bicarbonate ion concentration, when **metabolic** alkalosis or acidosis develops, or because of a change in the carbonic acid concentration, when **respiratory** problems cause a disturbance of the blood pH so that respiratory alkalosis or acidosis occurs.

In acidosis, the patient has a reduced consciousness, tachycardia develops, the blood pressure falls and signs of cyanosis develop. Ventricular fibrillation may develop—uncoordinated cardiac muscle contractions which arrest the circulation and result in sudden death. Alkalosis can also be a threat to life. Rapid diagnosis and administration of drugs to correct the pH are essential measures of intensive care (page 574).

Measurement of pH. The pH of the blood is determined most simply with a glass electrode (Fig. 3.9). Special kinds of glass are slightly permeable to hydrogen ions,

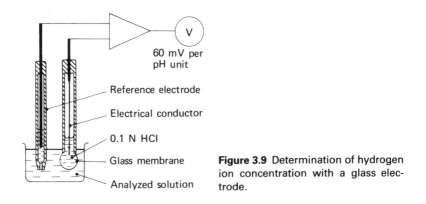

60 mV per
pH unit

Reference electrode

Electrical conductor

0.1 N HCl

Glass membrane

Analyzed solution

Figure 3.9 Determination of hydrogen ion concentration with a glass electrode.

and the potential across the membrane depends on the relative hydrogen ion concentration on each side. A calomel electrode is often used as the reference, because its potential is independent of the hydrogen ion concentration of the sample. The pH is a linear function of the potential difference, and one pH unit corresponds to 60 mV. The internal resistance of a glass electrode is high, 10^7–10^{10} ohms.

3.52	The normal pH of the blood is	
3.53	Above a pH of .... a state of .... exists.	7.4
3.54	Below a pH of .... a state of .... exists.	7.45 alkalosis
3.55	The pH of the blood is influenced by two physiological processes, namely, ... and	7.35 acidosis
3.56	The Henderson–Hasselbalch equation for the hydrogen ion concentration in blood plasma is: pH = 6.1 + ...	respiration metabolism

3.57	The hydrogen ion concentration of the blood is most easily determined with a	$\log \dfrac{[HCO_3^-]}{0.03^\cdot PCO_2}$
3.58	Measurement of pH with a glass electrode is based on the fact that certain glass membranes are .... to hydrogen ions, so that if the hydrogen ion concentration is different on each side of the membrane, a .... difference is set up across it. The potential difference is a .... function of the pH.	glass electrode
3.59	A person with acute gastritis has vomited repeatedly, losing large amounts of hydrochloric acid; .... (metabolic, respiratory) .... (alkalosis, acidosis) develops, which contributes to the patient's discomfort. After the patient ceases vomiting, he is advised to drink plenty of water to produce large volumes of urine. This corrects the acid-base disturbance by excretion through the kidneys.	slightly permeable potential linear
3.60	A healthy, lively infant cries violently over a long period. Hyperventilation results in excessive loss of carbon dioxide and .... develops, which leads to convulsions and spasms, after which the child falls asleep. The blood pH then returns to normal and the child recovers.	metabolic alkalosis
3.61	A patient with diabetes is careless and forgets to take insulin; formation of organic acids increases and .... develops; the unconscious patient is admitted to the hospital in a diabetic coma.	respiratory alkalosis
3.62	A patient that has taken an overdose of sleeping pills (or alcohol and certain narcotics) is admitted to the hospital in a deep coma. Because of the low tolerance of the respiratory center to drugs and toxins, its regulatory function is eliminated and the carbon dioxide tension rises, but there is no increased ventilation; as a result, ... develops. The condition is aggravated by the rising carbon dioxide tension, which exerts a narcotic effect on the respiratory center. Treatment with a ventilator and correction of the blood pH become necessary.	metabolic acidosis
		respiratory acidosis

CIRCULATION

The condition of the circulatory organs is examined by hemodynamic measurements and by recording the electrical activity of the heart muscle—electrocardiography. These methods are described here in greater detail, together with two therapeutic procedures for controlling the heart rhythm, namely, defibrillation and pacemaker therapy.

HEMODYNAMICS

The amount of blood that the heart pumps per unit time—the **cardiac output**—is the product of the heart rate and the stroke volume. The cardiac output for an adult at rest is about 5 liters/min; during exercise it is 20 liters/min or more. The heart rate is partly controlled by the autonomic nervous system; the sympathetic system increases the heart rate and the parasympathetic system reduces it, partly by hormone action, as described above (page 93). The stroke volume is determined by four factors, namely, the filling pressure, the compliance of the ventricular wall during diastole, the arterial pressure and the contractility of the ventricular wall—all factors that are dependent on several other physiological functions.

For a thorough clinical analysis of a patient's circulatory state, the heart sounds are recorded by **phonocardiography**, and the **blood pressure, blood flow** and **blood volumes** are measured.

3.63	The state of the circulatory organs is examined by .... measurements and by recording the heart's .... activity.	
3.64	Hemodynamics is the study of the blood's	hemodynamic electrical
3.65	Defibrillation and pacemaker treatment are two procedures used in treating disturbances of the heart	flow
3.66	The amount of blood pumped by the heart at rest is normally ....; this quantity is known as the	rhythm
3.67	The cardiac output is defined as the product of .... and	5 liters/min cardiac output

3.68	The heart rate is regulated by the ....,.... nervous system; the sympathetic system .... and the parasympathetic system .... the heart rate. The stroke volume is influenced by a number of physiological factors.	stroke volume heart rate
3.69	For a thorough analysis of the patient's hemodynamic condition, measurements are made of the ...., ... and ...., and the heart sounds are recorded by	autonomic increases decreases
		blood pressure blood flow blood volumes phonocardiography

Cardiac Catheterization

For an exact diagnosis of an organic heart defect, for example, valvular defect or a congenital deformity, it is necessary to perform measurements directly within the heart chambers. This can be done by inserting a catheter through peripheral vessels—a procedure known as cardiac catheterization.

A catheter consists of a flexible plastic tube about one meter long, with an external diameter of about 3 mm. The catheter can be radiopaque or it can be visualized in radiographs (x-ray pictures) by means of a metal guide wire. The position of the catheter can be monitored during catheterization by means of fluoroscopy or television radiography.

With the catheter it is possible to reach all the chambers of the heart and the nearby major vessels. Hemodynamic measurements of blood pressure and blood flow are made, blood specimens are taken for analyses of oxygen and carbon dioxide contents, heart sounds are recorded and a radiopaque medium is injected in order to visualize changes in the heart's anatomy. These examinations are of critical importance for the preoperative assessment of the patient's condition—to decide whether a heart operation should be performed and, if so, the best procedures. Catheterization during physical exercise can be performed by having the patient operate a bicycle ergometer in the supine position. The catheterization is carried out under sterile conditions to avoid infection. Because the vessels are insensitive to pain, local anesthesia of the skin at the site where the catheter is inserted is usually sufficient.

Types of cardiac catheterization

One or more of the following three catheterization techniques may be chosen, depending on which regions of the heart and which vessels are to be examined

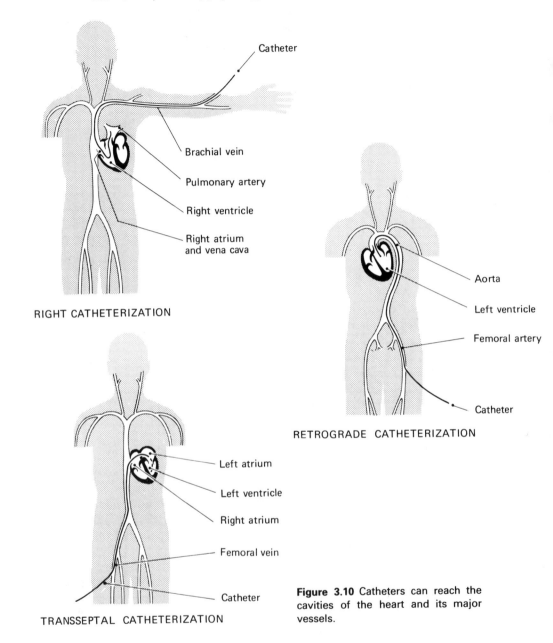

Catheter

Brachial vein

Pulmonary artery

Right ventricle

Right atrium
and vena cava

RIGHT CATHETERIZATION

Aorta

Left ventricle

Femoral artery

Catheter

RETROGRADE CATHETERIZATION

Left atrium

Left ventricle

Right atrium

Femoral vein

Catheter

TRANSSEPTAL CATHETERIZATION

Figure 3.10 Catheters can reach the cavities of the heart and its major vessels.

(Fig. 3.10). In all three, the catheter is preferably inserted by the **percutaneous technique** (Seldinger's method, Fig. 3.11). A peripheral artery or vein is punctured by means of a cannula, through which a metal or nylon guide wire is inserted a distance into the vessel. Over the guide, whose external diameter is

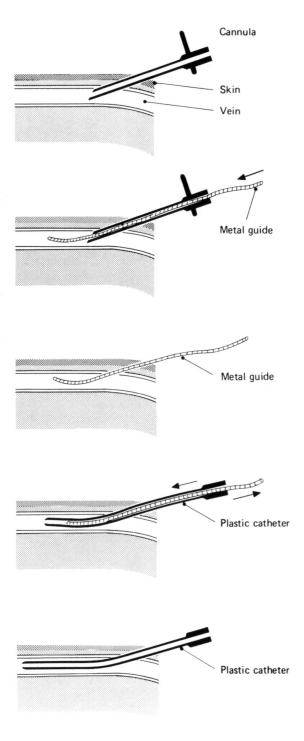

Cannula

Skin

Vein

Metal guide

Metal guide

Plastic catheter

Plastic catheter

Figure 3.11 Percutaneous technique for inserting a catheter.

slightly less than the internal diameter of the catheter, the catheter is passed into the vessel, after which the guide can be withdrawn. If the catheter diameter is comparable to that of the vessel, a cutdown is performed, in which the vessel is surgically exposed prior to insertion.

Right catheterization.   The catheter is inserted in an elbow vein and advanced through the venous system to the vena cava, into the right atrium and ventricle, and out into the pulmonary artery. It is of particular interest to obtain samples of mixed venous blood for determining the cardiac output from the right half of the heart (page 175). It is also important to measure the pulmonary artery pressure, which is elevated in mitral stenosis and in lung changes. By further advancing the catheter into a smaller lung artery, the catheter wedges into the artery and seals off the effects of arterial pressure. Then the catheter lumen measures a pressure closely corresponding to the pulmonary vein pressure, which is equal to the left atrial pressure. To find whether there is a stenosis, the pressure difference across each valve is measured by recording the pressure as the catheter is being withdrawn—a so-called pullback curve is plotted.

Retrograde catheterization.   The catheter is inserted into the left ventricle via a peripheral artery on the inside of the elbow or groin. Retrograde catheterization is performed chiefly to examine aortic and mitral valve defects. In the case of tight aortic stenosis, it is impossible to reach the left ventricle by retrograde catheterization, and transseptal catheterization is then required.

Transseptal catheterization.   A large-caliber catheter is inserted into the femoral vein in the right groin and advanced into the right atrium via the venous system and inferior vena cava. By means of a special needle which is inserted in the catheter, the atrial septum is punctured, and the catheter is inserted into the left atrium. Through this large-caliber catheter, a smaller one is inserted into the left ventricle. This technique is used for measuring the pressure in the left atrium through the large-caliber catheter and, at the same time, the pressure in the left ventricle through the smaller catheter, in suspected mitral stenosis, mitral insufficiency or aortic stenosis.

In suspected mitral valve defect, retrograde left ventricular catheterization is combined with transseptal left atrial catheterization for simultaneous measurement of pressure in the left atrium and ventricle.

Risks in cardiac catheterization

When experienced personnel use good technique, cardiac catheterization is relatively safe. One potentially serious complication, however, is ventricular fibrillation—a disturbance of the heart rhythm that leads to circulatory arrest (see page 196). The ECG is always monitored in order to display extrasystoles (page 196), a sign that indicates the threat of ventricular fibrillation. Extrasystoles often occur when the tip of the catheter touches the heart muscle. Since there is the possibility of ventricular fibrillation, resuscitation equipment must be immediately available. This should include a defibrillator, together with equipment for heart massage and artificial ventilation.

From an engineering viewpoint, we must examine the risk associated with an electric current passing through the catheter. Since the catheter is a good insulator, a current could pass through the saline-filled catheter to the tip, which might be in contact with a sensitive part of the ventricular muscle. Under these conditions, a current as small as 10μA might cause ventricular fibrillation. Thus, for all equipment in contact with the patient, not only must the case be electrically grounded, but also the connections to the patient must have very low current flowing through them. Under no circumstances—with the electric current switched on or off—should leakage current in the catheters be large enough to cause ventricular fibrillation.

Catheters made of conducting material have been made. These prevent a high current density at the tip, by diffusing the leakage current through the conductive walls. However, since many patients have a conducting pacemaker wire leading to the heart, all equipment must be designed for low leakage anyway and normal catheters are sufficient.

3.70	In cardiac catheterization, measurements can be performed directly in the . . . . and in neighboring major	
3.71	Catheterization is performed under . . . . (degree of cleanliness) conditions.	chambers of the heart vessels
3.72	The catheter is inserted under fluoroscopic observation by using . . . .; this is possible since the catheter is made	sterile
3.73	In catheterization, hemodynamic measurements of . . . . and . . . . are performed.	x-ray imaging radiopaque (x-ray attenuating)
3.74	Blood samples can be taken for chemical analysis of . . . . and . . . . tension.	blood pressure blood flow
3.75	By using an indwelling catheter, any change in the anatomy of the heart and vessels can be examined by . . . . immediately after injecting a	oxygen carbon dioxide

3.76	In right catheterization the catheter is inserted into a .... and passed through the vascular system into the .... atrium and .... ventricle and out into the	radiography contrast medium
3.77	Right catheterization and pressure measurement in the pulmonary artery are performed in suspected .... and	vein right right pulmonary artery
3.78	By right catheterization it is possible to obtain samples of mixed .... (arterial, venous) blood for determining the cardiac output.	mitral stenosis lung changes
3.79	In retrograde catheterization the catheter is inserted into the .... It is performed in suspected .... and	venous
3.80	In transseptal catheterization the catheter is placed in a .... and advanced through the vascular system into the .... atrium and through the .... to the	left ventricle aortic valve defect mitral valve defect
3.81	Transseptal catheterization and pressure measurement in the left atrium are performed in suspected .... and	vein right atrial septum left atrium
3.82	In catheterization the catheter is preferably inserted by a method known as the .... First, a .... is punctured with a cannula. Through this a .... is inserted. The catheter is passed over this and into the vessel; the .... is then withdrawn and the catheter is left in place.	mitral valve defect aortic stenosis
3.83	The occurrence of extrasystoles during cardiac catheterization is a sign of threatening .... Resuscitation equipment should therefore be immediately available. This should include a ...., and equipment for maintaining circulation and ventilation.	percutaneous technique (Seldinger's method) vessel guide guide

3.84	All apparatus in contact with a patient during cardiac catheterization must be designed to prevent .... from flowing through the catheter. Since the catheter is a good insulator an electric current will pass through the ...., which may be in contact with part of the heart muscle. This might cause .... It is particularly important to ensure that all apparatus is .... and that no current leaks can arise in the catheter.	ventricular fibrillation defibrillator
3.85	From the following conditions, calculate the current in a cardiac catheter that could produce ventricular fibrillation. In the case of an electrical shock, in which current passes from one arm to another in the chest—the most dangerous direction for a current in the body—a current of 50 mA can be fatal. Assume that this current is distributed uniformly over a 20 by 20 cm cross-section of the chest in the sagittal plane, and that the same current density in a catheter tip 3 mm in diameter could cause ventricular fibrillation, if the tip were in direct contact with a sensitive part of the heart muscle.	leakage current catheter tip ventricular fibrillation grounded
		about 9 μA

Phonocardiography

An objective analysis of heart sounds can be made by using a microphone as a pickup, amplifying the output and recording it simultaneously with an ECG curve. The microphone is normally placed on the chest in the same positions as in auscultation. A miniaturized microphone in the tip of a cardiac catheter can also be used for a more exact diagnosis.

Since heart sounds contain frequencies up to 500 Hz, an ordinary ECG pen recorder does not have adequate frequency response. Thus either the high frequencies must be shifted to a lower frequency range, or a special recorder with adequate frequency response must be used (page 209). A simple frequency analysis of the signal can be made by dividing the signal into a number of frequency bands—for example, 25, 50, 100, 200 and 400 Hz. Figs. 3.12 and 3.13 show examples of phonograms.

If computer analysis is desired, the signals are recorded on magnetic tape, thus allowing more advanced procedures of frequency analysis (Fig. 3.14). Such methods have not proved to be of practical importance since an analysis of the frequency components of murmurs is of no help in identifying the various types of valve defects.

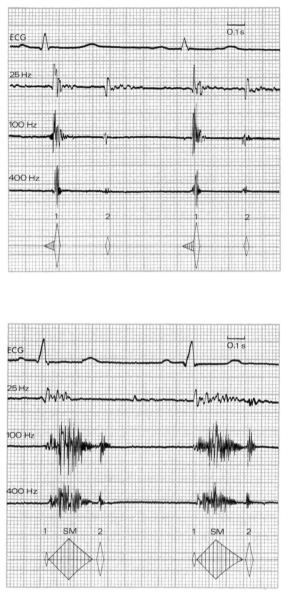

Figure 3.12 Normal phonocardiogram. The first and second heart sounds are clearly reproduced at the three frequencies 25, 100 and 400 Hz. To determine the timing of the heart sounds, an electrocardiogram (top) is recorded simultaneously. The findings in a phonocardiographic examination are often presented schematically as shown at the bottom of the figure.

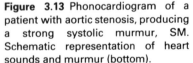

Figure 3.13 Phonocardiogram of a patient with aortic stenosis, producing a strong systolic murmur, SM. Schematic representation of heart sounds and murmur (bottom).

By means of phonocardiography it is possible to determine the exact time relations of the heart sounds in the cardiac cycle, any split sounds, variation during the breathing cycle and changes during physical effort. Although the diagnostic information yielded by phonocardiography does not differ essentially from that obtained by ordinary auscultation (see pages 127–32), the method is a valuable

Hz

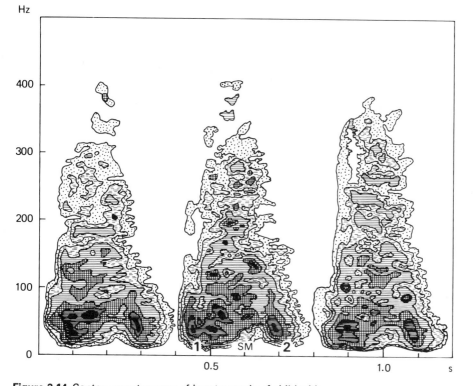

Figure 3.14 Contour spectrogram of heart sounds of child with pulmonary artery stenosis. The first (1) and second (2) heart sounds and the systolic murmur, SM, can be distinguished. Note the differences in the frequency content of the three heart beats. Since the causes of these differences are not known, they are of no diagnostic significance. (Drawn from Lowell et al., *Computer Analysis of the Phonocardiogram*, in Bernard L. Segal & David G. Kilpatrick, *Engineering in the Practice of Medicine*, Baltimore, Md., The Williams & Wilkins Company, 1967, by permission.)

supplement to other heart examinations because of the possibility of objective recording and analysis that it affords.

3.86	The procedure of picking up heart sounds with a microphone, amplifying and recording them is known as	
3.87	Microphones are placed on the . . . . or in a	phonocardiography

3.88	The heart sounds are registered by a recorder having an upper frequency limit of at least . . . . Hz.	chest cardiac catheter
3.89	Phonocardiography has the advantage that it is possible to replace the . . . . evaluation of auscultation with an . . . . recording method.	500
3.90	Of particular value is the possibility of determining exactly the . . . . relations of the heart sounds in the cardiac cycle, the presence of . . . . sounds and changes in the heart sounds during the . . . . cycle and during . . . . effort.	subjective objective
		time split breathing physical

Blood Pressure Measurement

For a thorough hemodynamic examination of the cardiovascular system, the indirect method of measuring blood pressure using a cuff, described earlier (page 133), is inadequate. Instead, a direct method is used in which the vessels are punctured.

All measurements of blood pressure must take into account differences in level due to body position. To eliminate differences in hydrostatic pressure, all measurements are made with the right atrium as a reference point. In a supine patient, the right atrium is assumed to lie in the point of intersection of a perpendicular line through the fourth intercostal space at the sternum and a horizontal line at the level of half the height of the thorax (Fig. 3.15).

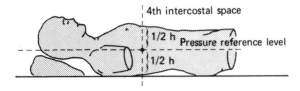

Figure 3.15 In pressure measurements in the vascular system, the level of the right atrium is chosen as the pressure reference.

For static measurements of blood pressure and calibration of pressure transducers, water or mercury manometers are used. The manometer often consists of a disposable plastic tube. When connected directly to a blood vessel, for example a vein, the manometer is filled with a 0.9 percent sterile solution of sodium chloride. This "physiological saline" can be injected into the blood stream. Then it is possible to flush the connecting tube and cannula with saline, to which heparin has been added to prevent coagulation of the blood. Pressure measurement with a liquid manometer has the advantages of simplicity and precision.

For dynamic pressure measurements, electromechanical pressure transducers must be used. These are usually located outside the patient and connected to a cannula or a catheter, which is inserted into the vessel—as is done, for example, in cardiac catheterization.

There are transmission problems associated with the use of fluid filled catheters in measuring blood pressure. The transducer's frequency response is greatly lowered when the catheter is connected. The mass of the transducer that moves with the pressure variations is increased by the mass of the liquid column, thus increasing the inertia of the system. This lowers the resonant frequency of the system and produces resonant peaks in the frequency response. The mass can be reduced by decreasing the internal diameter of the catheter, but this causes an increase in losses due to friction between the liquid column and the catheter wall. The friction induces damping, the magnitude of which must be adjusted to give the system the best possible frequency characteristic. An optimally damped system can accurately reproduce an arterial pressure wave if the system's upper limiting frequency is above 25 Hz (Fig. 3.16). A small leak or a small volume of air in the catheter, even a cubic millimeter or so in volume, increases the compliance, completely alters the catheter's transmission properties and introduces errors.

The dynamic properties of a catheter-transducer system are thus determined by the radius, r, and length, l, of the catheter and by the compliances (dV/dP) of the catheter, C_c, and transducer, C_t. The compliance is expressed as a change in volume per unit of pressure per meter, m^4/N (meter^4/newton), and that of the transducer as a change in volume per unit of pressure, m^5/N. The resonant frequency for a catheter-transducer system filled with water can be calculated roughly from the expression:

$$f_o = r/112[l(C_cl + C_t)]^{\frac{1}{2}}$$

and the damping factor of the system from the expression:

$$d = 7 \times 10^{-5}[l(C_cl + C_t)]^{\frac{1}{2}}/r^3$$

Good transducers should have a compliance greater than 2×10^{-14} m^5/N (corresponding to about 0.25 mm^3/100 mm Hg or 0.02 mm^3/kPa); with available catheters these give resonant frequencies above 20 Hz. A 1 mm^3 air bubble in the system will increase the compliance by about 1×10^{-14} m^5/N and will thus have a considerable effect on the resonant frequency and damping factor.

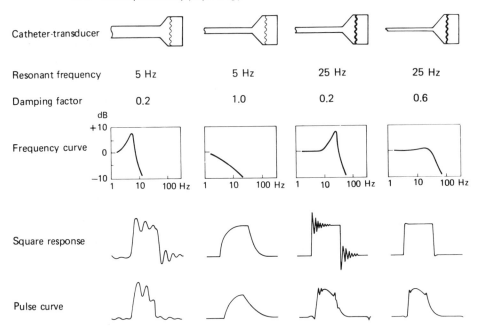

Figure 3.16 The transmission properties of a catheter–transducer system for pressure measurement are determined largely by the inner radius of the catheter, if the compliance of the transducer is low. In the first two cases on the left, the transducer membrane is flexible, and this gives too high a compliance. In the two cases on the right, the membrane is rigid, giving a low compliance; the damping factor is determined by choice of catheter dimensions.

Various types of pressure transducers are used with catheters, among them, wire strain gauge transducers, capacitive transducers (differential capacitors) and inductive transducers (differential transformers). To avoid the problems with pressure transmission in the catheter, miniaturized transducers have been designed, which are housed in the tip of a cardiac catheter having an external diameter of 3 mm. These utilize either a miniature strain gauge transducer, a differential transformer or a mechanical–optical system. In the last of these the illuminating and detector components are external and connected by fiber optics to the catheter tip.

Each systole generates a pulse wave in the arterial system that travels much more rapidly than the movement of the blood column. The blood flow velocity does not exceed 0.5 m/s, whereas the pulse wave normally travels at 5 m/s. The arterial walls, which contain smooth muscle, are elastic and able to gradually contract to some extent. The pulse wave velocity is dependent on the elasticity and contraction of the vessel and the blood pressure. The pulse wave is propagated in the vessel wall as a surface wave—like ripples on the water.

When the pulse wave reaches arterial branches, a part of it is reflected, causing minor oscillations in the pressure wave. The abrupt closure of the aortic valve also creates oscillations. The appearance of the pressure curve varies with the site of measurement. For example, the shape of the curve for the ascending aorta differs from that for the abdominal aorta (Fig. 3.17).

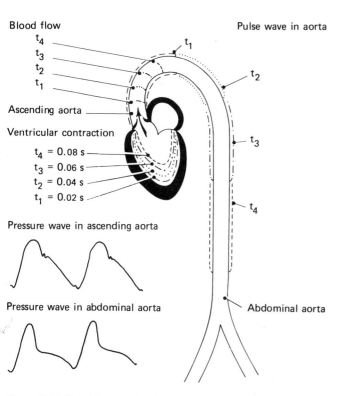

Blood flow

Pulse wave in aorta

t_4
t_3
t_2
t_1

t_1
t_2

Ascending aorta

t_3

Ventricular contraction

$t_4 = 0.08$ s
$t_3 = 0.06$ s
$t_2 = 0.04$ s
$t_1 = 0.02$ s

t_4

Pressure wave in ascending aorta

Pressure wave in abdominal aorta

Abdominal aorta

Figure 3.17 Blood flow and pulse waves in the aorta.

3.91	To eliminate the effect of differences in level, all measurements of blood pressure are related to the		
3.92	For static measurements and for calibrating pressure transducers a .... manometer is used.	right atrium	
3.93	In measurements with a pressure transducer via a cardiac catheter, the frequency characteristic of the system is largely dependent on the properties of the	liquid	

3.94	An optimally damped system is obtained by correctly relating the mass of the liquid column in the catheter to the catheter wall friction; this is done by selecting the right . . . . of the catheter.	catheter
3.95	Pressure transducers for measuring blood pressure generally utilize one or more of the following three types of transducer: . . . . , ... or	internal diameter
3.96	During systole a pulse wave generated by the heart is transmitted more . . . . (slowly, rapidly) than the blood column. The pulse wave travels at a velocity of about . . . . , whereas the blood flow velocity is less than	strain gauge transducer capacitive transducer inductive transducer
3.97	The velocity of the pulse wave is dependent on the . . . . of the vessel wall and the blood	rapidly 5 m/s 0.5 m/s
3.98	The aorta is capable of some . . . . , which affects the elasticity of the wall and the shape of the	elasticity pressure
3.99	The pulse wave is propagated as a . . . . wave.	contraction pulse wave
3.100	The pulse wave shape varies with the site of observation in the arterial system; to some extent this is due to . . . . in the system.	surface
3.101	By listening over the heart with a stethoscope and palpating the arterial pulse in the wrist, the time delay between systole and the pulse wave in the wrist can be observed. Try to estimate the delay for an adult: about . . . . seconds.	reflections
		0.2

Blood Flow Determination

A large number of procedures for measuring blood flow have been developed. For measurements in cardiology, two methods are in common use in connection with cardiac catheterization; one is based on the Fick principle, and the other is the indicator dilution method. Both are indirect methods and give the mean blood flow. There are less-used methods that give the instantaneous flow, for example, those based on electromagnetic induction or ultrasonic principles.

Indirect methods for determining mean blood flow

The Fick principle. The blood flow through an organ can be calculated by continuously infusing a substance into the blood or removing a substance from it and measuring the amount of the substance in the blood before and after its passage. The amount infused, I, or removed, per unit of time, is equal to the difference between the amounts in the blood arriving at, and departing from, the site of measurement. As the latter amounts can be expressed as the product of the flow, Q, and the concentrations, C_V and C_A, in the incoming and outgoing blood, respectively,

$$I = C_A Q - C_V Q, \text{ and}$$

$$Q = I/(C_A - C_V)$$

When the Fick principle is used for determining the cardiac output, the indicator substance used is the quantity of oxygen taken up in the lungs (Fig. 3.18). The oxygen consumption is determined by analyzing the exhaled air collected in a bag during a given time—about 10 min. The oxygen concentration of mixed venous blood is measured by taking samples from a central vein or the pulmonary artery through a cardiac catheter. For analysis of arterial blood, samples are taken from an artery—for example, one in the forearm.

The method can also be used for measuring the flow in other organs, such as the kidneys. In this case, the indicator substance can be injected intravenously, para-aminohippuric acid, PAH, is often used. Almost 100 percent of this is excreted by the kidneys, so the concentration in the renal vein is assumed to be zero; therefore, the vein does not need to be catheterized to obtain samples. The plasma flow value so obtained is known as the **renal clearance**:

$$\text{PAH clearance (ml/min)} = \frac{\text{PAH in the urine (mg/min)}}{\text{PAH in the arterial blood plasma (mg/ml)}}$$

A clearance determination is commonly performed in suspected renal disease.

Indicator dilution method. This technique can be used for determining blood flow. A known amount, M, of a dye, radioactive isotope, or cold saline is suddenly injected in a vessel. After mixing, the blood is continuously analyzed, resulting in a smooth curve, showing the concentration, c, of the indicator in the blood, plotted as a function of time. The integrated area under the curve is used in the following formula to calculate flow. M mg or calories (joules) of indicator is injected in the vessel with the flow rate Q ml/s. An increment of volume, dV, passes the sampling

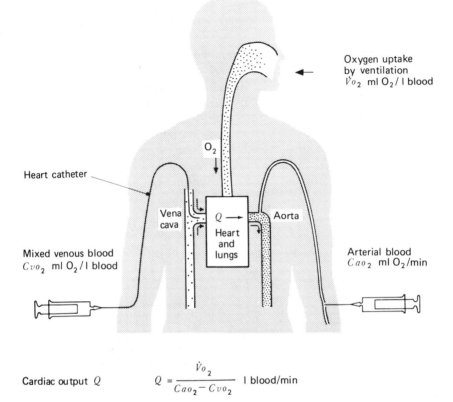

Oxygen uptake
by ventilation
$\dot{V}_{O_2}$ ml O_2/ l blood

Heart catheter

O_2

Vena
cava

$Q \longrightarrow$ Aorta

Heart
and
lungs

Mixed venous blood
C_{vo_2} ml O_2/l blood

Arterial blood
C_{ao_2} ml O_2/min

Cardiac output Q $\qquad$ $Q = \dfrac{\dot{V}_{o_2}}{C_{ao_2} - C_{vo_2}}$ l blood/min

Figure 3.18 The Fick principle for determining the cardiac output.

site in time, dt. The mass of dye, dM, contained in dV is the concentration, c, times the volume, hence $dM = cdV$. Dividing by dt, we obtain $dM/dt = cdV/dt$. But $dV/dt = Q$, therefore $dM = Qc\, dt$. Integrating over the time of the experiment, we obtain $M = \int_0^t Qc\, dt$.

Since minor variations in the flow, Q, produced by the heart beat are smoothed out, the flow may be considered to be constant, and

$$Q = M / \int_0^t c\, dt$$

A complicating factor is the occurrence of some recirculation, with the result that indicator substance is present in the sampling artery on the second time round the circuit, before the concentration has fallen to zero (Fig. 3.19). It is therefore necessary to extrapolate to zero concentration before integrating. As the concentration decreases exponentially with time, the extrapolation can be performed by fitting a straight line to the data plotted on semi-logarithmic coordinates.

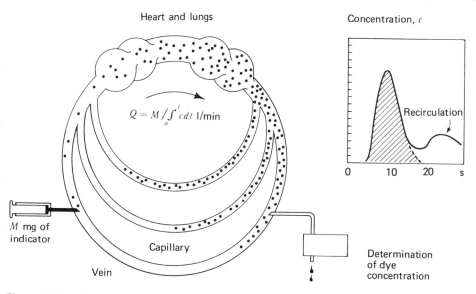

Figure 3.19 Indicator dilution method for determining the cardiac output.

The procedure varies with the indicator used. For dye, or a radioactive isotope, the blood is drawn from an artery through a cuvette (measuring chamber), where a detector continuously analyzes the blood. Disadvantages of these techniques are that a foreign substance is injected into the body, and that blood must be withdrawn. In the **thermodilution method**, when used for measuring the cardiac output, a bolus of about 10 ml of 0–20°C saline is injected into the right atrium. After mixing, the temperature curve is obtained from a thermistor in the pulmonary artery. This method can be used for many repeated measurements, since there is no buildup of foreign substance in the body. The error due to recirculation is negligible, since the temperature levels in the body remain nearly constant.

The indicator dilution method is easy to apply and in most cases gives reliable values of the cardiac output. An exception is cases of certain severe heart defects, such as congenital malformations, where the blood recirculates more rapidly than normal due to the presence of shunts between the right and left halves of the heart (Fig. 3.20). Examples of such shunts are holes in the wall separating the two halves; there are two types, namely **atrial septal defect** and **ventricular septal defect**. Another common shunt is patent **ductus arteriosus**—a communication between the aorta and the pulmonary artery persisting after birth. Although in these cases the cardiac output cannot be determined by the indicator dilution method, valuable diagnostic information can be obtained from the characteristic change in the shape of the curve (Fig. 3.20).

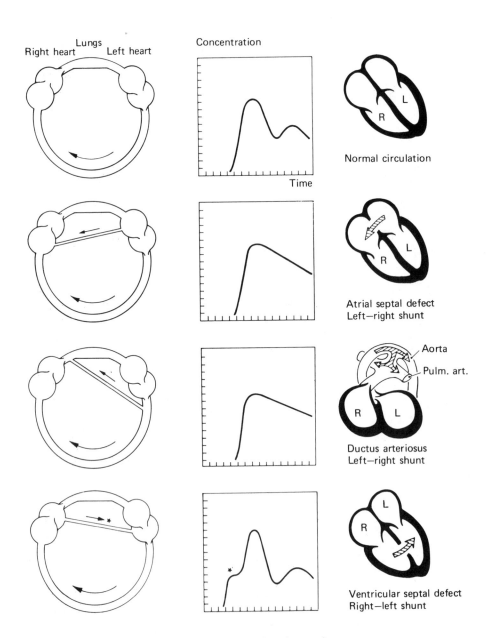

Figure 3.20 Congenital deformities with circulation shunts give indicator dye dilution curves having different shapes.

178

3.102	Indirect methods for measuring blood flow give .... (instantaneous values, mean values) of the flow.	
3.103	For the determination of blood flow through an organ by the Fick principle, a substance must be .... or .... the blood during its passage.	mean values
3.104	Measurement is made of the amount of the substance added to or removed from the blood per ...., and the .... of the substance in the blood before and after its passage through the organ.	added to removed from
3.105	If the amount infused or removed is I, and the concentration in the arterial and venous blood is C_A and C_V, respectively, the flow, Q, is given by the expression	unit time concentration
3.106	In the application of the Fick principle for determining the cardiac output, the .... is measured from the exhaled air and the .... are measured in mixed venous blood and in arterial blood.	$Q = I/(C_A - C_V)$
3.107	Mixed venous blood is obtained via a .... from the	oxygen consumption oxygen concentrations
3.108	The oxygen consumption is 250 ml per minute. Mixed venous blood has an oxygen concentration of 140 ml/liter of blood, and arterial blood 190 ml/liter of blood. The cardiac output is ...., which is a .... (low, high, normal) value.	cardiac catheter central vein or pulmonary artery
3.109	In the application of the Fick principle for measuring renal function, the indicator is injected intravenously and excreted .... through the kidneys; the concentration of the indicator in the .... (venous blood, arterial blood) is assumed to be zero. Catheterization .... (is, is not) required.	5 l/min normal

3.110	For determining the renal plasma flow it is necessary to know the amount of indicator .... per unit time and the concentration of the indicator in .... (venous, arterial) plasma.	completely venous blood is not
3.111	The plasma flow so determined is known as the renal	excreted arterial
3.112	For an indicator dilution curve, M is the amount injected, and c is the instantaneous concentration. The flow Q is given by the equation	clearance
3.113	For determining the cardiac output by the thermodilution method, a known amount of cold saline is injected into the .... The temperature is determined by a thermistor placed in the	$Q = M/\int_0^t c\,dt$
3.114	In determination of the cardiac output with the dye dilution method, a correction to the curve must be made because the blood .... during the sampling time; therefore an extrapolation to .... concentration is performed.	right atrium pulmonary artery
3.115	Two patients, A and B, have the following indicator dilution curves. Patient A has the .... (larger, smaller) cardiac output. Concentration Time	recirculates zero

3.116 A child with an extremely low physical work capacity and cyanosis at rest has the following indicator dilution curve. The curve shows that there is a disturbance caused by .... of the blood, and giving a .... (more rapid, slower) recirculation than normal.

larger

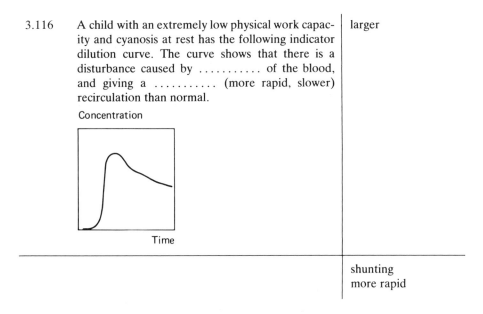

Concentration

Time

shunting
more rapid

Methods for measuring instantaneous blood flow

During thoracic surgery and animal experiments, when the larger vessels are exposed, it is possible to measure the instantaneous blood flow with certain methods based on electromagnetism, or hydrodynamics. As the hydrodynamic methods are similar to those used in engineering technology, they will not be dealt with here. Ultrasonic methods may be used to measure blood flow either on exposed vessels or in certain vessels through the intact skin.

The velocity in a vessel varies over its cross-section. At constant laminar flow the velocity profile is parabolic; the rate is a maximum on the axis of the vessel, and decreases with the square of the distance from the axis, reaching zero at the wall. In the case of turbulent flow the profile is blunter, a profile also obtained under other conditions—for example, in a tapering tube and in the case of oscillating flow. Thus, the beginnings of the aorta and pulmonary artery, into which the blood flows from the wider ventricles, have a turbulent, almost flat velocity profile.

Electromagnetic flow measurement is based on the fact that an electromotive force is induced in an electric conductor moving in a magnetic field. The conductor in this case is the blood, which has a high enough electric conductivity. When a magnetic field is applied across the vessel, parallel to a diameter, the flow of blood induces a potential difference directed along a diameter perpendicular to the magnetic field (Fig. 3.21). The potential difference, e, in volts is directly proportional to the mean velocity of the blood stream, v, in m/s, the flux density of

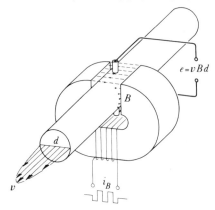

Figure 3.21 Electromagnetic flow measurement.

the magnetic field, B, in Wb/m^2 (T), and the internal diameter of the vessel, d, in m; thus:

$$e = vBd$$

As long as the velocity profile is axially symmetric, it can have any shape without causing error. This simplifies the medical application of the method.

The earliest electromagnetic blood flowmeters used permanent magnets, but this caused error due to electrode polarization, direct current amplifier drift and artifacts from heart and muscle biopotentials. For this reason alternating current magnetic fields are now generally used. The signal from the electrodes has the same frequency as the magnetic field and is amplitude-modulated by the variation in blood flow. To reduce interference due to inductive pick-up from the magnetizing current, a square wave may be employed. As the blood-flow signals contain frequencies up to about 20 times the heart rate—that is, up to a maximum of about 60 Hz, magnetic field frequencies of several times this rate are required for satisfactory operation.

The electromagnetic principle is also used in a catheter tip transducer, which may be advanced to the human ascending aorta, thus measuring regurgitation through the aortic valve.

Ultrasonic methods of measuring blood flow. Early ultrasonic flowmeters were based on the transit time principle. A piezoelectric crystal emitted a brief pulse of ultrasound, which propagated diagonally across the vessel. If the flow was in the same direction as the pulse, the pulse reached a receiving crystal sooner. Appropriate electronics could convert the change in transit time to velocity. The transit time flowmeter has been largely replaced by the Doppler type, shown in Fig. 3.22.

In the continuous-wave type, a 5–10 MHz oscillator excites a transmitting crystal, which emits a beam of ultrasound. The red cells reflect a small portion of

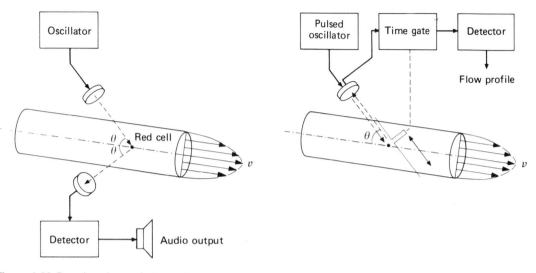

Figure 3.22 Doppler ultrasonic blood flowmeter. Left—simple, continuous-wave type. Right—pulsed type.

the energy to the receiving crystal. If the red cells move, the ultrasonic path lengthens, resulting in a Doppler frequency shift. The detector converts these frequencies into the audio range and provides an audio output, which provides much qualitative information on flow. For quantitative recording, an electronic frequency meter converts these signals. The blood velocity is given by the equation, $v = f_d c / 2 f_0 \cos \theta$, where f_d is the Doppler frequency shift, c is the velocity of sound, f_0 is the oscillator frequency and θ is shown in Fig. 3.22.

For qualitative demonstration of blood flow—for example, in the examination of pregnant women to decide whether the fetus is alive—this ultrasonic method has great potential. The beam is directed at the heart or umbilical cord of the fetus; the mother's blood flow can be distinguished from that of the fetus by the higher pulse rate of the fetus. The ultrasonic method is thus of value in patient supervision during delivery (page 611). These instruments are also used to locate flow obstructions in vessels close to the skin.

The pulsed flowmeter uses the same crystal for both transmitting and receiving. A single pulse is transmitted in a manner similar to a radar system. Echoes from various locations across the vessel are received sequentially in time. They are detected, analyzed for Doppler shift, then used to construct a velocity profile across the vessel. The process is repeated at a high rate, giving information on the shift of the velocity profile during the cardiac cycle. By integration over the flow profile, it is possible with a pulse flowmeter to determine the flow through a vessel; the instrument is, however, more complex than the continuous-wave type.

3.117	Blood flow can be measured using the electromagnetic principle, because blood has a high enough	
3.118	If v is the mean velocity, B is the magnetic flux density, and d is the vessel diameter, the induced electromotive force, e, is given by the formula	electrical conductivity
3.119	To avoid electrode polarization and biopotential artifacts, electromagnetic blood flowmeters use .... magnetic fields.	$e = vBd$
3.120	A Doppler ultrasonic blood flowmeter cannot be calibrated using saline, because there are no .... to reflect the ultrasonic energy.	ac (alternating current)
3.121	In addition to measuring mean flow, the pulsed Doppler ultrasonic blood flowmeter also displays the	red cells
3.122	For a qualitative assessment of blood flow, the Doppler ultrasonic method is of clinical value in the supervision of ....; here, the .... of the fetus is measured.	velocity profile
		deliveries pulse rate

Fluid and Tissue Compartments of the Body

The absolute volume of the body's fluid and tissue compartments (page 26) can be determined in some cases by an indicator dilution method. An indicator is injected that mixes uniformly in one of the compartments but does not pass into the others, and after mixing, samples are taken. The volume is obtained from the expression $V = M/C$, where M is the injected mass of the indicator and C is the concentration in the compartment.

The plasma volume is determined by means of an indicator having the property that it does not leave the bloodstream. Examples of such indicators are Evan's blue (a dye that binds to albumin, the blood protein), and albumin labeled with the radionuclide, ^{131}I. The red cell volume is measured with an indicator consisting of red cells labeled with the radionuclide ^{51}Cr. Since other blood cells have negligible volume, the sum of the plasma volume and the red cell volume equals the total blood volume.

The total amount of hemoglobin in the blood cells can be measured in a similar way. The method is based on the fact that carbon monoxide, CO, has a roughly 200 times greater affinity for hemoglobin than has oxygen. This is the reason that carbon monoxide, even in comparatively low concentrations, produces lethal poisoning by internal suffocation. In small quantities, carbon monoxide can safely be used as an indicator. The patient breathes in a small amount of carbon monoxide, which is completely taken up by the hemoglobin. After mixing in the body, the concentration of CO-hemoglobin is determined and the total amount of hemoglobin can be calculated.

The total amount of water in the body can be measured by using heavy water as an indicator; this can be analyzed by mass spectrometry or a density gradient method.

3.123	For determining the volume of the body's various water and tissue compartments, the . . . . method is used.	
3.124	In the volume to be measured, a known mass, M, of an indicator is injected, which mixes . . . . in the volume but does not pass into other body compartments. Samples are taken after . . . . and the . . . ., C, of the indicator in the sample is determined. The volume is calculated from the expression	indicator dilution
3.125	The indicator used is a . . . . or a radioactive or stable . . . ., that does not leave the compartment because of its size or because it . . . . itself to substances present in the compartment.	uniformly mixing concentration $V = M/C$
3.126	An indicator for determining the plasma volume must have a high enough . . . . not to pass through the vessel wall. Examples of indicators are . . . . and	dye isotope binds
3.127	The red cell volume can be measured with blood cells labeled with the radionuclide	molecular weight Evan's blue ^{131}I-labeled albumin
3.128	The total amount of hemoglobin in the body can be measured with . . . ., which must be inhaled. Its affinity for hemoglobin is . . . . times greater than that of oxygen.	^{51}Cr

3.129 The total body fluid can be measured with	carbon monoxide 200
	heavy water

Peripheral circulation

By measuring the blood flow to the extremities, it is possible to diagnose pathological changes in the peripheral arteries. Examples of such conditions are arteriosclerosis and other vascular diseases, which lead to impaired or arrested circulation (**obstructive** vascular diseases; obstruction or **occlusion**, complete blockage).

Impairment of the peripheral circulation lowers the work capacity in the extremities. If the circulatory impairment affects a leg artery, walking causes leg pains and the patient walks a short distance, limps a short time and then has to stop, because of intermittent oxygen deficiency in the leg muscles.

Sudden, total occlusion of an artery by an embolus causes severe pain and leads to gangrene (see page 27) if the part blocked off cannot be supplied by **collateral** arteries—that is, by alternative pathways in the arterial system—or if the circulation cannot be restored surgically within a few hours.

An exact diagnosis is of crucial importance for deciding whether a vascular operation should be undertaken to restore the circulation. The diagnosis is best made by radiography after injection of a contrast medium proximal to the pathological change, a technique known as arteriography (see page 391). At first, simpler methods, including oscillometry and plethysmography are sometimes used.

Oscillometry.   In this method the pulse-synchronous variations in volume in an extremity are recorded. A cuff similar to a blood-pressure cuff is applied round the extremity. Volume variations are recorded at different pressures in the cuff. Oscillometry provides an objective recording of what is subjectively felt when palpating the pulse.

The method has severe limitations because the pulse wave and blood flow are not directly correlated (see page 173). The pulse amplitude is dependent on the stroke volume, blood pressure and elasticity of the vascular system, parameters on which the blood flow is not primarily dependent. A comparative examination is made of the right and left sides; a difference of 15–25 percent or more is regarded as significant.

Plethysmography   means measuring changes in volume and includes **venous occlusion plethysmography** and **impedance plethysmography**, or **rheography**.

In occlusion plethysmography the increase in volume in an extremity is measured immediately after venous occlusion. The extremity, or a part of it, is placed in a plethysmograph chamber and the space between the skin and the chamber is made watertight, so variations of volume in the extremities are transmitted to a recording instrument (Fig. 3.23). The return venous flow from the

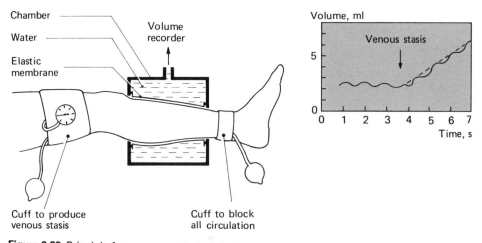

Figure 3.23 Principle for venous occlusion plethysmography.

extremities is arrested by venous stasis, produced proximal to the plethysmograph by pumping a blood-pressure cuff to a pressure of about 50 mm Hg (6.7 kPa). The increase in tissue volume per unit time represents the arterial blood flow to the extremities, provided that the flow is not hindered by the occluding pressure or by the rising venous pressure in the tissue enclosed in the plethysmograph, and provided that the arrest of the venous flow is complete. The method is based on a well defined physical phenomenon, and is the most reliable and the technically simplest one for quantitative determination of volume flow to an extremity.

In impedance plethysmography or rheography, the variation of electrical impedance in a tissue volume is recorded. The method is based on the fact that the arteries expand during systole, the segment cross-sectional area increases and the tissue impedance decreases. Interpretation of the measured results is complicated, however, by the fact that the conductivity is dependent on the blood velocity in a vessel—a phenomenon caused by the preferential orientation of the blood cells during flow. Impedance plethysmography can be used to compare volume pulsations in the two legs and thus provide an indication of unilateral occlusion. The method can also be used for relative measurements of ventilation and cardiac output.

3.130   One reason for measuring the peripheral circulation to an extremity is to diagnose . . . ., which may have caused calcification of the arteries.

3.131	Reduced peripheral circulation lowers the .... of the extremities.	arteriosclerosis
3.132	The impairment of the arterial blood flow causes .... during walking due to oxygen deficiency in the muscles.	work capacity
3.133	Also in complete blockage—that is, ..., of a minor or moderately large artery, need not lead to necrosis—that is, ...—because an adequate circulation may be provided by .... vessels (alternative pathways).	pain
3.134	A diagnosis of obstructive arterial disease is best made by radiography after injecting a contrast medium .... (proximal, distal) to the pathological change, a technique called	obstruction or occlusion tissue death collateral
3.135	In venous occlusion plethysmography the change in .... per .... due to the arterial flow is measured; this change occurs immediately after .... the venous return flow from the part of the body being measured.	proximal arteriography
3.136	Impedance plethysmography can be used for recording pulsatile changes in leg .... and for relative measurement of .... and	volume unit time closing off
		volume ventilation cardiac output

ELECTROCARDIOGRAPHY

The mechanical work of the heart is accompanied by electrical activity, which always slightly precedes the muscle contraction. The electrical activity can be studied by picking up potentials on the body surface. The potentials originate in the individual fibers of the heart muscle and are summated to give the waveforms of the electrocardiogram.

When the individual muscle fibers contract, potential changes occur on the surface. At rest the muscle fibers are polarized, the inside of the cell membrane being about $-90\,mV$ with respect to the outside. The potential is maintained by active transport of ions through the membrane; an ion pump works constantly so that sodium ions are transported to the outside of the muscle cell and potassium to the inside. During muscle contraction, an **action potential** is produced, which is due to a sudden change in the sodium ion permeability of the cell membrane, so that these positive ions enter the cell and cause the interior to go positive. During this rapid **depolarization**, a dipole field is created between the polarized and depolarized parts of the muscle fiber (Fig. 3.24). The contraction wave and the dipole field travel along the muscle fiber at a velocity of a meter or so a second. After about half a second, **repolarization** of the heart muscle fibers occurs and this is accompanied by a similar moving dipole field, but with reversed polarity.

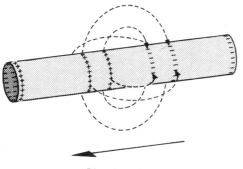

Direction of dipole field motion

Figure 3.24 The depolarization of a muscle fiber is accompanied by a dipole field, which travels along the muscle fiber at the same rate as the contraction.

The heart is composed of a large number of muscle fibers, which pass around the ventricles and atria in certain loops. These loops are in similar anatomic locations in different persons. The individual electric field vectors from each dipole are summed together to give a total resultant vector. Because the contraction spreads in the heart muscle mass in a regular temporal sequence, the resultant vector varies in magnitude and direction in a similar way in different persons (Fig. 3.25). Typical deviations occur in certain pathological conditions of the heart.

ECG lead systems

The potentials generated in the heart are conducted to the body surface. During each cardiac cycle the potential distribution changes in a regular, but quite complex way (Fig. 3.26). It is therefore essential to choose standardized electrode positions when recording electrocardiograms. The most common lead systems will be outlined.

Bipolar limb leads—standard leads I, II, and III. For each standard lead, potential changes between the measuring points shown in Fig. 3.27 are recorded.

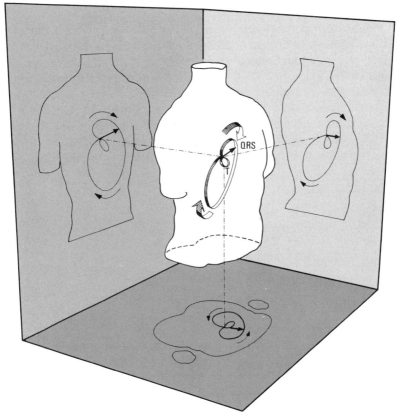

Figure 3.25 Electric field vectors of the heart projected on three planes.

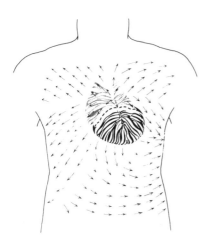

Figure 3.26 Electric field vectors recorded at the instant the heart's electrical activity is maximum (at the beginning of systole). The action potentials are propagating along the ventricular muscle fibers (solid lines) in the direction shown (dashed lines). This produces a body surface potential distribution with the most positive potential located below and to the left of the heart. Surface vectors indicate direction of the electric field, but not magnitude.

190

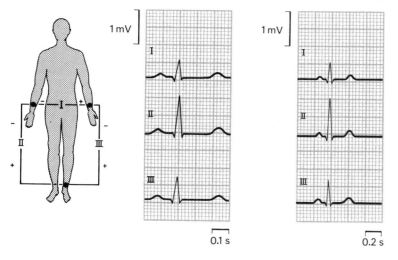

Figure 3.27 (left) Standard leads for recording an ECG. (center) European recording paper usually travels 50 mm/s. (right) U.S. recording paper usually travels 25 mm/s.

These curves record the difference between the potentials at two points, which are simultaneously varying; thus a differential amplifier is used. This simple lead system, which is the original one, is still the most commonly used.

Unipolar limb leads, aVR, aVL and aVF. Other views of the heart are obtained by connecting two equal, large resistors to pairs of limbs. The center of this resistive network feeds one terminal of the amplifier and the remaining limb feeds the other. See Fig. 3.28. The leads are named for the remaining limb, aVR

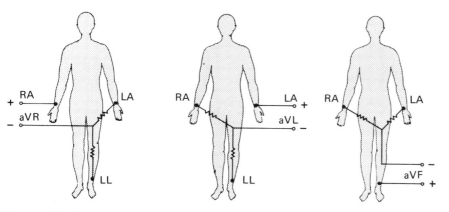

Figure 3.28 Unipolar leads. RA = right arm, LA = left arm, LL = left leg.

(augmented voltage right arm), aVL (augmented voltage left arm), aVF (augmented voltage foot).

Unipolar chest (precordial) leads, $V_1, \ldots V_n$, etc.   To obtain more detailed information on potential variations in different parts of the heart, electrodes are placed on the chest, close to the heart at the anatomic points shown in Fig. 3.29. An indifferent electrode is formed by connecting three equal large resistances to the left arm, right arm and left leg. The arrangement in which such a resistance network is used as the indifferent lead is known as the Wilson system. The other lead is connected sequentially to the electrodes shown in Fig. 3.29.

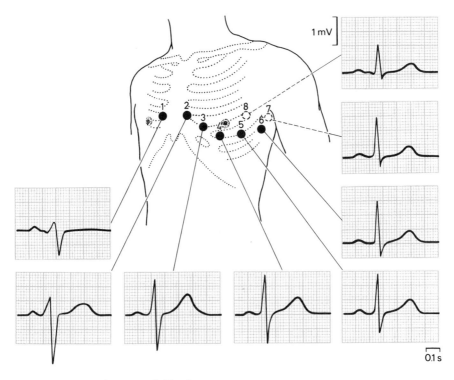

Figure 3.29 Unipolar precordial leads.

It is routine practice in cardiology to use 12 leads, the 3 standard bipolar leads, the 3 unipolar limb leads, and chest leads, 1 through 6.

Corrected orthogonal leads—Frank lead system.   In order to obtain a three-dimensional view of the heart, a number of orthogonal systems have been developed. With the aid of torso models, empirical tests have been performed with resistance networks, in which the heart vector is resolved into three mutually perpendicular signal components. These are chosen in the transverse, X, craniocaudal, Y, and dorsoventral, Z, directions. The resistance network is connected to certain geometrically and anatomically defined electrode positions on the body—for example, those shown for the Frank system in Fig. 3.30. Because of anatomic variations in different individuals, there is a variability of ± 20 percent in the estimated size of the heart's equivalent dipole. Orthogonal leads are used in vectorcardiography and in certain kinds of automatic data analysis of electrocardiograms.

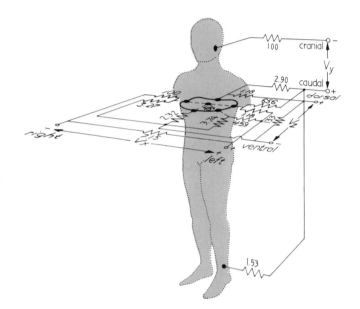

Figure 3.30 Frank lead system for resolving the ECG vector into three orthogonal components.

The information content of the signals obtained with orthogonal leads is considered to be just as great as for the conventional 12 leads; for it has been possible to reconstruct the conventional leads from the orthogonal ones to a high degree of accuracy.

| 3.137 | A muscle fiber is normally polarized so that the inside of the cell membrane has a .... potential with respect to the outside. | |

3.138	When the muscle fiber contracts, ... potential is generated because the cell membrane is	negative
3.139	During depolarization, a dipole field is generated that travels along the muscle fiber at a velocity of about	an action depolarized
3.140	The action potentials from all the muscle fibers of the heart summate to produce a resultant electric .... In normal persons it varies in .... and .... during the cardiac cycle, in a fairly regular manner.	1 m/s
3.141	The pickup locations for the standard bipolar leads are between I: ...., II: .... and III:	vector magnitude direction
3.142	In unipolar limb leads the pickup locations are between an indifferent electrode and the following extremity: aVR: ...., aVL: .... and aVF:	I: l. arm—r. arm II: l. leg—r. arm III: l. leg—l. arm
3.143	For chest leads, the indifferent electrode is a point connected through equal resistances to the right arm, left arm and left leg. This is known as the .... system and each lead is then denoted by the symbol	aVR: r. arm aVL: l. arm aVF: l. leg
3.144	If the patient is connected with an empirically tested resistance network in order to resolve the heart's dipole field into three mutually perpendicular components, this is known as an .... lead system.	Wilson V_n
		orthogonal

Heart rhythm and arrhythmias (rhythm disturbances)

Pacing centers in the heart muscle initiate the heart beat. The heart thus has its own system for generating and conducting action potentials—unlike the skeletal muscles, which are controlled entirely from the central nervous system.

In the wall of the right atrium, near the entry of the vena cava, is the **sinus node**, which generates impulses at the normal rate of the heart, about 70 beats per minute at rest. The rate is governed by the autonomic nervous system, being increased by the sympathetic and decreased by the parasympathetic system (see page 88). The action potential contracts the atrial muscle and the impulse spreads through the atrial wall during a period of about 0.04 s to the **AV node** (atrioventricular node). This node is located in the lower part of the wall between the two atria. The AV node delays the spread of excitation for about 0.11 s. Then a special conduction system carries the action potential to the ventricular muscle (Fig. 3.31). This system consists of a short common part (the bundle of His), two bundle branches on each side of the septum, and fine Purkinje fibers which arborize in the ventricular muscle.

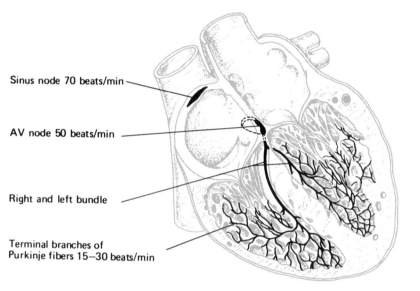

Sinus node 70 beats/min

AV node 50 beats/min

Right and left bundle

Terminal branches of
Purkinje fibers 15–30 beats/min

Figure 3.31 The conduction system of the heart.

The atria and ventricles are thus functionally linked only by the AV node and the conduction system. The AV delay is provided, so the atrial contraction can complete the ventricular filling before these contract.

The AV node, other parts of the conduction system and the heart muscle can also initiate excitation which results in ventricular contraction. This occurs in pathological conditions where the impulses from the sinus node are not conducted. The pulse frequency is, however, lower for the AV node, about 50 beats per minute, and it decreases further in the periphery of the conduction system; in the ventricular wall the frequency is about 20 beats per minute. If the normal conduction system is disturbed, the pulse rate will therefore be slower than the normal sinus rhythm. This state is known as **heart block**. There are different kinds of heart block, depending on the severity of the conduction defect and the anatomic location of the lesion:

- **1st degree AV block** where only the conduction time is prolonged.

- **2nd degree AV block** where some of the pulses are conducted from the atrium.
- **3rd degree AV block** or **total block**, where the atrium and the ventricle beat asynchronously. In sudden attacks of total block, the patient generally loses consciousness—so-called **Adams–Stokes** attacks.
- **Bundle block** (right-sided or left-sided) where the stimulus is not conducted normally to the respective ventricle. The spread of the contraction in the ventricles occurs abnormally over a longer period.

Some kinds of block result in greatly impaired heart function—for example, patients with Adams–Stokes attacks. They can be treated successfully with a pacemaker. This consists of an electrical pulse generator, which is connected to the heart muscle (see page 219).

There are a number of other kinds of arrhythmia. Most common is the occurrence of **extrasystoles**, which occur due to premature depolarization of the heart muscle. There are three kinds of extrasystole, **atrial**, **nodal** and **ventricular**, depending upon the site of depolarization. Atrial extrasystoles frequently occur in normal persons—"my heart stops" or "my heart turns over." It is characteristic of atrial extrasystoles that they do not increase in number during physical effort. Ventricular extrasystoles are commonly called premature ventricular contractions (PVC's). In heart patients they have a more serious implication, since they may immediately precede serious arrhythmia, leading to circulatory arrest. When electrocardiograms are employed for monitoring in intensive care, an alarm may be set to ring if more than a certain number (say three) of PVC's occur per minute (see page 586). Nodal extrasystoles originate in the AV node and the wave of excitation spreads in both directions.

In **atrial flutter** the rhythm is regular but the atrial rate is high: 250–350 beats per minute. In **atrial fibrillation** the rhythm is completely irregular and the rate is 300–500 beats per minute. The ventricles cannot keep up with this high frequency but beat more slowly, and thus maintain some circulation.

Ventricular fibrillation is a dangerous condition. The ventricular muscle contracts so rapidly and irregularly that the ventricles fail to fill, and circulatory arrest follows. The patient loses consciousness in 10–15 s and, unless the condition is corrected, dies within a few minutes from oxygen deficiency in the brain. **Asystole**, the failure of the heart muscle to contract, is another type of circulatory arrest. In both cases, external heart massage and artificial ventilation must be given immediately (page 554). Ventricular fibrillation can often be corrected by defibrillation—that is, by passing large electric current through the heart (see page 217).

Electrocardiography is the most important method of examination for an exact diagnosis of any form of arrhythmia.

| 3.145 | The heart beat is normally generated by the part of the atrial muscle known as the . . . . It has a normal rate of about . . . . beats/min. | |

3.146	The sinus rhythm is controlled by the autonomic nervous system, the sympathetic system .... the pulse rate, and the parasympathetic system .... it.	sinus node 70
3.147	Too rapid a heart rate is known as .... and too slow as .... (see page 122).	increases decreases
3.148	Atrial contractions are conducted to the ventricles via the .... and the	tachycardia bradycardia
3.149	The spread of excitation from the atria to the ventricle is delayed about .... seconds, which allows time for the ventricles to complete their .... before contracting.	AV node conduction system
3.150	If either the conductivity to the AV node or the conduction system is interrupted, the ventricles will beat at a ..... rate than the atria.	0.11 filling
3.151	If the AV node controls the ventricles, the frequency will be about ..... beats/min. If a lesion blocks the conduction system further in the periphery, the rate will be ....; for contractions generated in the ventricular wall, it will be about ..... beats/min.	slower
3.152	In a 1st degree block the conduction time is	50 slower 20
3.153	In a 2nd degree block .... (all, some, no) impulses are conducted from the atria.	prolonged
3.154	In a 3rd degree block, total block, the atria and ventricles beat .... (synchronously, asynchronously).	some
3.155	An Adams–Stokes attack is a sudden	asynchronously
3.156	A heart condition that can result in sudden death is .... (atrial flutter, atrial fibrillation, ventricular fibrillation), because it leads to circulatory arrest.	total block (3rd degree block)
3.157	Adams–Stokes attacks can be successfully treated with a	ventricular fibrillation

3.158	A patient consults a physician for heart trouble. The ECG shows that the atria beat regularly but that some ventricular contractions are absent. The diagnosis is	pacemaker
3.159	The patient is admitted to a hospital for examination and on one occasion suddenly loses consciousness. Another ECG shows that the ventricular rhythm is quite independent of the atrial rhythm. The patient has had an .... attack because the 2nd degree block changed to	2nd degree block
3.160	A ventricular extrasystole is also known as a ...., abbreviated to	Adams–Stokes total block (3rd degree block)
3.161	A patient with severe heart disease—valvular defect and enlarged heart—had a series of PVC's, closely followed by ventricular fibrillation; this led to circulatory .... and unconsciousness within about .... (time). The patient would have died in .... (time) from .... (secondary cause of death) if treatment had not been given immediately.	premature ventricular contraction PVC
3.162	A high-school student entered military service and began to smoke more heavily. He felt on occasions that his heart "stopped." He anxiously consulted a physician who recorded an ECG. The examination succeeded unusually well, since the patient had an extrasystole at the time. The ECG showed that the extrasystole was of .... origin. No treatment was given, but the student was advised to give up smoking.	arrest 15 seconds a few minutes oxygen deficiency in the brain
3.163	Arrhythmias are diagnosed by	atrial
		electrocardiography

Analysis of ECG curves

Figure 3.32 shows a normal electrocardiogram. The curve is divided, with the conventional alphabetical notation, into the **P wave**, corresponding to atrial depolarization and contraction, the **QRS complex**, corresponding to ventricular depolarization, the **S–T interval**, corresponding to ventricular contraction, and the **T wave,** corresponding to ventricular repolarization.

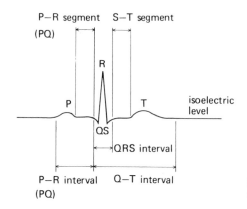

P–R segment (PQ)
S–T segment

R

P   T   isoelectric level

QS

QRS interval

P–R interval (PQ)   Q–T interval

Figure 3.32 Normal lead II ECG curve with notation.

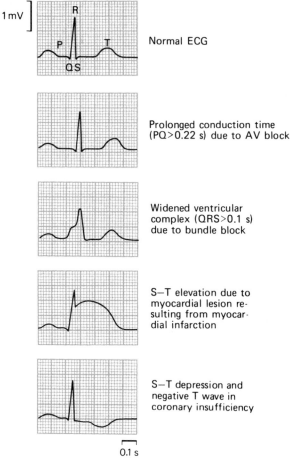

1 mV

R
P   T
QS

Normal ECG

Prolonged conduction time (PQ>0.22 s) due to AV block

Widened ventricular complex (QRS>0.1 s) due to bundle block

S–T elevation due to myocardial lesion resulting from myocardial infarction

S–T depression and negative T wave in coronary insufficiency

0.1 s

Figure 3.33 Some common ECG changes.

199

The interpretation of the electrocardiogram is based on time and amplitude analyses of the curve. The conduction time is determined by measuring the interval from the beginning of the P wave to the first sign of ventricular depolarization—that is, the Q or R wave (if the Q wave is not clearly formed, as is often the case). This P–R interval is normally 0.12–0.22 s. A longer interval indicates obstruction of the spread of the excitation from atria to ventricles, AV block (Fig. 3.33). The width of the QRS complex is normally 0.07–0.10 s. An increase in width indicates an interruption in that part of the conduction system which distributes the excitation in the ventricular wall; the condition is known as bundle block, which can be on the right or left side.

In a myocardial infarction there are characteristic ECG changes which can confirm the diagnosis. The electrocardiogram also changes typically in the days following the infarction, so repeated recordings may be informative. The ECG changes are dependent on the extent and site of the infarction; because of their location some infarcts are difficult to detect.

In **coronary insufficiency**, that is, deficient blood circulation in the coronary arteries, the S–T interval is shortened and the T wave is sometimes inverted, because the oxygen deficiency of the heart muscle interferes with repolarization. The ECG changes increase during physical effort; to cause larger changes the ECG can be recorded while the patient pedals a bicycle ergometer. This produces an **exercise ECG** (see page 227).

A number of general principles for interpreting ECGs are based on a knowledge, and functional analysis, of the electrical activity in the various parts of the heart. For the most part, however, specialized clinical interpretations are based on empirical knowledge, without using the theoretical understanding of the ECG changes. The interpretation is therefore subjective, and ECGs are frequently classified differently by different investigators.

3.164	ECG diagnosis is based on an analysis of the . . . . and . . . . relations of the ECG curve.	
3.165	For the following ECG curve, enter the conventional alphabetical notation of the waves.	time amplitude

3.166	The P wave is generated during .... (depolarization, repolarization) and contraction of the	Normal ECG
3.167	The QRS complex corresponds to .... at the beginning of contraction of the	depolarization atria
3.168	The T wave is produced during .... of the	depolarization ventricles
3.169	A 55-year-old somewhat obese man has been living under stress. During physical effort, he is troubled by pains in the heart region, which radiate along the ulnar side of the left arm. The physician in his examination room records the illustrated ECG. This shows the following pathological changes	repolarization ventricles
3.170	The patient is referred to a specialist at a cardiology laboratory and a new ECG is taken, but with the same result. The illustrated exercise ECG was therefore taken using a bicycle ergometer. This shows .... and an .... which indicate	none

3.171	The patient was advised to lose some weight, take regular exercise and lead a less hectic life. He disregarded these instructions, however, and a year later became suddenly ill with abdominal and chest pains, and was admitted to the hospital in a state of shock. The illustrated ECG indicates	ST depression inverted T wave coronary insufficiency
3.172	The patient had further heart attacks while in the hospital, but after several weeks he was discharged with his condition improved. Before discharge the following ECG was recorded. This shows that there was still . . . . and . . . . Diagnosis: permanent myocardial lesion with . . . . block and . . . . block.	myocardial infarction
		prolonged conduction time widened ventricular complex 1st degree AV bundle

Measurement Considerations for Electrocardiography

Although the ECG signals have neither an exceptionally low amplitude nor a large frequency range, a special recording technique is required. The amplitude of the QRS complex is about 1 mV. For faithful reproduction, an amplifier band-width of 0.05–100 Hz is required. Difficulties arise when we try to transfer these body signals to recording equipment.

ECG electrodes

At frequencies below 100 Hz, most of the body tissues have an impedance which may be regarded as purely resistive. At low frequencies the blood has a higher conductivity than the non-liquid tissues due to the electrolyte it contains; for muscle, lung, liver and other such organs the conductivity ranges between one tenth and one half of that for the blood, and for fatty tissue it is still lower. In ECG recording, however, the electrical properties of these tissues are not of major importance; it is the low conductivity of the outermost horny layer of the skin that presents the greatest problems.

The conductivity of the skin is dependent largely on its moistness. A typical ECG electrode on dry skin has a contact impedance with a resistive component of about 100 kΩ and a capacitive component of about 0.01 μF. To improve the contact, an electrode paste containing an electrolyte solution is applied between the skin and the electrodes. In this way the resistive component, R, is reduced to about 10 kΩ and the capacitive component, C, is increased to about 0.1 μF. The impedance can be further reduced by special procedures, such as scraping the horny layer or perforating the corium. Perforation is accomplished by pressing a grater-like electrode against the skin, multipoint electrodes (Fig. 3.34).

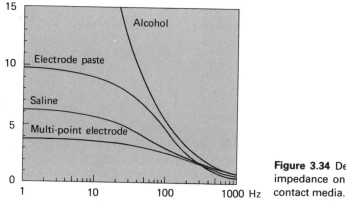

Impedance, kΩ

Figure 3.34 Dependence of electrode impedance on frequency, for various contact media.

For measurements of the electrode impedance an ac method must be used. With dc, there is marked polarization of the electrodes in contact with the electrolyte and the skin, and a back electromotive force is generated, which lowers the current through the electrodes and gives a computed apparent value of the resistance that is many times too great.

The electrode impedance varies not only with the moistness of the horny layer but also with the skin's fat content, its blood supply, the electrode's contact pressure and many other factors that are difficult to control. The amplifier must be capable of handling these variations in impedance.

3.173	The skin's impedance is ....:..... (higher, lower) than that of the rest of the body. The skin impedance is dependent largely on the .... of the horny layer.	
3.174	To obtain good contact between the electrode and the skin, the gap is filled with an electrode paste containing .... It is then possible to reduce the electrode resistance R to about .... and increase the electrode capacitance C to about	higher moistness
3.175	A patient's electrode impedance is measured with an ordinary, battery powered ohmmeter. A high value of 80 kΩ is found, and a new measurement with another of the instrument's measuring ranges gives a value of 120 kΩ. The method resulted in a large error. The use of dc resulted in ...., and a .... force was generated in the electrodes, producing a high apparent value of the impedance. The change in the recorded value when a different measuring range was used was due to a change in current, and this affected the magnitude of the	electrolytes $\approx 10\,\text{k}\Omega$ $\approx 0.1\,\mu\text{F}$
		polarization back electromotive polarization

ECG amplifiers

The input impedance of an ECG amplifier must be very much higher than the electrode impedance for faithful reproduction. For a direct connection with standard leads I, II and III, the input impedance usually exceeds 10 MΩ. When a resistive network is used—for example, with Wilson or Frank leads, a buffer amplifier is usually placed before the resistance network, to avoid loading the electrode impedance.

The upper frequency limit should be at least 100 Hz. The pen inertia of many pen recorders limits the system frequency response to about 50 Hz, which somewhat lowers the fidelity of the QRS complex.

The lower frequency limit should extend down to 0.05 Hz, which corresponds to a time constant, $\tau = 3$ s, which follows from $f = 1/2\pi\tau$. A shorter time constant distorts the P and T waves, which may result in incorrect diagnosis. If the time constant is much larger than 3 s, the recovery time of the amplifier will be too long if driven into saturation. This often occurs when switching from one lead to another, due to the change in dc offset potential between different pairs of electrodes.

One problem encountered when recording the ECG is interference from the electric field of the power lines. This is minimized by using a differential amplifier, which amplifies the difference signals from the heart, but rejects the common mode signals from the power lines (Fig. 3.35). The amplifier's common mode

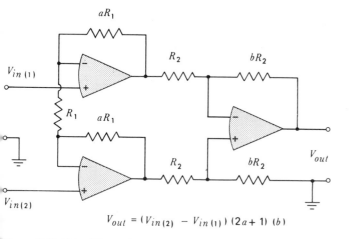

$$V_{out} = (V_{in\,(2)} - V_{in\,(1)})\,(2a+1)\,(b)$$

Figure 3.35 This differential amplifier amplifies the differential signal, rejects the common mode signal and has a very high input impedance.

rejection (interference reduction factor) usually exceeds 60 dB (1000 : 1). In addition, the patient must be connected to ground, and this is usually done using an electrode on the right leg. However, a simple direct earth connection is less safe and may cause interference. The problem usually arises from the capacitive coupling, $C = 5 - 10$ pF, between the patient and power lines in the vicinity (Fig. 3.36). The patient will then be connected to the power lines via a voltage divider, consisting of the capacitance, C, and the electrode impedance, Z_G. Thus, over the entire body and at the two inputs to the amplifier there will be an ac common mode voltage. Under ideal conditions, this ac interference would be completely suppressed by a differential amplifier. This is not achieved in practice because the electrode impedances, Z_R, Z_L and Z_F, are unequal, with the result that the voltage division in these and the corresponding stray capacitances in the amplifier inputs, C_R, C_L and C_F, are not constant. A differential amplifier does not guarantee total suppression of interference.

A most effective way of eliminating interference is to add an auxiliary amplifier in a feedback circuit, as shown in Fig. 3.37. This "driven right leg ground" circuit

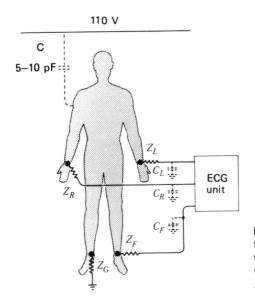

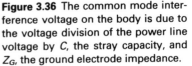

Figure 3.36 The common mode interference voltage on the body is due to
the voltage division of the power line
voltage by C, the stray capacity, and
Z_G, the ground electrode impedance.

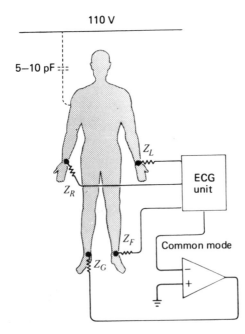

Figure 3.37 In the amplifier using the
driven right leg ground, if the body
common mode voltage is different
from zero, the ECG unit senses this
difference, the auxiliary amplifier
greatly amplifies the difference and
using negative feedback, drives the
body to zero common mode voltage.

actively drives the common mode interference voltage to a very low value.
   Grounding the patient presents some risks. If the body comes into contact with
a 110 V wire, a dangerous current could pass through it to ground. The current for

causing ventricular fibrillation in a healthy person for wires touching the body surface is considered to be greater than 50 mA. A current as low as 0.5 mA can be felt, however, and this should be the maximum value to which the patient should be exposed; it is easy to design equipment to meet this requirement. It is considerably more difficult to ensure safety when parts of the equipment enter the heart, for example, cardiac catheters. Because the high current density at the tip might cause ventricular fibrillation, the current should then be limited to $10\,\mu A$. It is necessary to limit the current to ground. In the case of the driven right leg ground, this is accomplished by limiting the current output from the auxiliary amplifier.

Cables to the patient electrodes form open loops, and stray magnetic fields can induce interference into these loops. The area of the loops should be kept as small as possible. Both electric and magnetic field interference can be minimized by avoiding operation near electrical apparatus and power lines.

To eliminate interference from muscle potentials—which arises when the patient cannot relax—a low-pass filter with an upper limiting frequency of 20 Hz can be inserted in the circuit. This distorts the electrocardiogram, however, and the fact that a filter has been used during the recording must be noted on the curve.

No electrocardiogram is complete without a 1 mV calibration signal. This is entered on the curve by using a push button.

3.176	The input impedance of an ECG amplifier is usually .... and must be high compared to the electrode impedance, which is generally	
3.177	When ECG electrodes are to be connected to a resistance network, as when the Wilson or Frank coupling is used, a .... amplifier is inserted in the circuit to avoid loading the electrode impedance.	10 MΩ 10 kΩ
3.178	The upper limiting frequency for a good ECG amplifier and recorder should be at least .... Hz and the low frequency time constant about .... seconds.	buffer
3.179	To reduce the interference a .... amplifier is used.	100 3
3.180	A differential amplifier alone is not sufficient to limit interference. Due to the .... (capacitive, inductive) coupling between the patient and the power lines, there is an alternating common mode voltage between the patient and	differential

3.181	In order to ground the patient more effectively, an auxiliary amplifier is connected in a .... circuit so that the patient is actively driven to ground potential.	capacitive ground
3.182	Because the driven right leg amplifier current is ...., the patient is not exposed to danger-ous currents.	feedback
3.183	The limiting value for the perception of current for wires on the body surface is about	limited
3.184	The current through a cardiac catheter should be limited to	0.5 mA
3.185	A new piece of equipment has been delivered to a cardiac catheterization laboratory. It is not intended for direct connection to the patient. When deli-vered, it operates well, but when it is running there is ac interference in the electrocardiogram. The equip-ment designer, who is present during the catheteri-zation, wishes to help solve this engineering prob-lem and connects the patient to ground by connect-ing his right leg to the ground terminal of the power lines. To the designer's distress, not only does the interference increase, but ventricular fibrillation develops and the patient loses consciousness. Two mistakes have been made. First, the new equipment produced interference in other equipment in the laboratory. Since ECG recorders are usually fitted with an auxiliary amplifier to suppress .... conducted interference, the interference from the new apparatus was probably .... Second, when the patient was connected directly to the power lines ground terminal, a .... current of probably more than .... was generated via the cardiac catheter.	10 μA
3.186	No ECG curve is complete without a calibration signal having an amplitude of	capacitively inductive leakage 10 μA
		1 mV

Recording and Transmission of ECG

The methods for recording ECG data have varying complexity. The units used for routine purposes are directly connected to the patient's body via amplifiers. These usually permit simultaneous recording from several leads, which reduces the time required for recording. For special purposes, more advanced methods have been developed, such as vectorcardiographic presentation methods and telemetry for wireless transmission of ECG signals. Data-reducing systems utilize automatic techniques of different levels of sophistication, from simple rhythm and pulse detectors for intensive care monitors, to methods for diagnostic interpretation, applying computer technology.

ECG recording units

A recording unit should enable the ECG signal to be recorded on a medium that is available for immediate inspection and that can be stored for long periods. In addition, the high-frequency components of the signal should not be cut off.

A recorder employing light-beam galvanometers and photographic paper is occasionally used in specialized applications, such as the cardiac catheterization laboratory. Since this has problems in chemical development of the paper, the most common recorder in the US uses a mechanical galvanometer, driving either an ink pen, or a heated stylus. The mechanical mass of these types makes it difficult to reach the required frequency response of 100 Hz. Better from this aspect are the recorders using a jet of liquid instead of a pen. Liquid-jet recorders of this type

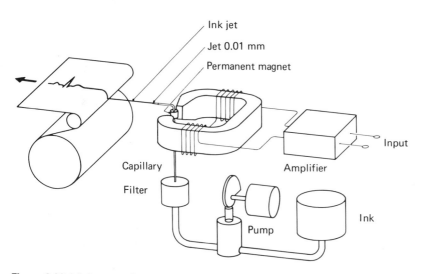

Figure 3.38 Ink-jet recorder—so-called Mingograph. High upper frequency limit about 1000 Hz, obtained by means of small dimensions of glass capillary and permanent magnet.

are known as Mingographs (from the Latin *micturire*, to urinate). A liquid jet from a glass capillary is directed by means of an electromagnetic system onto recording paper, which is fed at a constant speed (Fig. 3.38). Galvanometers of this type have a natural frequency of about 800 Hz, and signals with frequencies below about 500 Hz are recorded with a high level of accuracy.

Electronic presentation systems for ECG

For monitoring purposes, for example, during examinations and in intensive care units where the electrocardiogram need not be stored, cathode ray tubes with long persistance phosphor or television picture tubes with a memory function are used. Cathode ray tubes are also used in vectorcardiography.

As Fig. 3.26 shows, the potential distribution over the chest is closely related to the de- and repolarization of the heart muscle. Even with chest electrodes arranged in a circle around the thorax, information can be lost.

Attempts have therefore been made to obtain a picture of the potential distribution during the various phases of the cardiac cycle by a technique known as display electrocardiography. The potential distribution can be examined by using 70 electrodes on the chest—7 rows in the craniocaudal direction by 10 columns in the transverse direction. The potential differences between adjacent electrodes then control the light intensity of corresponding areas on a cathode ray tube. To facilitate analysis of certain phases of the cardiac cycle, for example, the QRS complex, signals can be gated on during particular short intervals; the rest of the cardiac cycle is then not reproduced. The progression and regression of myocardial infarction are best examined during the S-T interval. The images obtained have a variability and complexity that cannot be interpreted in terms of the usual electrocardiographic theory. The value of the method for routine diagnosis remains to be established. One disadvantage is that a complicated technique yields an image that cannot be evaluated by engineering methods but requires subjective interpretation. The method thus does not provide an opportunity for data reduction.

Vectorcardiography

An ECG curve obtained with one standard lead provides scalar information; several curves recorded simultaneously with leads in different directions contain vectorial information. This vectorial information is not exploited in conventional, scalar interpretation. At the present stage of ECG diagnosis, it is reasonable to assume that the heart activity can be represented by a single, resultant dipole. Thus vectorcardiography offers the possibility of reducing ECG data to a form that might ease the analysis.

By means of an orthogonal lead system, the spatial relations of the heart vector can be displayed on an oscilloscope. This is accomplished by resolving the signal into three images, corresponding to the frontal, sagittal and transverse planes. To enable the determination of loop direction and time, the signal is intensity-modulated with a saw-tooth voltage; the loop is thus divided into a number of arrow-shaped segments (Fig. 3.39). In compliance with recommended standards

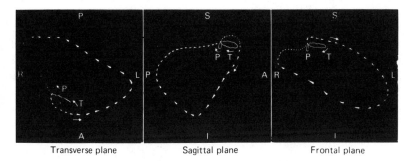

Figure 3.39 Normal vectorcardiogram. (R, Right; L, Left; P, Posterior; A, Anterior; S, Superior; I, Inferior).

the saw-tooth frequency is chosen in multiples of 200 Hz so that the time interval between the loop segments is 5 ms or a fraction of 5 ms. Some instruments reverse the direction of the saw-tooth, resulting in comet-like loop segments. A Polaroid camera photographs the oscilloscope screen to provide a permanent record.

A normal vectorcardiogram consists of three loops corresponding to the P, QRS and T waves. The vectorcardiogram is dominated by the QRS complex, which corresponds to the depolarization of the ventricular muscle. The loop is normally directed to the left, caudally and somewhat dorsally (Fig. 3.25). The repolarization of the heart ventricles produces a small T loop, normally directed caudally and somewhat ventrally, and making an angle of 0–30° to the QRS loop. In pathological conditions, the loops are altered in a characteristic fashion—for example, as shown in Fig. 3.40 for an infarction. The QRS and T loops may not be

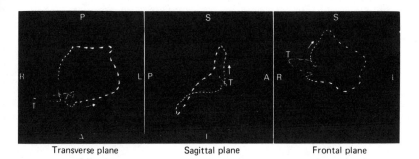

Figure 3.40 Vectorcardiogram in a case of myocardial infarction, showing irregularities of the heart vector.

closed loops, ending in a point, but may together form a composite loop; for the standard leads the S-T segment then does not reach the iso-electric line.

One disadvantage of the vectorcardiographic technique is the difficulty of obtaining a clear presentation in three planes. The parts of the vectorcardiogram that in the standard leads are represented by small deviations from the iso-electric line, are difficult to observe, as they do not differ greatly from the end point of the vector. (The iso-electric line in the standard leads is represented in the vectorcardiogram by the end point of the vectors.) Also it is difficult to make exact time determinations, and this is the method's greatest drawback. Although from the aspect of information theory there is less redundancy in the vectorcardiogram than in a 12-lead electrocardiogram, it is difficult to interpret. The method has not been extensively adopted for routine clinical use; only with automatic data processing for interpreting ECGs can the advantages of a vectorcardiographic analysis be realistically exploited.

3.187	In vectorcardiography, the heart's dipole field is reproduced on an oscilloscope by representing the magnitude and direction of the resultant heart vector in three planes, namely, the ...., ... and	
3.188	In vectorcardiography an .... lead system must be used.	frontal plane sagittal plane transverse plane
3.189	With the standard lead system, the large loop corresponds to the .... (P, T wave, QRS complex, S-T interval), which in the cardiac cycle corresponds to .... (atrial, ventricular) .... (depolarization, repolarization).	orthogonal
3.190	The iso-electric line in the standard lead system is represented in the vectorcardiogram by the	QRS complex ventricular depolarization
		endpoint of the vectors

Telemetry and storage of ECG data

To enable ECGs to be recorded over periods of several hours, and during normal activities, the signal can either be recorded on a portable tape recorder or it can be telemetered to a receiver nearby. In telemetry, transmission is usually accomplished by means of a frequency-modulated carrier wave and the signal may be recorded on magnetic tape. In the USA, early telemetry units used the FM broadcast band, 88–108 MHz. Now the FCC has allotted a special band for patient monitoring at 450 MHz. Other countries have other bands. The range can be up to a hundred meters or so, though much less in buildings of steel or reinforced concrete construction. Recording by such methods is usually made with only one pair of chest electrodes.

In addition to monitoring patients in the coronary care unit, the method can be used for diagnosing intermittent disorders of heart rhythm and function. It can also be applied in stress examinations—for example, on vehicle drivers and pilots in critical situations and on military personnel.

Reduction of ECG data

With some of the above recording units, the amount of data that can be collected is so great that the interpretation cannot be performed conventionally by examining each cardiac period. The interpretation would require as much of the physician's time as is needed for the recording. Since by far the majority of ECG periods are normal and identical, data reduction is essential for extracting the diagnostically significant changes. This can be accomplished in a number of ways. By means of comparatively simple electronic logic circuits, the changes in rhythm and frequency outside the normal preset limits are sensed and recorded on an ECG recorder. Automatic data processing can also be used. One of the principle aims in the design of technical aids in medical diagnosis, is to accomplish an appropriate reduction of data.

3.191	For recording ECGs over long periods and while the patient is engaged in his normal activities, the signals may be recorded on . . . . , either on portable recording equipment or by telemetry.	
3.192	Recording of ECGs over a long period is of value in diagnosing . . . . disorders of rhythm and function and for . . . . examinations.	magnetic tape
3.193	With modern equipment for ECG recording, such large amounts of data can be collected that it is often necessary to use . . . . methods to make interpretation practical.	intermittent stress
3.194	By means of electronic logic circuits, it is possible to trigger the separation and recording of ECG complexes having a rhythm and/or frequency lying outside the . . . . preset on the apparatus.	data reduction
		normal limits

Computer Analysis of ECG

The heart's electrical signals, which have a simple and rhythmically recurring waveform, are well suited for analysis by automatic methods. Automatic data processing has important applications in medicine, since ECG diagnosis is one of the most common methods of examination and the analysis of curves is a time-consuming routine.

Computer interpretation of ECGs (Fig. 3.41) includes:

- amplifying, possible transmission over telephone lines, filtering and analog-digital conversion
- identification of waveform features by pattern recognition, and mathematical analysis of the signal for determining various parameters, including amplitude and time relations, and usually also a number of vectorcardiographic parameters.
- classification and interpretation of the electrocardiogram on a statistical basis

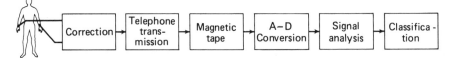

Figure 3.41 Typical steps in computerized ECG interpretation.

Signal recording. Greater demands are made on signal recording for computer analysis than for the usual reading of ECG waves. This is due to the ability of the human brain to disregard, for example, occasional disturbances and drift of the baseline—artifacts that can confuse the computer analysis. No data processing technique can yield good interpretations from poor raw material. Essential requirements are correct electrode technique, limitation of interference in picking up the signals and high-fidelity tape-recording techniques. If noise is introduced by telephone transmission, filtering may be required.

FM tape recorders are usually employed in order to obtain accurate reproduction at low frequencies. A frequency response of 0.05–200 Hz is commonly used. To avoid loss of information, the signal is then sampled at a rate of 500 samples/s and with an amplitude resolution of 0.1 percent.

Signal analysis. The first step in a computer analysis is wave recognition. Some systems acquire data from the conventional 12-lead scalar ECG, some utilize the Frank vectorcardiogram and some use data from both. As an example, the vectorcardiographic system is described, which for each of the three component leads computes the derivatives of voltage with respect to time. The QRS wave contains higher frequency components than other waves; thus the onset of the QRS complex waveform is recognized by comparing the computed spatial velocity of the waveform with a standard spatial velocity template. The comparison is implemented by sliding the template relative to the waveform of interest until the difference between the waveform and the template is minimized in a least squares sense, thereby achieving temporal alignment. The standard template used in this technique is based upon an average of hundreds of normal and abnormal QRS complexes where the QRS onset had been visually identified. After the QRS complex is identified, the onset and end of P, QRS, and T waves are defined by measuring amplitudes and derivatives.

Over 300 measurements may be abstracted from each tracing. The variables are of six types: voltage amplitudes; maximum amplitudes; angles; Q, R, S, and T wave durations; time of peak amplitude; and wave areas expressed in units of $mV \times ms$. Since this set of measurements is highly redundant, an initial screening is used to reduce their number.

Computer classification. One form of computer classification utilizes decision-tree type computer analysis. In this method, the computer mimics the methods of cardiologists. The computer measures various durations, amplitudes and polarities of conventional 12-lead tracings in a structured, branching sequence, following standardized criteria accepted by cardiologists. The computer can never perform more accurately than the cardiologist it seeks to mimic, since the cardiologist is considered 100 percent correct and serves as the ultimate judge of the computer's performance.

An improvement in computer classification is obtained in one system by requiring the physician requesting the ECG to choose one or more tentative diagnoses from the following set: normal cardiovascular status, coronary artery disease, hypertensive cardiovascular disease, valvular or congenital heart disease, pulmonary disease, primary myocardial disease, or other diseases not related to the cardiovascular system. The computer utilizes a prior probability table associated with each choice and Bayes' theorem to calculate the posterior probability of 12 diagnostic categories, which include identification and location of myocardial infarct, ventricular hypertrophy, conduction defect, etc.

This multivariate classification technique is able to correctly classify more than 85 percent of the cases documented by clinical diagnosis (clinical, laboratory and autopsy information). This compares with less than 70 percent correctly classified by conventional 12-lead tracings read by cardiologists. Thus this multivariate classification technique using prior probabilities appears superior to either readings by cardiologists or decision-tree type computer analysis systems that mimic the methods of cardiologists.

The value of computer analysis in ECG diagnosis is twofold. First, there are the benefits of automation, which not only is of importance in medical treatment, but also enables ECG diagnosis to be used to a greater extent in preventive medicine. Second, a subjective interpretive procedure is replaced by an objective statistical analysis and classification. With accumulated experience, more reliable estimates can be obtained for the probability of correct diagnosis.

3.195	Computer analysis of ECGs is performed in three stages, namely: 1 . . . ., 2 . . . . and 3	
3.196	Computer analysis requires ⌐tter signal recording than manual reading of ECGs because the human brain—unlike computers—can disregard . . . . more easily.	signal recording signal analysis computer classification
3.197	The first stage in signal analysis consists of . . . .; here use is made of the fact that the QRS complex contains . . . . than other waves in the electrocardiogram.	artifacts
3.198	When the waves have been identified, certain scalar quantities can be determined, namely, ..., ... and . . . . relations for P, QRS, and T waves.	wave recognition higher frequency components
3.199	If, for the myocardial infarction patient in question 3.171, the wave areas expressed in mV × ms of the heart vectors is determined, a . . . . (higher, lower) value would be obtained than for a normal subject.	time amplitude angle
3.200	The computer analysis yields the best diagnosis when the requesting physician is required to choose a . . . . from one of seven broad categories.	higher
3.201	This enables the computer to use a prior probability table associated with each set and use . . . . theorem to calculate the posterior probability of . . . . diagnosis categories.	tentative diagnosis
3.202	The 12 diagnostic categories include . . . ., ..., and	Bayes' 12
3.203	The performance of computer classification methods should be compared with clinical diagnoses (. . . . ., ..., and . . . . information) rather than compared with readings by cardiologists.	myocardial infarct ventricular hypertrophy conduction defect

3.204	The importance of computer ECG analysis is twofold. First, there are the benefits of . . . ., which opens up new possibilities for . . . . examinations. Second, a subjective interpretive procedure can be replaced by an . . . . analysis, which can give the . . . . of correct diagnosis.	clinical laboratory autopsy
		automation preventive medical objective statistical probability

CARDIAC DEFIBRILLATION

Some cardiac arrhythmias can be treated by passing a brief electric shock through the heart. Ventricular fibrillation can often be stopped before circulatory arrest has caused irreversible brain damage due to oxygen deficiency. Likewise, atrial fibrillation and atrial flutter can often be stopped by defibrillation.

Ventricular fibrillation may be caused by an external electric shock, which occurs near the peak of the T wave—the vulnerable period when the ventricle is repolarizing. It may also be caused when a PVC occurs during this same vulnerable period; in this case the heart electrocutes itself. Fibrillation has been likened to a dog chasing its tail, with continuous travel of the waves of depolarization and repolarization. During defibrillation, a large electric shock causes simultaneous depolarization of all cardiac muscle fibers. When they recover, normal pacing resumes. An energy of 50–500 Ws (joules) has been found most effective, with the current passing through the heart along its longitudinal axis. Defibrillation can be performed externally via two electrodes placed on the chest (Fig. 3.42), or internally on the exposed heart during an operation. With an electrode about 50 cm^2 in area, the resistance through the thorax is about 100 Ω. For internal defibrillation on an exposed heart the resistance is lower, about 50 Ω.

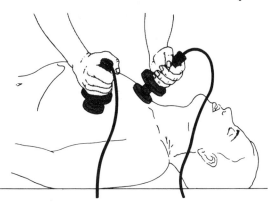

Figure 3.42 External cardiac defibrillation.

There are three types of defibrillators. They use alternating current, direct current and double pulses. The alternating current defibrillator is only of historical interest, since it requires a large amount of energy for defibrillation; this injures the cardiac muscle and may cause infarction. The pulse duration for an alternating current defibrillator is about 0.1 s.

In direct current defibrillation, a capacitor is charged to produce pulse times of a few milliseconds. In typical cases, a $16\,\mu\mathrm{F}$ capacitor is charged to 7 kV. The required pulse duration, about 5 ms, can be obtained by connecting an inductance of about 0.1 H in series. Lower energies are required for dc than for ac defibrillation, and there is therefore less risk of myocardial damage. At first a value of 100 Ws (J) is tried, and if this is unsuccessful, it is increased to 200, and then possibly to 400. For internal defibrillation on the exposed heart during an operation, less energy is required.

Defibrillation with double pulses has been demonstrated; two pulses separated by a short interval are used. The first pulse defibrillates all excitable cells, but does not affect those cells in a refractory (not capable of being stimulated) state. The second pulse defibrillates the cells that were refractory to the first pulse, but which have become excitable. At the end of the second pulse, all cells are depolarized. By stimulation of all cells in their excitable phase, the total energy required is lower. For example, for the exposed canine heart, successful defibrillation was obtained with 40 V, 20 ms pulses separated by a 100 ms interval. The mean energy was 2.0 Ws (J) for this double pulse method, whereas conventional, single pulse defibrillators require 15 Ws (J). This method has not been adopted clinically.

Paradoxically, a shock with an energy that stops ventricular fibrillation is also capable of causing it. For if the shock occurs during the vulnerable period of the T wave, ventricular fibrillation can be initiated. Therefore, in the treatment of atrial flutter and fibrillation, it is necessary to synchronize the defibrillation with the ventricular cycle. The R spike of the heart's action potentials is picked up, delayed, and used to synchronize the defibrillation pulse.

The large current used in defibrillation causes powerful contractions of the chest muscles. If the patient is unconscious, this is of minor importance, but in a conscious patient it causes great discomfort, and for this reason atrial defibrillation is usually performed under general anesthesia.

The conversion of atrial fibrillation to a normal rhythm by defibrillation is usually called **cardioversion**.

3.205	The heart arrhythmias, ventricular fibrillation, atrial fibrillation and atrial flutter can be treated by means of a brief electric shock through the heart with an energy between . . . . and . . . . The method is called . . . .

3.206	Ac defibrillation is unsuitable because .... energy is required and this can cause damage to the	50 Ws (J) 500 Ws (J) defibrillation (cardioversion)
3.207	In direct current defibrillation, a pulse with a dura-tion of about .... is used. The pulse is generated by means of a	high myocardium (heart muscle)
3.208	An electric current pulse of the magnitude used in defibrillation can also cause ventricular fibrillation if the pulse occurs in the vulnerable period of the .... wave. Therefore, in defibrillation of atrial arrhythmias, the defibrillation pulse is syn-chronized by using the .... of the ECG.	5 ms capacitor discharge
3.209	In external defibrillation, the electrodes are applied to the .... For a conscious patient, car-dioversion is usually performed .... to avoid patient discomfort due to .... of the chest muscles.	T R spike
3.210	In internal defibrillation of an exposed heart, the required energy is considerably .... (lower, higher). The thorax muscles .... (contract, do not contract).	chest under general anesthesia contractions
		lower do not contract

PACEMAKER THERAPY

In diseases where the ventricular rate is too low, it can be increased to normal by using an electrical pulse generator, known as a **pacemaker**. The various rhythm disturbances that result in block and Adams–Stokes attacks (see page 196), represent a serious pathological condition. The patients become invalids because of the constant risk of suddenly losing consciousness. With conventional drug therapy, the mortality within a year is 50 percent. Pacemaker therapy lowers this figure to 15 percent, and leads to a considerable improvement in the patient's mental and physical wellbeing.

Energy requirements. Like all muscle tissue, the heart can be stimulated with an electric shock. The minimum energy required is about 10 μWs (μJ); as a safety precaution, a level about 10 times this is used. Typically, a pulse of 5 V, 10 mA and 2 ms is used.

Too high a pulse energy may provoke ventricular fibrillation, which can be caused by a pulse of about $400\,\mu$Ws, if it occurs during the vulnerable period of the T wave. In addition, because of the limited battery life, pacemaker design should avoid unnecessarily high pulse energy.

The pulse type is important. A dc pulse causes a tissue reaction around the electrodes. This is greatest at the anode, where the muscle tissue is converted to connective tissue and the electrode surface is corroded. These problems are minimized by placing a capacitor in series with one electrode, so that equal charges flow in both directions.

The energy for a pacemaker is usually supplied by mercury batteries. These have a long storage time, a high electrical capacity per unit volume, and maintain a nearly constant voltage while discharging more than 90 percent of their energy. The energy may be transmitted to a pacemaker, using a radio frequency field, or inductively, using a low frequency electromagnetic field. However, this is not practical, since most patients do not like to be dependent on an external device. Periodic cardiac or respiratory movements can be utilized to generate electric energy. A piezoelectric crystal, coupled mechanically to these organs, can generate enough energy to drive a pacemaker, but this method has not been adopted. One source of pacemaker power is the use of radionuclides. As these decay, they generate heat, which is converted to electricity by thermocouples. These have been implanted in a number of patients and should last 10 years, instead of the 2 years typical for mercury batteries.

Also, lithium-iodine batteries will probably become an important source of energy for pacemakers; a life of 10 years appears to be possible.

3.211	To produce ventricular contraction with an electric pulse, an energy of about .... is required, but as a safety precaution, an energy level .... times higher is usually used in pacemaker therapy.	
3.212	Too high pulse energy is risky because it may cause .... if the pulse occurs during the vulnerable part of the .... wave.	$10\,\mu$Ws $(\mu$J$)$ 10
3.213	Ventricular fibrillation can be caused by an energy of about .... μWs.	ventricular fibrillation T

3.214	The commonest source of energy for pacemakers is the .... because this has a .... life, high capacity per unit .... and an ideal	400
		mercury battery long volume discharge characteristic

Types of pacemaker

For all types of pacemakers, the stimulating electrodes are placed in or near the heart. The location of stimulation varies, however, and also the type and synchronization of the pulse rate, which may be classified as follows:

- constant pulse rate
- variable, manually adjustable pulse rate
- ventricular synchronous pulse rate
- atrial synchronous pulse rate

In the simplest pacemaker design, the impulse frequency is constant—usually 70 impulses/min, corresponding to the normal sinus rhythm. This pacemaker is suitable for patients with either a stable, total AV block, a slow atrial rate or atrial arrhythmia. Figure 3.43 shows an example of a simple electronic circuit using an "astable multivibrator" as the pulse generator.

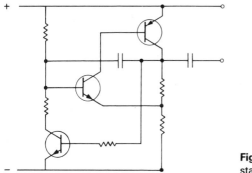

Figure 3.43 Pacemaker circuit for constant impulse frequency.

Pacemakers with a manually adjustable impulse frequency have been designed; in the case of an external pulse generator, the rate is easily changed by a control knob on the generator; with a completely implanted unit, the rate is changed by rotating an external magnet over the unit. However, experience has shown that for psychological reasons, patients are unwilling to control their own pulse rate. Therefore, the method has not been adopted for routine permanent implantation, but is primarily intended for testing suitable pacemakers in patients with recently implanted or existing electrodes, before permanent implantation is performed.

Pacemakers with a constant frequency have several disadvantages. One obvious shortcoming is that the heart rate cannot be increased to match greater physical effort. Another is that stimulation with a fixed impulse frequency results in the ventricles and atria beating at different rates. This varies the stroke volumes of the heart, which causes some loss in cardiac output. A fixed pulse frequency can also cause problems in patients with an unstable block; the heart is then periodically paced by the SA node, with resulting interference between the ventricular contractions evoked by the pacemaker and the atria. Some pacemaker impulses fall in the vulnerable period of the T wave for atrial-generated ventricular contractions. This increases the risk of ventricular fibrillation, even if an attempt is made to keep the pulse energy low enough to prevent this complication.

Patients with only short periods of AV block can be supplied with a ventricular synchronized pacemaker or a demand pacemaker (ventricular inhibited pacemaker). These do not compete with the normal heart activity. The single transvenous electrode placed in the right ventricle both senses the R wave and delivers the stimulation; thus no separate, sensing electrode is required. An R wave from an atrial-generated ventricular contraction triggers the ventricular synchronized pacemaker, which provides an impulse falling in the later part of the normal QRS complex. This ensures that the pacemaker does not interfere with the sinus rhythm. If atrial-generated ventricular contractions are absent, the pacemaker provides impulses at a basic frequency of 70 impulses/min. The demand pacemaker provides impulses only when the atrial-generated ventricular contractions are absent, thus conserving energy.

About 70 percent of all patients are supplied with ventricular synchronized or demand pacemakers. Their disadvantage is that the atrial and ventricular contractions are not synchronized. An improvement of about 10 percent in cardiac output can be obtained by atrial synchronization.

Atrial synchronization requires the most advanced type of pacemakers. The atrial activity can be picked up by a sensing electrode placed in the loose connective tissue in the mediastinum, as close as possible to the dorsal wall of the atrium. This should result in an amplitude of at least 1.5 mV. The P wave is amplified in the pacemaker and after a delay of 0.12 s, a pacemaker impulse stimulates the ventricle. The pacemaker is synchronized to the atrium between 50 and 150 impulses/min, but has a maximum frequency of 150 impulses/min, so it will not increase further, even if atrial flutter or fibrillation should develop. If the P wave is not detected, or does not occur, the pacemaker has a basic frequency of 50 impulses/min. Figure 3.44 shows a block diagram for such an atrially synchronized pacemaker. This type is used for young active patients with a mostly stäble block.

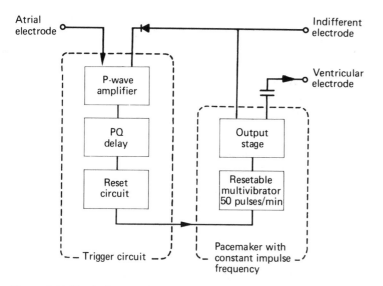

Figure 3.44 Block diagram for atrial synchronous pacemaker. With normal sinus rhythm, the pacemaker frequency is synchronized with the heart; when the sinus rhythm is absent, the pacemaker generates a constant frequency of about 50 impulses/min.

Atrial and ventricular synchronous pacemakers are more sensitive to external electromagnetic interference than the simpler types are, because they incorporate an action-potential amplifier. Electric shavers, car ignition systems and microwave ovens are examples of interference sources that affected the older types of pacemakers, but the newer pacemakers incorporate low-pass filters in the amplifier input circuit to reduce this problem. (Pacemaker patients should neither have diathermy treatment (see page 631), nor be exposed to airport security metal detectors.)

3.215   The ability to manually adjust the impulse frequency is primarily used for .... pacemakers intended for implantation in patients with recently implanted or existing electrodes.

3.216	A pacemaker with constant impulse frequency is used in patients with stable, total A V block, where it is unnecessary to avoid the risk of .... between ventricular contraction generated by the pacemaker and by the atria.	testing
3.217	In an atrial synchronous pacemaker, the .... wave is picked up from the atria, and after delay, is used to generate the pacemaker impulses, which are thus .... with the atrial activity, so long as this is present. If it ceases, ventricular contractions are produced at the .... of the pacemaker.	interference
3.218	An atrial synchronous pacemaker is used in young patients with mostly stable block, to avoid interference between the ventricular contractions generated by the .... and the .... For if the pacemaker impulse should fall in the vulnerable period of an .... generated T wave, there is a risk of ...., which leads to	P synchronous basic frequency
3.219	A ventricular synchronous pacemaker is used in patients with occasional A V block. When the ventricular contraction is atrial-generated, the pacemaker generates synchronous impulses in the later part of the ...., and therefore the .... period of the T wave is avoided. During periods of block, the pacemaker generates impulses with a .... and the circulation can then be maintained satisfactorily.	atria pacemaker atrially ventricular fibrillation circulatory arrest
3.220	The demand pacemaker is blocked during normal	QRS complex vulnerable basic frequency (70 impulses/min)
3.221	External electromagnetic fields can .... a pacemaker. This applies particularly to types provided with .... for synchronization, using the heart's action potentials.	atrial rhythm
3.222	Because of the risk of electromagnetic interference, pacemaker patients should neither be given .... treatment, nor be inspected by	interfere with an amplifier

3.223

A patient has been troubled for 6 months by reduced physical work capacity and slow heart rate, and at all examinations the above ECG changes were recorded. A pacemaker is chosen . . . . (with constant frequency, that is atrial synchronous, that is ventricular synchronous) because the diagnosis is

. . . .

diathermy
airport metal
detectors

with constant
frequency
stable,
total AV block

Implantation of pacemakers

The pacemaker is connected to the heart by means of cables and the electrical connection is made through electrodes. The electrodes can be placed in contact with the heart muscle or in the heart cavities. Only one electrode needs to make direct contact with the heart for stimulation; the other can be on the pacemaker case, or implanted subcutaneously near the heart. It is true that the required current will then be somewhat greater than if two electrodes are placed side by side in the myocardium.

Formerly, the thorax was opened in order to suture the electrodes on the outside of the myocardium and the pacemaker was placed in the abdomen. However, many patients were so weakened by the disease, that the mortality due to the added trauma of the operation was high.

Now, under local anesthetic, a flap of skin just below the right clavicle is opened. The transvenous pacemaker is placed in this pocket and the cable threaded through a vein in the shoulder or neck, passed via the superior vena cava and through the right atrium until the electrode is at the tip of the right ventricle. The position of the electrode can be checked during its insertion fluoroscopically or by connecting the cable to an ECG unit—a characteristic change in the signal appears as the electrode passes through the valve system between the atrium and the ventricle. An electrode for picking up the atrial activity can also be inserted without opening the thoracic cavity. By means of a mediastinoscope inserted from the jugular fossa, a passage is made in the loose connective tissue surrounding the atria. Figure 3.45 shows the position of a pacemaker, cables and electrodes.

An external pacemaker is connected via cables that pass through the skin. This arrangement is unsuitable for permanent use, because infection will eventually work its way along the cables and enter the body.

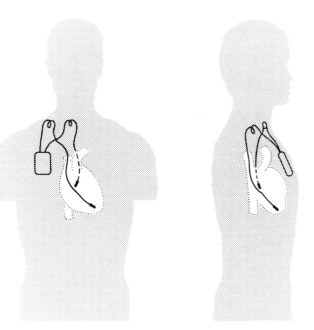

Figure 3.45 Transvenous pacemaker with leads.

    The electrodes and cables must be made of special materials. For electrodes in contact with tissues, noble metals are used to prevent corrosion and tissue reaction. Because of the risk of material fatigue due to the heart movements, 100,000 beats a day, special, highly flexible cables have been designed. Thin coils of special steel are encased in silastic rubber, which is a material chosen to prevent clotting in the veins.

3.224	A pacemaker electrode can be inserted without a major surgical operation, by passing a cable through a neck vein via the .... (vessel), through the .... atrium and into the .... ventricle.	
3.225	Electrode position can be checked by .... and by connecting the cable to an	superior vena cava right right
3.226	A cable for picking up atrial activity can be inserted with the aid of a mediastinoscope, which is introduced from the	fluoroscopy ECG unit

3.227	Connection of an external pacemaker by passing a cable through the skin, has the disadvantage that it causes a	jugular fossa
		risk of infection

PHYSICAL WORK CAPACITY

There are a number of reasons for determining the physical work capacity. In the diagnosis of heart diseases, especially coronary insufficiency, it is important to be able to subject the patient to a physical work load of known magnitude, since the typical pathological changes—ST depression in the ECG—often appear only during effort. An objective determination of the work capacity is also made in examination of patients with heart and lung diseases that impair the circulation or respiration. The physical condition is also determined, to follow the results of physical exercise, not only in connection with athletics, but also for rehabilitation and in pre-operative examinations of a patient, for judging whether the physical condition is good enough for the patient to undergo a major operation.

The best method for determining the work capacity is provided by the bicycle ergometer. The patient operates the bicycle at a given speed at a known instantaneous load. The method has several advantages over others (climbing stairs or running on a treadmill): the load is readily adjusted to the desired value and can be determined accurately, and a number of physiological parameters can be recorded simultaneously, such as the ECG, breathing rate and oxygen uptake through the lungs. Work capacity tests can also be performed during cardiac catheterization; here, the patient operates the bicycle in the supine position.

The bicycle ergometer can be loaded mechanically with a brake band, which is loaded with a known force; it is then important for the patient to maintain the required speed, 60 rev/min, so that the work load is constant. When electric braking is used, the load is inversely proportional to the pedaling rate, which automatically results in constant work, even if the pedaling rate varies by ±20 percent.

Exercise tests are performed in different ways, depending on the individual medical requirements and the patient's state of health. If this permits the maximum load to be used, the load is increased by multiples of 30 or 50 W every six minutes (for example, 50, 100, 150 and 200 W) up to a heart rate of about 170 beats/min. To provide a measure of a person's physical work capacity the load usually stipulated is that which, extrapolated or interpolated, gives a pulse rate of 170 beats/min.

Men aged 20–60 years, in normal health, should be able to manage 150–200 W, and women 65–130 W.

The heart reaches its maximum cardiac output at a pulse rate that is specific for the individual, and the body's work capacity is then also the maximum. The maximum heart rate may be limited by impaired oxygen uptake in the lungs; this situation is obviously of diagnostic value. The oxygen uptake during the exercise test should be 2.5–3.5 liters/min for men and 1.1–2.2 liters/min for women.

3.228	The physical work capacity is determined with a	
3.229	Patients with suspected coronary insufficiency are subjected to physical work load in order to provoke an . . . . in the ECG.	bicycle ergometer
3.230	The work capacity is reduced mainly in diseases of the . . . . and	ST-depression
3.231	Determinations of the physical condition by exercise tests are performed not only for athletic purposes but also for examining whether the patient's condition is good enough for him to undergo a major	circulatory organs respiratory organs
3.232	On an electrically braked bicycle ergometer the . . . . (load, pedaling rate) is adjusted to the instantaneous . . . . so that the . . . . is kept constant.	surgical operation
3.233	The pedaling rate should normally be	load pedaling rate work load
3.234	A man aged 20–60 in normal health should be able to manage . . . . and a woman	60 rev/min
3.235	The maximum work capacity is usually determined primarily by the . . . . , and secondarily by the	150–200 W 65–130 W
		cardiac output respiration

REFERENCES

BELLVILLE, J. W. and WEAVER, C. S. *Techniques in Clinical Physiology; A Survey of Measurements in Anesthesiology*. New York (Macmillan) 1969. 532 pages.

BLACKBURN, H. *Measurement in Exercise Electrocardiography*. Springfield (Thomas) 1969. 488 pages.

COBBOLD, R. S. C. *Transducers for Biomedical Measurements: Principles and Applications*. New York (Wiley) 1974. 486 pages.

COMROE, J. H. JR. *Physiology of Respiration: An Introductory Text*. Chicago (Year Book) 1974. 316 pages.

COMROE, J. H. JR. et al. *The Lung, Clinical and Pulmonary Function Tests*. 2 ed. Chicago (Year Book) 1962. 390 pages.

CROMWELL, L. et al. *Biomedical Instrumentation and Measurements*. Englewood Cliffs (Prentice Hall) 1973. 446 pages.

GEDDES, L. A. *Electrodes and the Measurement of Bioelectric Events*. New York (Wiley) 1972. 364 pages.

GEDDES, L. A. *The Direct and Indirect Measurement of Blood Pressure*. Chicago (Year Book) 1970. 196 pages.

GEDDES, L. A. and BAKER, L. E. *Principles of Applied Biomedical Instrumentation*. New York (Wiley) 1975. 479 pages.

GOLDMAN, M. J. *Principles of Clinical Electrocardiography*. Los Altos (Lange) 1976. 400 pages.

GUYTON, A. C. *Basic Human Physiology: Normal Function and Mechanisms of Disease*. Philadelphia (Saunders) 1971. 721 pages.

GUYTON, A. C. *Textbook of Medical Physiology*. Philadelphia (Saunders) 1976. 1100 pages.

McDONALD, D. A. *Blood Flow in Arteries*. Baltimore (Williams & Wilkins) 1974. 496 pages.

NETTER, F. H. *The CIBA Collection of Medical Illustrations*, Vol. 5, *Heart*, Summit, New Jersey (CIBA Pharmaceutical Company) 1969. 295 pages.

PIPBERGER, H. V. et al. Clinical Application of a Second Generation Electrocardiographic Computer Program. *Am. J. Cardiol.* Vol. 35 (1975) pp. 597–608.

RAY, C. D. *Medical Engineering*. Chicago (Year Book) 1974. 1256 pages.

RESNEKOV, L. et al. Ventricular Defibrillation by Monophasic Trapezoidal-Shaped Double-Pulses of Low Electrical Energy, *Cardiovasc. Res.* Vol. 3 (1968) pp. 261–264.

RUSHMER, R. F. *Cardiovascular Dynamics*. Philadelphia (Saunders) 1976. 576 pages.

SCHALDACH, M. and FURMAN, S. *Advances in Pacemaker Technology*. New York (Springer-Verlag) 1975. 554 pages.

SELZER, A. *Principles of Clinical Cardiology*. Philadelphia (Saunders) 1975. 735 pages.

TAVEL, M. E. *Clinical Phonocardiography and External Pulse Recording*. Chicago (Year Book) 1972. 322 pages.

WEBSTER, J. G. (Ed.). *Medical Instrumentation: Application and Design*. Boston (Houghton Mifflin) 1978. 719 pages.

<table>
<tr><td>

chapter 4

</td><td>

Clinical
Neurophysiology

</td></tr>
</table>

The nervous system is the body's principal regulatory system and pathological processes in it often lead to serious functional disturbances. The symptoms vary greatly, depending on the part of the nervous system affected by the pathological changes.

There are two essentially different groups of diseases, which are diagnosed and treated in two distinct specialties: **neurology** and **psychiatry**. Neurology is the study of organic nervous diseases. These have symptoms due to objectively observable changes in the brain, spinal cord, peripheral nerves or muscles—changes that can be seen with the naked eye or under the microscope, or recorded by electrophysiological measurements. Psychiatry is the study of those diseases that, at least initially, do not present objectively observable pathoanatomic changes.

Neurological diagnosis is a highly specialized science, which is based on a thorough knowledge of the anatomy and physiology of the nervous system. Part of the diagnosis is performed by using electrical methods of examination. Because of the complex nature of these techniques, it has become necessary to set up special laboratories of clinical neurophysiology. In these the electrical activity—the **action potentials** and the **synaptic potentials**—are recorded. The electrical activity of the brain is recorded in order to diagnose, for example, epilepsy. The action potentials of the skeletal muscles are recorded to determine the causes of muscular paralysis, which can be due either to damage of the nerve supplying the muscle or to a primary muscle disease. When the function of a nerve is impaired, its action potentials and its conduction velocity are measured—for example, in order to locate the nerve lesion and to give the neurologist an indication as to whether the nerve should be moved by means of surgery in order to avoid further functional deterioration.

Question		Answer
4.1	In a disease of the nervous system, the symptoms vary widely depending upon the . . . . of the pathological process in the nervous system.	
4.2	A neurological disease is due to . . . . observable changes in the nervous system.	location
4.3	In a mental disease, there . . . . (is, is not) objectively demonstrable damage to the nervous system.	objectively
4.4	For the diagnosis of neurological diseases, examinations are carried out at neurological clinics, where an important method of measurement uses . . . . techniques.	is not
4.5	Muscular paralysis may be due to damage to the . . . . or to the	electrical
4.6	In the investigation of a pathological condition with reduced motor power in a muscle, the neurologist performs an examination of its . . . . , and of the supplying nerve's . . . . and	nervous system muscles
4.7	One method used in examining the central nervous system is to record the . . . . of the brain.	action potential action potential conduction velocity
		electrical activity

THE CENTRAL NERVOUS SYSTEM—EEG

The brain generates rhythmical potential changes, which can be picked up with electrodes either from the scalp or directly from the cerebral cortex. These potentials originate in the individual neurons of the brain, are summated as millions of cells discharge synchronously and appear as a surface waveform—the **electroencephalogram, EEG**. For picking up, amplifying and recording the EEG potentials, essentially the same procedures are used as in electrocardiography. An important difference between the two methods is that the physiological mechanisms that produce the ECG waveform are largely known, whereas the synchronizing mechanisms that generate the different EEG waveforms are less well known. Therefore, EEG curves can only be clinically interpreted on a purely empirical basis.

The neurons, like the other cells of the body, are electrically polarized at rest. The interior of the neuron is at a potential of about −70 mV relative to the exterior. This potential is chiefly due to the active transport of the positive K^+ ions to the interior of the neuron. When a neuron is exposed to a stimulus above a certain threshold—whether electrical, chemical, mechanical or thermal—a nerve impulse, which is seen as a change in membrane potential, is generated and spread in the cell. This is due to a sudden increase in the Na^+ ion permeability of the membrane, which results in depolarization of the membrane. Shortly afterwards, repolarization occurs.

Different types of membrane potentials are generated in the neuron. In the nerve fiber (axon) the all-or-nothing law applies; thus, when a certain threshold of stimulation is exceeded, an impulse is generated and conducted at a certain velocity throughout the length of the fiber. The conduction velocity depends on the diameter of the fiber (page 20).

In the body of a neuron, two different potentials are generated via synapses (page 21)—that is, by stimulation from the end fibers of other neurons in contact with the neuron in question. The excitatory postsynaptic potential, EPSP, stimulates and the inhibitory postsynaptic potential, IPSP, inhibits (Fig. 4.1). The

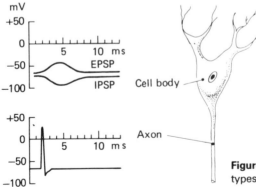

Figure 4.1 In the neuron, different types of potentials occur.

synaptic potentials do not spread very far, and the amplitude rapidly decreases with distance from the point of stimulation. A number of nerve fibers may each generate an EPSP too small to stimulate a neuron, yet the summation of these potentials will generate an impulse.

The membrane potential of an individual neuron in the cerebral **cortex** cannot be detected on the scalp because of the thickness of the intervening tissues. For measurable potentials to be generated, the activity from millions of neurons must be synchronized. Such synchronization is controlled by **subcortical** centers, probably from the brain stem, but the mechanism is still not fully understood. The peak-to-peak amplitude of the waves that can be picked up from the scalp is normally $100\,\mu$V or less, while that on the exposed brain is 10–20 times greater, 1 mV. The frequency content ranges from less than 1 to 50 Hz. The nature of the waves varies over the different lobes of the brain and is dependent on the level of wakefulness and sleep. There are large individual differences.

4.8	The resting potential of the inside of the neuron is about . . . . (voltage).	
4.9	When a nerve impulse is generated, ... of the membrane occurs, and a . . . . is set up which spreads throughout the neuron, and it causes current flows, which produce measurable potential changes in the surrounding tissue.	-70 mV
4.10	The duration of the membrane potential varies in different parts of the neuron and, as Fig. 4.1 shows, ranges from 1 to 5 . . . . (unit).	depolarization membrane potential
4.11	For a discharge to be generated in a neuron, the stimulus must exceed a certain	ms
4.12	A neuron can be stimulated by various kinds of energy: . . . . , ... , ... and	threshold
4.13	Electroencephalography and words derived from it—for example, electroencephalogram—are abbreviated	electrical chemical mechanical thermal
4.14	The amplitude of waves picked up from the scalp is normally . . . . and that of waves picked up from the cerebral cortex	EEG

4.15	EEG waves include frequency content ranging from .... to	$100\ \mu\text{V}$ 1 mV
4.16	EEG waves are produced by .... electrical activity in the neurons of the cerebral cortex.	< 1 Hz 50 Hz
4.17	The synchronization is controlled by the	synchronized
4.18	The appearance of EEG waves .... (varies, does not vary) in different normal persons.	brain stem (subcortical centers)
		varies

Recording Techniques

There are a number of systems for electrode placement on the scalp. Figure 4.2 shows the international standard 10–20 electrode placement system, so named because the positions of the electrodes are based on intervals of 10 and 20 percent of the distance between specified points on the scalp. Reference points used are the root of the nose and the ossification center (bump) on the occipital bone, which can usually be easily felt. From these points, the skull perimeters are measured in the transverse and median planes, and these perimeters are divided into 10 and 20 percent intervals to determine the electrode locations. Three other electrodes are placed on each side equidistant from the neighboring points, as shown. The electrodes are kept in place with elastic bands. To obtain good electrical contact,

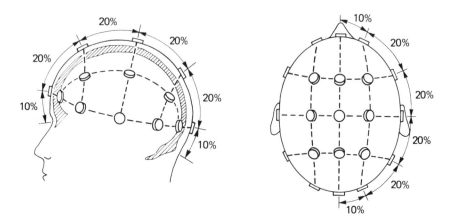

Figure 4.2 Placement of the 21 electrodes used in the international 10–20 system.

the scalp is cleaned, lightly abraded, and electrode paste applied between the electrode and the skin. The contact impedance should be less than 10 kΩ. In the case of unconscious and some conscious patients, needle electrodes inserted in the scalp are often used.

An EEG, like the ECG (page 189), can be recorded by **bipolar** or **unipolar** (monopolar) techniques. In the bipolar technique, the difference in potential between two adjacent electrodes is measured, whereas in the unipolar technique, the potential of each electrode is measured with respect to an indifferent electrode. This can consist of electrodes on the chin, ear, or back of the neck, but then slight interference is picked up from adjacent muscles and the ECG. It is better to connect all the other electrodes through equal resistances to create the indifferent electrode, in the same way as in the Wilson ECG system. The two systems give EEGs containing essentially the same information, but they are used together for practical reasons to help locate pathological changes (Fig. 4.3).

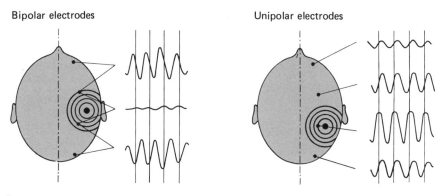

Bipolar electrodes   Unipolar electrodes

Figure 4.3 Both bipolar and unipolar electrode systems are used to facilitate the location of foci, that is, cortical areas from which abnormal waves spread. The phase relationship of the waves indicates the position of the focus and in some cases, enables the velocity at which the waves spread to be calculated.

The potential picked up on the scalp from a certain cortical center of activity decreases roughly with the square of the distance. Therefore, the electrical activity picked up by each electrode in a unipolar system and by each pair of electrodes in a bipolar system largely represents the cortical activity below or between the electrodes. The position of each electrode is not critical because the generated potential spreads out in the intervening bone and soft tissues: positions within ±1 cm on the scalp are satisfactory.

4.19   EEG signals can be picked up with either a
.... or a .... system.

4.20	With bipolar leads, the potential difference between two .... electrodes is measured.	bipolar unipolar
4.21	With unipolar leads, the potential of each electrode is measured with respect to an .... electrode which is usually formed by connecting equal resistances to the .... electrodes.	adjacent
4.22	The two types of electrode systems are used together to help .... pathological changes.	indifferent other scalp
4.23	The potential picked up on the scalp from a cortical center of activity decreases with the .... (power) of the distance, and therefore, each electrode picks up mostly the .... activity.	locate
4.24	The electrode impedance in an EEG system should be .... (magnitude).	square adjacent
		$< 10\ k\Omega$

Wave Types

The electrical activity that can be recorded from the scalp varies both in frequency and amplitude. Under certain circumstances—for example, in certain normal mental states (different levels of consciousness) and pathological conditions, such as epilepsy—definite patterns are seen in the EEG signals (Fig. 4.4). Under normal conditions there is generally an inverse relationship between amplitude and frequency: if the frequency increases, the amplitude usually decreases. This is because an increased cerebral activity leads to a more desynchronized activity of the nerve cells, rather than a synchronized discharge of large groups of cells.

The normal wave types are labeled with the Greek letters. For historical reasons, the sequence of the letters does not correspond to the frequency ranges of the waves: alpha waves were discovered first, and waves with both higher and lower frequencies were discovered later.

Alpha waves have frequencies between 8 and 13 Hz and a mean amplitude of $50\ \mu V$. They appear over the occipital lobes in the awake, mentally relaxed state with the eyes closed. When the eyes are opened, the alpha activity disappears and waves of a higher frequency and lower amplitude appear (Fig. 4.5). If the patient falls asleep, the alpha activity disappears entirely. The wave characteristics—their time dependence, noise content and frequency spectrum—display large individual differences; in about 10 percent of all normal subjects no typical alpha activity can be recorded.

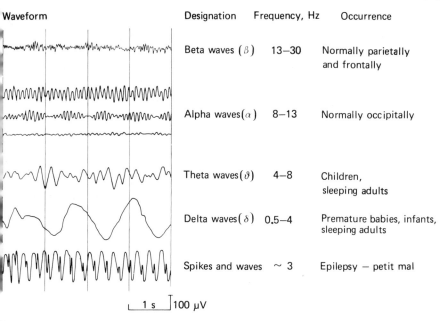

Waveform	Designation	Frequency, Hz	Occurrence
	Beta waves (β)	13–30	Normally parietally and frontally
	Alpha waves(α)	8–13	Normally occipitally
	Theta waves(ϑ)	4–8	Children, sleeping adults
	Delta waves(δ)	0.5–4	Premature babies, infants, sleeping adults
	Spikes and waves	~ 3	Epilepsy — petit mal

1 s] 100 μV

Figure 4.4 Some examples of EEG waves.

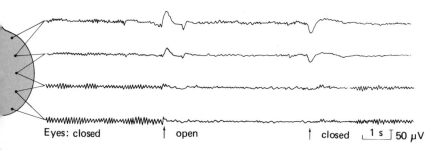

Eyes: closed ↑ open ↑ closed   1 s] 50 μV

Figure 4.5 Normal EEG illustrating the extinction of alpha rhythm that occurs when the eyes are opened.

Beta waves have higher frequencies, 13–30 Hz. They appear over the parietal and frontal lobes.

The frequency range of the **theta waves** is 4–8 Hz. They appear in adults during light sleep and in children.

Delta waves contain all the EEG activity below 4 Hz. They appear in adults during deep sleep, in premature babies and in infants.

An example of a pathological waveform, **spikes and waves**, is shown in Fig. 4.4. This waveform occurs during attacks of epilepsy. There are many other waveforms: they vary widely in appearance, and sometimes appear as transients, with a duration of 80–200 ms, in otherwise normal recordings.

The EEG waves may be altered by pathological processes in the cerebral cortex or brain stem. Extinction or damping of the electrical activity in the cortex can be due to a tumor, which presses on the neurons and destroys them, or to oxygen deficiency caused by a circulatory disturbance such as bleeding or embolus.

If tumors or scars from previous damage are present in the cortex, these can cause nearby neurons to generate abnormal electrical activity. All the processes in the brain stem that affect the level of consciousness also affect the shape of the EEG waves by modifying the synchronization of the cortex cells. For example, drowsiness, sleep and different levels of consciousness cause the changes shown in Fig. 4.6.

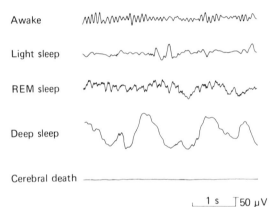

Awake

Light sleep

REM sleep

Deep sleep

Cerebral death

|_1 s_| 50 µV

Figure 4.6 EEG activity is dependent on the level of consciousness.

4.25	The electrical activity recorded from the scalp usually does not have a characteristic . . . . or	
4.26	Distinct types of waves normally appear only at certain levels of . . . . and in certain	amplitude frequency
4.27	The amplitude and frequency generally bear an . . . . relation to each other; this is because an increase in cerebral activity is associated with . . . . (synchronized, desynchronized) discharges in the neurons of the brain.	consciousness (wakefulness) diseases

4.28	Normal EEG activity is divided according to the frequency range of the waves; the following four types are distinguished: ...., ..., ... and	inverse desynchronized
4.29	Alpha waves appear when .... (awake, asleep), mentally .... (relaxed, excited), and with the eyes .... (open, closed).	β: 13–30 Hz α: 8–13 Hz θ: 4–8 Hz δ:< 4 Hz
4.30	Alpha waves appear over the .... lobes.	awake relaxed closed
4.31	Alpha waves display large .... between individuals, and are absent in .... percent of all normal human subjects.	occipital
4.32	Beta waves appear over the .... lobes and over the .... lobes.	differences 10
4.33	Theta waves appear in adults during .... (light, deep) sleep and in	parietal frontal
4.34	Delta waves appear in adults during .... sleep and in .... and	light children
4.35	The spike-and-wave complex is an example of a .... waveform.	deep infants premature babies
4.36	Pathological waveforms can vary greatly in duration, sometimes occurring only as .... in otherwise normal recordings.	pathological
4.37	A tumor that exerts pressure on brain tissues so that the neurons die, or oxygen deficiency due to a circulatory disturbance, can result in .... or .... of the brain's electrical activity.	transients
4.38	Abnormal electrical activity in the cortex can be caused by a .... or a .... from previous damage.	damping extinction

4.39	The shape of EEG waves is also affected by pathological processes in the brain stem, which influence the	tumor scar
		level of consciousness

Provocation of EEG

Since pathological waveforms appear only occasionally, it is useful to be able to provoke them in the laboratory. This may be done by hyperventilation, sleep and flashes of light.

During hyperventilation, the carbon dioxide tension in the blood is reduced and respiratory alkalosis develops (page 157). The stimulus threshold for neurons in the cerebral cortex, as well as for other cells of the body, is then lowered, and there is a greater probability that pathological waveforms will be evoked during the examination.

The fact that some epileptic seizures occur during sleep can also be utilized to provoke pathological waveforms.

However, the simplest method is to expose the patient to short light pulses from a stroboscope, typically 10 Mlx (megalux) pulses of 20 μs duration. If the frequency of the light pulses is increased from 1 to 25 Hz, there will normally be a frequency at which the alpha wave activity synchronizes with the pulses; the appearance of pathological waveforms during the first attempt at photostimulation may be a sign of epilepsy. In some cases epileptic attacks can be provoked by such photostimulation.

4.40	Provocation of pathological EEG waves is diagnostically necessary because they occur only	
4.41	Three ways in which pathological EEG waves can be provoked are ...., ... and	occasionally
4.42	Provocation by hyperventilation is based on the development of .... (respiratory, metabolic) .... (acidosis, alkalosis) and resultant lowering of the ....of the neurons; this increases the probability of pathological discharges.	hyperventilation sleep light flashes
4.43	The use of sleep as a provocation method is based on the fact that .... seizures often occur during sleep.	respiratory alkalosis stimulus threshold

4.44	Technically the simplest method of provocation is by stimulation with	epileptic
4.45	If the light pulse frequency is gradually increased, a frequency will normally be reached at which there is synchronization with the	light flashes
4.46	The occurrence of pathological waveforms during light flash stimulation may be a sign of	alpha wave activity
		epilepsy

Clinical Use of EEG

Electroencephalography is used chiefly in the examination of epilepsy, brain damage, brain tumors and other organic brain injuries, and sometimes for determining the level of consciousness—for example, depth of anesthesia and sleep—and for demonstrating brain death.

Epilepsy

Epilepsy is a symptom of brain damage. This may have been caused during birth delivery or, later in life, by head trauma (injury), received in a traffic accident or during boxing. It may also be due to a brain tumor. Epilepsy is thus not itself a disease; an epileptic seizure can be provoked in any person by passing a brief electric shock through the brain. This knowledge is used in electric shock treatment during psychiatric therapy.

Epileptic attacks are fairly common, occurring in about 0.5 percent of the population.

Epilepsy is characterized by synchronous discharges of large groups of neurons, often including the whole brain. There are two major types of attack: **grand mal** and **petit mal**. In grand mal there are large discharges, lasting from a few seconds to several minutes, and usually spreading to all parts of the central nervous system, including the spinal cord. If the discharges originate in the brain stem, they spread so rapidly that the patient immediately loses consciousness, spasms occur and ventilation is impaired, with resulting cyanosis, passage of urine, etc.

A grand mal seizure is often preceded for half a minute or so by an **aura**, a set of symptoms that the patient recognizes and that enables him to prepare for the seizure by lying down. The aura is associated with the onset of discharges in a **focus** in the cerebral cortex. The nature of the aura depends on the location of the focus. If it is situated in the visual center in the occipital lobe, the patient experiences a flash of light, and if it is in the acoustic center in the temporal lobe, he hears a noise or roar. There may also be olefactory and gustatory sensations and strange mental phenomena. If the focus is located in motor centers in the cerebral cortex, the patient has spasms and twitches in individual groups of muscles, known as **jacksonian attacks**. If the discharges spread, as is commonly the case, a grand mal seizure develops, and unconsciousness follows. The EEG waves in a grand mal attack are the same over the whole cortex.

In a petit mal attack there is abnormal EEG activity with a very characteristic pattern (Fig. 4.4). The seizure usually lasts for 1–20 s. At the same time there may be attacks of depressed or otherwise disturbed consciousness, but the person is then able to resume whatever he was doing before the seizure.

Focal epilepsy can sometimes be cured by surgical removal of the focus in the cortex. **Electrocorticography** provides the only way to locate the focus, since no observable anatomical changes are present. The cortex is exposed, and a number of electrodes are placed in or on it. By examining the electrical output of these electrodes, the location of the focus is determined, and that part of the cortex containing the functional lesion is removed by suction. Epilepsy is usually treated with drugs.

4.47	The EEG is used clinically in examinations for suspected .... and ...., and for determining the level of	
4.48	Epilepsy is a ...., not a	epilepsy brain tumor consciousness
4.49	Epilepsy is a symptom of a brain	symptom disease
4.50	The brain lesion can have been caused during ...., by head .... or by a	lesion
4.51	An epileptic attack can be induced in a normal person by means of an	delivery trauma brain tumor
4.52	Epilepsy is characterized by a .... discharge of large groups of neurons in the central nervous system.	electric shock

4.53	 The above EEG changes are a sign of	synchronous
4.54	A grand mal seizure spreads throughout .... (the whole, parts) of the central nervous system, and the patient then becomes .... and has	epilepsy (petit mal)
4.55	A petit mal seizure usually lasts only	the whole unconscious spasms
4.56	An epileptic seizure is often preceded by motor and sensory phenomena—known as an .... This is due to discharges in the cortex at a certain site, which is called a	a few seconds
4.57	The nature of the aura is dependent entirely on the .... of the focus.	aura focus
4.58	Epilepsy can sometimes be treated surgically, and the focus is then located by	location
		electrocorticography

Brain tumors

Brain tumors can affect the EEG in two ways. If the tumor displaces the cortex and if it is large enough, the electrical activity will be absent in that part of the hemisphere, since no electric potentials originate in the tumor itself. An extinguished or damped EEG over a certain part of the cortex can thus be a sign of a tumor, but there are other possible causes—for example, a major hemorrhage. A more common symptom than extinction is the induction by the tumor of synchronous discharges in adjacent nervous tissues, and then low-frequency, high-amplitude EEG waves are recorded.

A tumor can also provoke an epileptic attack. The EEG is only one of many diagnostic aids that can be used for examining brain tumors.

4.59	Brain tumors affect the EEG, by . . . . nor-mal waves and provoking . . . . waves.

extinguishing
(damping)
pathological

Level of consciousness

The appearance of the EEG changes with the level of consciousness. Diminished mental activity usually results in EEG waves that have a lower frequency and a larger amplitude. There are exceptions; for example, under conditions of stress and sudden disappointment, theta waves appear for 10–20 s or so. It has already been mentioned that, when the eyes are opened, the alpha activity is extinguished; this also occurs as a result of, for example, acoustic and mental stimuli, as during mental arithmetic.

The EEG has made valuable contributions to the study of the sleep physiology. In the drowsy state, alpha activity is recorded; these waves decrease in amplitude and intermittently cease, and as sleep comes on are replaced by periods of low amplitude theta waves (Fig. 4.6). As the depth of sleep increases, the EEG undergoes changes in a series of stages until, in deep sleep, it consists of irregular theta and delta waves over the whole scalp. Deep sleep is characterized by deep and heavy breathing, constant low values of blood pressure and pulse, possibly snoring, and absence of eye movements and absence of dreams. This level of sleep is fairly regularly interrupted by periods of REM (rapid eye movement) sleep lasting from 5 to 30 minutes. EEG waves similar to those in the wakened state appear.

REM sleep coincides with periods of dreaming. It is characterized by fluctuating blood pressure and pulse rate, rapid eye movements and penile erection, even during dreams that have no sexual content. About one quarter of sleep is REM sleep. It is considered essential for mental health.

The EEG displays characteristic features during general anesthesia. As shallow anesthesia develops, the brain wave frequency decreases and the amplitude increases; theta and delta activity appear. As the depth of anesthesia increases, the amplitude gradually decreases; this can be used as an objective means of recording the depth of anesthesia. Attempts have been made to utilize EEG signals for administration of anesthetics so as to maintain a suitable depth of anesthesia automatically—servo anesthesia. The method has not been generally adopted, however, because the EEG signal varies between different patients, and the level of reliability has not been high enough.

In the case of certain brain lesions that increase the pressure in the skull, the brain dies, and the brain's electrical activity stops (Fig. 4.6). An EEG showing a permanent absence of brain waves is evidence of **brain death**, even though the respiration and circulation may be maintained by intensive care.

4.60	In persons with normal health, a reduction in mental activity is generally accompanied by .... (an increase, a decrease) in frequency and .... (an increase, a decrease) in amplitude of the EEG waves.	
4.61	1 s 100 µV From a normal patient, the above EEG wave is recorded during the night. Characterize the waves by determining the frequency and indicate the patient's mental state (see Fig. 4.6).	a decrease an increase
4.62	1 s 100 µV Same question as 4.61	10 Hz α waves awake mental relaxation eyes closed
4.63	1 s 100 µV Same question as 4.61.	6–2 Hz θ and δ waves deep sleep
4.64	In sleep during the onset of shallow anesthesia, the EEG waves .... (decrease, increase) in frequency, and the amplitude	irregular (20 Hz) REM sleep
4.65	As the depth of anesthesia increases, the .... (frequency, amplitude) gradually falls.	decrease increases
4.66	The EEG is extinguished in	amplitude
		brain death

Automatic Signal Analysis of EEG

An EEG examination yields large amounts of data—for example, it is common to record analog values in 16 leads for a half an hour or so. Diagnostically valuable information can appear for just a fraction of a second in any of the leads. Therefore, the examination of EEG waves is a time-consuming procedure and efforts have been made to develop automatic methods for data reduction in order to ease the evaluation.

In other applications, automatic analysis of experimental data is based on a knowledge of the underlying physical processes. For the EEG, this has not yet been possible, because the mechanisms underlying the EEG waves have been largely unknown. Therefore, in automatic analysis, attempts have been made to simulate the empirical interpretation procedure; this is done by analyzing the frequency and amplitude during short intervals in each lead, and by comparing these parameters and the phase between different leads.

The EEG signal has an irregular form which can be described in statistical terms. There are two waveforms of interest. In the first, the observed signal has statistically regular features (for example, normal alpha or beta rhythm) and the signal can be regarded as a stationary, stochastic process. In the second type, specific transients such as isolated pulses or complex bursts (for example, spikes and waves) are observed. A number of techniques for analyzing these processes have been developed.

Analysis of stationary processes

The stationary processes are characterized primarily by their spectral properties. They can be examined in various ways—for example, by determining the spectral density by Fourier analysis, measurement of autocorrelation functions and subsequent calculation of the spectrum, and by means of spectrum analyzers furnished with a number of narrow-band filters.

Determination of spectral density by Fourier analysis.   Figure 4.7 shows the frequency spectrum of an EEG. The spectral density is determined by Fourier analysis on a computer using the FFT (Fast Fourier Transform). If a high frequency resolution is desired with this method, there will be a relatively large statistical error in the spectral density. Details in the curve are not useful for interpretation, since their origin is unknown and there are large individual differences between normal subjects.

Determination of spectral density by correlation analysis and parameter estimation.   In spectral analysis using the autocorrelation function $\psi_{11}(\tau)$, this function is calculated from the expression:

$$\psi_{11}(\tau) = \frac{1}{T} \int_{-T/2}^{T/2} x(t)x(t+\tau)\, dt$$

Relative amplitude

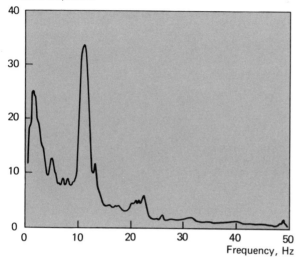

Frequency, Hz

Figure 4.7 Frequency spectrum of a normal EEG with a maximum in the alpha region.

where the observed signal, x, varies with time t, and where τ is a delay which is given continuously increasing values to measure the degree of a regular relationship between the signal value and the same signal delayed by time, τ. The integration time, T, should be chosen as high as possible, consistent with the assumption of stationarity. In practice, values of 20–60 s are used.

A cross correlation analysis can be performed to measure the degree of interdependence between the signals from two or more channels. The crosscorrelation function $\psi_{12}(\tau)$ is calculated from the expression:

$$\psi_{12}(\tau) = \frac{1}{T} \int_{-T/2}^{T/2} x(t)y(t+\tau)\, dt$$

where x and y are the signals in the two leads as a function of time t, and τ is the delay which is given continuously increasing values to measure the degree of a regular relationship between the signals from the two channels.

Autocorrelograms from the occipital and parietal EEG leads, recorded for a period of one minute are shown in Fig. 4.8. The damped periodic form of the curves shows that the EEG signal contains almost periodic components. However, if the interval between the two correlated signals is increased, the correlation between these almost periodic components becomes steadily weaker.

A method for computer analysis of EEG signals has been designed, in which the autocorrelogram is the point of departure. The result is a description of the spectral density with the aid of, normally, 10 parameters—the so-called power and frequency parameters which the program estimates from the data. With these, the spectral density can be obtained as the sum of a number of spectral components, each of which results in a peak in the resulting spectral diagram. The

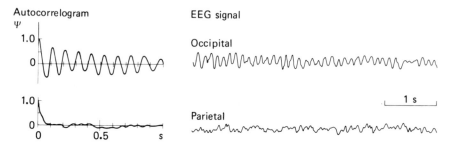

Figure 4.8 Normalized autocorrelogram for alpha activity recorded from the occipital and parietal leads for 1 minute.

frequency parameters indicate the resonant frequency and bandwidth for these components, while the power parameters correspond to the power content and are a measure of the asymmetry of the spectrum. The low-frequency components are usually described by two parameters, namely, bandwidth and power content. Most EEG's require three components, designed δ, α and β, where the δ component contains the low-frequencies, while the other two represent higher frequencies. The names are associated with known properties of the spectrum, the α component having a resonant frequency of about 10 Hz and the β component one of about 20 Hz.

Continuous frequency analysis with band-pass filters. In computer processing to identify random or periodic pathological changes in EEG signals, it is necessary to choose a number of parameters that can be studied as a function of the whole period of recording. This is most simply accomplished by dividing the signal into frequency bands with band-pass filters and recording the signals passing through the respective filters. With this technique, using tuned electrical filters, there is, however, the possibility of artifacts due to ringing in the filters; if these are made too selective, noise sets up oscillations having a frequency equal to the tuned frequency of the filters.

Data can be compressed for ready inspection by integrating the variance of the signals that are separated by the different tuned filters. The signal amplitude is squared, integrated and written out on a pen recorder. The slopes of the curves provide a measure of the activity in the respective frequency bands (Fig. 4.9). The ratio between the slopes—the variance index—is a measure of the change in activity. The method has certain practical advantages; for example, an objective numerical result can be obtained as a measure of the respective activities, and the values for quite a long observation period can be compressed into a single readily inspected curve. In an ordinary EEG recording about 60 m of paper are used, whereas the results of an analysis of variance can be presented on a single sheet. With this method, however, diagnostically significant details in the waveforms are lost, and therefore conventional recording is also necessary.

$$\int_{0}^{t} V^{2} dt$$

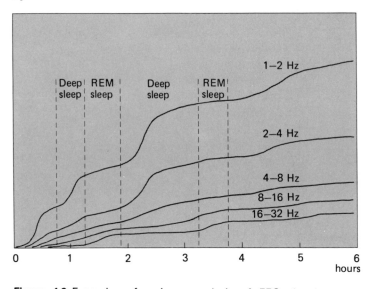

Figure 4.9 Examples of variance analysis of EEG signals obtained during a 6-hour period of sleep. During deep sleep, the EEG activity of lower frequencies predominates, and during REM sleep, higher frequencies.

Analysis of transients. Transients in the EEG can be of great diagnostic significance. For example, spike-and-wave complexes can occur sporadically, but last for a short time. The human brain has a greater capacity than automatic methods for recognizing patterns; particularly important is the ability to exclude artifacts from the curves by inspection. For this reason, automatic methods have been primarily used for separating out the parts of the EEG signal that are likely to contain useful information and that should then be examined visually. This reduces the data by excluding the normal parts, which are quantitatively greater in length, but diagnostically irrelevant.

A simple and, from the data processing viewpoint, economically feasible means of detecting transients, is to determine when the EEG signal and its first and second derivatives cross the zero base-line (Fig. 4.10). At these instants, pulses are generated; the time relations between them can be used to identify various waveforms of diagnostic interest. However, because of the large individual differences in the EEG signal waveforms, the criteria for inclusion must be rather wide; this means that large amounts of normal data must be examined visually.

Methods have been developed for detecting transients by means of signal matched filters. Computers or analog equipment may be used. This procedure will probably be widely adopted for spike detection, when it is economically feasible to apply it in several recording channels on-line.

EEG signal

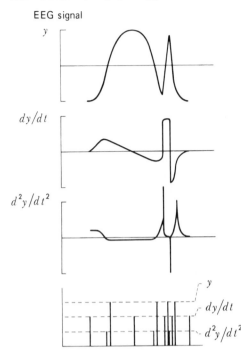

Figure 4.10 Pattern recognition of spike-and-wave complex by means of the time relations between zero-crossings for the signal and its first and second derivatives.

EEG display systems

With the usual graphic presentation of EEG curves it is not possible to observe the areal distribution of the signal amplitude and phase over the hemispheres. There are, however, a number of methods by which this can be accomplished—for example, by successively deflecting the beam of a cathode ray tube to a position corresponding to the position of the EEG electrodes on the scalp, and by intensity modulating to show the potential variation of each electrode. This enables the details of the potential distribution to be observed. The disadvantage of this procedure, as with other, similar display techniques in which plots of isopotential lines, isophase lines, etc., are produced, lies in the difficulty of obtaining a permanent record suitable for simple visual inspection.

None of the analytical methods for automatic EEG signal analysis tested so far has been able to replace visual examination of the curves and interpretation by an experienced specialist.

4.67	The evaluation of an EEG curve is based on an analysis of the . . . . and . . . . of the waves during a short interval in each lead, and a comparison of these parameters and of the . . . . between different leads.

4.68	In an automatic signal analysis it is necessary to look for .... relationships, since the mechanisms underlying the production of EEG waves are largely	amplitude frequency phase
4.69	Stationary segments of EEG signals can be analyzed by determining the spectral density using .... analysis and .... analysis.	empirical unknown
4.70	A continuous signal analysis over long periods of time can be performed by frequency analysis with the aid of	Fourier autocorrelation
4.71	A technically simple method for detecting EEG transients is to determine the time relations between the zero-crossings of the signal, of its .... and of its	band-pass filters
4.72	Transients can also be detected with	first derivative second derivative
4.73	By means of a two-dimensional display of EEG data, details of the potential distribution can be examined, but there are practical difficulties in obtaining a permanent	signal matched filters
4.74	Automatic methods of analysis .... (can, cannot) replace visual examination of EEG curves and their clinical interpretation.	record
		cannot

PERIPHERAL NERVES AND MUSCLES

Reduced motor power, muscular **paresis**, or total muscular **paralysis**, can be due to a lesion in the parts of the nervous system that supply the muscle, or to a pathological process in the muscle itself (Fig. 4.11). The pathological picture varies with the location and type of lesion. If the motor cortical centers in the brain are destroyed (as in cerebral hemorrhage) or the conducting pathways in the spinal cord are damaged (as in multiple sclerosis, MS), the muscle cannot be voluntarily contracted, but the muscular activity can still be provoked by means of reflexes. If the spinal cord neurons that supply the muscle are destroyed (for example, by poliomyelitis) or if the peripheral nerve is severed, reflexes cannot be elicited. Such a **denervated** muscle can be made to contract soon after the injury

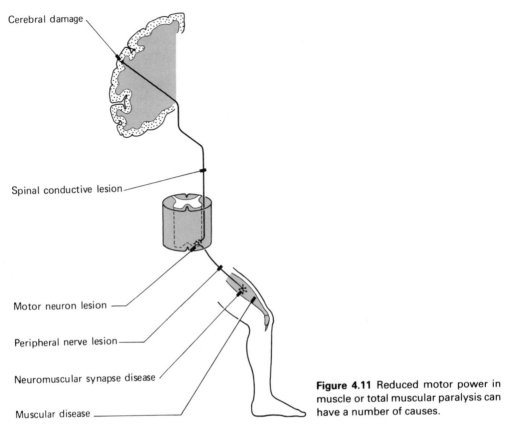

Cerebral damage

Spinal conductive lesion

Motor neuron lesion

Peripheral nerve lesion

Neuromuscular synapse disease

Muscular disease

Figure 4.11 Reduced motor power in muscle or total muscular paralysis can have a number of causes.

by electrical stimulation; ultimately, however, the muscle **atrophies** and is converted to connective tissue. Moderate pressure on a peripheral nerve (exerted by a herniated disc or some other form of pinching action) leads to a reduction in motor power due to impairment of nerve impulse conductivity. In addition, there will be sensory disturbances: pain, numbness and reduced sensibility. A pathological process in the end-plates of the nerve fiber, the neuromuscular synapses (as in myasthenia gravis), leads to loss of power and abnormally rapid fatigue, even though the nervous system and the muscular system are otherwise intact. Loss of power also occurs in diseases of the actual muscle (for example, in progressive muscular dystrophy, a hereditary disease with a poor prognosis). Another disease of the muscles (myotonia) leads to abnormally heightened excitability, with the result that the muscle cannot be relaxed after voluntary contraction.

A neurophysiological diagnosis of nervous and muscular diseases is based on recording of the muscles' electrical action potentials, **electromyography**, **EMG**, measurement of **conduction velocity** in motor nerves, and recording of the peripheral nerves' action potentials, **electroneurography**.

4.75	Muscular paresis may be due to a lesion or disease either in the . . . . or in the	
4.76	The pathological picture varies with the anatomic . . . . of the lesion.	muscular system nervous system
4.77	In lesions of the motor cortical centers or of the conducting pathways of the spinal cord, the muscle cannot be contracted . . . ., but muscular activity can be elicited by	location
4.78	When the neurons that supply either the muscle or the peripheral nerve are destroyed, muscular contraction can only be elicited artificially by . . . . of the muscle.	voluntarily reflexes
4.79	A muscle whose nerves have been severed will be paralyzed. The muscle is then said to be	electrical stimulation
4.80	Such a muscle will	denervated
4.81	Moderate pressure on a nerve may lead to diminished . . . . in the corresponding muscle; this is due to impaired	atrophy
4.82	Pressure on a peripheral nerve results in the following sensory disturbances: . . . ., ... and	motor power impulse conductivity
4.83	Poliomyelitis, myasthenia gravis and progressive muscular dystrophy are diseases that result in the same symptom, reduced or abolished . . . ., while these pathological processes have different anatomic	pain numbness reduced sensibility
4.84	EMG is the abbreviation for	motor power locations
		electromyography

Electromyography

In contraction of skeletal muscle, action potentials are generated in the individual muscle fibers, just as they are in the cardiac muscle (page 189), but in skeletal muscle, repolarization takes place much more rapidly, the action potential lasting only a few milliseconds. The electrical activity of the underlying muscle mass can be observed by means of surface electrodes on the skin. However, it is of greater diagnostic interest to record the action potentials from individual motor units, and this is done by inserting a needle electrode into the muscle (Fig. 4.12). The

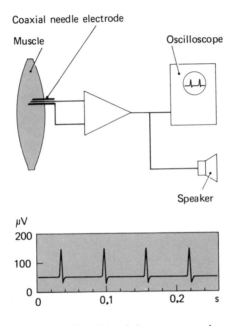

Figure 4.12 Principle of electromyography.

amplifier and recorder should have a bandwidth of at least 20–5000 Hz. In addition to an oscilloscope, a speaker may be included so that as the needle is inserted, its position can be monitored by listening to the clicks caused by the action potentials.

In voluntary contraction of skeletal muscles, the muscle potentials range from $50\,\mu V$ to 2 mV and last for 2 to 10 ms. The values vary with the anatomic position of the muscle and the size and location of the electrode. The maximum discharge frequency is 60 Hz. In a relaxed muscle, there are normally no action potentials.

In the case of a nerve lesion, there is a loss of contraction in some motor units, while the remaining ones function at normal frequency.

By recording action potentials from different muscles, the area supplied by the damaged nerve can be defined and the approximate site of the lesion determined.

In myasthenia gravis, the amplitude of the impulses gradually decreases during contraction, due to too rapid fatigue of the neuromuscular synapses. In some diseases split "polyphasic" waveforms occur.

Of special interest are the discharges, **fibrillations**, that occur spontaneously in a denervated muscle a couple of weeks after the injury has been inflicted. These denervation potentials have a lower amplitude ($<100 \mu V$) and a shorter duration (≈ 1 ms) than normal action potentials. The fibrillations are not under voluntary control. Unlike the action potentials of motor units, they occur in individual muscle fibers. Denervation of a muscle can only be disclosed by demonstrating fibrillations electromyographically.

4.85	In contraction of a skeletal muscle, action potentials are generated in the	
4.86	The action potentials of the motor units can be picked up with .... electrodes.	motor units
4.87	The action potential has an amplitude of ...., a duration of ...., and a maximum frequency of .... The recording apparatus must be capable of reproducing frequencies over a range of at least	needle
4.88	The frequency of the action potential in the relaxed muscle is .... Hz.	$50 \mu V–2$ mV 2–10 ms 60 Hz 20–5000 Hz
4.89	A patient has had numbness in the left little finger and reduced motor power during abduction and adduction (page 41) of the left fingers. Electromyography shows loss of motor units, which points to a .... (muscular disease, nerve lesion).	0
4.90	The area supplied by the damaged nerve in the previous question can be determined by means of an electromyographic examination of various .... of the hand and forearm; the lesion is found to be located somewhere in the ulnar nerve.	nerve lesion

4.91	In a road accident, a blow on the outside of the arm fractures a person's right arm. He is unable to extend the wrist or fingers of the hand. Two weeks later fibrillations are recorded from all muscles supplied by the radial nerve. These muscles have thus been . . . . , due to nerve damage caused by the accident.	muscles
4.92	The denervation potentials demonstrated in the previous case have a . . . . (lower, higher) amplitude and a . . . . (shorter, longer) duration than normal action potentials.	denervated
		lower shorter

Conduction Velocities in Motor Nerves

To be able to treat a traumatic nerve lesion, its exact position must be determined. This cannot be done by electromyography, since the nerve function must be examined directly in the various segments of the nerve.

The measurement of conduction velocity in motor nerves is technically simple and usually indicates the location and type of the lesion; only in special cases is it necessary to resort to electroneurography, which is technically more difficult to perform.

To measure conduction velocity, the nerve is stimulated with a brief electric shock having a pulse duration of 0.2–0.5 ms. The stimulation is produced via electrodes placed on the skin over the nerve. This elicits impulses in the nerve fibers, and when the excitation reaches the muscle, this contracts with a short twitch. Since all nerve fibers are stimulated at the same time, and since the conduction velocity is normally about the same in all the nerve fibers, there is practically synchronous activation of all the muscle fibers. The action potential of the muscle is picked up with surface or needle electrodes, and displayed on an oscilloscope, together with the stimulating impulse (Fig. 4.13). The elapsed time, the **latency**, between the stimulating impulse and the muscles' action potential, is composed of the time for the impulse to be conducted by the nerve and the time for transmission of the impulse in the nerve-end branches and neuromuscular synapses (page 21). In order to determine only the conduction velocity in a given nerve segment, the latencies must be measured for stimulation proximal and distal to the desired nerve segment. The conduction velocity in the nerve segment is given by the distance between the two points of stimulation divided by the difference in the two latencies.

The conduction velocity can be reduced, or the conductivity can be abolished, over a short segment of the nerve, while remaining normal proximal and distal to

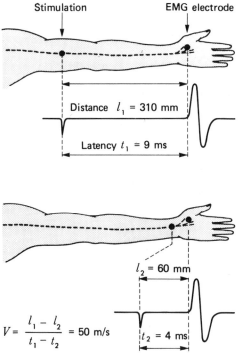

$$V = \frac{l_1 - l_2}{t_1 - t_2} = 50 \text{ m/s}$$

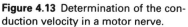

Figure 4.13 Determination of the conduction velocity in a motor nerve.

the lesion. In fairly severe injury, the conduction velocity can be reduced, or the conductivity can be totally abolished, over the whole distance distal to the lesion. The conduction velocity is normally 50 m/s; values below 40 m/s are pathological.

4.93	The exact position of a nerve lesion can be determined by measuring nerve	
4.94	To measure conduction velocity, the nerve is stimulated by electrical impulses of short duration via electrodes placed on the .... over the nerve, and the action potentials evoked in the .... are recorded.	conduction velocity
4.95	Conduction velocity is given by the .... between the two points of stimulation, divided by the .... in the two latencies, for stimulation proximal and distal to the desired nerve segment.	skin muscle

4.96	A person has long been troubled by numbness in the little finger of the left hand and some loss of power in the hand itself. The conduction velocity in the ulnar nerve is measured and found to be normal, about .... (velocity), throughout the nerve except for a short segment in the elbow, where it is 20 m/s, a .... value. Diagnosis: local .... due to pinching of the nerve in the elbow between the ulna and humerus. An operation is performed, in which the nerve is moved to a more protected position on the anterior side of the arm.	distance difference
4.97	A person sleeps in a drunken stupor on a park bench. The wooden bench presses on the outside of the arm for several hours. The patient awakens with total paralysis of the radial nerve, and measurement of conduction velocity over the lesion showed a value of .... (<40 m/s, 0 m/s), that is, nervous impulses .... (are conducted slowly, are not conducted). Since nerve fibers regenerate at a rate of about 1 mm a day, the patient should recover after about .... (time).	50 m/s pathological nerve damage
		0 m/s are not conducted 1 year

Electroneurography

The activity in the peripheral nerves can be examined by stimulating the nerve electrically and picking up the resulting nerve impulses with a fine needle. To avoid nerve damage, specially designed needles must be used; they should have a tip diameter of less than 0.01 mm and be tapered to a maximum shank diameter of 0.2 mm, at a distance greater than 1 mm from the tip. The stimulus is a brief electric shock applied to the skin over the nerve, using surface electrodes, and action potentials are usually picked up proximal to the site of excitation (Fig. 4.14). Both sensory and motor nerve fibers can be examined in this way. If the conduction velocity in different fibers is altered, the amplitude and waveshape of the nerve action potentials are also altered, and these changes are a diagnostically more valuable measure of nerve function than are absolute values of the conduction velocity. Electroneurography is technically more difficult to perform than the measurement of motor nerve conduction velocity and is used only in cases where the latter does not provide reliable information.

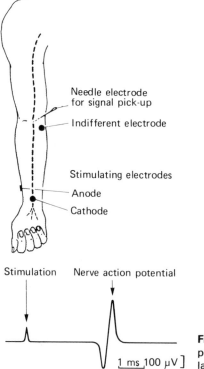

Needle electrode
for signal pick-up

Indifferent electrode

Stimulating electrodes

Anode

Cathode

Stimulation   Nerve action potential

1 ms 100 µV]

Figure 4.14 Measurement of nerve potential for median nerve after stimulation of the wrist.

4.98	In electroneurography, the . . . . elicited in a nerve fiber after stimulation are measured.	
4.99	In electroneurography, stimulation is performed using short electrical impulses via . . . . electrodes and the action potentials are picked up with . . . . electrodes.	action potentials
4.100	With electroneurography, it is possible to determine the conduction velocity in both . . . . and . . . . nerve fibers.	surface (skin) needle
4.101	Diagnostically more important than the absolute value of the conduction velocity is the . . . . of the action potentials, since this changes characteristically in various pathological states.	sensory motor
		waveshape

NEUROPHYSIOLOGICAL MEASUREMENT TECHNIQUES

The problems of measurement technique in neurophysiology are similar to those in electrocardiography; however, the amplitude of the electrical signals is often lower and the electrode impedances higher, resulting in greater demands on the neurophysiological apparatus.

Electrodes

There are two types of electrodes, namely, surface electrodes, which are applied to the skin, and needle electrodes, which are inserted into muscles or nerves to obtain localized recordings.

A surface electrode consists of a disc, 0.5–2 cm in diameter. It is made of a metal that gives a low polarization voltage, for example, silver electrolytically coated in a sodium chloride bath so that contact is obtained via a layer of silver chloride, an Ag–AgCl electrode. Surface electrodes are applied to the skin, which has been cleaned of oil, with a thin layer of electrode paste as is done in picking up ECG signals (page 203). The electrodes are kept in place by means of elastic bands, suction, plastic tape or adhesion. Surface electrodes usually have a resistance of $< 10\,k\Omega$. To avoid errors in EEG recording, the electrode impedance is determined from the voltage division of an ac voltage, applied across the electrode and a series coupled resistor. A surface electrode picks up the electrical activity from all the underlying tissues. Therefore, the origin of the signals cannot be accurately located.

There are two types of needle electrodes: unipolar and coaxial (Fig. 4.15). The unipolar electrode consists of a fine needle which, except for the actual tip, is covered with an insulating layer. The reference for a unipolar electrode is a surface electrode placed on the skin. A coaxial electrode consists of an insulated

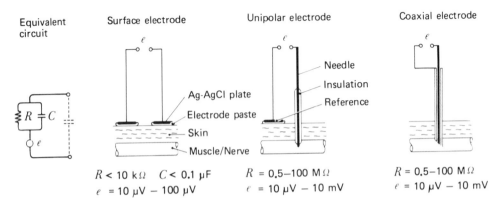

Figure 4.15 Electrode systems for picking up neurophysiological potentials.

wire threaded through a hyperdermic needle, which has an oblique tip for easy penetration.

Unipolar needle electrodes range in diameter from 0.001 to 0.2 mm, and coaxial electrodes from 0.2 to 0.5 mm. Because of the small contact area with the tissue, the impedance is high, generally 0.5–100 MΩ.

For recording the action potentials from a single nerve, a microelectrode must be used. In a glass microelectrode, the central conductor consists of an electrolyte solution, which fills a tapered glass tube; the high impedance at the tip is largely resistive. If a microelectrode is made of metal, the capacitive component of the tip impedance will be large, due to polarization at the metal surface. For both microelectrodes, there is a shunt capacity (indicated by a broken line in Fig. 4.15), which often requires that a special amplifier be used.

With needle electrodes it is possible to pick up action potentials from selected nerves and muscles—and individual motor units—and this offers greater diagnostic possibilities than does recording with surface electrodes.

Amplifiers

The recording of neurophysiological phenomena calls for a special amplifier technique because of the nature of the signals picked up and the type of electrodes used. The signals have a low amplitude, 10μV–10 mV, and the electrodes have a high impedance, 10 kΩ–100 MΩ.

The amplifier should not load the signal source, because of the risk of electrode polarization. For low frequencies, enough current flows during one-half cycle to charge up the capacitor, C, shown in Fig. 4.15. The capacitor voltage (back electromotive force), subtracts from the measured biopotential, e, thus distorting the waveform. This process, called polarization, can be minimized by keeping the current low, which is accomplished by having a high amplifier input impedance. The magnitude of the polarization is primarily dependent on the current density in the area of contact between tissue and metal electrode.

The use of microelectrodes places extreme demands on the input stage of the amplifier, not only so that the current drawn through the electrode will be low, but also so that the maximum base current (grid current in a vacuum-tube amplifier) will be low enough, $<10^{-11}$ A, to avoid damage to the system on which the measurements are to be made—for example, a neuron.

Input impedances of $>10^9 \Omega$ are required, for they must be at least two orders of magnitude higher than the electrode impedances.

Another difficulty is that the measurements are performed on a system in which external interference signals are many times stronger than the signals to be recorded. The interference may enter the amplifier input circuit as a result of capacitive, inductive or resistive coupling (Fig. 4.16).

In capacitive coupling, C, there is electric field interference from nearby power-lines. This interference can be reduced by using shields, differential amplifiers (page 205) and auxiliary amplifiers for active grounding (page 206).

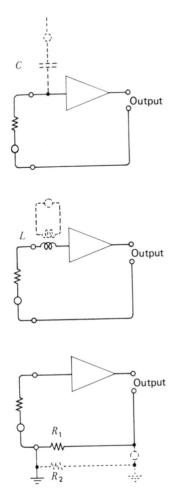

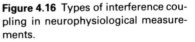

Figure 4.16 Types of interference coupling in neurophysiological measurements.

In inductive coupling, L, the interference is induced by magnetic fields passing through loops in the input circuit; this form of interference can be eliminated only by reducing the fields and keeping the areas of the loops small.

Resistively generated interference occurs in the case of incorrect ground connections—for example, as shown in the lowest circuit in Fig. 4.16. By grounding both the electrode system and the amplifier, a ground loop is formed with two resistances, R_1 and R_2, creating a voltage divider for any interference induced in the loop. Even if R_1 is small, large potentials can be generated in it due to the high current in the low impedance loop. In order to avoid ground loops, grounding should be performed at only one point.

When using high impedance electrodes, the input circuit should contain driven shields (Fig. 4.17). If the shields were connected to ground in the conventional

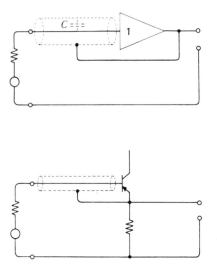

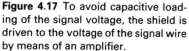

Figure 4.17 To avoid capacitive loading of the signal voltage, the shield is driven to the voltage of the signal wire by means of an amplifier.

way, the signal would be attenuated due to the capacitance C between the shield and the wire, and the higher frequencies would be cut off. For example, a capacitance of 100 pF at 10 kHz gives an impedance of about 0.2 MΩ, which is considerably lower than the electrode impedance 0.5–100 MΩ. To avoid this attenuation, the shield around the signal wire is driven to the same potential as the signal wire itself, by means of an impedance-converting amplifier—for example, an emitter follower. The effect of the capacitance is greatly reduced and attenuation of the signal is avoided.

4.102	Electrodes for picking up neurophysiological phenomena are of two types: .... and	
4.103	Surface electrodes are applied to the .... with a layer of .... to reduce the contact impedance to <..........	surface electrodes needle electrodes
4.104	Needle electrodes are of two types: .... and	skin electrode paste 10 kΩ
4.105	Because of the small area of contact between needle electrodes and tissue, these electrodes have a high impedance, typically	unipolar coaxial

4.106	An amplifier connected to needle electrodes must have a very high . . . ., to reduce the load on the electrodes, which for metal electrodes might result in	0.5–100 MΩ
4.107	The magnitude of the polarization for a given electrode material is dependent primarily on the . . . . at the surface of contact between electrode and tissue.	input impedance polarization
4.108	In polarization a . . . . force is generated.	current density
4.109	This back electromotive force subtracts from the desired biopotential, thus distorting the	back electromotive
4.110	Interference can enter the input circuit of an amplifier by three types of coupling: . . . ., ... and	waveform
4.111	Capacitive interference can be eliminated by . . . . the input circuit, using a . . . . and using	capacitive inductive resistive
4.112	An auxiliary amplifier for active grounding is used to eliminate interference due to the . . . . field.	shielding differential amplifier active grounding
4.113	Interference due to inductive coupling can be minimized only by decreasing the . . . . and reducing the area of . . . . in the input circuit.	electric
4.114	Resistively generated interference arises through incorrect	interfering magnetic fields loops
4.115	To avoid capacitive loading of an input circuit, the wire's shield is driven to the same potential as the . . . . by means of an . . . . amplifier.	grounding
		wire impedance-converting

Recording of neurophysiological data

The choice of recording method is dependent on the frequency range of the signals examined and the presence of any interference. Mechanical recording devices of the fluid jet type (page 209), or of the moving coil galvanometer type, similar to those used in electrocardiography, are used when the upper frequency limit of these mechanical systems is satisfactory, for example, in electroencephalography, where the signals do not contain frequencies over 50 Hz. In electromyography and electroneurography and in the measurement of motor nerve conduction velocities, the frequency range of the signals is higher, with a maximum of about 30 kHz, and therefore cathode ray oscilloscopes are often used. The recording must then be performed photographically—for example, with Polaroid cameras. Electrostatic recorders, working on a principle similar to the Xerographic method, can record at these frequencies on specially prepared paper.

Special problems arise when the signals to be recorded contain so much noise that they cannot be directly displayed. This is often so in the case of **evoked potentials,** which are responses provoked by stimulation in one way or another. Evoked potentials in the EEG can be elicited by visual or acoustic stimuli (page 240). In electroneurographic recording they are generated by electrical stimulation (page 256). In order to display such a signal, which is mixed with a large component of noise, averaging techniques are used, in which the stimulating impulse serves as a time reference. One simple method is to photograph the signals on an oscilloscope, with repeated exposure of the same film, the light intensity being chosen so that each sweep just barely darkens the film. During repeated sweeps, which are synchronized by means of the stimulus impulse, the places on the film where exposures are superimposed will be more intensely darkened. After a hundred or so sweeps, the signals can be distinguished easily from the lightly exposed noise.

A better display of the signal in the presence of noise is obtained using an average response computer. Each evoked response is divided into a series of time intervals, say 400. In real time, interval one's analog value is converted into a digital value and added to the previous value stored in memory location one (which is zero, at the beginning). This is repeated for all 400 intervals, to complete the processing for the first evoked response. The second evoked response is similarly added to the first, and so on up to the number desired, say 100. Then each memory location contains the sum of all responses for a particular instant of time. Evoked responses are all in the same direction, are directly summed and therefore are proportional to N, the number of responses. Background noise has random directions and sums as $\sqrt{N}$. Thus the signal-to-noise ratio is improved by the factor $N/\sqrt{N} = \sqrt{N}$.

There are also analog computers for averaging, in which values are stored on capacitors charged via field effect transistors. The result after averaging can be displayed on an oscilloscope as a smoothed curve which is largely cleared of the noise that was present in each individual signal. A block diagram for such a system with the associated electronics for interference suppression, is shown in Fig. 4.18.

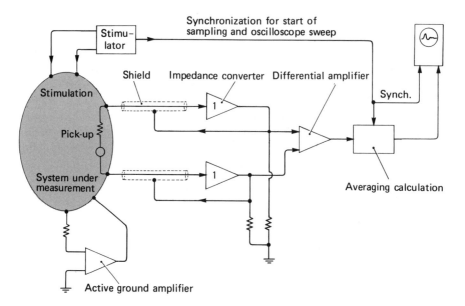

Figure 4.18 Example of an experimental arrangement using an average response computer for calculating the mean value of evoked potentials.

REFERENCES

AIDLEY, D. J. *The Physiology of Excitable Cells.* Cambridge (Cambridge University Press) 1971. 468 pages.

FORSTER, F. M. *Clinical Neurology.* St. Louis (Mosby) 1973. 208 pages.

KILOH, L. G. and OSSELTON, J. W. *Clinical Electroencephalography.* Washington, D.C. (Butterworth) 1966. 147 pages.

NETTER, F. H. *The CIBA Collection of Medical Illustrations,* Vol. 1, *Nervous System.* Summit, NJ (CIBA Pharmaceutical Co.) 1972. 168 pages.

STRONG, P. *Biophysical Measurements.* Beaverton, Ore. (Tektronix) 1970. 499 pages.

THOMPSON, R. F. and PATTERSON, M. M. *Bioelectric Recording Techniques, Part B, Electroencephalography and Human Brain Potentials.* New York (Academic Press) 1974. 327 pages.

chapter 5

Clinical Chemistry
and Hematology

Most pathological processes result in chemical changes in the internal environment of the body. The changes can often be demonstrated by analysis of various samples. Clinical chemistry has become one of the most important supportive medical sciences, not only for making **diagnoses** but also for **checking treatment** and for making a **prognosis** (page 102).

Samples taken from various parts of the body and under different conditions are examined. The most common substance for analysis is **blood**. This would be expected, since the most important function of blood is to serve as a transport medium—many pathological processes in the body lead to chemically demonstrable changes in the blood. Deviations from the normal composition of **urine** also reflect many pathological processes; this is because urine is a filtration product of blood. Other common substances for analysis are the **gastric juice**, the **feces** and the **cerebrospinal fluid**, which surrounds the central nervous system (pages 79 and 82). Thus, it is the body fluids that are most frequently examined; only rarely are chemical analyses of biopsy specimens of tissue performed.

In this chapter, examples are given of the clinical applications of chemical analyses. Some facts concerning the origin of blood, urine and other commonly examined substances are presented. The normal composition of these is given, as are the changes that occur in certain pathological processes. Some of the most common analytical procedures are also described. First, however, some general remarks are presented on how the results of analyses are evaluated in relation to what may be regarded as normal, and on the difficulties encountered when attempting to establish normal values.

Normal values

It is often difficult in medicine to state what is normal and what is abnormal. For example, it is a matter of opinion whether a person 2 meters in height is abnormal—nor is it of much medical interest how the classification is made. What is beyond doubt, however, is that the person is taller than the average (mean) for the population. We can also express in statistical terms how much a person's height differs from this mean. The situation is similar for practically all chemical analyses: the limiting values for what is normal cannot be established exactly. It is necessary to assess the analytical results from a statistical point of view.

A number of biological variables show a **normal distribution**. This is the case for body height: if the number of persons is plotted as a function of body height, a normally distributed frequency curve (gaussian curve) is obtained (Fig. 5.1). Similar curves are sometimes obtained for the concentration of certain substances in the blood or urine for a large number of normal subjects. Similarly, normal distribution curves are obtained if the same analysis is repeated many times on one and the same sample.

Number of observations

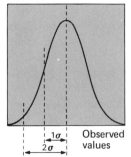
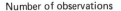
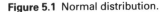

Observed values

Figure 5.1 Normal distribution.

In the case of a normally distributed variable, it is easy to express statistically how a certain analytical value is related to the mean for the normal population. We use the standard deviation $\sigma = [\Sigma(x - m)^2/(n - 1)]^{1/2}$, where x is the observed value, n the number of observations and $m = \Sigma x/n$, the arithmetical mean. In a normally distributed variable, 95.5 percent of the observed values fall within the range $\pm 2\sigma$. In clinical chemistry the **normal range** is usually given as the mean $\pm 2\sigma$.

Often, however, biological variables are not normally distributed. This is particularly the case when the mean lies near a limit that cannot be exceeded. Thus, the survival time after treatment for a malignant tumor disease has a skew distribution. The same is the case for many laboratory tests in clinical use. For example, the number of white blood cells per cubic millimeter has a skew distribution in a normal population. The erythrocyte sedimentation rate, ESR, in millimeters per hour (page 288) is another example. Skew distributions complicate the statistical analysis and the setting of normal limits. Often, however, skew distributions can be treated as if they were normally distributed by using the logarithms of the values instead of the values themselves (Fig. 5.2).

Number of observations

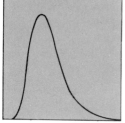

Observed
values

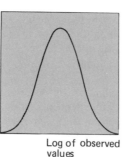

Log of observed
values

Figure 5.2 A skew distribution may often appear normal if the logarithms of the observed values are used.

It is thus impossible in the individual case to distinguish with absolute certainty between normal and abnormal. We can only examine the results of the chemical analyses from a statistical viewpoint. The farther the result of a test for a disease lies outside the normal range, the mean $\pm 2\sigma$, the greater is the probability that the patient is ill; the closer the result of a test is to the mean, the less probable it is that the patient has the disease.

Question	Answer
5.1 A patient consults a physician for general tiredness, lack of energy, thirst and passage of large quantities of urine. The urine is found to contain sugar (glucose), and the blood glucose level is too high. The clinical chemistry examination thus confirms the tentative ...., made when the history was taken, namely, that the patient is suffering from diabetes mellitus.	

5.2	In the subsequent care of the patient, clinical chemistry analyses of the patient's urine and blood are used for a	diagnosis
5.3	A patient with rheumatic fever feels that he has improved in the last month. The patient's ESR, however, is very high. This laboratory finding indicates that the patient has not yet recovered, and that his .... is such that a relapse of the disease is probable.	check of the treatment
5.4	In clinical chemistry examinations, the samples obtained from the patient may consist of ...., ..., ... juice, ... and .... fluid.	prognosis
5.5	A medical examination is performed at a company with a thousand employees. For each laboratory test with normal limits set at $\pm 2\sigma$, the physician will find that about .... percent of the healthy persons will fall outside these limits.	blood urine gastric feces cerebrospinal
5.6	If, in the medical examinations in the previous question, 10 mutually independent laboratory examinations were performed on the same persons, about .... percent of the healthy persons will have at least one test outside the normal range. (For the reader interested in probability calculations; others should memorize the answer.)	5
		40

MEDICAL DIAGNOSIS WITH CHEMICAL TESTS

In this section a brief account is given of the origin and composition of the various substances analyzed by chemical tests. This knowledge is necessary in order to understand the changes that occur when pathological processes are present in the body. Some examples are also given of how the pathological processes can be diagnosed and followed by means of chemical analyses.

BLOOD

The liquid part of the blood, the **blood plasma**, and the formed elements, the **blood cells**, are analyzed during a chemical examination. The blood plasma accounts for about 60 percent of the blood volume, and the blood cells occupy the other 40 percent.

The study of the blood-forming organs and their diseases is called **hematology**. This includes the study of the microscopic appearance of the blood cells and the changes that occur in pathological states.

To understand the significance of the composition of the blood and its pathological changes, it is necessary to know the most important functions of the blood:

To the cells of the body, the blood transports the products of digestion from the intestines, and oxygen from the lungs.

From the cells of the body, the blood transports the products of combustion to the excretory organs—carbon dioxide to the lungs and a large number of low molecular weight substances to the kidneys, intestines and skin.

The blood is part of the body's regulatory system and conveys information—among other things, through hormones from the glands of internal secretion—so that the function of the other organs is effectively coordinated and the internal chemical environment will be optimal for the cells of the body.

The blood is part of the body's system of defense against infection by microorganisms and foreign substances.

The blood has the ability to coagulate, so as to prevent bleeding to death and to enable tissue wounds to heal.

Blood Plasma and Blood Serum

Blood plasma contains both low and high molecular weight substances. The low-molecular weight substances consist of organic substances and electrolytes, while the macromolecular substances consist mainly of proteins.

The plasma is obtained by centrifuging a blood sample that has been prevented from coagulating by adding an anticoagulant. During centrifugation, the heavy blood cells become packed at the bottom of the centrifuge tube and the plasma can be removed. The plasma is a somewhat viscous, light-yellow liquid that is almost clear in the fasting state.

The blood serum is obtained by centrifuging a blood sample that has been allowed to clot. During coagulation a dissolved macromolecular substance, **fibrinogen**, is converted to insoluble **fibrin** (page 292). Fibrin consists of invisible fibers that hold the clot together. Blood serum is thus the liquid part of clotted blood.

5.7   The liquid part of the blood is known as . . . .

5.8	Blood plasma is obtained by . . . . blood that has been prevented from coagulating.	plasma
5.9	Blood serum is . . . . from which the . . . . has been removed.	centrifuging
5.10	Blood serum is obtained by centrifuging blood that has been allowed to	plasma fibrinogen
5.11	The study of blood-forming organs and their diseases is known as	clot
		hematology

Electrolytes in the blood

The most abundant positive ions in the body are sodium, potassium and calcium. The most abundant negative ions are phosphate, chloride and bicarbonate. The correct concentrations of ions are necessary for the normal function of the cells and the body (Table 5.1).

The ion concentrations vary over wide limits at different places in the body; for example, most potassium is located intracellularly and most sodium extracellularly.

Sodium is the most abundant **extracellular** positive ion. It plays a central role in the body's electrolyte and fluid balance. Changes in sodium ion concentration are usually accompanied by changes in the water balance; this is because the body tends to keep constant both the fluid volume and the sodium ion concentration in the extracellular space (page 26). The responsible regulatory organs are the adrenal glands, which control the excretion of sodium and water through the kidneys by means of a hormone (aldosterone).

An increase of the sodium concentration in the blood serum occurs in **dehydration**, in certain types of **renal damage** that cause edema (accumulation of fluid interstitially, page 28) and in **adrenocortical hyperfunction**, that is, increased secretion of hormone by the adrenal glands, as occurs in Cushing's syndrome.

A reduction in the sodium ion concentration occurs in **diarrhea** (in which the body loses sodium), in types of **renal damage** that cause increased excretion of sodium and in **adrenocortical hypofunction** (inadequate output of hormone), as in Addison's disease.

Potassium. The correct potassium ion distribution is of vital importance for cell function—most potassium is located **intracellularly**. For example, serum must have a correct potassium concentration for normal nerve cell conduction and for normal muscle cell contraction.

Of particular importance is the effect on the heart muscle; if the potassium concentration in the serum exceeds a certain level, there is risk of cardiac arrest due to prolonged diastole—**asystole**.

There is an increased serum potassium concentration, **hyperkalemia**, in certain types of **renal damage** and in several diseases, among them **adrenocortical hypofunction**, **shock** and **acidosis**.

A depressed potassium level, **hypokalemia**, is found in **adrenocortical hyperfunction**—thus, this situation is opposite to that for sodium.

Calcium has several functions in the body. Besides being a component of the **skeleton**, which includes about 1 kg of calcium, it occurs extracellularly in ionic form. The correct calcium ion concentration is important for nerve and muscle cell function—calcium is antagonistic to potassium. If too much calcium ion is given in an intravenous injection, there is risk of affecting the heart, with consequent circulatory arrest—just as in the case of increased potassium ion concentration—though calcium produces **fibrillation** whereas potassium produces asystole

Calcium is also of importance for the permeability of cell membranes and for the **clotting** of **blood** (page 291).

Phosphate. Phosphorus metabolism is linked with calcium metabolism. This would be expected since the substance that endows the **skeleton** with its hardness is hydroxyapatite—calcium phosphate.

The body tends to keep the product of the calcium and phosphate ions in the plasma constant. This is controlled in part by a hormone from the parathyroid gland. In increased excretion of parathyroid hormone, **hyperparathyroidism**, the serum calcium level is raised and the serum phosphate level lowered. In hypoparathyroidism the opposite situation prevails. Hyperparathyroidism results in decalcification of the skeleton, and often renal damage through the formation of kidney stones.

Bicarbonate ions are essential for maintaining the correct hydrogen ion concentration in the body. Bicarbonate ions are part of a buffer system, which acts according to the Henderson–Hasselbalch equation (page 157). Thus, in **acidosis** and **alkalosis**, it is of great importance to determine the bicarbonate ion concentration. It can be expressed as either the "standard bicarbonate" value or the "base excess" value. They are used for quantifying acid base disturbances in, for example, intensive care (page 575).

Chloride. The chloride ion is the most abundant negative ion in the extracellular fluid. Less is known about mechanisms of chloride balance than the other abundant ions, but it is nevertheless an important measurement. Among other things, it provides useful information bearing on the presence of other positive ions in blood; i.e., chloride is displaced by the positive ions of organic acids which are not routinely measured. The presence of low chloride and low bicarbonate ion concentration is indirect evidence of the presence of organic acid negative ions.

Table 5.1 Example of electrolytes in the serum

Ion	Normal values		Examples of diagnostic use	
	mEq/l*	SI units mmol/l	Elevated values	Lowered values
sodium	138–148	138–148	renal damage, adrenocortical hyperfunction, dehydration	renal failure, adrenocortical hypofunction
potassium	3.6–5.1	3.6–5.1	adrenocortical hypofunction, shock, acidosis	adrenocortical hyperfunction
calcium	4.3–5.3	2.2–2.7	hyperparathyroidism	hypoparathyroidism, reduced absorption
phosphate	2.2–5.0	0.7–1.6	hypoparathyroidism	hyperparathyroidism
bicarbonate	22–30	22–30	metabolic alkalosis	metabolic acidosis
chloride	95–110	95–110	respiratory alkalosis, hyperparathyroidism	diabetic acidosis, lactic acid acidosis, persistent vomiting

* mEq/l = milliequivalent per liter; equivalent = moleweight/valence

5.12	Abundant positive ions in the body are ...., ... and	
5.13	The most abundant negative ions are ...., ... and	sodium (Na$^+$) potassium (K$^+$) calcium (Ca^{++})
5.14	Most sodium is located ....-cellularly and most potassium ....-cellularly.	phosphate (PO$_4^-$) chloride (Cl$^-$) bicarbonate (HCO$_3^-$)
5.15	After eating salty food we become thirsty. This is because the body tends to maintain a constant	extra intra
5.16	In a patient with extensive burns, there is tissue destruction, with the result that potassium leaks from the cells into the blood. The kidneys are unable to compensate for this by increased excretion of potassium. The patient has cardiac arrest due to	sodium ion concentration (1 g NaCl binds 0.1 liter of water)

5.17	In certain hypersensitive reactions accompanied by edema—for example, in the larynx, which results in difficulty in breathing—calcium ions are given intravenously. This must be done slowly so as not to risk producing .... due to a sudden increase in the blood's calcium ion concentration.	asystole
5.18	A patient undergoes an operation for toxic goiter. The parathyroid glands are also removed by mistake. After the operation the patient suffers from increased excitability of the nerves and muscles, which results in a tendency for spasms. This is due to hypoparathyroidism, deficiency of parathyroid hormone, which results in a lowering of the .... concentration in the serum.	ventricular fibrillation
5.19	The "standard bicarbonate" value is determined in suspected disturbance of the .... balance.	calcium ion
		acid-base (acidosis or alkalosis)

Low-molecular weight organic substances in blood serum

The low-molecular weight organic substances in the blood serum consist of **nutrients**, which are taken up by the intestine, or which are mobilized from the body's store, and of **waste products**, which are formed during metabolism in the cells. A large number of these substances can be readily analyzed, and they provide valuable information on both normal and pathological changes in metabolism (Table 5.2).

Carbohydrates are absorbed in the intestine in the form of simple types of sugar, monosaccharides. Of these, **glucose** is clinically the most important. A fasting person normally has a **blood glucose concentration** of 60–110 mg/dl—the unit, mg/dl, expresses the number of mg of examined substance per 100 ml (SI units: 3.3–6.1 mmol/l).

Part of the glucose in the blood is burned in the cells to yield carbon dioxide and water. Some glucose is stored in the liver and muscle, by formation of **glycogen**, or animal starch. Glycogen is one of the most important of the body's reserve supply of nutrients and serves as a quickly mobilizable source of carbohydrate.

In untreated diabetes mellitus, which is mainly due to a relative deficiency of insulin, the blood glucose level becomes elevated. A lowered blood glucose level occurs in hyperinsulinism—that is, when there is too much insulin produced, due, for example, to an insulin-producing tumor in the pancreas.

Table 5.2   Example of some low-molecular weight substances in blood serum

Substance	Normal values		Examples of diagnostic use	
	mg/dl	SI units	Elevated values	Lowered values
glucose	60–110	3.3–6.1 mmol/l	diabetes	hyperinsulinism, starvation
triglycerides	20–150	0.23–1.7 mmol/l	diabetes hyperlipoprotein- emia	
cholesterol	80–300	2.1–8.0 mmol/l	diabetes, arteriosclerosis	disturbed intestinal absorption, liver damage
ketone bodies	1–5		diabetes, starva- tion, fever	
creatinine	0.8–1.3	70–115 μmol/l	renal failure, dehydration	pregnancy, reduced muscle mass
urea	20–45	3.3–7.5 mmol/l	renal failure, dehydration	
bilirubin	<1.2	<20 μmol/l	biliary stasis, liver damage, hemolytic state	

Fats   are transported in the blood in different ways. They can occur in the form of small fat droplets, or as fatty acids or as converted fat-like compounds. Fat also occurs in the blood as lipoproteins—fat compounds linked to the proteins. The fats pass through the intestinal wall without completely breaking down (or the fats are resynthesized after resorption) so that they are taken up by the lymph ducts in the intestines as finely divided fat droplets and pass into the blood via the thoracic duct (page 61). After a fatty meal the blood serum becomes opalescent (cloudy) due to the presence of these fat droplets. The fat droplets, which consist mainly of triglycerides, are taken up by the fatty tissues and by the liver. From the fat deposits, free fatty acids can be mobilized as required. Fat normally burns to yield carbon dioxide and water. More than one half of the body's calorie requirements are furnished by combustion of the free fatty acids.

Part of the fat circulating in the blood is taken up by the liver, where it is partially metabolized, with the formation of various compounds. One of these is **cholesterol**, a substance that is the primary material for the synthesis of a group of compounds known as **steroids**. These include the adrenal and sex hormones. Most cholesterol is oxidized to cholic acids and excreted by the liver, through the bile ducts to the duodenum. There they serve an important detergent function of importance in the absorption of fat.

To demonstrate disturbances in fat metabolism, the serum concentrations of **triglycerides** and **cholesterol** are determined. Of particular interest is the fact that elevated cholesterol values are considered to be a causal factor in the development of arteriosclerosis—a disease that begins with deposition of fat in the vessel walls.

In disturbed combustion of glucose, as occurs in untreated diabetes, the body mobilizes other energy sources. There is combustion of fat, but this is incomplete and organic acids are formed. The patient develops metabolic acidosis (page157). The substances formed are known as **ketone bodies**, which is a collective name for acetone and the closely related compounds, acetoacetic acid and β-hydroxybutyric acid. The ketone bodies are excreted in the urine. Normally, neither blood nor urine contains demonstrable amounts. Elevated values are found in diabetes and in other conditions where there is fat metabolization, such as fever states and starvation (see questions 2.66 and 2.67).

Nitrogen-containing substances in the serum. The proteins in food are broken down to **amino acids** before they are absorbed in the small intestine. The amino acids, of which there are a score or so different ones, are used in the synthesis of the body's proteins. In addition, amino acids are used for the synthesis of other nitrogen-containing substances, such as **creatine**. This is a key substance utilized in muscular contraction. Elevated creatine values are observed in certain serious muscle diseases, for example, myasthenia gravis, progressive muscular dystrophy and poliomyelitis. The end product of creatine metabolism is **creatinine**, which is excreted in the urine. Because creatinine is formed in constant amounts every day and is excreted only through the kidneys, it is possible to determine the degree of the renal damage by measuring the concentration in the serum. Elevated creatinine values are thus seen in renal failure, since the kidneys then are unable to maintain adequate excretion. Elevated values are also seen in dehydrated patients. Lowered values are observed in pregnancy and in patients with reduced muscle mass.

Since amino acids cannot be stored in the body, any excess must be broken down. This occurs in different ways; one way involves a metabolic cycle in the liver, in which the amine group is removed and metabolized to **urea** while the rest of the molecule is burned as though it were carbohydrate. Urea is excreted through the kidneys. Thus, in renal damage, elevated values of urea in the serum are obtained.

Bile pigment. In the breakdown of **hemoglobin**—the pigment of the red blood cells—several other colored substances, **bile pigments**, are formed. These are of importance in the diagnosis of liver diseases.

Hemoglobin consists of a protein component, **globin**, and a low molecular weight component, the **heme** group, which is red in color. The heme component is liberated when the hemoglobin is broken down and is converted to **biliverdin**, a green pigment, which is then converted to **bilirubin**, a reddish-yellow pigment. The breakdown takes place in the reticuloendothelial system, RES, which consists of certain cells in locations such as the spleen, liver and bone marrow (page 343).

Bilirubin is taken up by the liver and excreted in the bile in a water soluble form as bilirubin glucuronide (Fig. 5.3). In the intestines these products are converted to the colorless **urobilinogen** and the yellowish-brown pigment,

urobilin, which gives the feces their typical color. A portion of these substances is taken up from the intestines and excreted in the urine; they do not, however, normally give the urine its color; only in pathological conditions can they give a color change.

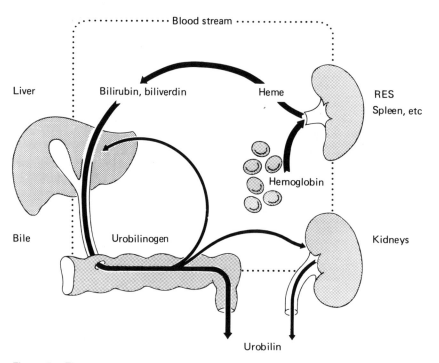

Figure 5.3 The bile pigment consists of breakdown products of the heme group of the hemoglobin.

In liver damage or biliary stasis due to the presence of gallstones or tumors in the bile ducts, disturbances occur in the metabolism of bile pigment. In total obstruction, the feces are grayish-white and the urine is port colored due to the increased excretion of bile pigment through the kidneys. The patient develops **jaundice** because of the increased amount of bilirubin in the blood.

Even in the normally functioning liver and bile ducts, the amount of bilirubin in the serum can be elevated due to excessive breakdown of blood cells—so-called **hemolytic states** (page 288).

5.20	The blood sugar level on a fasting stomach is normally . . . .

5.21	A person travels through several time zones in an east–west direction; he becomes tired during the day and finds it difficult to sleep at night. This is because the liver rhythm is out of phase. The liver maintains the original 24-hour rhythm for several days, both when building up glycogen, that is . . . ., which is formed from . . . . in the blood, and in the reverse process when the latter substance is mobilized to the blood stream. This results in low . . . . values during the daytime, which results in tiredness, and high values at night, with consequent difficulty in sleeping.	60–110 mg/dl (3.3–6.1 mmol/l)
5.22	Fat normally burns to form . . . . and	animal starch glucose blood glucose
5.23	Read questions 2.66 and 2.67. Both patients smelled of acetone because of disturbed metabolism. There was incomplete burning of	carbon dioxide water
5.24	Certain hormones are derived from cholesterol. These are known as	fat
5.25	A patient with renal damage is treated using an artificial kidney. After treatment, the blood is analyzed to determine the level of an active breakdown product of creatine, known as	steroids
5.26	In the patient in the previous question, it is also possible to determine the concentration of a substance that is the end product of a metabolic cycle in which amino acids are broken down. That substance is	creatinine
5.27	Read question 1.251. The patient's jaundice is caused by an increase in the . . . . level in the blood serum.	urea
		bilirubin

Plasma proteins

The most important macromolecular substances in the blood plasma are the proteins **albumin**, **globulins** and **fibrinogen**. Globulins are a mixed group comprising more than a score of different proteins. Plasma proteins have different functions in the body. Many of them are formed in the liver, such as albumin and fibrinogen. Some plasma proteins are synthesized in other organs, for example, gamma globulin is formed by the reticuloendothelial system, RES, under the influence of phagocytic cells circulating in the blood (page 343). The total amount of plasma protein is normally about 7 g/dl (SI—70 g/l) of plasma (Table 5.3).

Table 5.3 Some data on the proteins in serum

Substance	Amount g/dl	SI units g/l	Molecular weight	Function
total	7	70	—	
albumin	4.4	44	65,000	maintenance of colloid osmotic pressure, nutrition
globulins (>20 different)	2.5	25	40,000–900,000	varying (gamma globulins—antibody defense)
fibrinogen (in plasma)	0.3	3	400,000	blood clotting

The proteins in the serum can be separated by electrophoresis (page 308). This is possible because the protein molecules have different electric charges and their migration velocity in the electric field is therefore different. An electrophoresis curve is shown in Fig. 5.4. As is seen, albumin constitutes the bulk of the plasma protein. Far right are the gamma globulins; which are the body's antibodies—substances which are used as specific defenses against infections (page 344). The peaks which appear between albumin and gamma globulin in electrophoresis are from a variety of substances. They are, however, of diagnostic interest; in pathological conditions—for example, tumor diseases—special macromolecular substances appear in this group.

Colloid osmotic pressure. The plasma proteins are of fundamental importance for the fluid balance of the body. The presence of macromolecular substances in the blood results in a **colloid osmotic pressure**, which is required to maintain a certain blood volume and to produce a circulation of the interstitial fluid (page 26).

The colloid osmotic pressure exists because the capillary walls are semipermeable. They allow low-molecular weight substances, such as water, electrolytes and certain organic compounds, to pass through, but they are impermeable to macromolecular substances. The colloid osmotic pressure is about 25 mm Hg (≈ 3 kPa), and is generated chiefly by albumin. This is not only because albumin constitutes the bulk of the plasma proteins, but also because it has a lower

Amount of substance

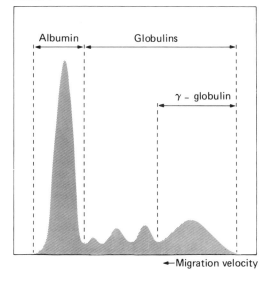

Albumin Globulins

γ – globulin

←—Migration velocity

Figure 5.4 Electrophoresis of normal blood serum.

molecular weight than the other plasma proteins. Albumin thus makes a relatively larger contribution to the colloid osmotic pressure, since this is proportional to the number of molecules per unit volume.

The hydrostatic pressure in the vessels opposes the colloid osmotic pressure. The colloid osmotic pressure tends to draw fluid from the interstitial tissue space—which has a low content of macromolecular substances—and tends to prevent fluid from leaving the blood stream. The hydrostatic pressure in the capillaries, which is generated by heart contractions, acts in the reverse direction. On the whole, the pressures normally balance one another so that the blood volume is kept relatively constant.

If the plasma protein concentration falls below a certain critical level, the colloid osmotic pressure will be too low and water will leave the blood stream and collect interstitially—causing **edema**. Clearly, the determination of the total protein concentration in the serum is an important diagnostic test. For example, in surgical treatment it is of fundamental importance to monitor serum proteins to ensure that the colloid osmotic pressure is maintained. This can be done by giving blood or albumin which is extensively used for restoring the colloid osmotic pressure in the case of blood loss and hence countering shock (page 557).

Circulation of the interstitial fluid is produced by differences in hydrostatic and colloid osmotic pressure in the capillaries (Fig. 5.5). On the arterial side, the hydrostatic pressure, about 30 mm Hg (4 kPa), exceeds the colloid osmotic pressure and fluid is expelled through the semipermeable capillary walls. On the venous side, fluid is drawn back into the capillaries because here the colloid osmotic pressure is greater than the hydrostatic, which can reach 15 mm Hg (2 kPa). A small portion of the interstitial fluid is taken up by the lymph ducts.

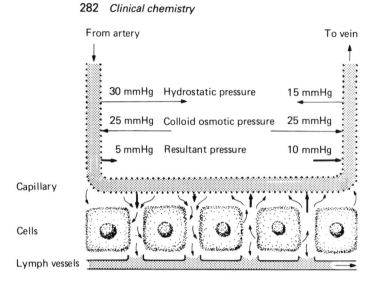

From artery   To vein

30 mmHg   Hydrostatic pressure   15 mmHg

25 mmHg   Colloid osmotic pressure   25 mmHg

5 mmHg   Resultant pressure   10 mmHg

Capillary

Cells

Lymph vessels

Figure 5.5 Circulation of the interstitial fluid is due to differences between the hydrostatic and colloid osmotic pressure. To convert from mm Hg (shown) to kPa (SI units), multiply by 0.133, or see scales on Fig. 2.17.

5.28	Albumin, globulins and fibrinogen are the body's most important	
5.29	A patient suffers a blood loss and no blood for transfusion is available. There are two infusion liquids to choose between, isotonic saline (0.9 percent NaCl) and albumin. To ensure normal circulation, the blood volume must be maintained. For this reason .... is given.	plasma proteins
5.30	If in the previous question isotonic saline had been given, it would immediately have passed out into the .... space and there produced .... (collection of fluid in this space).	albumin
5.31	A patient has an exceptionally low resistance to infections. Electrophoresis performed on the plasma disclosed the cause, namely, a low .... level.	interstitial edema
		gamma globulin

Enzyme concentration

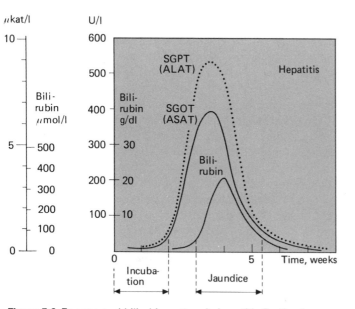

Figure 5.6 Enzyme and bilirubin pattern in hepatitis B—the rise lasts several weeks.

Enzyme concentration

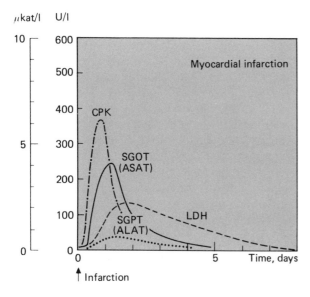

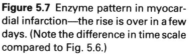

Figure 5.7 Enzyme pattern in myocardial infarction—the rise is over in a few days. (Note the difference in time scale compared to Fig. 5.6.)

283

Enzyme diagnosis. In tissue damage, certain enzymes are liberated from the cells, and the enzymes can then be detected in the blood. Normally, such enzymes are present in high concentrations only inside the cells, not in the blood.

The enzymes are catalysts which make possible the biochemical processes in the cells. The enzymes thus manage the body's **metabolism**. A distinction is made between **catabolism**, which involves breakdown of substances with the resultant liberation of energy, and **anabolism**, which consists of synthesis of the substances requiring energy.

Nearly all protein in the cells consists of enzymes. The body's cells have different functions and contain different amounts, and to some extent also different types, of enzymes. Since they are liberated in tissue damage, by determining the concentration and type of enzymes present in the blood, it is sometimes possible to obtain an indirect indication of where in the body the tissue damage is located. The time during which they appear in the blood is different for different diseases. Diagnostic information can thus be obtained by following the enzyme pattern during the course of the disease.

The enzyme values are measured in different ways. The old measure is the unit U, which is defined as the enzyme activity that under standardized conditions converts 1 μmol of substrate in one minute. The SI-unit is **katal** (catalytic unit), which is defined as the enzyme activity that converts 1 mole of the substrate in one second.

Examples of enzyme patterns in hepatitis and myocardial infarction are given in Fig. 5.6 and Fig. 5.7 on page 283. The increase in the enzyme level lasts 10 times longer in hepatitis than in myocardial infarction (different time scale). Moreover, in hepatitis the increase in SGPT (glutamic-pyruvic transaminase), new term ALAT (alanine-amino-transferase) is greater than in SGOT (glutamic-oxalacetic transaminase), new term ASAT (asparate-amino-transferase); the reverse is true in myocardial infarction. It is of diagnostic interest that an increase in the enzyme level in the blood takes place earlier than an increase in bilirubin—which produces jaundice. In myocardial infarction, LDH (lactic dehydrogenase) reaches a maximum some hours later than SGOT (ASAT) and falls more slowly. The fastest rise and decline occur for the enzyme CPK (creatine phosphokinase).

Some enzymes are specific for certain tissues. For example, an elevated activity of acid phosphatases is a strong indicator of prostate carcinoma. Similarly, OCT (ornithine-carbamyl transferase) is specific for liver damage.

5.32	Metabolism consists of catabolism, in which .... is liberated, and of anabolism, in which the substances are .... in the cells.

5.33	Cell metabolism takes place with the aid of ...., which constitute practically all of the cell's	energy synthesized
5.34	When the cells are damaged, enzymes are liberated and pass into the	enzymes protein
5.35	Enzymes liberated from different cells in the body display unequal enzyme patterns; that is, different enzymes appear in the blood with different .... and for different	blood stream
5.36	A patient has been unusually tired during the past week. The examining physician finds nothing abnormal but takes a blood sample to see whether the enzyme pattern can give a clue. He suspects hepatitis B because of abnormally high .... and .... levels—the former is even higher than the latter. A week later the patient's skin becomes yellow, indicating jaundice, which confirms the suspected diagnosis.	concentrations durations
5.37	A patient has been abnormally tired during the past 24 hours and complains of chest pains. The ECG is normal. Since the diagnosis is difficult, samples are taken for SGOT (ASAT), SGPT (ALAT), LDH, and CPK. Twelve hours after the patient fell ill, all show elevated values, with SGOT (ASAT) and CPK the most elevated. In spite of the negative ECG findings the diagnosis is probably	SGPT (ALAT) SGOT (ASAT)
		myocardial infarction

Blood Cells and Blood Diseases

The blood cells have important functions in the body. The erythrocytes, or red blood cells, transport oxygen and carbon dioxide. The leukocytes, or white blood cells, are part of the body's defenses against infections and foreign substances. The thrombocytes, or blood platelets, are involved in clotting of the blood. A large number of pathological states can develop in the blood cells, some of which are described below.

In the examination of the blood cells, a number of purely chemical methods are used; in the first place, however, hematological methods are used in which the blood cells are examined under the microscope. Determinations are made of the number of white cells, the relative distribution and number of different white blood cells and the occurrence of any abnormal forms, for example, immature stem cells. In addition to the microscopic examination of the blood, samples are taken from the sites in the bone marrow where the blood cells are formed (bone-marrow punctures).

Erythrocytes

The red pigment in the blood cells consists of **hemoglobin**, a red protein with the ability to bind oxygen and carbon dioxide. The blood cells consist of hemoglobin surrounded by a thin membrane. The blood must contain a certain amount of hemoglobin if an adequate transport capacity is to be maintained (page 153).

The amount of hemoglobin in the blood may be too high or too low. These states may be due to temporary changes in the fluid balance or to more profound disorders. The temporary disturbances in fluid balance are **dehydration** (occurs in loss of liquids, for example, after diarrhea or disturbed fluid supply) and **edema** (occurs when too much liquid is given intravenously after an operation). **Polycythemia** is a chronic disease which results in an absolute increase in the amount of hemoglobin in the blood—the body produces too many red blood cells. The most common disorder, however, is **anemia**, blood deficiency, when the blood contains too little hemoglobin.

If the hemoglobin concentration is too high or too low, it is necessary to decide whether it is due to a temporary disorder, in which the patient has a correct amount of hemoglobin relative to the body volume, or whether there is an absolute change in the amount of hemoglobin. In these cases, the patient's medical history is of critical importance for the interpretation of the laboratory findings.

Anemia is accompanied by a number of general symptoms such as headache, tiredness and giddiness.

Anemia can be due to different factors. One obvious cause is bleeding, for example, after operations and accidents. Bleeding from the gastrointestinal tract is also common, and may be due to, for example, peptic ulcer or tumor; however, the source of bleeding may be difficult to find even with a thorough diagnostic examination. Since iron is part of the hemoglobin molecule, iron deficiency is a common cause of anemia, especially in women, who regularly lose blood through menstruation. Other deficiency diseases and absorption disorders can also cause anemia, such as a deficiency of vitamin B_{12}, which causes pernicious anemia (page 353). Finally, anemia occurs as a secondary feature of a large number of diseases: chronic infections (for example, tuberculosis), various forms of carcinoma and nephritis (inflammation of the kidneys).

The amount of hemoglobin in the blood is easy to measure by photometry. The normal **Hb value** for men is 13–17 g/dl (130–170 g/l), and for women 12–16 g/dl (120–160 g/l).

The blood cells make up a portion of the total blood volume. Since the red cells are so much more numerous than the white, a reliable indicator of red cell disorder can be obtained by determining the volume percentage of these in the blood. This **hematocrit value**, or packed cell volume, is obtained by centrifuging a blood sample in a capillary tube. The cells are then packed in the bottom and the volume percentage is determined by measuring the relative height of the packed cells and the plasma with a scale. The normal range of hematocrit for men is 42–54 (%), and for women 37–47. The hematocrit is easy to determine and has a smaller methodological error than determination of the hemoglobin content.

The number of red blood cells is also counted and this can be done under a microscope. The diluted sample is placed in a counting chamber of known volume on the stage of the microscope. Men normally have 4.5–5.5 million/μl, and women 4.0–5.0 million/μl. The number is increased in dehydration and polycythemia and decreased in anemia and dilution of the blood. Such dilution occurs after an operation, when a plasma substitute, such as dextran is given.

Since microscope counting is time consuming, most red blood cell counts are performed on an automatic blood cell counter. The method is based on the fact that red cells have a higher electrical resistivity than the saline solution in which they are suspended. A diluted blood sample is drawn through a small orifice ($<100 \mu$m), while the electrical conductivity is measured across it by means of two electrodes placed in the solution on opposite sides, Fig. 5.8. Since the column

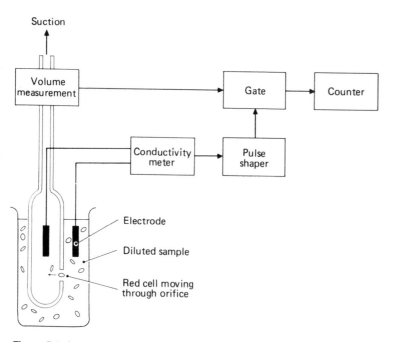

Figure 5.8 Automatic blood cell counter.

of saline within the orifice constitutes the greater part of the resistance between the electrodes, each single red cell moving through the orifice will produce a sudden increase in resistance, which will be detected as an impulse in a conductivity meter. The number of impulses is counted for a certain volume displacement through the orifice, and this gives the red cell count.

While the diameter of the red blood cells can also be determined, it is usually of greater interest to measure the mean corpuscular volume, the mean corpuscular hemoglobin and the mean corpuscular hemoglobin concentration.

Hemolysis. The plasma normally does not contain hemoglobin, but may do so in pathological conditions. This occurs when some red cells are **hemolyzed**—that is, the hemoglobin has escaped through the cell membranes into the plasma. Hemolysis can result from a number of causes; for example, it may be due to the effect of **toxins** (bacterial toxins, snake venom), of specific substances called **hemolysins**, or of **hypotonic solutions**, that is, solutions with a lower ion concentration than that of normal plasma.

In some of the **hemolytic anemias**, the blood cells have an increased tendency to hemolyze. In normal blood, 50 percent of the cells hemolyze at a sodium chloride concentration of 0.44–0.48 percent (an isotonic sodium chloride solution is 0.9 percent). The osmotic pressure difference between the inside of the blood cells and the surrounding fluid is then so great that the cells swell and the membranes rupture. In hemolytic anemia, the resistance to rupture is lowered, and therefore hemolysis occurs at higher than normal salt concentrations.

Erythrocyte sedimentation rate, ESR. If blood mixed with a substance that prevents clotting is drawn up in a glass tube and left for an hour or so, the blood cells gradually settle. Over the cells, plasma collects. The height of the plasma column constitutes a measure of the rate of sedimentation, which is expressed in millimeters per hour. The normal range of ESR for men is 1–15 mm/h and for women 1–20 mm/h. The ESR is increased in pregnancy and in a number of diseases, including infections and often in cancer.

The sedimentation rate is an indirect measure of the tendency of the blood cells to form so-called **rouleaux**— clumps of cells like a roll of coins. The more the cells are packed together, the greater is the formation of rouleaux and thus the higher the ESR. The increase in rouleau formation may be due to a raised concentration of macromolecular substances in the plasma—for example, fibrinogen, certain globulins, and plasma substitutes (dextran).

White blood cells

The number of white blood cells and the relative distribution of the different types of cells changes in pathological processes. Normally there are 3,500–9,000 per μl; of these, neutrophilic unsegmented rod-shaped granulocytes comprise 2–5%, neutrophilic segmented granulocytes 45–70%, eosinophilic granulocytes 1–4%, basophilic granulocytes 0–1%, lymphocytes 20–45% and monocytes 4–8%. The determination of the relative numbers of different white blood cells is known as the **differential count**. It is performed by examining a stained smear of blood on a microscope slide.

In infections, the number of white blood cells is increased; however, the relative distribution varies depending on whether the infection is acute or chronic. Neutrophilic leukocytes render certain foreign substances harmless, and their number is raised in acute infections. Lymphocytes transport and produce certain antibodies (page 346) and they are increased in infections, especially chronic ones. In hypersensitive reactions, there is an increased number of eosinophilic granulocytes, which renders the antigen-antibody complex harmless (page 347).

In **leukemia**, blood cancer, immature forms of leukocytes appear in the blood. They are liberated prematurely from the bone marrow. At the same time, the number of leukocytes is often greatly increased. There are different forms of such pathological conditions—common to them all is the fact that their cause is largely unknown.

The number of white blood cells may also be reduced, **leukopenia**. This condition can occur as a result of toxic effects, for example, in hypersensitivity to drugs. The patient's resistance to infections is lowered, as would be expected from the role of the white cells in the specific infection defense mechanism (page 344).

5.38	The study of the blood-forming organs, including normal and pathological changes in the microscopic features of the blood cells, is known as	
5.39	The formed elements of the blood, the blood cells, consist of . . . . , ... and	hematology
5.40	In a complete hematological analysis, an examination is made not only of the circulating blood cells but also of changes in the	erythrocytes (red cells) leukocytes (white cells) thrombocytes (platelets)
5.41	A previously healthy child has severe diarrhea for a couple of days and becomes dehydrated due to the fluid losses. The child is admitted to the hospital where, among other things, a routine examination of the blood is performed. An Hb value is found that is abnormally . . . . (high, low).	bone marrow

5.42	During a patient's physical examination a physician finds a hard, firm, palm-sized formation, located in the abdomen on the left side below the costal arch. The patient's skin is an intense red and the mucous membranes are also red. By palpating the abdomen, the physician finds that the spleen is enlarged. He suspects polycythemia, and this is confirmed by a laboratory examination. The hematocrit, hemoglobin and red cell count are too .... (high, low).	high
5.43	A female patient has recently been suffering from weakness, shortness of breath on exertion, and giddiness. Routine examination of the blood gives the following values: hematocrit 21%, Hb 6 g/dl and red cell count 2.1 million/μl. Diagnosis:	high
5.44	A child falls into a fresh-water lake. When brought to land some minutes later, he is unconscious and application of the mouth-to-mouth resuscitation and heart massage are in vain. At the autopsy, water is found in the lungs and the blood plasma is an intense red. Water has thus been taken up by the lungs and diluted the blood, which lowered the osmotic pressure of the plasma. This led to .... of the blood cells.	anemia
5.45	A child falls into the sea (salt concentration 3 percent). When he is brought to land some minutes later, he is unconscious, but is resuscitated by the mouth-to-mouth method. The child presumably breathed in water which diluted the blood, but this has not caused hemolysis of the blood cells because during the dilution, the osmotic pressure of the blood plasma .... (increased, decreased).	hemolysis
5.46	At a medical health examination, a man 50 years old is found to have an ESR of 47 mm/h, which is too .... (high, low). He is examined further, because there is the possibility of .... or	increased
5.47	A child has tonsilitis, with high fever for a number of days. Blood tests show 20,000 leukocytes per μl; the patient thus has leukocytosis—that is, too .... (many, few)	high infection cancer

5.48 A patient has been troubled over the last 6 months by tiredness, thumping of the heart, shortness of breath and feeling of heaviness in the left side of the abdomen. He has had intermittent attacks of fever. Blood tests show 100,000 leukocytes per μl with immature forms. Diagnosis:	many white blood cells
	leukemia (blood cancer)

Bleeding Diseases and Blood Clotting

There are a number of different bleeding diseases. They have many causes, which can be divided into three groups: disorders of the blood vessels, especially the capillaries, changes in the thrombocytes (blood platelets) and defects in the mechanism for blood clotting. There are also conditions in which the blood clots in the vessels in an abnormal way, so that diseases involving thrombosis (page 29) occur. The conditions are very complicated and they are dealt with here only superficially.

The normal course of hemostasis is the following. In an injury in which bleeding occurs, reflex vasoconstriction results in a reduction of the blood supply. In addition, the thrombocytes circulating in the blood agglutinate (clump together), and adhere to the walls of the damaged capillaries. The thrombocytes liberate certain substances which pass out into the blood plasma. This initiates a chain of chemical reactions, which ends with clotting of the blood and the arrest of bleeding—the healing process can then start.

Disorders of the blood vessels occur in certain hereditary diseases, in allergic reactions (page 351), in toxic effects (bacterial toxins, side effects of drugs, etc.) and in deficiency diseases (lack of vitamin C).

Thrombocyte disorders consist of a reduced number of blood platelets, **thrombocytopenia**, or pathological changes in existing platelets. Thrombocytopenia can be due to hypersensitivity to drugs (quinine, etc.) and to ionizing radiation (bone-marrow damage, see page 400). In a thrombocyte disorder, the clotting time is normal (5–10 min), but the bleeding time is prolonged. The bleeding time is determined by making an incision 0.8 mm deep in the skin and observing the time taken for bleeding to cease. The normal range is 1–5 min.

Clotting of the blood occurs via a complex chain of reactions, which can be simply expressed by the following stages. Coagulation begins with the liberation of a platelet factor from the thrombocytes. When this passes out into the blood plasma, it converts the **prothrombin** located there into **thrombin**. The thrombin converts the **fibrinogen** to **fibrin**. The whole reaction requires the presence of a number of components in the plasma, including **calcium ions**. The final stage of the coagulation process occurs when the fibrinogen dissolved in the blood plasma changes into insoluble fibrin. The fibrin consists of fine fibers, which form a network which encloses the blood cells.

If any of the various factors are absent, the clotting time is affected. It is determined by direct observation of a blood sample which is swung slowly to and fro until it clots. The normal range of clotting time is 5–10 min.

Usually, the amount of prothrombin is also determined. The prothrombin is synthesized in the liver, and requires the participation of vitamin K, which in turn is formed and absorbed in the intestines. Both in liver damage and in intestinal absorption damage, the prothrombin (clotting) time may be prolonged because of the reduced amount of prothrombin. This analysis is performed by determining the clotting time of the plasma when other clotting factors are at their optimal concentration. The prothrombin activity is expressed as a percentage of the normal value; the normal range is 80–120 percent.

Hemophilia is a **hereditary deficiency** of one of the plasma proteins needed for normal blood clotting. Patients with this disease bleed profusely after injury and may develop spontaneous hemorrhage, particularly into the joints. They are treated with a concentrated preparation of the clotting protein. This can be prepared by techniques that rely on differential solubility at varying temperature or by chemical fractionation.

5.49	A patient dies from cerebral meningitis. At autopsy, numerous hemorrhages are found in most of the internal organs. The cause is that bacterial toxins have been carried through the blood stream to these organs, resulting in damage to the	
5.50	In a reactor accident, a technician is exposed to radiation, about 400 rad (4 Gy). The same day he falls ill, with weakness and vomiting, but recovers after a couple of days. Two weeks later, he has loss of hair, increasing weakness and fever. Many punctiform hemorrhages are seen on the skin and mucous membranes. This latter sign is due to the fact that the radiation damaged the bone marrow, so that .... developed.	blood vessels (capillaries)

5.51 A patient with gallstone attacks is to have an operation. The case history suggests that a gallstone has lodged in the common duct (page 52), so that the bile is prevented from flowing into the intestines. Absorption of vitamin K, which is soluble in fat, is diminished, and the formation of prothrombin in the liver is inhibited. Laboratory examinations show a prolonged .... The patient is given an injection of vitamin K the day before the operation; this is essential to prevent hemorrhage during and after the operation.	thrombocytopenia (reduced number of platelets)
	prothrombin time

URINE

Urine is a filtration product of blood plasma. The composition of urine therefore reflects that of the blood, and urinalysis can often be used for diagnosing diseases that result in changes in the blood chemistry. Urine tests are also useful in examining renal function.

Renal Function

Two major functions of the kidneys are:

- Excretion of waste products formed during metabolism
- Regulation of the fluid and electrolyte balance in the body

The urine is formed by three processes: **filtration** of blood plasma, active **secretion** of certain substances and **reabsorption** of certain other substances so that they are restored to the blood. The urine is formed in the functional units of the kidneys, known as **nephrons**. Each kidney contains about 1 million nephrons. The nephron consists of two parts, the **glomerulus** (plural glomeruli), in which the filtration takes place, and the **tubule** (plural tubules), in which the active secretion and reabsorption occur.

A nephron is shown schematically in Fig. 5.9. Blood flows from the artery to the capillary loop within the glomerulus. The capillary wall is semipermeable and thus normally impermeable to the macromolecular substances in the blood plasma. Because the hydrostatic pressure in the capillary loop is greater than the colloid osmotic pressure, the low molecular weight substances and water are forced out. This glomerular filtrate is taken up by the capsule surrounding the capillary loop. About 1,000 liter/day of blood pass through the glomerular capillaries, resulting in the production of about 100 liter/day of glomerular

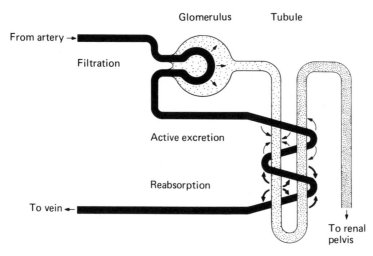

Glomerulus   Tubule

From artery →

Filtration

Active excretion

Reabsorption

To vein ←

To renal
pelvis

Figure 5.9 The urine is generated by filtration in the glomeruli
and by active secretion and reabsorption in the tubules.

filtrate. This passes down through the tubules, which are surrounded by blood
capillaries. The cells in the tubule walls have an active capacity for secreting
certain substances and reabsorbing others—particularly water. In this way the
urine is concentrated so that the amount leaving the kidneys is only a liter or so a
day.

Some substances are almost completely reabsorbed in the tubules. Examples
are glucose and sodium chloride. The kidneys cannot, however, maintain
concentration gradients between blood and urine above certain threshold values.
Whether large amounts appear in the urine thus depends on the concentration in
the blood plasma. If, for example, the blood sugar level exceeds about 160 mg/dl
(9 mmol/l), reabsorption by the tubules is not complete and glucose appears in the
urine. This can happen in diabetes, when the blood sugar level is often elevated.
The amount of sodium chloride in the urine is to a large extent dependent on the
intake in the food. If the supply is low, the threshold value is not exceeded and the
urine contains only traces.

Other substances are actively secreted to some extent or reabsorbed only to a
small degree. Examples are urea, uric acid and phosphates and therefore these
substances appear in the urine in high concentrations.

A few substances are totally excreted, so that the blood that flows through the
kidneys is completely cleared of them; one example is PAH (page 175).

| 5.52 | The kidneys have two major functions: . . . . of waste products of metabolism and . . . . of the fluid and electrolyte balance in the body. | |

294

5.53	The urine is a filtration product of	excretion regulation
5.54	Normal glomerular filtrate consists of blood plasma cleared of	blood plasma
5.55	Glomerular filtrate is formed in the .... (anatomic unit).	macromolecular sub- stances (proteins)
5.56	As the glomerular filtrate passes through the tubules, some substances are actively ...., while others are actively	glomeruli
5.57	The amount of glomerular filtrate is about .... liter/day; the amount of urine leaving the body is about .... liter/day.	reabsorbed secreted
5.58	The glomerular filtrate is concentrated by reabsorption in .... (anatomic unit).	100 1
5.59	Glomeruli and tubules together form the functional unit of the kidney, known as a	tubules
5.60	Glucose and sodium chloride are totally reabsorbed in tubules, only if the blood concentration is below a	nephron
5.61	PAH is .... excreted.	threshold value
		totally

Composition of the Urine

As the urine reflects the composition of the blood plasma, urinalysis can be used in the diagnosis of diseases that are accompanied by metabolic disorders. Table 5.4 gives normal values for some substances that occur in the urine, with the diagnostic implications when deviations occur. Many hormonal disorders produce changes in the urine. This would be expected from the previous description of hormonally caused changes in electrolyte composition of blood plasma (page 272) and glucose concentration (page 275). In tissue breakdown—for example, in cases of burns—the amount of potassium and creatinine in the urine increases as a direct result of the liberation of these substances from the tissues. In liver and biliary tract diseases, there are disturbances in the plasma concentration of bile pigments (page 277) and their breakdown products, and these disturbances can easily be detected in the urine. In gout, the uric acid synthesis is increased, and this leads to the formation of crystals in the joints, which cause pain; at the same time the uric acid level in the urine is increased. (Uric acid is a breakdown product of nucleic acids—the carriers of the genes in the cells; uric acid also forms in another way in the body.)

Table 5.4   Some examples of substances in the urine

Substance	Normal values		Examples of diagnostic use	
	Old units	*SI units mmol/day*	*Elevated values*	*Lowered values*
Na$^+$	50–200 mEq/day	50–200	adrenocortical insufficiency	adrenocortical hyper-function, diet low in salt, diarrhea
K$^+$	35–100 mEq/day	35–100	tissue destruction (burns)	
glucose	≈0.01 g/dl	≈1	diabetes mellitus	urinary tract infection
urea	≈30 g/day	≈500		
uric acid	<1 g/day	<6	gout	renal failure
creatinine	0.8–1.6 g/day	7–14	tissue destruction	renal failure, reduced muscle mass
urobilinogen	small		hemolytic and hepatic jaundice	obstructive jaundice
protein	0		renal damage	

Pathological processes in the kidneys often alter the composition of the urine. Protein sometimes appears in the urine, **proteinuria** (often, but less correctly, known as albuminuria). This is because protein passes from the blood plasma into the urine due to damage to glomeruli or tubules. Such damage can be due to inflammation of the glomeruli or toxic processes in the tubules. Protein can also appear due to the growth of bacteria in the urinary tract.

In severe renal failure, there is a drop in the daily amounts of substances excreted by the kidneys. The plasma creatinine level is of diagnostic interest, since in renal damage the creatinine level in the blood plasma increases (page 277).

Microscopic examinations of the urine are also performed—so-called **urine sediment analysis**. The urine is centrifuged and the precipitate is placed on an object glass under the microscope. A search is made for, among other things, red and white blood cells and epithelial cells that have separated from the walls of the urinary tract. The presence of red cells in the urine is known as **hematuria**; this can be a sign of inflammation of the kidneys. White blood cells occur in various bacterial infections in the kidneys or urinary tract.

Clearance. Glomerular function can be measured quantitatively by a clearance determination. "Clearance" is defined as the volume of plasma that is completely cleared of a substance in one minute. In other words, clearance is the volume of plasma—expressed, for example, in milliliters—that contains the amount of a substance excreted per minute in the urine. Clearance can be measured using PAH, which has a concentration in the renal vein assumed to be zero (page 175).

Clearance can also be measured using substances that have a nonzero concentration in the renal vein, provided tubule reabsorption and secretion are about equal. Such substances are inulin and creatinine. The clearance is determined from the creatinine concentration in the plasma, C_p, the creatinine concentration in the urine, C_u, and the urine volume, V, excreted in time, t, as follows

$$\text{Clearance} = \frac{C_u V}{C_p t}$$

The normal range of creatinine clearance is 65–110 ml/min for a person having a body surface area of 1.73 m^2, if the creatinine formed in the body is used—the so-called endogenous creatinine clearance.

5.62	A child is to be given a medical examination for various obscure symptoms. The parents are informed that the child must be in a fasting condition when the samples are taken. The child, who does not understand that he must not have any food, eats much candy secretly. The blood glucose level rises so that at the time the samples are taken, it is 180 mg/dl (10 mmol/l). The threshold value for the kidneys is .... (exceeded, not exceeded) and the urine therefore .... (contains, does not contain) quite large amounts of glucose.	
5.63	The child is admitted to the hospital and samples are taken again. The blood glucose level is then 80 mg/dl (4.4 mmol/l), which is .... (normal, abnormal).	exceeded contains
5.64	When military inductees are having their physical examinations, one man is found to have glucose in the urine. Questioning reveals that he has recently been troubled by increased thirst and large amounts of urine, and has been listless and tired. .... (disease) is strongly suspected.	normal

5.65	Two causes of protein appearing in the urine are .... and	diabetes mellitus
5.66	From a patient with hepatitis in an early stage, samples of the urine are taken, and examined for bilirubin glucuronide. Look at Fig. 5.3 and decide whether bilirubin glucuronide can or cannot be found in the urine. Answer:	damage to glomeruli or tubules bacteria growth in urinary tract
5.67	A patient with complete occlusion of the biliary tract due to a pancreatic tumor has constant jaundice. Look at Fig. 5.3 and decide whether the amount of urobilin in the urine is .... (greatly increased, slightly increased, not demonstrable).	can be found
5.68	A man who is overweight has severe pain in one of his big toes. No fever. The physician suspects gout and this is confirmed by urine tests. An elevated value for .... is found.	not demonstrable
5.69	A child is ill for a couple of days from tonsilitis and has high fever. A couple of weeks later the patient is troubled with headache, reduced amounts of urine and swelling of the face. The patient has glomerulonephritis—inflammation of the kidneys —secondary to the throat infection, due to hemolytic streptococci (page 326). Tests show that the urine contains .... (substance); this condition is called	uric acid
5.70	In an examination of the patient's urinary sediment, red blood cells are found; this condition is called	protein (albumin) proteinuria (albuminuria)
5.71	A man with a history of hypertension (too high blood pressure) over several years has edema (accumulation of fluid interstitially) and hematuria. The condition is due to acute renal failure. The creatinine level in the blood plasma is .... (elevated, lowered) and the creatinine level in the urine is .... (elevated, lowered).	hematuria
		elevated lowered

GASTRIC AND INTESTINAL JUICE AND FECES

Before food substances are absorbed, they are broken down by the process of **digestion**. This breaking down is accomplished by a number of **enzymes**. The enzymes act at different degrees of acidity, and the pH level varies from one part of the gastrointestinal tract to another: acid in the stomach and weakly alkaline in the small intestine. Undigested food remains are removed through the **feces**; most of which normally consist, however, of **bacteria** that grow in the intestines. Some substances are actively excreted by the intestines.

Carbohydrates in the diet usually contain a large percentage of starch. Starch is broken down into disaccharides by **amylase**, also known as diastase, which is secreted partly by the salivary glands, and partly by the pancreas. The remaining portion of carbohydrates is largely disaccharides (sucrose, lactose, maltose). Different enzymes break down the disaccharides into monosaccharides (glucose, galactose, fructose), that can be absorbed.

Fats are broken down partly by **lipase** from the pancreas. For absorption, **bile** is also required; this emulsifies the fat into a finely divided form, so that it can pass through the intestinal epithelium. Fat droplets are taken up by the lymph ducts in the intestinal wall and conveyed via the thoracic duct (page 61) out into the blood.

Proteins are broken down by, among other things, the enzymes **pepsin**, which forms in the stomach, and **trypsin**, which is excreted by the pancreas. The gastric juice also contains enzymes which split protein. The proteins are absorbed as amino acids.

Gastric and intestinal disorders

Many pathological processes can afflict the gastrointestinal tract. The **digestion** is disturbed by changes in the composition of the gastric and intestinal juices. In other diseases, the **resorption** is impaired by damage to the intestine. Common conditions are tumors, which may cause, among other things, **mechanical obstruction** to the passage of the digestive products. **Bleeding** may be suggestive of a tumor and can be disclosed by analysis of feces (guaiac test). Bleeding also has other causes, such as peptic ulcer. The origin of the bleeding is sometimes very difficult to locate.

There are various types of disturbances of the stomach's hydrochloric acid production. **Hypersecretion**—increased production of hydrochloric acid—is common in duodenal ulcer. **Hyposecretion**—reduced production of hydrochloric acid—may occur in gastritis (inflammation of the stomach) and in stomach cancer. **Achlorhydria**—total arrest of hydrochloric acid production—can arise in diseases associated with hyposecretion. Achlorhydria is usually present in pernicious anemia, when the gastric mucosa (mucous membrane lining the stomach) atrophies probably as a result of an autoimmune pathological process (page 352). The ability of the gastric mucosa to produce hydrochloric acid is measured by chemical analysis of gastric juice, obtained with a probe inserted into the stomach. To obtain standardized conditions, the secretion of gastric juice is stimulated by a large dose of histamine. This is conveyed by the blood stream to the cells of the gastric mucosa which produce hydrochloric acid.

When the digestive or absorption disorders are so great that the body is unable to utilize the constituents of food, a pathological state known as **maldigestion** and **malabsorption** arises. (Often the causes are not distinguished, "malabsorption" being used to cover a number of diseases.) The most common cause of maldigestion is inadequate production of bile and pancreatic juice. Maldigestion, in common with malabsorption, leads to emaciation and muscular atrophy, due to deficient uptake of proteins and fats. Osteoporosis, decalcification of the skeleton with resulting increased risk of fracturing the bone, also occurs.

In maldigestion and malabsorption, the feces are rich in fat—they then become voluminous, shiny from the fat, grayish-white and foul-smelling. They float in water because of the high fat content. The condition is known as **steatorrhea**. Fat determination in the feces should not give higher values than 6 g/day.

5.72	The saliva contains an enzyme, amylase (diastase), which breaks down	
5.73	Gastric juice contains pepsin, which breaks down	starch
5.74	Gastric juice also contains . . . . acid.	protein
5.75	Pancreatic juice contains enzymes which break down . . . . , ... and	hydrochloric
5.76	A patient has in the last month been troubled alternately by constipation and diarrhea. The guaiac test on the feces is positive—that is, the feces contain traces of	carbohydrates fats proteins
5.77	The patient is therefore sent for an x-ray examination with a tentative diagnosis of	blood
5.78	In gastritis (inflammation of the stomach) and stomach cancer, there may be hyposecretion, that is	tumor

5.79	A patient with pain in the pit of the stomach 3–4 hours after a meal has too great a production of hydrochloric acid, that is, ... , which points to	too low a production of hydrochloric acid
5.80	Achlorhydria means	hypersecretion duodenal ulcer
5.81	A patient has become emaciated and listless due to muscular atrophy, and has multiple (a number of) vertebral fractures, which cause pain due to compression of nerves. An examination shows that the foul-smelling feces are grayish white and float on water. The condition is due to pancreatic malfunction, which results in	total arrest of hydrochloric acid production
5.82	Chemical examination of the feces in the previous question confirms the presence of steatorrhea—that is, the feces contain excess	maldigestion (malabsorption)
		fat

CEREBROSPINAL FLUID

The whole brain and spinal cord are surrounded by a layer of liquid, **cerebrospinal fluid**. This is formed within the lateral ventricles of the brain—about 0.5 liter is secreted per day. The fluid passes out via the third ventricle, through a narrow channel, and then out via the fourth ventricle into the fluid space around the brain and spinal cord. The fluid is absorbed by special formations which are located in the dura mater. The cerebrospinal fluid serves to protect the sensitive parts of the central nervous system from trauma.

Samples of cerebrospinal fluid can be taken by **lumbar puncture**, that is, by inserting a hypodermic needle between the third and fourth lumbar vertebrae. The fluid normally has the lowest protein content of any fluid in the body. This is due to the fact that a blood-fluid barrier effectively prevents blood proteins from passing out into the fluid. In inflammations—for example, meningitis (inflammation of the cerebral meninges)—and in tumors of the central nervous system, the protein content increases because this barrier cannot be maintained.

The fluid normally contains no red blood cells and only a few white cells. In certain brain hemorrhages, in inflammations and in tumors, red blood cells may occur, or white ones can increase in number. Therefore, a microscopic examination of the cerebrospinal fluid is performed in suspect diseases of these types.

5.83	The fluid surrounding the brain and spinal cord is known as	
5.84	In a child with whooping cough, the condition spreads to the cerebral meninges and meningitis results. He has severe headache, weakness, vomiting and a stiff neck—that is, a cramp in the neck muscles. The lumbar fluid contains pus—that is, it contains .... and is rich in .... (substance).	cerebrospinal fluid
		white blood cells protein

METHODS OF CHEMICAL ANALYSIS

A wide variety of analytical methods are used in clinical chemistry. This is due to the considerable differences in the substances to be analyzed: inorganic electrolytes, low molecular weight organic substances and macromolecular substances. The substances that are more or less routinely analyzed number more than one hundred. In addition, the concentration range varies widely, from < 0.1 mg/liter to > 100 g/liter. A particular substance may also display large variations in properties; for example, an enzyme activity in the blood may rise a thousandfold in a pathological condition.

The analytical methods used should be specific for the substance analyzed; that is, there should be no interference from any of the innumerable other substances present in the sample. In addition, the analytical method should be rapid, economic and suitable for automation. The analytical methods in most common use may be classed as **optical**, **electrochemical** and **chromatographic**. The **radioimmunological** method, described in Chapter 6, is often used in clinical chemistry.

Methods of Optical Analysis

Light can be both absorbed and emitted by materials. This occurs to different extents depending on the wavelength, and on the chemical and physical properties of the material. Most of the analytical methods used in clinical chemistry are based on this fact. Two different methods are described below: **absorption photometry** and **emission photometry**.

Absorption photometry

Quantitative absorption photometry is based on the principle that the light absorption of the test substance bears a known relation to the concentration of the substance. The sample is usually pretreated by the addition of reagents. Different chemical processes are used; for example, the substance may be linked with a pigment or converted to a suitably colored substance. The color need not be visible to the naked eye, since absorption measurements can be made using either ultraviolet or infrared light. Absorption photometry is by far the most common analytical method in clinical chemistry. For example, it is used for determining the concentration of practically all low molecular weight organic substances.

A quantitative determination is performed by measuring the light absorption of the prepared sample (Fig. 5.10). Light from a lamp is made monochromatic by

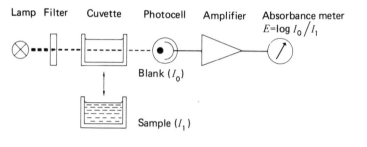

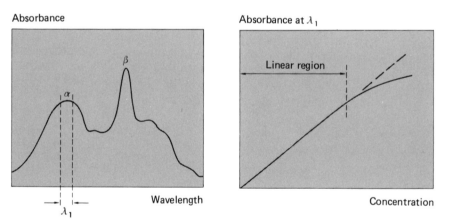

Figure 5.10 Principle of absorption photometry.

filtration (or by some other suitable technique) and is passed through a cuvette (cell) containing the sample solution. By means of a photoelectric circuit, the light transmission, I_1, is measured. The light transmission I_0 is also measured with the cuvette filled with reagent solution containing none of the analyzed substances, a **blank value** is thus obtained. According to Lambert–Beer's law,

$$I_1 = I_0 10^{-\varepsilon x c}$$

where c is the concentration (kg/m^3), x the pathlength of the cuvette (m) and ε, the extinction coefficient (m^2/kg). (We may consider the extinction coefficient to be the apparent area that one kilogram of the substance blocks for the light wavelength in question. The greater this apparent cross-sectional area is for a substance, the greater is the probability that a photon will be absorbed by a molecule of the substance.) The concentration, c, of the substance is calculated from the **absorbance**, also called the **extinction**, E,

$$E = \log I_0/I_1 = \varepsilon x c$$

The choice of wavelength in absorption photometry is critical. Thus, the wavelength used must be one where the absorption of the analyzed substance is high relative to that of the reagent solution or other substances present in the sample. Furthermore, the wavelength should be chosen so that the part of the absorption curve used is almost horizontal. This avoids errors, due to the fact that the light is not completely monochromatic. For example, the absorption peak β in Fig. 5.10 is not used even though it is higher than the peak α. By using the peak α, a more accurate determination can be made, since it is possible to work mainly at a plateau of the curve. The relationship between concentration and absorbance is usually assumed as linear, thereby simplifying calculations.

Nonlinear relationships between concentration and absorbance can be due to two causes: physical and chemical. The physical causes, which are the more common, are usually due to the light not being sufficiently monochromatic relative to the shape of the absorption curve; this causes a shift in the peak wavelength, as the light is selectively filtered by the sample.

The chemically produced nonlinear relationship may be due to the fact that the color reaction is affected by the presence of other substances (salt error, protein error) or that the color reaction does not behave strictly stoichiometrically, that is, that side-reactions occur so that the reaction does not follow any simple formula.

Emission photometry

Light can be emitted in different ways. Two analytical procedures used in clinical chemistry are based on light emission. In a method known as **flame photometry**, the sample is heated, and in **fluorometry**, the sample is irradiated with ultraviolet light.

Flame photometry.   The sample is heated in an open flame, which results in the emission of certain narrow-band wavelengths from the excited ions (Fig. 5.11). The sample is divided into fine droplets by passing oxygen past the opening of a capillary tube containing the sample—as occurs in an atomizer spray nozzle. A combustible gas, such as acetylene, is then added. The mixture is burned and the light emitted is filtered so that only a limited wavelength range, corresponding to

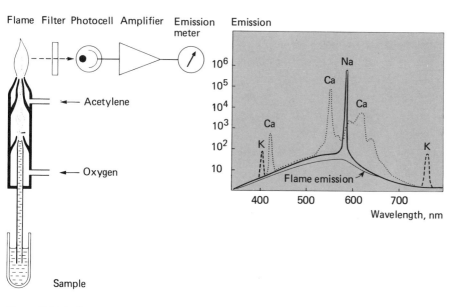

Figure 5.11 In flame photometry, the sample is heated in an open flame and the intensity of the emitted light is determined in a narrow wavelength range.

the emission line of the analyzed substance, is incident on a photocell. The current output of the cell is proportional to the concentration of the substance in the sample

Flame photometry is used mainly for analyzing sodium, potassium, calcium and lithium. Sometimes lithium is used as the calibration substance in the analysis of the other three substances; in this case, a known amount of lithium is added to the sample and the light intensity of the substance under analysis is measured relative to that of the lithium. In this way errors due to, for example, varying flame temperature are eliminated.

Fluorometry is performed by illuminating the sample at a wavelength that is absorbed by it (absorption peak) and measuring the excited intensity at a different wavelength (fluorescence peak), (Fig. 5.12). At low concentrations, the intensity of the emitted light is proportional to that of the absorbed light; that is, the ratio between fluorescing and absorbed light intensity is independent of concentration; at higher concentrations, however, the relationship is more complex. The calculation of the concentration of the substance under analysis is therefore more complicated than in flame photometry. Usually, determinations are made after calibration with standard solutions of known concentrations.

Fluorometry is used for analyzing substances present only in low concentrations, for example, certain hormones and vitamins.

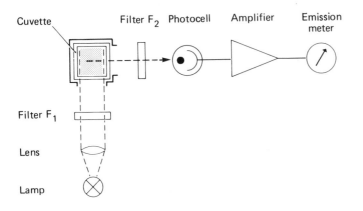

Figure 5.12 Principle of fluorometry. The filter, F_1, transmits only the wavelength band at which the sample has an absorption peak. The filter, F_2, transmits only the wavelength band corresponding to the fluorescence peak.

5.85	Two methods of optical analysis often used in clinical chemistry are .... and	
5.86	In absorption photometry, the substance under analysis takes part in a chemical reaction, in which a compound is formed that has a high .... within a certain wavelength range.	absorption photometry emission photometry
5.87	The wavelengths usually lie within the .... range, but they can also lie within the .... or .... wavelength range.	light absorption
5.88	Two types of emission photometry are used in clinical chemistry, ... and	visible ultraviolet infrared
5.89	In flame photometry, the sample is sprayed into a flame and the light emission is determined within a narrow	flame photometry fluorometry
5.90	The light intensity in flame photometry bears the following mathematical relation to the concentration of the substance:	wavelength range

5.91	In fluorometry, a determination is made of the light intensity emitted by the sample, when illuminated with light of a different	direct proportionality
5.92	Fluorometry is used mostly for analyzing fluorescing substances present in low concentrations, for example, ... and	wavelength
5.93	Flame photometry is used for analysis of . . . ., ..., ... and	hormones vitamins
5.94	The analytical method in most common use in clinical chemistry is	sodium potassium calcium lithium
		absorption photometry

Methods of Electrochemical Analysis

Among the methods of electrochemical analysis are **potentiometry**, **polarography** and **electrophoresis**.

Potentiometry. One form of potentiometry is the earlier described method for pH measurement (page 158), in which the potential is determined across a glass electrode with a selective sensitivity for hydrogen ions.

In the same way, several other ions, such as calcium and potassium, can be analyzed with ion specific membranes. The measuring circuit employed is similar to that shown in Fig. 3.9. For each decade change in ion activity, a potential change of about 60 mV is obtained for monovalent ions, and about 30 mV for divalent ions.

An advantage of the method is that of the total concentration only the physiologically active part is measured. A disadvantage is that the specificity of the membrane is not ideal, that is, other ions than that measured add to the potential, resulting in a certain error.

Some organic compounds can also be analyzed by such a potentiometric method by detecting an ionic product of a specific enzyme reaction. For example, urea can be determined by measuring with an ammonium electrode the ammonium ion released during breakdown by the enzyme urease.

Polarography. A polarographic method for determining oxygen tension was mentioned earlier (page 154). It is based on measurement of the current when a certain potential is applied to a platinum electrode in contact with the sample.

A similar method can be utilized for analyzing a number of organic compounds by means of specific enzyme reactions. A coenzyme or a reaction product is determined polarographically on a noble metal electrode, and they are an indirect measure of the substrate itself. Thus, the redox reaction accompanying the enzymatic breakdown of the substrate causes a change in the current at the electrode. The change in current is a linear function of the concentration of the analyzed compound if the enzymatic reaction is made to proceed in a first order reaction.

For example, glucose can be analyzed by means of glucose oxidase and lactate by cytochrome b_2 as enzymes. The method has the advantage of requiring little preparation of the blood sample and this results in a short analysis time; this is of importance in certain clinical conditions involving critically ill patients.

Electrophoresis is a method for separating and analyzing macromolecular substances such as plasma proteins. The method is based on the fact that the molecules carry electric charges and therefore migrate in an electric field. One form of the procedure is **zone electrophoresis**, which is illustrated in Fig. 5.13. The

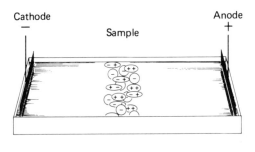

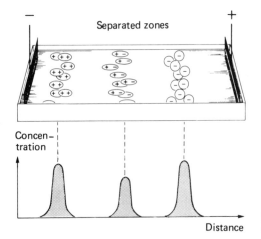

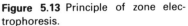

Figure 5.13 Principle of zone electrophoresis.

charges are due to basic and acidic groups on the surface of the protein molecules which, in a given environment, give the molecules a certain net charge. The magnitude and sign of the net charge determines to some extent the migration velocity in an applied electric field. The migration velocity is also dependent on the viscosity of the solvent. The pH of the solution has an indirect influence, since it determines the degree of dissociation of the charged groups and thus also the net charge of the protein molecules.

A substance, *i*, migrates in time, *t*, through a distance, *l*, in a field of field strength, *E*:

$$l = u_i E \cdot t$$

where u_i is the electrophoretic mobility, a constant characteristic of each substance. Experimental measurement of this quantity can be used for classifying, for example, plasma proteins.

Electrophoresis can be performed in different ways. In **free electrophoresis** only a buffer solution is used as a medium for the electric field. One disadvantage is that the separation is countered by convection movements in the liquid, caused by local density gradients. The convection can be reduced by having the electrophoresis occur in thin layers—for example, in a filter paper saturated with buffer solution, so-called **paper electrophoresis**, or in a gel, **gel electrophoresis**. These procedures have the advantage that when separation is complete, the substances are easily drawn off from the paper strips or collected fractions of the gel.

Another variant of the procedure is **immunoelectrophoresis**, in which the separated macromolecular substances are identified by antigen-antibody reactions (page 355).

5.95	Three methods of electrochemical analysis in clinical chemistry are ...., ... and	
5.96	Calcium ion activity determination with an ion specific membrane is an example of	potentiometry polarography electrophoresis
5.97	In polarography, a quantitative measurement is performed by measuring the .... (current passing through, potential across, resistance of) an electrode immersed in the test solution.	potentiometry

5.98	In electrophoresis, macromolecular substances are analyzed by determining their .... in an electric field.	current passing through
5.99	The macromolecular molecules migrate through the electric field because they have a net charge due to the presence of .... and .... groups.	migration velocity
5.100	The net charge is dependent on the .... of the solution.	acidic basic
5.101	In electrophoresis, the distance that a substance migrates is proportional to the ...., ... and	pH
5.102	Free electrophoresis has the disadvantage that the separation process can be disturbed by	field strength time electrophoretic mobility
5.103	To reduce convection, two other forms of electrophoresis can be used, namely, ... and	convection
		paper electrophoresis gel electrophoresis

Chromatography

Chromatography is a method for separating closely related chemical substances. It is based on differences in the migration velocity of the substances between a stationary phase and a mobile phase. The difference in migration velocity is due to a difference in solubility in the two phases.

The stationary phase consists of a solid substance or a liquid, which is rendered immobile by means of a porous solid medium. The mobile phase is either a liquid, **liquid chromatography**, or a gas, **gas chromatography**. The two methods are used for separating substances that can be brought into solution or into gaseous form. The sample is added to the mobile phase; the various components will travel faster in the mobile phase if their solubility is lower in the stationary phase. The different components can be characterized by the rate of flow:

$$R_f = \frac{v_i}{v_s}$$

where v_i is the velocity for the component i, and v_s the velocity for the mobile phase.

The principle of chromatography is shown in Fig. 5.14. The column may consist of a glass tube packed with a substance capable of taking up a large amount

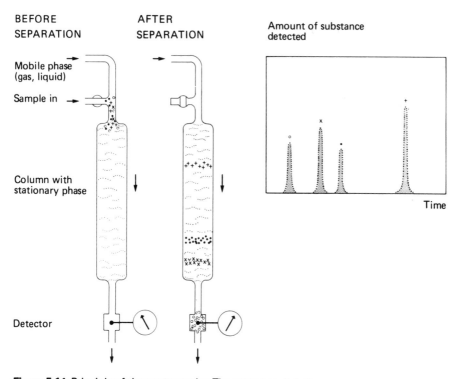

Figure 5.14 Principle of chromatography. The components in the sample separate as a result of their different migration velocities when the mobile phase passes over the stationary phase.

of the stationary phase. In liquid chromatography, water is generally used as the stationary phase; this can be supported by absorption in a suitable medium—for example, cellulose. In gas chromatography, the stationary phase is a liquid with a high vaporization temperature in an inactive porous medium. In liquid chromatography, the mobile phase is an organic solvent, and in gas chromatography it is usually helium. After the sample is introduced and passes through the system, the components are separated according to their relative solubility in the mobile and solid phases. The process can be followed by means of a detector placed in the outflow of the column. There are various detection techniques—for example, those based on measurement of thermal conductivity or density, or on photometric principles.

With liquid chromatography, many substances can be analyzed, for example, amino acids and drugs used in sleeping pills. Gas chromatography is used for analyzing substances that can be vaporized, for example, steroids (page 276) and aromatic acids in the urine, which appear in many diseases (for example, phenylketonuria, a congenital disorder that must be diagnosed at birth so that treatment can be introduced before brain damage results).

5.104	In chromatography, methods of separation and analysis are based on the difference in .... between a mobile and a stationary phase.	
5.105	Differences in migration velocity are due to the difference in .... of substances under analysis in the stationary and mobile phases.	migration velocity
5.106	A quantitative measure of migration velocity is the quantity R_f defined as the ratio between the velocities for the .... and the	solubility
5.107	Based on the form in which the sample travels through the column, two forms of chromatography are distinguished: .... and	analyzed component mobile phase
		liquid chromatography gas chromatography

AUTOMATED ANALYTICAL METHODS

Routine analytical methods in clinical chemistry are well suited for automation. The number of analyses of the same type is large—at major hospitals a hundred or so determinations of the more common types of analyses are performed daily—for example, blood sugar and hemoglobin. For analyses performed only 10–20 times a day, automation can still be advantageous; for those performed occasionally, the manual routine is usually retained.

The automated procedure has several advantages over manual handling. A **greater capacity** for performing more tests is immediately available, while at the same time personnel are freed for other, more demanding, tasks. The **cost** per analysis is lower if the increased capacity is utilized. **Greater reliability** is obtained due to, for example, the lower risk of confusing samples, and of incurring reading and writing errors. The **accuracy** of analysis can often be improved. The precision is higher because of exact measurements of volume and more accurate control of time and temperature, etc. The absolute accuracy can be controlled better because the methodological error can be checked daily by inserting standard samples in series with patient samples. (In the case of some automated analytical procedures, however, simplification of the processes can lead to analytical errors.) It should, in principle, also be possible to **shorten the time** between ordering the analyses and presentation of the results to the referring physician; in practice, simple manual analyses can be carried out at a speed that meets existing medical needs, and the introduction of automation is not justified simply on grounds of greater rapidity.

Laboratory automation includes a number of steps. For complete automation, all the stages must be carried out with no manual intervention; however, considerable gains in reliability and economy of effort can still be achieved with automation of only some of the following procedures:

- The sample is divided among different types of analyses.
- A certain carefully adjusted amount of sample is measured for each analysis.
- The wet analytical process is carried out to completion, which includes addition of reagent and any dialysis or filtration, and thermostating. The wet analytical process is performed by the principle of **continuous flow** (AutoAnalyzer principle) or by **discrete analysis**.
- The quantitative measurement of the analytical value is performed, and this is usually obtained as an analog electric signal.
- The analog measurement value is converted so that it is expressed in customary units.
- The analytical results are sorted and written out, together with the patient identification; this must be done in such a way as to facilitate interpretation by the physician requesting the laboratory examinations.
- The methodological errors are determined by statistics.

Automatic analysis by continuous flow

When using the principle of the AutoAnalyzer (proprietary name of Technicon, Inc.), the analyzed liquid samples are advanced by a rollerpump through a long plastic tube (Fig. 5.15). The reagent solutions are mixed in a system consisting of several converging tubes. The sample can be dialyzed through a thin membrane, thus leaving the macromolecular substances behind. The reaction mixture is thermostated and finally, the quantitative measurement is performed by a photometric technique.

The samples from different patients are thus passed in successive order through the same tube system. To reduce carryover—that is, contamination of a particular sample with the one ahead in the tube, as would occur if the flow profile were parabolic—air bubbles are introduced into the tube system so that the liquid column in the tube is broken up into short segments. This results in better separation of adjacent samples because an almost rectangular flow profile is obtained.

The principle of the AutoAnalyzer has advantages and disadvantages. The system can easily be adapted for almost any type of analytical reaction in which

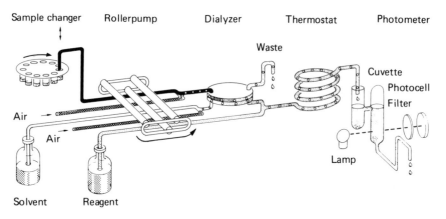

Sample changer Rollerpump Dialyzer Thermostat Photometer

Waste

Cuvette
Photocell
Filter

Air

Air

Lamp

Solvent Reagent

Figure 5.15 Principle of the AutoAnalyzer. The rollerpump continuously pumps the sample liquid, air, solvent and reagent by peristaltic action of rollers on the plastic tubes. Exact amounts of samples—for example, blood serum—are sucked through a pipette, dipped for a certain time into sample tubes placed in the sample changer. The air bubbles in the plastic tubes separate the liquid columns into short segments to prevent mixing of successive samples. In the dialyzer, the substances under analysis are separated from the macromolecular substances in the sample. Thermostatic control is obtained by leading the liquid column into a spiral glass tube immersed in a regulated water bath. The required analysis value is measured in the photometer and recorded, for example, on a pen recorder.

photometry can be used—absorption photometry, flame photometry or fluorometry. The operating costs are low. One shortcoming is that contamination cannot be entirely ruled out in spite of the separation by air bubbles. This also limits the rate of analysis, which is normally one sample or so per minute. Because of shortage of time, the dialysis process cannot be carried to equilibrium, and it is necessary to assume that the examined samples are dialyzed at the same rate as the standard solutions used.

Identification of the samples is based on the sequence principle—the same order out as in. This complicates the insertion of "acute" samples—that is, ones for which the result is needed urgently. Even with these disadvantages, the method is widely used. Nearly 80 percent of the analytical results of a clinical chemistry laboratory can be obtained with AutoAnalyzers. To analyze a single sample for many of its constituents, 12 systems similar to that shown in Fig. 5.15 are typically operated in parallel.

Automatic analysis with discrete samples

To avoid the disadvantages associated with continuous methods of analysis, to enable the samples to be identified by some technique other than sequence, to reduce contamination of adjacent samples, to increase the speed of analysis, and to facilitate the introduction of acute samples in an analytical series, various automatic analysis units using discrete systems have been developed. At least three groups of discrete analyzers may be identified.

High volume multichannel analyzers (Hycel Mark X, Hycel 17, Ortho Accuchem, and Vickers Multichannel 300) use chemical methods that are essentially those used in manual techniques. In fact, analysis is performed in test tubes that must be thoroughly cleaned by the automated instrument between tests. Samples can be processed in several parallel channels; thus, a high analytical capacity can be achieved. Cost per sample is comparable with that of AutoAnalyzer systems.

Centrifuge analyzers (American Instruments RotoChem, Electronucleonics GeMSAEC, Union Carbide CentrifiChem) use centrifugal force to add, transfer, and mix reagent and sample. Samples are processed in parallel cavities in a modified centrifuge head, which contains, along its outer wall, an optical cuvette for each sample. Figure 5.16 shows the GeMSAEC Fast Analyzer transfer disk and shows the arrangement of sample and reagent cavities at rest and during acceleration. High volume analysis is possible; rates of up to 420 samples per hour are demonstrated. Cost per sample is low because micro volumes of reagent are used.

Instruments discussed above operate in a batch mode. That is, all samples are treated in the same way and assayed for the same constituents.

Random test order is offered by the DuPont Automatic Clinical Analyzer, ACA. The individual test reagents are prepackaged in a plastic pack (with optical coding to indicate the individual chemical test) which, after sample and diluent additions and mixing, becomes an optical cuvette. Tests may be run in any order. Test results are printed on an optical image of the patient sample identity card. Sample throughput is not as high (approximately 100 samples/h), as some instruments, but with 30 tests available, the ACA is quite versatile. Cost per sample is higher because of specialized reagent preparation.

AUTOMATIC DATA PROCESSING IN CLINICAL CHEMISTRY

Many of the processing problems in clinical chemistry laboratories can be solved by using computers. The **calculation** of the analytical results from the analog measurement values can be centralized. Reliable continuous **sample identification** can be achieved, thus avoiding errors due to handling mistakes. Mention has been made above of the possibility of performing continuous **statistical checks** of the analytical results so as to follow the accuracy of the analytical method. The **printout** of the analytical results can be organized so as to ease the hospital staff's task of interpreting the results. For example, abnormal values are printed out in a distinctly different way from the normal ones. Clarity of presentation is obtained by printing out the earlier and the current values for each patient, compiled in the right time sequence and by marking significant changes.

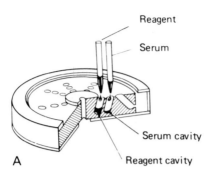

Reagent

Serum

Serum cavity

Reagent cavity

A

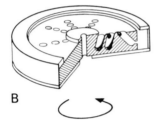

B

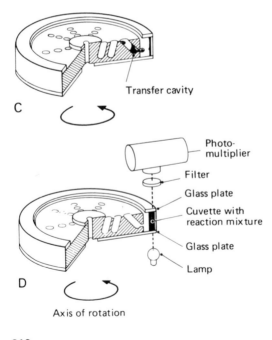

Transfer cavity

C

Photo-
multiplier

Filter

Glass plate

Cuvette with
reaction mixture

Glass plate

Lamp

D

Axis of rotation

Figure 5.16 GeMSAEC Fast analyzer transfer disk. (A) Sample and reagent are measured into chambers where they remain separate and unmixed at rest and during rotation at low speed. (B) As speed is increased, both liquids begin to move radially into outer chamber of transfer disk. (C) Liquids flow rapidly out of transfer disk and into cuvettes in the cuvette rotor. (D) The reactant solutions are held against the outer walls of the cuvette and air bubbles are displaced from the mixtures by centrifugal displacement. Optical measurements may now begin.

316

Data processing can be performed off-line or on-line. The off-line technique has the disadvantage that results cannot be obtained until the whole series of analyses has been carried out. Nor are the process-regulating capabilities of the computer exploited. The on-line technique affords a better opportunity for efficient use of available analytical equipment and, on the whole, leads to a shorter time between sample input and communication of the analytical results to the ward.

Human error is the most serious source of unreliability in clinical chemistry. The reliability is comparatively low; it has been estimated that, at a major hospital, about 7 percent of the analytical results communicated to the wards contain at least one type of error. Confusion of samples, reading errors and errors in manual transfer of data are the commonest causes. Automation is the most important measure for increasing accuracy. The risk of incorrect identification of the samples as they are obtained from the patients still presents a problem.

The aim of an automated laboratory goes beyond just providing results of requested analyses. An attempt is also made to obtain an optimal combination of analyses of samples; for example, many determinations beyond those requested are often performed at no additional cost—and should initial tests suggest logical successive tests, these may be automatically proposed. With the increasing resources for data collection that are provided by modern techniques, such an expanded service is possible.

5.108	With automated methods for clinical analysis, increased . . . . (analytical capacity, analytical accuracy) and reduced . . . . (risk of confusion, analysis times) are achieved.	
5.109	Automated analysis affords a good opportunity for continuous control of daily production by statistical calculation of the	analytical capacity risk of confusion
5.110	The wet chemical analysis process can be automated in two different ways: according to the principle of . . . . and according to the principle of	methodological error
5.111	In the continuous flow principle, the uptake of samples, mixing of solvents and reagents, dialysis, thermostatic control and photometry are performed by feeding through a	continuous flow (AutoAnalyzer principle) discrete samples
5.112	In discrete sample automatic analyses, samples are separated by placing them in separate	tube system

5.113 More reliable calculation of analysis results, better statistical analysis, more reliable sample identification and better display of printed-out clinical chemical data can be obtained by	test tubes
	automatic data processing

RADIONUCLIDE METHODS

Radionuclides (radioactive isotopes) are used clinically for measuring certain organ functions and for visualizing organs. Accounts are given here of how the thyroid gland and renal function can be examined and, on page 449, of how the visualization is performed.

Thyroid gland function.   The thyroid gland takes up a large amount of the iodine entering the body—iodine is included in the hormones secreted by the thyroid gland, and any disturbance of the thyroid gland alters its iodine uptake. This fact can be used in the quantitative measurement of the degree of the disturbance. An oral dose of 10–30 μCi (SI units 0.4–1 MBq)* of ^{131}I is given as NaI and after 24 hours the amount of radioactivity taken up by the thyroid gland is measured.

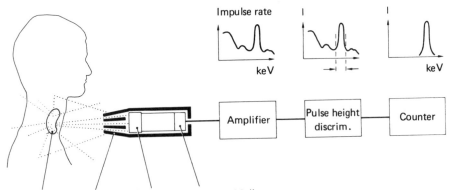

Thyroid gland   Collimator   Scintillator   Photomultiplier

Figure 5.17 Measurement of thyroid gland uptake of ^{131}I. The curves show the spectral distribution of impulses before and after pulse height discrimination.

* Ci = curie, $3.7 \cdot 10^{10}$ disintegrations/s; Bq = Becquerel = s^{-1}.

Normally, 7–30 percent of the administered dose is present in the thyroid gland; higher values point to hyperthyroidism (page 74) and lower values to hypothyroidism (page 74).

The amount of radionuclide taken up is measured with a scintillation detector placed in front of the patient's neck (Fig. 5.17). The detector is furnished with a lead collimator to eliminate radiation not coming from the thyroid gland.

The impulses recorded by the detector are discriminated with a pulse height analyzer. Only the γ-radiation emitted by the ^{131}I is counted. Impulses of other energy are excluded—for example, those appearing in the surrounding tissue due to Compton scattering of secondary radiation from the thyroidal ^{131}I.

Renal function. By means of a method similar to that used in thyroid examination, the function of each kidney can be determined separately. Two scintillation detectors are directed at the kidneys on the dorsal side of the body. The patient is given a radioactively labeled substance that is excreted only through the kidneys—that is, a substance with a high renal clearance, such as ^{131}I-labeled Hippuran.

The count rates from the scintillation detectors are displayed on a two-channel recorder. The outputs normally reach a maximum about 5 min after intravenous injection of the ^{131}I-labeled substance, and then decrease as the urine drains down into the bladder. From these curves—**renograms**—it is possible to determine the blood flow, tubular secretion and excretion of urine for each kidney separately.

5.114	The function of certain organs can be examined by measuring what fraction of an administered radioactive substance the organ has	
5.115	The thyroid gland normally takes up the radionuclide	taken up
5.116	The kidneys take up	^{131}I
5.117	The radioactivity taken up is measured by means of a . . . . detector.	^{131}I-labeled Hippuran
5.118	After amplification of the electrical impulses from the scintillation detector, these are usually analyzed by a . . . . in order to lower the sensitivity of the recording apparatus to emitted secondary radiation.	scintillation

5.119	A patient that in recent months has been suffering from pounding heart, anxiety, loss of hair and diarrhea is examined by giving ^{131}I and determining the thyroid gland activity. The uptake of the radionuclide was found to be 75 percent. Diagnosis:	pulse height discriminator
		hyperthyroidism

REFERENCES

BARON, D. N. *A Short Textbook of Clinical Biochemistry.* Philadelphia (Lippincott) 1973. 247 pages.

BURTIS, C. A. et al. Increased Rate of Analysis by Use of a 42-cuvette GeMSAEC Fast Analyzer. *Clin. Chem.* Vol. 17 (1971). p. 686.

HARPER, H. A. *Review of Physiological Chemistry.* Los Altos (Lange) 1975. 570 pages.

HENRY, R. J., CANNON, D. C. and WINKELMAN, J. W. *Clinical Chemistry; Principles and Technics.* Hagerstown, Maryland (Harper & Row) 1974. 1629 pages.

MAYNARD, C. D. *Clinical Nuclear Medicine.* Philadelphia (Lea & Febiger) 1969. 280 pages.

PITTS, R. F. *Physiology of the Kidney and Body Fluids: An Introductory Text.* Chicago (Year Book) 1974. 307 pages.

QUIMBY, E. H., FEITELBERG, S. and GROSS, W. *Radioactive Nuclides in Medicine and Biology.* Philadelphia (Lea & Febiger) 1970. 390 pages.

RAY, C. D. (Ed.). *Medical Engineering.* Chicago (Year Book) 1974. pp. 743–782.

THOMAS, H. E. *Handbook of Biomedical Instrumentation and Measurement.* Reston, Va. (Reston) 1974. 550 pages.

WILLARD, H. H., MERRITT, L. L. and DEAN, J. A. *Instrumental Methods of Analysis.* Princeton, New Jersey (Van Nostrand) 1965. 784 pages.

chapter 6

Clinical Microbiology and Immunology

Many pathological conditions are caused by microorganisms. It is often necessary to determine their types and properties, for proper treatment to be given. There are two essentially different ways in which this can be done: by demonstrating that the patient has the **infectious agent** itself or by demonstrating that the patient has developed **specific immunity** to it.

Pathogenic microorganisms are demonstrated by analyzing various specimens from the patient. The specimens are examined by culturing on certain culture media. The shape, size and smell of the colonies grown are noted, as well as what type of media and environment that the microorganisms require for the culture. As a guide to the choice of treatment, resistance determinations are sometimes performed—that is, quantitative measurements of the resistance of the microorganisms to certain drugs.

Specific immunity is demonstrated by examining the patient's serum—**serological diagnosis**. This determines the presence of antibodies—that is, specific antitoxins to different pathogens.

This chapter surveys some common diagnostic examination procedures used in a clinical microbiology laboratory. First, the various pathogenic microorganisms are presented. It is also important to know the methods for sterilization and disinfection, and for preventing transfer of infections, which are applied not only in microbiology but also in all other fields of medical care. Finally, some important areas of immunology are covered: principles of vaccination, information about a group of diseases having an immunological causation and principles of serological diagnosis; some particular aspects of immunology are mentioned in the context of blood and transplantation (Chapter 7).

The term "clinical microbiology" is preferable to "clinical bacteriology" which remains in use for historical reasons. But the latter term does not cover the diagnosis of diseases caused by all microorganisms because many of those known today are not included among the bacteria. "Clinical microbiology" is more appropriate since it also includes **virology**, the science and study of virus diseases, **mycology**, the science and study of fungal diseases, and the science and study of protozoa and other parasites.

Question		*Answer*
6.1	Diseases caused by microorganisms can be diagnosed in two ways, by direct demonstration of the . . . . and by demonstrating that the patient has developed specific . . . . to it.	
6.2	The infectious agent in a disease can sometimes be identified by means of	infectious agent (microorganism) immunity
6.3	In a resistance determination, the resistance of the microorganisms to certain . . . . is determined.	culturing
6.4	In serological diagnosis, certain diseases can be identified by examining the patient's	drugs
6.5	The science of virus diseases is known as	blood serum
6.6	The science of fungal diseases is known as	virology
		mycology

CLINICAL MICROBIOLOGY

From a medical aspect, microorganisms may be divided into two groups, namely, **pathogenic**, giving rise to disease, and **nonpathogenic**, not giving rise to disease. This division is, however, not absolute. Many bacteria that occur normally in one place can produce a pathological state in another part of the body. The higher animals live in symbiosis with many bacteria; for example, in addition to nondigestible, nonabsorbable matter such as cellulose, feces contain bacteria that have developed in the intestines and that participate in the breakdown of food and the formation of certain substances, such as vitamin K. If, however, bacteria enter the abdominal cavity through a lesion in the intestinal wall, peritonitis—inflammation of the peritoneal membrane—immediately develops (Question 1.252); this can lead to death if left untreated. Similarly, in the mouth there is a rich flora of bacteria, which cause infection if they enter an articular cavity (arthritis), or into bone (osteomyelitis). In the vagina, there is a bacterial flora that maintains a low pH; this serves as a protection against other bacteria, which may be pathogenic. To evaluate the findings in bacterial cultures, it is necessary to know the origin of the specimen. It is important to take the specimen with the correct technique in order to avoid contamination with bacteria from another source.

From a biological standpoint, the pathogenic microorganisms can be divided into **protozoa**, **fungi**, **bacteria** and **virus** and other groups.

6.7	A nonpathogenic bacterium .... (does, does not) produce	
6.8	A soldier receives a bullet wound in the abdomen. The bowel contents, which are rich in bacteria, enter the abdominal cavity and peritonitis, ..., develops (cf, Question 1.252) because the bacteria that are .... (pathogenic, nonpathogenic) in the intestines are .... in the abdominal cavity. At the operation, care must be taken to suture all bowel lesions to prevent further escape of the intestinal contents into the abdominal cavity.	does not disease
		inflammation of the peritoneal membrane nonpathogenic pathogenic

Protozoa are single-celled animals and the most highly developed of the pathogenic microorganisms. Protozoa cause a number of tropical diseases. In northern climates **malaria** is rare, but **toxoplasmosis**, which is usually asymptomatic, is more common. The latter is an infectious disease often located in the lymph nodes and lymphoreticular system. Protozoa pass through a developmental cycle with certain species as the host organisms. For example, the malarial protozoa are dependent on certain species of mosquito to complete the life cycle, and the disease can therefore be combated by exterminating the mosquito.

Fungi occupy an intermediate position between plants and animals. Their metabolism is similar to that of the lower animals, but externally they resemble plants. The most common fungal diseases are skin diseases, but deep infections can also occur. In addition, fungal infections occur as a complication of prolonged antibiotic therapy, when internal organs can be attacked. Fungal diseases are known as **mycoses**.

Bacteria are the microorganisms that have been most carefully investigated. There are about 2,000 different types of bacteria, but the great majority are nonpathogenic. Bacteria are present everywhere in nature—in the atmosphere, in the sea and in the soil. Only some 100 types can produce diseases in animals and man.

Bacteria are classified according to different principles. Morphologically, (morphology, the science of the form and structure of organisms) bacteria are divided according to shape: spherical—**cocci**; rod-shaped—**bacilli**; and spiral—**spirilla**.

Cocci can grow in pairs; then they are called **diplococci**. This is the case for the bacteria responsible for gonorrhea and for certain forms of cerebral meningitis. Cocci can also grow in chain-like structures—**streptococci**, which occur in some throat infections. Finally, they can grow in grape-like clusters—**staphylococci**, which are common in a number of diseases including wound and skin infections, ear, nose and throat infections, pyelonephritis and pneumonia.

Among the diseases caused by bacilli are tuberculosis, leprosy and diphtheria. The intestines normally contain many rod-shaped bacteria, the vast majority of which are anaerobic. **Salmonella bacteria** and other types may cause a pathological condition.

Syphilis is caused by a spiral bacteria known as a **spirochete**.

Bacteria are usually about 1 μm in size, but some spiral bacteria are more than 10 μm long.

An important way of classifying bacteria is to determine their **staining properties**. Some cannot be stained at all. Or they may be beyond the resolution of a microscope. These are viewed by dark-field microscopy—they are illuminated from the side, and because of the difference in refractive index in relation to the surrounding aqueous solution, they scatter light and appear as shining particles against a dark background. Other bacteria can be stained, and some even retain a stain if they are subsequently treated with acids; these are said to be **acid-fast**. One common acid-fast bacillus causes tuberculosis. Similarly, by virtue of their ability to retain certain stains after washing with alcohol or acetone, bacteria can be divided into two groups known as **gram positive** (which retains a purple stain) and **gram negative** (which loses the purple stain and takes the red color of the counterstain).

The difference in staining properties reflects other functionally more important differences between the bacteria than only enabling a diagnosis to be made. For example, the acid-fast property of the tubercle bacilli means that the bacteria can resist the hydrochloric acid environment of the gastric juice, which would otherwise render many bacteria harmless. Intestinal tuberculosis was therefore a common disease before milk was pasteurized or the cows became "reaction-free"—that is, free from tuberculous infectious agents. The infectious agent is easily transferred to man from tuberculous foci in the udder and carried in the milk.

A discriminating feature of medical importance is the bacterias' need for oxygen; **aerobes** require oxygen to grow, **anaerobes** cannot grow in the presence of oxygen, and **facultative** bacteria do not require oxygen and can grow in its presence. Most bacteria are aerobic. An example of an anaerobe is the tetanus bacterium, which is common in soil, especially in the presence of horse manure. Because of the anaerobic nature of the bacteria, tetanus infection usually does not occur in the presence of air even where there are very extensive lesions. In the cases of puncture wounds—for example, one caused by stepping on a nail or by animal bites—air cannot penetrate the wound channel and there is a risk of tetanus infection; vaccination is therefore necessary. Tetanus infection is a dangerous condition with an often fatal outcome.

Rickettsia are an intermediate form between bacteria and viruses. They are spread by lice, fleas, ticks and mites, and produce a number of diseases, including Rocky Mountain spotted fever and typhus.

Viruses   are the smallest and least developed of the microorganisms. With a size of 20–300 nm, they cannot be seen under the ordinary light microscope, and they pass through bacteria filters. Therefore, virus diseases can be transmitted experimentally through cell-free filtrates. Viruses can only multiply in living cells; they are said to be obligate intracellular parasites.

They can be oblong with spiral structure, helical, or cubic.

In the systematic classification of virus, the shape is used as the basis. Other characteristics are the type of nucleic acid (carrier of the genetic traits) that the virus contains, the number of protein units, which are linked to the nucleic acid, and whether the virus has a capsule.

Table 6.1 Some common diseases caused by microorganisms, their incubation times and location of the infectious agents in the body

Disease	Microorganism	Incubation time	Site
malaria	malarial plasmodium	10–12 d	blood
dermatophytoses	fungi		skin
gonorrhea	diplococci	2–6 d	sexual organs, eyes
epidemic cerebral meningitis	diplococci	1–3 d	cerebral meninges
erysipelas	hemolytic streptococci	3–5 d	skin
impetigo	hemolytic streptococci		skin
sore throat	hemolytic streptococci		throat
ear inflammation	hemolytic streptococci		middle ear
scarlet fever	hemolytic streptococci	2–5 d	skin, throat, etc.
impetigo	staphylococci		skin
ear, nose and throat infections	staphylococci		airways
pneumonia	staphylococci		lungs
pyelonephritis	staphylococci		kidneys, urinary tract
food poisoning	staphylococci		gastrointestinal tract
endocarditis	staphylococci		heart valves
osteomyelitis	staphylococci		bone marrow
paratyphoid fever	salmonella bacteria	2–5 d	gastrointestinal tract, etc.
tetanus	tetanus bacteria	1–2 w	wound lesions
tuberculosis	tubercle bacilli	6–8 w	lungs, gastrointestinal tract, cerebral meninges, kidneys skin, etc.
leprosy	leprosy bacilli	6–10 y	skin, internal organs
measles	rubeola virus	9–11 d	skin, mucous membranes, internal organs
German measles	rubella virus	~14 d	lymph nodes, skin
chickenpox	varicella virus	~14 d	skin (mainly children)
shingles	varicella virus		skin (mainly adults)
smallpox	variola virus	11–12 d	skin
hepatitis A	hepatitis virus	3–5 w	liver
hepatitis B (from inoculation as in blood transfusions, etc.)	hepatitis virus	2–6 mo	liver

This systematic classification is unsuitable for diagnostic work. Instead, viruses are grouped according to the symptoms they produce. Several **exanthem viruses** can cause diseases accompanied by skin eruptions, for example, measles, German measles, smallpox, chickenpox and shingles. **Respiratory viruses** produce influenza, viral pneumonia (a special form of pneumonia) and psittacosis (a form of pneumonia spread by certain parrots and other birds). **Neurotropic viruses** produce poliomyelitis, encephalitis (page 77), viral meningitis and rabies, diseases that produce disorders of the nervous system. A number of these viruses, for example, polio, echo and coxsackie viruses reproduce in the intestinal tract, and they are therefore also classified as **enteroviruses. Hepatitis viruses** produce infections of the liver. Hepatitis A was formerly known as infectious hepatitis and hepatitis B was formerly known as serum hepatitis.

Some viruses can produce tumors, though all tumors are not due to viruses.

6.9	Pathogenic organisms can be divided into four groups ...., ..., ... and	
6.10	Protozoa are single-celled ...., which are the cause of a number of .... diseases.	protozoa fungi bacteria viruses
6.11	Fungi produce a number of .... diseases.	animals tropical
6.12	In size most bacteria are of the order of ...., and viruses	skin
6.13	Bacteria can be divided on the basis of their shape into ...., ... and	$1\,\mu$m 100 nm
6.14	The spherical ones are called	spherical rod-shaped spiral
6.15	The rod-shaped bacteria are called	cocci
6.16	Spirilla bacteria are .... shaped.	bacilli
6.17	Bacteria can also be classified on the basis of their .... properties.	spiral
6.18	An example of acid-fast bacilli is	staining
6.19	The terms gram positive and gram negative denote different .... of bacteria.	tubercle bacillus
6.20	Exanthem viruses cause diseases with	staining properties
6.21	Respiratory viruses are located in the	skin eruptions

6.22	Poliomyelitis, encephalitis and rabies are caused by .... viruses.	respiratory tract
6.23	Enteroviruses propagate in the	neurotropic
6.24	A patient has bleeding from the gastrointestinal tract that is difficult to locate and is given a number of blood transfusions. He recovers after an operation for gastric ulcer but four months later becomes ill again, with fatigue and jaundice. The patient has been infected with .... viruses during the blood transfusion.	intestinal tract
6.25	A man who had spent some time in the tropics has intermittent fever every three days lasting 3–4 hours (Fig. 2.19). The physician immediately suspects malaria and takes blood specimens during the fever attack. Microscopic examination discloses the infectious agent, which consists of .... (the group of microorganisms).	hepatitis B
6.26	A military barracks has a shower room with a floor consisting of permanently damp wooden slats. On these thrive the microorganisms that cause athlete's foot. Some time after exposure, the disease appears as inflamed skin and irritation between the toes. This condition is caused by .... (latin name for the fungal disease).	protozoa
6.27	In a family, the mother has a sore throat, a 14-year-old child has a purulent skin eruption, a child of 10 years has scarlet fever and an infant has diarrhea. The physician immediately suspects that the various diseases are due to the same infectious agent, a hemolytic strepto-........... He also suspects that the father may be the carrier of the infection, and this was confirmed by bacteriological examination of specimens from his throat. The same infectious agent can thus produce diseases with different locations in the body and therefore give different .... (signs of disease). The whole family is treated with antibiotics, since this bacterium is capable of producing more serious pathological conditions, including rheumatic fever and nephritis (inflammation of the kidneys).	mycosis

6.28	A person who has vacationed in a subtropical area becomes ill a month after returning home, with increasing severe fatigue, headache, pain in the pit of the stomach and liver region and nausea. After a week or so the eyeballs turn yellow. One diagnostic consideration should be	coccus symptoms
		hepatitis A

MICROBIOLOGICAL CULTURE TECHNIQUES

Infectious diseases are diagnosed in essentially two ways. One method is to demonstrate in the patient the occurrence of a specific immunity to the disease in a way described below in the section on immunology. Since immunity does not develop for a week or longer, this diagnosis cannot be made at the onset of the illness, and often not until the convalescent stage.

The second method can often be applied and gives the diagnosis earlier. This consists of different culture procedures. By taking specimens from the patient, the infectious agent is transferred to a series of culture media, where it propagates. By isolating the infectious agent and studying the growth, it can be classified. In some cases, for example in the case of gonorrhea, the infectious agent can be observed directly by microscopic examination of stained preparations. These are produced from secretions obtained from the patient; to verify the diagnosis, cultures are also made.

Specimen-taking technique

All specimens for cultures from patients are taken in sterile specimen vessels. The use of a swab permits the specimen to be taken without the risk of contaminating it and without contaminating the hands. The type of vessel for specimen-taking varies with the purpose of the examination. For specimens from mucous membranes—for example, from the throat and urethra—the end of the stick is furnished with a twisted tuft of cotton for picking up the secretion; it is known as a cotton swab. In the case of fecal specimens, the rod is shaped as a small glass spatula on which a small amount of feces can easily be picked up. For dispatch by mail, the specimen is sometimes packed in a chilled cooler to prevent growth from occurring before the specimen reaches the laboratory.

Bacteriological specimens are collected from a number of sources. For example, they may consist of **sputum, urine, feces, gastric washings, blood** and **pus** from wounds. At the bacteriological laboratory a small amount of the specimen is transferred to various culture media.

Culture media

Most pathogenic bacteria can be cultured outside the human body, if they are offered suitable media. Only a few bacteria require such special conditions that the culture must be performed by inoculation in animals. Viruses require living media.

The basic medium for cultures of pathogenic bacteria consists of meat bouillon, peptone (breakdown product of proteins) and salts. To this basic medium can be added growth-promoting substrates, such as blood, blood serum and ascitic fluid (fluid collecting in peritoneal cavity), or growth-inhibiting substances, which depress growth of certain bacteria so that others can be isolated. An example is gentian violet, which inhibits staphylococci. The various culture media are added to agar, a macromolecular carbohydrate which gives the medium a suitable, relatively firm, gelatinous consistency. The substrate is sterilized and poured into Petri dishes or test tubes.

From the specimen vessel a small quantity of the specimen is transferred to agar plates with a platinum loop that has been sterilized in a flame and then cooled. This is drawn in a streaking pattern over the agar plate so as to obtain sufficient spread. This enables individual bacteria to grow into isolated uniform colonies.

The culture is usually incubated at 37°C in a thermostatically controlled environment and sometimes in special gaseous environments—for example, anaerobe cultures (oxygen-free atmosphere) or culture in the presence of carbon dioxide. The culture time is usually 24 hours, though it can be considerably longer for bacteria with slow growth.

The gross appearance of colonies of bacteria provides one basis of classification, and a further grouping can be performed by microscopic examination of stained samples from the colonies. It is also noted on which media bacteria are able to grow, by transferring specimens from colonies by means of platinum loops to agar plates with other substrates—**reinoculation** (Fig. 6.1). In some cases liquid

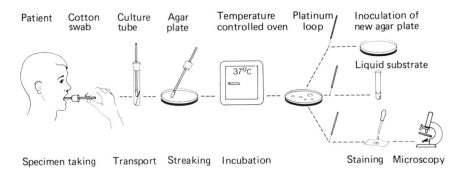

Figure 6.1 Bacteriological culture technique.

substrates are used—for example, solutions of different kinds of sugar for classifying the bacteria on the basis of their ability to break these down.

The medium and the culture procedures are chosen according to the type of test and the tentative diagnosis. It is therefore important to know the clinical context—for example, streptococcus infection or tuberculosis—when choosing the medium and the culture technique.

6.29	Infectious diseases can be diagnosed in two main ways, namely, by demonstrating the presence of either an . . . . or of	
6.30	Pathogenic microorganisms are usually demonstrated by isolating the infectious agent and identifying it by repeated . . . . ; only occasionally can the microorganisms be identified by direct . . . . . , ... of stained preparations, which are prepared from secretions obtained from the patient.	infectious agent (microorganism) immunity
6.31	To prevent the contamination of the specimen with other microorganisms, the specimen is taken under . . . . conditions.	culturing microscopy
6.32	Specimens for culture are obtained from a number of sources, for example, they may consist of . . . . , ... , ... , ... , ... or	sterile
6.33	Cultures are usually performed on plates with a nutrient medium to which a macromolecular carbohydrate known as . . . . has been added as a supporting substance.	sputum urine feces gastric washings blood pus
6.34	A specimen for bacteriological examination usually contains several types of bacteria. Pure cultures can be obtained by distributing the material on solid media so that the individual . . . . are located at a safe distance from each other. They then produce isolated	agar

6.35	Bacteria are classified by observing the appearance of ...., by staining samples from the colonies and viewing these under a ...., by examining the growth on, or in, different .... and by examining the bacteria's ability to .... certain substances, such as sugars.	bacteria colonies
6.36	The transfer of bacteria from one colony to a new agar plate is known as .... and is performed with a flamed	colonies microscope media break down
6.37	Examples of different growth-promoting substrates used for classifying bacteria by culturing are ...., ... and	reinoculation platinum loop
6.38	To facilitate isolation of certain bacteria, additives are sometimes used that .... the growth of other bacteria. Such additives are often stains.	blood blood serum ascitic fluid (abdominal fluid)
		inhibit

Determination of bacterial resistance. To be able to choose the right medicine—that is, the right **chemotherapeutic agent** (synthetically prepared chemical compound) or **antibiotic** (originally a compound prepared from another microorganism, hereafter included in the term "chemotherapeutic agent"), the sensitivity of the pathogenic microorganism to these should be known. The sensitivity can vary for a given type of bacteria. It can also decrease during the course of a disease in a patient so that the bacteria become **resistant** to the drug. "Resistant" means that a microorganism can overcome the effect of a chemotherapeutic agent. A drug chosen for treatment should be one for which the microorganism has a low resistance.

Resistance is determined by culturing microorganisms in the presence of various chemotherapeutic agents. Bacteria from at least 10 different colonies on an agar plate are suspended in broth. After dilution, this is poured on to a large blood-agar plate; the excess liquid is absorbed and the plate left to dry. On the plate a number of pieces of filter paper impregnated with various chemotherapeutic agents are placed. As a result of diffusion, the concentration of the chemotherapeutic agent will decrease with the distance from the center of the filter paper. Bacterial growth is inhibited in a zone around each piece (Fig. 6.2). The size of the zone of inhibition reflects the sensitivity of the bacterial strain to the chemotherapeutic agent in question. The diameter of the zone is proportional to the logarithm of the inverse of the concentration that is just needed to obtain inhibition.

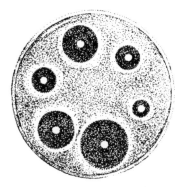

Figure 6.2 Resistance determination
with antibiotic test paper. The bacterial
strain is most sensitive to the antibiotic
in the bottom right area (5 o'clock).

6.39	The ability of a microorganism to overcome the effect of a chemotherapeutic agent (and antibiotics) is known as	
6.40	The resistance of a microorganism is determined by culturing it in the presence of a chemotherapeutic agent and observing the .... at which growth is just inhibited.	resistance
6.41	In a resistance determination, bacteria are cultured on a blood-agar medium. A varying concentration of the agent is obtained by allowing it to .... from a piece of filter paper impregnated with it.	concentration
6.42	Bacterial growth is inhibited around the piece of filter paper, and the diameter of the zone in which there is inhibition is .... (proportional to, inversely proportional to, proportional to the logarithm of, inversely proportional to the logarithm of) the inverse of the concentration required to obtain inhibition.	diffuse
		proportional to the logarithm of

Culture in animals. Most pathogenic bacteria can be cultured on non-living media, but sometimes they must be inoculated into animals. This applies particularly to tubercle bacilli. Although these can be cultured on Löwenstein-Jensen agar, tests in the guinea pig may be occasionally required to confirm the diagnosis.

The guinea pig is highly susceptible to tuberculosis. The specimen is treated with 6 percent hydrochloric acid for 10 minutes to kill microorganisms that are not acid-fast. After washing and centrifuging, the sediment is injected in the right thigh muscle of the guinea pig. After 6 weeks the animal is sacrificed and examined for tuberculous foci in the lymph nodes. The diagnosis is confirmed by microscopic examination of specimens from these foci.

Culture of viruses. Laboratory diagnosis of viral diseases is performed in essentially the same way as for bacterial infections, namely, by isolating and identifying the infectious agent and demonstrating specific immunity in blood serum. The practical procedure for the handling of viruses varies; they cannot be cultured on dead media. Viruses require living media—either living animals or tissue cultures. A tissue culture consists of cells taken from an organ of an animal and treated so that they remain living and multiply in a suitable nutrient solution and environment. By using different types of tissue cultures, viruses can be classified in a similar way to that using selective media in bacteriology. The time required for classifying by means of cultures varies from a couple of days to weeks or months. Viral diagnosis is difficult, expensive and time-consuming.

6.43	Viruses can be cultured only in . . . . cells.	
6.44	For culturing viruses, ... cultures are often used.	living
6.45	A tissue culture consists of . . . . from animals. The cells remain living in a suitable	tissue
6.46	Viruses can be typed by studying the growth in tissue cultures with different kinds of	cells nutrient solution
		cells

Growth curves. Bacteria reproduce by division. If there are sufficient nutrient substances, growth proceeds regularly, with renewed division after a constant interval. This varies according to the type of bacteria. For **coliform bacteria**, the usual intestinal bacteria, it is 20 minutes. If a number of bacteria are added to a liquid nutrient solution, the growth is exponential. Thus, if $\alpha = (dB/dt)/B$, where B is the amount of bacterial substance, the amount after time, t, is given by the expression $B_t = B_0\, e^{\alpha t}$. In this formula $\alpha = \ln 2/T = 0.693/T$, where T is the time required for the number of bacteria to double.

This uninhibited growth obviously cannot proceed undisturbed for a long time; a deficiency of nutrient substances will soon result in inhibition, and the accumulation of toxic products in the culture medium will be a further factor in the replacement of the **exponential phase** in the growth by a **stationary phase**, in which there is no increase in the number of bacteria.

Some bacteria can form **spores**, which occur during a resting state. The spores are highly resistant to heat, drying and disinfection. Spore formation presents a problem in sterilization because of their high tolerance to unfavorable environmental conditions.

6.47	Assume that a new mutation of a single coli bacterium could utilize all the organic substances in a human subject, about 10^5 g, as substrates. Assume, moreover, that the mixture of the organic material does not hinder growth during the exponential phase. After how long will the bacteria have used all the substrate and entered the stationary phase? One bacterium weighs 10^{-12} g. The time between two divisions of a bacterium, the generation time, is 20 minutes.	
6.48	Some bacteria form a resting state, when they are known as	19 hours ($\alpha = 2.08$)
		spores

STERILIZATION AND DISINFECTION

Modern medical care is based to a large extent on **asepsis**—that is, on the fact that instruments used and parts of the patient treated are kept as free as possible from microorganisms. This is accomplished by **disinfection** of the operative area and site where specimens are taken and by **sterilization** of instruments and other equipment.

The term "sterilization" refers to different procedures by which all microorganisms, including bacterial spores, on the objects in question are killed. In disinfection, the number of pathogenic microorganisms is reduced as far as practicable.

Careful disinfection can thus never replace sterilization. Instruments and dressings for use during operations, delivery and punctures must be sterile. They are often packed in paper or plastic in order to facilitate their transport under non-sterile external conditions. The packed objects have a limited shelf life, and the time is dependent on the type of packaging: textiles 1 month, paper 1–6 months and nylon, glass and metal 1 year, if tightly closed.

Sterilization

In sterilization, the only methods that can be used are ones that kill all microorganisms. The effectiveness of different sterilization methods is dependent on the amount of microorganisms present, and effective **mechanical cleaning** is a necessary procedure when preparing apparatus, etc. for sterilization. Sterilization can be performed according to three different principles: heat sterilization, chemical sterilization and radiation sterilization.

Heat sterilization

Sterilization with heat is the simplest, most effective and inexpensive method for use in medical care. Two different procedures are used, depending on the tolerance of the material concerned: **autoclaving**, which should always be used where possible, and **dry sterilization**.

Autoclaving is sterilization with saturated steam under pressure—that is, at a temperature over 100°C. The objects being sterilized are packed in double-thickness paper wrappers, nylon foil or cloth, so that steam can pass through but so that they can be stored and handled afterwards without becoming unsterile.

The objects are packed loosely in the autoclave so that they occupy only four fifths of its volume, thus facilitating circulation and heat transfer. The air is withdrawn during the **pre-vacuum period**. During the **sterilizing period** steam is introduced under pressure; the apparatus is heated to 120°C (corresponding to 1.0 atm, SI 100 kPa) for at least 15 min, or to 144°C (corresponding to 3.0 atm, SI 300 kPa) for at least 2 min. Sterilization is followed by a **post-vacuum** period, when steam is withdrawn so as to dry the autoclaved apparatus.

Most autoclaves have automatic programs, giving a choice of temperature and time. Short times are preferred, but as this implies a high temperature, which can damage the objects, it is often necessary to choose longer times and lower temperatures. To ensure that the autoclaving is being correctly performed, the pressure and temperature are recorded by a pen recorder throughout the autoclaving process. The curves are examined after each sterilization. In addition, the efficiency is checked every two weeks and after repairs—by spore tests; all spores in the test strips used must be killed. For a routine check that the material has actually undergone sterilization, packages are furnished with indicator tape, which changes color during autoclaving.

Dry-heat sterilization involves heating at atmospheric pressure. It is continued for half an hour at 180°, 1 hour at 170° or 2 hours at 160°C—the times are the periods during which the objects have been maintained at the respective temperatures. To obtain a uniform temperature, the dry-heat sterilizer is often provided with a circulation fan.

Dry-heat sterilization is a less reliable method than autoclaving. Large temperature differences can arise within a dry-heat sterilizer, as a result of the way in which the objects are packed. Many materials do not tolerate dry-heat sterilization—for example, textiles, rubber objects or ones packed in paper. Nor should dry-heat sterilization be used for certain sharp instruments (knives, scissors, hypodermic needles) because the edges are blunted at high temperatures.

Chemical sterilization

Many chemical compounds can be used for sterilization. The compounds are **gases** or **liquids**.

Gas sterilization can be performed with ethylene oxide at temperatures between 30° and 60°C and at pressures that depend on the partial pressure of the ethylene oxide. The exposure period is about 10 hours. Prior to gas sterilization the objects must be kept in an environment with a constant atmospheric humidity so as to obtain an optimal level of humidity. The residual ethylene oxide must be ventilated after sterilization, and the objects must therefore be stored in well ventilated premises. Ethylene oxide autoclaves are difficult to operate and the method is unsuitable for hospitals. It is mostly used in industry, for example, for sterilizing disposable material that does not tolerate a high temperature.

Gas sterilization can also be performed with formalin gas, but the method has similar disadvantages to that for ethylene oxide; special apparatus for formalin sterilization of endoscopes and anesthetic apparatus have been developed, however.

Liquid sterilization can sometimes be performed with buffered **glutaric aldehyde**. The objects are immersed in the liquid for several hours. Glutaric aldehyde is poisonous and after sterilization the objects must be thoroughly rinsed in sterile water.

Radiation sterilization

Ionizing radiation in high doses provides an effective means of sterilization. Gamma radiation from ^{60}Co is generally used but high-energy electron radiation from linear accelerators may be used. With the ^{60}Co method, 2.5–3.2 megarad is given (SI unit 25–32 kGy). The objects, which are packed in containers, are conveyed continuously round the radiation source on a conveyer belt so that most of the radiation is efficiently utilized and the containers are irradiated from all directions. Despite the long irradiation time—about 24 hours—the capacity is high.

Disinfection

In disinfection, the number of pathogenic microorganisms is reduced, but not all of them are killed. Disinfection is accomplished with **heat** and **chemical agents**. Objects that may be infected—for example, bedpans—must be disinfected at the earliest opportunity after use, and before cleaning. Before an operation, the patient's skin in the surgical field is disinfected. Likewise, before putting on the sterile gloves, the surgeon disinfects his hands as a precaution, in case the gloves should tear during the operation.

Heat disinfection   is accomplished by boiling in water at atmospheric pressure, usually for at least 5 minutes. Some bedpan rinsers and washing units have special programs which disinfect at the same time as they perform mechanical cleaning.

Chemical disinfection   is carried out with a number of different agents. Active substances are chosen according to the tolerance of the objects and the infectious agent in question. For disinfection of objects, agents containing **phenol** and some cleaning component are often used. These may be combined into a special soap. These substances destroy the membranes of the microorganisms. For disinfection of the skin, 70 percent alcohol may be used, which denatures the proteins of the microorganisms; hexachlorophene or surface active components are sometimes added. For disinfecting the hands before operations, soap containing hexachlorophene is used.

Because of the resistance of the virus in hepatitis, in suspected cases of this disease, heat disinfection or a 5 percent solution of chloramine should be used.

6.49	Keeping instruments and relevant parts of the patient free from microorganisms as far as possible is known as	
6.50	Aseptic conditions are achieved by means of two measures, namely . . . . and	asepsis
6.51	In sterilization the microorganisms are	sterilization disinfection
6.52	In disinfection the microorganisms are	killed
6.53	An essential measure before sterilization is	reduced in number

6.54	Sterilization can be accomplished in essentially three ways, namely, ... , ... and	mechanical cleaning
6.55	Heat sterilization, in turn, can be performed by two methods, namely, ... and	heat sterilization chemical sterilization radiation sterilization
6.56	In autoclaving, sterilization is performed with saturated . . . . at an elevated	autoclaving dry-heat sterilization
6.57	In autoclaving, the temperature used is . . . . -. . . . . corresponding to a pressure of . . . . -. . . . . and the time required is then	steam temperature (pressure)
6.58	The autoclaving procedure has three stages: . . . . , ... and	120–144°C 1–3 atm (100–300 kPa) 15–2 min
6.59	During the pre-vacuum procedure, ... is withdrawn, and during the post-vacuum period . . . . is withdrawn.	pre-vacuum period sterilization period post-vacuum period
6.60	In dry-heat sterilization, the objects are heated for . . . . (time) at . . . . (temperature).	air steam
6.61	In gas sterilization, several compounds can be used such as . . . . and	2, 1 or $\frac{1}{2}$ h 160, 170 or 180°C
6.62	Gas sterilization with ethylene oxide can be performed at temperatures in the range	ethylene oxide formalin
6.63	Gas sterilization with ethylene oxide is . . . . (suitable, unsuitable) for use in hospitals.	30–60°C
6.64	For liquid sterilization, ... is used; this is . . . . (poisonous, not poisonous).	unsuitable
6.65	In sterilization with gamma radiation, the radiation source is . . . . The dose is . . . . -.	buffered glutaric aldehyde poisonous
6.66	Disinfection can be performed by two principles, namely, with . . . . or	^{60}Co 2.5–3.2 megarad (25–32 kGy)

6.67	Heat disinfection is performed by boiling in .... (substance) at .... (pressure).	heat chemical agents
6.68	Phenol soap, 70 percent alcohol, chloramine solution and hexachlorophene are used for	water atmospheric pressure
6.69	The procedure in which the number of pathogenic bacteria is reduced is known as	disinfection
6.70	The procedure when all microorganisms are killed is known as	disinfection
		sterilization

HOSPITAL HYGIENE

The spread of infection in hospitals is a serious and difficult problem. In many places special staff appointments in hospital hygiene have been established to minimize the chance of spreading infection. The infectious diseases that prevail in the hospitals are known as **hospital infections** or **nosocomial infections** (Greek—nosokomeion, hospital).

Spread of infection

Most of the infectious agents that emanate from an ill patient die in an unfavorable environment; the few microorganisms that manage to keep alive until they reach a new host organism ensure the continued existence of the disease on earth. The infection is spread from the **source of infection** via **infection routes** to **objects of infection**. Spread can be prevented by combating the disease in all three stages.

The source of infection can be patients that are severely ill, those that are mildly ill and on their feet, or those who are healthy carriers. In the case of the seriously ill, the infectious microorganisms are present in great numbers; the risk of infection is, however, usually easy to control, since the patient is confined to bed and all the staff are aware of the risk. The mildly ill represent a greater risk, for they often move around within the hospital and outside. Healthy carriers are the most important carriers of infectious agents for many diseases, for example, scarlet fever and poliomyelitis.

The severity of the disease in an infected patient is dependent on his resistance. A person with a low resistance is most severely affected by a new infection, while a person with some resistance can be suffering from the disease without displaying clinical symptoms of it. The detection of healthy carriers so that they can be treated and possibly isolated often entails a comprehensive, time-consuming and expensive investigation of many persons in a community group.

Routes of infection include **human contact, water, food, atmosphere** and **animals**. Infection via animals, water and food is rare in hospitals. The most common route is human contact, especially via the hands—good hand hygiene is the most important preventive measure. Airborne infection also occurs. An example of airborne infection is that of viral upper respiratory infection, which is spread by droplets among staff and patients. Other infections may be transmitted to hospital dust, and spread with this to the wards. To interrupt this infection route, suitable clothing for personnel is important, as is correct hospital ventilation. It is important to isolate certain infected patients, such as those with tuberculosis.

The susceptibility of the object of infection to infectious diseases is dependent on a number of factors, such as the **degree of immunity**, and **general state of health** and on the **amount of infectious agents** involved in the exposure.

The reason that hospital infections are so serious a problem is the concentration in hospitals of many patients in poor general health, and this increases the susceptibility to infections. Patients that are particularly susceptible to infection—for example burn patients—may be isolated so as to avoid exposure to the risk of infection.

6.71	An infectious disease is spread from an . . . . via one or more . . . . to an	
6.72	Of these steps the disease can be combated in	infection source infection routes object of infection
6.73	The source of infection can be a patient that is . . . . ill, ... ill or	all
6.74	The greatest risk is generally incurred by the	severely mildly healthy
6.75	Possible infection routes are . . . . , ... , ... , ... and	healthy infection carriers

6.76	At a military barracks, epidemic cerebral meningitis is detected. An attempt is made to eradicate the disease by prophylactic sulfa treatment of the whole unit, but this fails. Only by reducing the size of the unit and thus increasing the distance between individuals are new cases prevented. The infection route is then made more difficult since it takes place through	human contact water food atmosphere animals
6.77	The susceptibility of an object of infection is dependent on, among other things, the ...., ... and the amount of	the atmosphere
		degree of immunity general state of health infectious agent

Hospital infections

In a hospital there is an accumulation of sick people with reduced resistance to infection. Hygiene cannot be effectively maintained. Infection spreads rapidly and there are favorable conditions of growth for resistant infectious agents. Many microorganisms have the ability to modify their living conditions according to changes in their environment. This applies particularly to staphylococci, tubercle bacilli, and such bacteria as proteus and pseudomonas, all of which may develop resistance to various chemotherapeutic drugs over a period of years (page 332).

Urinary tract infections are clinically important in this context, especially when there is need to catheterize patients (placing a catheter in the urethra). Today attempts are made to avoid this in order to prevent the transfer of infection.

In addition, **infections of clean surgical wounds** are not uncommon; they account for about one quarter of all cases of hospital infections.

Another clinically important nosocomial infection is **hepatitis B**, which is spread via blood transfusions and via syringes and other instruments that are not properly sterilized. It is sometimes necessary to suspend all surgical transplantation work and all dialysis treatment of kidney patients for a period in order to avoid hepatitis B infections of both patients and staff.

6.78	A hospital infection is also called a .... infection.

6.79	Some reasons that hospital infections present so serious a problem are that patients have a low . . . ., it is difficult to maintain effective . . . . and some bacterial types rapidly develop great . . . . to chemotherapeutic drugs.	nosocomial
6.80	Clinically common diseases from the nosocomial aspect are . . . ., ... and	resistance to infection hygiene resistance
		urinary tract infections infections of clean surgical wounds hepatitis B

IMMUNOLOGY

The body defends itself against microorganisms in two essentially different ways: a nonspecific defense mechanism and a specific immunity that develops against the special microorganisms entering the organism.

The **nonspecific defense mechanism** includes a number of **mechanical barriers** to the environment. The most important protection is the skin itself, which is usually effective in preventing microorganisms from penetrating into the body. The respiratory epithelium has the special function of transporting all kinds of particles, including microorganisms, against the incoming airstream; this is accomplished by means of a wavelike movement of the epithelial cells, which are furnished with cilia (page 13).

The nonspecific defense mechanism also includes the important function that some cells possess of engulfing and ingesting foreign bodies, such as bacteria, a process known as **phagocytosis**. There are several kinds of phagocytic cells at different sites in the body. These cells belong to the organ system usually called the **reticuloendothelial system**, **RES**. This is not located in a particular organ but is interspersed in the different tissues, including the liver, spleen and lymph nodes. The phagocytic function is also possessed by the granulocytes and monocytes of the blood. On contact between a phagocytic cell and an invading microorganism, a depression forms in the surface of the phagocyte. The depth of the depression increases rapidly and the whole microorganism is soon entirely engulfed. Two different mechanisms can be evoked depending on the type of phagocytic cell: either the microorganism is dissolved completely or there is only partial breakdown, leaving many residues. It is generally considered that these remains are used to form antibodies (page 346), which are included in the specific immunity (Fig. 6.3).

Bacteria   White blood cells

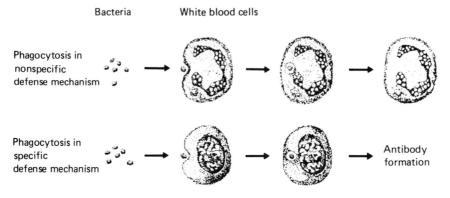

Phagocytosis in
nonspecific
defense mechanism

Phagocytosis in
specific
defense mechanism

Antibody
formation

Figure 6.3 White blood cells in the blood are capable of phagocytosing microorganisms—the process serves important functions in nonspecific and specific immunity defense mechanisms.

The nonspecific defense mechanism also uses chemical means. The skin has a certain bactericidal action because of its low pH of about 3.5, due to the secretion of lactic acid by the sweat and fat glands. The bactericidal action of gastric juice has been dealt with above (page 325). In the secretion from the intestinal membranes and the mucous membranes of the nose and in the saliva, there is an enzyme, **lysozyme**, that exerts a general bactericidal effect. In the cells, too, where viruses propagate, there is a substance called **interferon**, which has the property of inhibiting the synthesis of virus.

The **specific infection defense mechanism** is of particular microbiological interest and is dealt with more thoroughly in the following. It leads to the production of **antibodies** against some of those substances, **antigens**, that are characteristic of the types of microorganisms in question. The body thus becomes more or less immune to these microorganisms. The body can be stimulated to produce antibodies by **vaccination**—the injection of, for example, killed microorganisms. The ability to stimulate the formation of such antibodies is present not only in the substances of which the microorganisms are composed but also in many other macromolecular substances in our environment that can cause **allergic** diseases. In fact, under abnormal conditions, antibodies are formed even against some of the body's own substances—a process known as **autoimmunization**—an **autoimmune disease** thus appears. The presence of antibodies, of which there are many in the blood serum, is studied by **serological** methods.

6.81   The body defends itself against microorganisms in essentially two ways, namely, with a .... and a .... infection defense.

6.82	The skin and the movements of the cilia of the respiratory epithelium are nonspecific .... barriers against microorganisms.	nonspecific specific
6.83	Mechanical nonspecific infection defense mechanisms also include the property possessed by certain cells of engulfing and ingesting microorganisms; this is called	mechanical
6.84	Phagocytic cells are of different types and they are distributed in the various organs of the body. For example, they are found in the ...., ... and	phagocytosis
6.85	Besides the cells in these organs, the .... and .... circulating in the blood have a phagocytic function.	liver spleen lymph nodes
6.86	In phagocytosis, either the microorganisms can entirely .... or else some residues can remain that are used by the body to form ...., which are part of the specific defense mechanism.	granulocytes monocytes
6.87	The secretion of lactic acid by the skin, the production of hydrochloric acid by the stomach, the secretion of the enzyme lysozyme and the cells' ability to form interferon are part of the nonspecific .... infection defense.	dissolve antibodies
6.88	The pH of the skin is about ...., which gives a certain .... effect.	chemical
6.89	The pH of gastric juice is about .... (page 52).	3.5 bactericidal
6.90	The specific defense mechanism consists of the fact that the body produces antitoxins, called ...., against some of the macromolecular substances called .... which are characteristic of the microorganisms in question.	1.0
6.91	The body can be stimulated to form special antibodies by	antibodies antigens
		vaccination

ANTIGENS AND ANTIBODIES

As a mnemonic for distinguishing the terms "antigen" and "antibody" one should remember the meaning of **gene**, the hereditary factor. We were born with the genes, it is the primary factor. Antigens are substances that are usually foreign to the individual, hence the name, which denotes something that is contrary to the inherited properties of the individual (anti, against). However, an antigen is any substance that will elicit an antibody response, and may come from within the body. Antigens must first come into contact with immunocompetent cells before antibodies can form.

Antigens are the substances that can stimulate animal organisms to produce antibodies, which are specific against the antigen. Antigens are macromolecular substances. They consist either of proteins or of polysaccharides; pure lipids possess no property of eliciting antibody formation. For a substance to be able to behave as an antigen, it must have a molecular weight above 5,000. The antigen properties generally increase with the molecular weight.

Only rarely—and then it must be considered as a pathological state—can the substances found in the individual itself elicit formation of antibodies (see page 352 under "autoimmune diseases").

Antibodies are proteins that appear in blood serum after exposure of antigens, for example, during or after an infectious disease. There are also antibodies that are attached to certain cells in the body—lymphocytes and monocytes. A distinction is therefore made between **humoral immunity** (in the serum) and **cell-mediated immunity**.

Antibodies in the serum are present in a protein fraction known as gamma globulins. The molecular weights of these exceed 100,000. Antibodies do not appear until 1–3 weeks after the antigen has been supplied. The formation takes place with the participation of the reticuloendothelial system, RES, and of the phagocytic cells circulating in the blood and lymph (Fig. 6.3).

The formation of cell-mediated immunity is governed by an organ known as the **thymus** (behind the sternum). Its activity is greatest in early life, when the body is learning to identify the individual's own macromolecular substances, such as proteins and polysaccharides, so that the immune response is not developed against them. Cell-mediated immunity resides predominantly with a specific population of lymphocytes.

Cell-mediated immunity is of greatest importance in autoimmune diseases (page 352) and in the rejection of foreign tissues in transplantation (page 526), while humoral antibodies are most important in other immunological mechanisms—for example, in defense against infections.

When an antigen is first supplied, for example, when a foreign substance is injected into the body, there is only a moderate formation of antibodies. When the antigen is administered again after a week or more, the antibody formation increases greatly, and on the third occasion it is still greater. This fact is exploited in vaccination, when two or three injections are given to achieve adequate protection. After a month, the amount of antibodies in the serum usually begins to decrease unless antigens are supplied again; but the extent of the reduction depends on the nature of the antigen. After certain infections, for example, children's diseases, antibodies to these remain in the individual for the rest of his life.

The purpose of the formation of antibodies is to render the antigen harmless, and this can be effected in different ways. Bacteria can be clumped—by a process known as **agglutination**—after which they are eliminated by phagocytic cells. In addition, an antigen cell can be dissolved, a process known as **lysis**. This can occur, for example, with blood cells—hemolysis (page 288). Finally, there is **precipitation**, for example, of toxins, which then lose their properties (Fig. 6.4). An

Antigen   Antibody   Precipitation of antigen

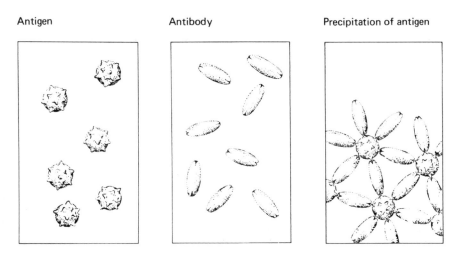

Figure 6.4 Precipitation of antigen by antibodies, presented schematically.

antigen–antibody complex forms, which is harmless—it is taken care of by the eosinophilic granulocytes (cf, pages 24 and 289).

6.92	Antigens are macromolecular substances that can stimulate the body to form	
6.93	Macromolecular substances, such as proteins or polysaccharides, but not lipids, can be	antibodies
6.94	Antigens are substances that are usually .... to the individual.	antigens

6.95	A distinction is drawn between humoral immunity, which occurs in ...., and cell-mediated immunity, which is associated with the body's	foreign
6.96	In the autoimmune diseases and in the rejection reaction involved in transplantations, the .... immunity is of the greatest importance.	blood serum cells
6.97	In defense against infections, ... immunity is of importance.	cell-mediated
6.98	The antibodies in blood serum belong to a protein fraction known as	humoral
6.99	Antibodies do not appear in blood serum until .... (time) after exposure to the antigen.	gamma globulins
6.100	After exposure to a new dose of antigen, the formation of antibodies .... (gradually decreases, is constant, greatly increases).	1–3 weeks
6.101	If a new dose of antigen is not supplied, the amount of antibodies in blood serum generally decreases after .... (time).	greatly increases
6.102	Antibodies act through clumping of bacteria, known as ...., the dissolution of the cells, known as .... or by separating out toxins, known as	about 1 month
		agglutination lysis precipitation

Immunization

When there are enough antibodies in the blood serum, the individual is not susceptible to the disease in question; **immunity** is said to have been induced. Immunization can be obtained in two ways, **passively** and **actively**.

Passive immunization is achieved by supplying the organism with preformed antibodies. Natural passive immunization occurs during fetal life as the antibodies from the mother's blood are transferred to the fetus via the placenta (page 596). For example, the newborn child is not susceptible to measles if the mother has previously had the disease. After some months, the amount of antibodies falls to a level that can no longer afford protection to the child.

Passive immunization to prevent disease is produced by injecting purified gamma globulins. These are prepared from blood obtained at deliveries, from blood that because of its age cannot be used for transfusion, or, in special cases, from blood obtained from patients that have had the diseases against which antibodies are required. The reason that blood from a normal population can be used is that most persons have antibodies to the commonest diseases in sufficient quantity for immunity to be transferred by the purified gamma globulins.

Examples of diseases that can be treated with the gamma globulins for preventive and therapeutic purposes are measles, mumps, whooping cough and hepatitis A.

Active immunization or **vaccination** is the process by which the individual himself is stimulated to form antibodies. This can be accomplished by supplying antigen from pathogenic organisms in essentially three ways: with a living but **attenuated infectious agent**, with a **killed infectious agent** or with an **inactivated toxin** derived from the infectious agent. The type of vaccine is chosen according to the agent's mode of attack on the organism.

Vaccination with attenuated living infectious agent generally provides longer immunity than vaccination with killed infectious agent. Much work has therefore been devoted to preparing attenuated microorganisms which, though capable of infecting the vaccinated individual, cannot produce a serious pathological state. BCG vaccination against tuberculosis and a special form of polio vaccination are examples of such vaccinations. Vaccination against smallpox—the first disease that could be prevented by active immunization—is similar to this method. It is not a product of the smallpox virus itself that is used, but a living infectious agent of cowpox—a closely related disease, which can also attack man. Because of the similarity between the cowpox and smallpox viruses, vaccination with the former produces immunity to the latter.

Where the infectious agent can overcome the nonspecific defense mechanisms as a result of properties that are directly linked to the infectious agent itself, a vaccine is chosen that is prepared from the agent. This is the case for typhus and paratyphoid fever. A vaccine against these diseases consists of bacteria that have been killed by heat treatment.

Vaccination with inactivated toxins can be chosen when the pathogenic microorganisms themselves do not harm the individual; the effect is obtained instead via secreted toxins (bacterial poisons). For example, this is the case in diphtheria and tetanus. Tetanus vaccine consists of a **toxoid**—that is, toxin obtained from tetanus bacteria that have been inactivated with formalin. This inactivation does not interfere with the toxin's ability to act as an antigen.

6.103	Immunization can be effected in two ways: . . . . and	
6.104	In passive immunization the individual is given preformed	actively passively
6.105	Antibodies are prepared from human blood serum, where they are included in the . . . . fraction.	antibodies
6.106	In active immunization, the individual is stimulated to produce	gamma globulin
6.107	Active immunization is performed by supplying inactivated . . . . or . . . . infectious agent or . . . . infectious agent.	antibodies
6.108	Immunization against hepatitis A is obtained by . . . . immunization.	toxin killed attenuated
6.109	In tetanus vaccination, a . . . . is injected.	passive
6.110	In vaccination against typhus and paratyphoid fever, ... are injected.	toxoid (inactivated bacterial toxin)
6.111	In BCG vaccination, ... are injected	killed bacteria
6.112	In smallpox vaccination, the living virus of . . . . is injected; this is immunologically closely related to smallpox.	attenuated living bacteria
6.113	There is a pathological state known as agamma-globulinemia (cf, a-, page 5, and -emia, page 24), in which the gamma globulins are absent from the blood serum. Based on what has been said in this chapter, what characteristics do you think these patients exhibit?	cowpox
		great susceptibility to infections

IMMUNOLOGICAL DISEASES

A number of diseases are caused by disturbances of the immunological system. The **allergic** diseases are due to such disturbances, as are the **autoimmune** diseases. The inability of the body to prevent tumors from developing in tumor diseases is probably largely also due to an incorrect immunological response of the individual; this is the subject of intensive investigations in **tumor immunology**.

Allergy

Allergic diseases are characterized by the development in the individual of an abnormally increased immunological reactivity. Two types of reaction can be distinguished, namely, those with an **immediate hypersensitive reaction** and those with a **delayed hypersensitive reaction**.

Allergic diseases are caused through repeated exposure of the individual to an antigen, with the result that he becomes **sensitized**. This sensitization implies increased reactivity during renewed exposure to the antigen; the immunological reaction then occurs, followed by allergic symptoms.

Immediate hypersensitive reactions can be localized or generalized. Examples of such reactions of the localized type are allergic hay fever, nettle rash, some forms of dermatitis and asthma. These conditions arise suddenly in the sensitized individual during renewed exposure to the antigen. In some cases it is difficult to determine the nature of the antigen since it can consist of very specific substances, with no characteristic location and association with objects, plants or animals. In other cases it is easy to identify the inciting antigen—for example, pollen can produce hay fever and cats can cause asthma.

In a generalized immediate hypersensitive reaction, **anaphylactic shock** can arise. This is a potentially dangerous condition. Within a few minutes of exposure to the antigen, the patient develops severe respiratory symptoms due to broncho-spasm (page 57), circulatory collapse due to falling blood pressure, often a rash over the whole body and sometimes vomiting and diarrhea. This intense generalized reaction in the form of anaphylactic shock is rare; it sometimes occurs after injection of a drug (for example, penicillin) or as a result of an insect sting (wasp).

Delayed hypersensitive reactions appear in susceptible individuals after repeated contact with the sensitizing substance. The reaction consists of contact dermatitis, which is manifested as reddening of the skin, and possibly formation of vesicles and swelling. A delayed hypersensitive reaction is used diagnostically for demonstrating past or current tubercular infection: the positive tuberculin reaction is a delayed hypersensitive reaction.

6.114	When the individual has developed abnormally increased immunological reactivity, a pathological state known as . . . . develops.

6.115	Allergic diseases develop when the susceptible individual is repeatedly exposed to an . . . . ; the individual then becomes	allergy
6.116	Allergic hay fever, nettle rash, some forms of eczema and asthma are examples of . . . . hypersensitive reactions.	antigen sensitized
6.117	The tuberculin test is an example of a . . . . hypersensitive reaction.	immediate
6.118	A patient some years previously had been given penicillin injections over a long period for an infectious disease, and recovered. To combat an acute throat infection, the physician gives a penicillin injection. Within a minute or so, severe respiratory distress develops, with pallor, cold sweat and a dazed state; a rash covers the whole body and there is diarrhea and vomiting; he dies in a quarter of an hour of . . . . (diagnosis). The first injections caused sensitization of the patient.	delayed
		anaphylactic shock

Autoimmune diseases

A state in which immunological reactions develop against the individual's own tissue is known as **autoimmunity**. The reaction can be directed against a particular organ, **organ-specific autoimmune diseases**, or against a number of organs, **systemic autoimmune diseases**. Antigens can consist of macromolecular substances on cell membranes, within the cell cytoplasm (page 12) or in the cell nucleus.

In autoimmune diseases, antibodies are generally present both in the serum—humoral antibodies—and bound to cells, where they are usually attached to the lymphocytes of the blood. It is, however, the cell-mediated immunity that is the pathogenic component of the immune reaction, while the humoral antibodies for the most part only reflect a general immunological reaction tendency.

The mechanism underlying an autoimmune disease is not fully known. One important factor is cell damage in an organ with resulting liberation of macromolecular substances, which then stimulate antibody formation. Another possibility is that macromolecular substances in the cell undergo changes whereby they acquire a structure so foreign to the organism that they can function as antigens. A probable contributory factor is an abnormally increased immunological reactivity of the organism. A virus infection in an organ can possibly result in its developing an autoimmune pathological state directed against the organ itself.

Organ-specific autoimmune diseases. The autoimmune mechanism can affect different organs. Examples of diseases that involve blood cells are **hemolytic anemia**, a blood deficiency disease due to an abnormally increased hemolysis (page 288) of the red blood cells, and **thrombocytopenia**, an increased bleeding tendency, due to a reduction in the number of blood platelets through agglutination (page 347).

In **sympathetic ophthalmia**, the sound eye is affected some weeks after mechanical damage to the other eye. The mechanism is obviously as follows: the trauma liberates an antigen from the damaged eye; cellular antibodies are then formed, which attack the corresponding substance in the sound eye, with resulting blindness in both eyes.

In the digestive organs, a number of autoimmune pathological states can arise. In patients with **ulcerative colitis** (page 55, question 1.250), antibodies have been observed that react specifically to the mucous membrane of the colon. **Pernicious anemia**, blood deficiency due to a lack of vitamin B_{12}, is thought to be caused by an autoimmune reaction that affects the mucous membrane of the stomach, and this leads to impaired absorption of this vitamin.

Motor nerve tissue can also be attacked; the muscle disease **myasthenia gravis** (page 252) is considered to be an example.

Finally, an example of an autoimmune disease in organ parenchyma (page 11) is **chronic thyroiditis**. Antibodies form that react specifically with thyroid gland tissue, leading to reduced thyroid function and hence **hypothyroidism** (page 74).

Systemic autoimmune diseases are characterized by the involvement of many different organs. Antibodies to a number of different tissues and cell components can be observed. These diseases are also called **collagenoses**. Examples are **rheumatoid arthritis** and lupus erythematosus, a disease with a poor prognosis if left untreated.

6.119	The condition in which the immunological reaction of the body is directed against a tissue of the same individual is known as	
6.120	Macromolecular substances on the cell membranes in the cell cytoplasm or in the cell nucleus can constitute . . . . in autoimmune diseases.	autoimmunity
6.121	The most important antibodies in autoimmune diseases are . . . . (cell-mediated, humoral).	antigens

6.122	Hemolytic anemia, thrombocytopenia, sympathetic ophthalmia, ulcerative colitis, pernicious anemia, myasthenia gravis and chronic thyroiditis are examples of .... autoimmune diseases.	cell-mediated
6.123	Rheumatoid arthritis and lupus erythematosus are examples of	organ-specific
		systemic autoimmune diseases

Tumor immunology. Tumor tissue has antigenic properties. Specific antibodies can thus be produced in the organism and produce an immunity to the tumor. This has been demonstrated in animal experiments; likewise it has been shown that certain substances can nonspecifically increase the animal's capacity to react immunologically against its own tumor.

Because of the existence of the many autoimmune pathological conditions in man, it is also probable that treatment of tumors might be performed according to some immunological principle. There is also much evidence that the resistance to tumors, and also the healing capacity after surgical treatment and radiotherapy, are due in a large measure to cell-mediated immunity.

Experiments to produce immunity in man with vaccine consisting of tumor extracts are at present considered to entail risks of transferring the tumor with some virus, and it has therefore still not been possible to perform such experiments.

SEROLOGY

The presence of an antibody for a certain antigen can be determined with serological methods. Antibodies are demonstrated by different methods, depending on the nature of the infectious agent. In the case of bacterial antigens, use is made of the phenomenon of **agglutination**, that is, the property of antibodies whereby they cause bacteria to clump. If dissolved antigens are present, an attempt is made to use **precipitation**—whereby antibodies form insoluble compounds with corresponding antigens, so that precipitation occurs. If the antigen–antibody complex does not cause precipitation, **complement fixation** can be used.

Serological reactions can be used for two essentially different purposes. First, a patient's disease can be diagnosed indirectly by demonstrating the formation of antibodies in serum—as antigens a number of known infectious agents, such as killed bacteria, may be used. Second, unknown infectious agents— for example, bacteria that have been isolated from patients—are identified by studying their reaction to a number of sera containing known antibodies.

In serological diagnosis, it is necessary to measure the amount of an antibody; this is done by **titration**. The specimen is diluted and the highest dilution at which the serological reaction can still be observed is noted. When performing the dilution, it is usual to halve the serum content at each step. Thus, if the first dilution is 1/10 the subsequent dilutions will be 1/20, 1/40, 1/80 . . . etc. The titer is expressed as the reciprocal of the dilution. If, for example, precipitation is observed at 1/160 but not at 1/320, the titer is 160.

Agglutination is obtained when antibodies react with large particles which have the character of antigens, for example, bacteria, fungi and red blood cells. An example of such a common agglutination reaction is **Widal's reaction**, when the antibody content is determined for a patient's serum, by using suspensions of known killed bacteria. First, a geometric series of dilutions of the examined sample is prepared, as indicated above, so as to obtain a number of samples with descending serum concentration. The bacterial suspension is added and the test tube series is kept at 37–50°C for an hour or so and then at room temperature or in the cold overnight. Agglutination can be observed as a typical precipitate at the bottom of the test tubes, which differs in appearance from sedimented bacteria alone. In other cases the agglutination is studied on a slide under the microscope.

Precipitation occurs when bivalent antibodies are specifically bound to multi-valent antigens to such an extent that large enough aggregates are obtained for precipitation. The amount of the precipitate is dependent on the proportions of antigen and antibody. The precipitation is greatest when antigen and antibody are present in equivalent amounts.

Complement fixation is used in those antigen-antibody reactions where there is no precipitation. Complement fixation in an antigen-antibody reaction is based on the consumption of a nonspecific factor called the complement. By demonstrating that the complement has been used up, it can be inferred indirectly that there has been a reaction between an antigen and an antibody.

First the complement present in the examined blood serum is inactivated by heating. A small, exactly known amount of complement and antigen are then added. If the examined serum contains antibodies for the antigen in question, no complement can be observed after a period of incubation.

The presence or absence of complement is examined in a **hemolytic** system consisting of sheep-blood cells and antibodies to these. If complement is added to this system, hemolysis occurs; if no complement is added, there is no hemolysis. An example of a common complement fixation reaction is the Wassermann reaction, W.R., in syphilis.

6.124	Serological reactions can be used for two essentially different purposes. First, they can be used for indirect diagnosis of a patient's disease by demonstrating that .... have been formed in the blood serum; in this case a number of known .... are used as antigens.	
6.125	Second, serological reactions can be used to determine unknown .... by studying how they react with a number of sera containing known	antibodies infectious agents
6.126	In a serological titration, the titer is expressed as the	infectious agents antibodies
6.127	When antibodies react with large particles that have the character of antigens, ... occurs.	reciprocal of the dilution
6.128	Widal's reaction is an .... reaction in which killed .... are used as the antigen.	agglutination
6.129	When bivalent antibodies are specifically bound to multivalent antigens to a sufficient extent, ... occurs.	agglutination bacteria
6.130	For an antigen-antibody reaction to be possible, the presence of a thermolabile factor known as the .... is required.	precipitation
6.131	In a complement-fixing reaction, an antigen-antibody reaction is demonstrated indirectly by observing that the .... is consumed.	complement
		complement

Radioimmunological assay. Serological methods are used for quantitative analysis of such substances that occur only in minute amounts in the body. For example, the method greatly facilitates the analysis of hormones. The radioimmunological method is based on the principle that the analyzed substance acts as an antigen in a serological reaction. Quantitative analysis is possible since one antibody only binds a certain amount of antigens. The fraction of the antigen binding capacity is determined after the sample has reacted with a known amount of antigens.

The procedure may be as follows. Two components are required. (1) A serum, for example, from a rabbit, containing antibodies against the particular hormone to be analyzed. The hormone thus acts as an antigen. (2) A test solution with the same antigen as that to be analyzed, but labeled with a radionuclide, such as ^{125}I. The sample is mixed with the serum with the known antigen binding capacity. The mixture is incubated so that the antigen is bound to the antibodies. The test solution with the labeled antigen is added in excess. Consequently, the antigen-antibody complex will contain antigens both from the sample and radioactive antigens. The antigen-antibody complexes are precipitated, for example, by adding alcohol. After centrifugation and washing, the activity of the precipitate is measured with a scintillation detector. The higher activity in the precipitate the lower was the hormone concentration in the sample.

TECHNICAL ASPECTS OF MICROBIOLOGICAL DIAGNOSIS

Automated laboratory diagnosis

Automated identification of bacteria presents much greater difficulties than automatic chemical laboratory diagnosis. This is because identification in bacteriological work is largely based on observation of the shape, size and staining properties of the microorganisms and on the gross appearance of the bacteria colonies—that is, the gathering of visual information. This is difficult to perform automatically with the present methods for pattern recognition. It is therefore improbable that in fully automated bacteriological diagnosis, the present methods of identification will be used. It will probably prove more economical to replace the whole identification procedure, or those parts of it that involve the collection of visual information, with other methods based on procedures of chemical analysis.

In the manual procedure, the choice of diagnostic route is largely determined by the findings obtained during the earlier procedure; in the automatic procedure, these decision processes will probably be reduced or eliminated entirely, because many more parallel analysis channels will be used. This implies a preference to perform a large number of superfluous parallel studies than to choose those motivated by the findings obtained at an earlier stage.

Such fully automated systems for bacteriological identification have still not been developed. The systems that have now been planned rely to a large extent on manual procedures and require the collaboration of bacteriologists. Only the actual handling of the bacterial cultures has been automated—for example, spreading on agar media, staining for microscopic examination, addition of reagents for agglutination determinations, and dilution for such reactions. Specially trained personnel will still be required to read out the results and choose the bacterial colonies for further diagnostic procedures.

It is possible to mechanize the processes that require determination of the ability of the bacteria to grow in or on different media. In liquid media, growth is demonstrated by photoelectric determination of the opalescence of the medium. On solid agar media, the number and size of the colonies can be determined by optical scanning procedures, although this does not enable a detailed classification of the appearance of the colonies to be made. Agglutination and precipitation can also be recorded photoelectrically.

The classification of bacteria by studying their immunological properties can be automated by using antibodies that are bound to substances that fluoresce. The procedure is as follows: the bacteria are applied to a slide, a solution of fluorescing antibodies is added and the preparation is washed and examined under a special microscope with illumination by ultraviolet light. If the bacteria fluoresce with the wavelength that is characteristic of the stain, the bacteria are of the type corresponding to the special antibodies used. The method has been applied in identification of the hemolytic streptococci that cause rheumatic fever and nephritis. Screening—that is, mass examination of large population groups—with such automatic methods is an urgent measure, since such bacterial infections should be treated with antibiotics in order to reduce the frequency of complications, such as rheumatic fever or nephritis (Question 6.27).

Data processing in clinical microbiology

Microbiological diagnosis is based on the observation of a number of biological phenomena, such as growth of bacteria in colonies, microscopic appearance and the results of serological tests. These observations provide a basis for a bacterial diagnosis. A compilation of these findings is a purely intellectual process, which is at present not practicable with computer techniques.

Because of the limited extent to which it has been possible to automate microbiological diagnosis, the use of computer techniques for administrative routines is confined to the collection and handling of the primary results. The result is a print-out of the bacteriological report lists.

The gathering of information can be accomplished by mark sensing on punch cards, which are then dealt with by the usual techniques.

REFERENCES

BELLANTI, J. A. *Immunology*. Philadelphia (Saunders) 1971. 584 pages.

DAVIS, B. D. *Microbiology; Including Immunology and Molecular Genetics*. Hagerstown, Maryland (Harper & Row) 1973. 1584 pages.

GOOD, R. A. and FISHER, D. W. *Immunobiology*. Stamford (Sinauer) 1971. 305 pages.

HOEPRICH, P. D. *Infectious Diseases; A Guide to the Understanding and Management of Infectious Processes*. Hagerstown, Maryland (Harper & Row) 1972. 1392 pages.

HUMPHREY, J. H. and WHITE, R. G. *Immunology for Students of Medicine*. Philadelphia (Lippincott) 1970. 498 pages.

JAWETZ, E. *Review of Medical Microbiology*. Los Altos (Lange) 1976. 550 pages.

LEWIN, R. *In Defense of the Body: An Introduction to the New Immunology*. Garden City (Anchor) 1974. 146 pages.

ROITT, I. M. *Essential Immunology*. Philadelphia (Lippincott/Blackwell) 1974. 264 pages.

chapter 7

Blood and Transplantation

Biological tissues generally cannot be transplanted from one person to another. This is due to subtle differences in the chemical structure of cell membranes that are immunologically recognizable by the recipient or host. The host develops a defense reaction to the foreign tissue graft after a few weeks, and the graft cells are killed. For transplantation to be possible there must be an extremely close **immunological compatibility** between the host and donor tissues.

Unlike most other tissues, blood can be transferred under certain conditions. There are fewer and less significant differences in the structure of the red cell membrane from one individual to another, so transfusions of blood are much more successful than transplantation of organs such as the kidney and heart. Successful blood transfusion requires that the proper donor blood be used. Some of the laboratory problems in this donor selection, as well as other practical problems, are described in this chapter. The principles of the laboratory tests of typing and preserving other organs for transplantation are briefly presented. The surgical problems associated with transplantation are touched on in Chapter 10.

359

BLOOD

The practice of transfusing blood is now widely applied. **Whole blood,** i.e., blood in the same form as it was taken from the donor's veins, or various components of blood, such as **red blood cells, platelets, plasma,** or concentrates of **specific plasma proteins** is given. Approximately 6–8 million transfusions are given each year in the United States alone. About half of these are given as whole blood. After sudden blood loss, such as loss during surgical operation, accident, or delivery of a baby complicated by hemorrhage, transfusions of whole blood are the chief means of preventing or arresting **shock** (page 557) which otherwise might cause death.

In internal medicine, transfusions of whole blood are given to patients with sudden spontaneous bleeding such as **hemorrhage** from the gastrointestinal tract (ulcers and tumors) or from the genitourinary tract (tumors of the kidneys and urinary bladder). Cases of **anemia** are treated by transfusion of a more concentrated suspension of red blood cells which is prepared by removing most of the plasma from the whole blood. The red blood cells of some newborn infants are damaged by antibodies which have been transmitted from the mother. They are treated by exchange or **replacement transfusion.** All of the infant's blood is removed and replaced with blood from a normal donor.

Some **treatment apparatus** such as heart-lung machines (page 563) and artificial kidneys (page 578) that are connected to the patient's circulatory system must first be primed with blood before use. This blood then mixes with the patient's own blood during the treatment procedure.

Question		*Answer*
7.1	For it to be possible to transplant a tissue from one person to another, there must be an extremely close .... compatibility between donor and host.	
7.2	If this immunological compatibility is absent, the host or recipient develops an immunological .... to the foreign tissue after some weeks and it is	immunological
7.3	Unlike most other tissues, which require good immunological compatibility, ... can be transfused if certain conditions are observed.	defense reaction rejected
7.4	On arrival at hospital, a patient who has been involved in a road accident is pale, in a cold sweat and dazed and his blood pressure is low. A blood transfusion is given to arrest the .... (pathological condition) that has developed.	blood

7.5	A patient who has periodically been troubled by pain in the pit of the stomach, especially $\frac{1}{2}$–1 hour after meals, has the last few days also felt exhausted and dizzy, and the feces have been black and tarry in consistency. Chemical analysis of the feces shows that they contain much blood. A radiographic examination of the gastrointestinal tract is made and a large gastric ulcer—an ulcer in the stomach—is found (cf, Fig. 8.10). The hemoglobin value is 5.2 g/dl (52 g/l), which is about 40 percent of normal (see page 286). Several blood transfusions are given as treatment for the patient's .... (condition) which is due to .... in the stomach.	shock
		blood deficiency (anemia) bleeding

BLOOD-GROUP SEROLOGY

A knowledge of blood group systems is essential for successful blood transfusion. The term **blood group** refers to subtle chemical variations in the red cell membrane structure. A person's blood group (that is, the structure of his own red cell membranes) is **inherited** and unchangeable, a fact that is utilized in paternity tests and in forensic (legal) medicine, as in the identification of blood stains. There are a dozen or more blood-group systems, all of which are inherited independently of each other.

An individual's blood can be classified according to his **type** in each of these systems. (For example: group A, Rh positive.) The reason for the existence of the blood groups is unknown—they have no known positive function in the body. They become important, however, when we attempt to transfuse blood from one person into the circulation of another because they are **antigenic** (page 346) and may provoke antibody formation in the recipient. The relative importance of the various blood group systems in transfusion practice is determined by whether the chemical variants in membrane structure are strongly or weakly antigenic, or in other words, how often they provoke antibody formation. Only the ABO and Rh systems must be considered in selecting blood for transfusion in 99 percent of cases.

7.6	Paternity tests are valid because a person's blood group is ....

7.7	During transfusion, different blood groups are .... and may provoke .... formation in the recipient.	inherited
7.8	In 99 percent of transfusions only the .... and .... systems must be considered.	antigenic antibody
7.9	Blood group systems are determined by chemical variations in the	ABO Rh
		red cell membrane

Blood groups

If donor blood carrying a specific antigen, such as Rh antigen, is transfused in error to a patient who does not have this antigen on his own red cells, that is the patient is Rh negative, an antibody (page 346) develops in the patient's plasma after several weeks. We say the patient has been immunized to the blood group antigen. The antibody is a protein and has the chemical characteristics of a gamma globulin (page 280). If donor blood carrying this same antigen is injected a second time, a **hemolytic transfusion reaction** will occur. The antibody in the patient's plasma combines with the antigen on the membrane of the donor red cells and damages them. The damaged red cells are then removed by the spleen and liver. The antigen-antibody reaction also may cause anaphylactic shock, which may be fatal (page 351). The patient experiences anxiety, pain in the chest, back, and abdomen, headache, nausea, and vomiting, difficulty in breathing, and symptoms related to fall in blood pressure.

In the ABO system it is not necessary to give a first transfusion of blood to provoke antibody formation. A short time after birth anti-A and anti-B antibodies develop naturally if these antigens are not present on the individual's own red cells. These antibodies are **naturally occurring**. They are regularly found in the plasma of all normal individuals after the age of 6 months. These antibodies can cause red cell destruction even at the time of the first blood transfusion if the wrong donor blood is used.

Anti-A and anti-B antibodies are often called **isoagglutinins**. The term **agglutinin** denotes the fact that, in the test tube, these antibodies can cause agglutination (clumping) of red cells suspended in saline solution. The individual red cells are linked together by antibody molecules in a lattice-work fashion. The large aggregates can be seen with the naked eye. The prefix **iso-** denotes the fact that this antibody recognizes differences between individuals belonging to the same species, in this case, man.

7.10	If blood with certain blood-group antigens is transfused into an individual that does not have this antigen, ... to the foreign blood-group antigen form after a week or so.	
7.11	If a second transfusion of blood with the same antigen is given, the antibodies may clump the transfused blood cells: the antibodies are therefore called	antibodies
7.12	Naturally occurring antibodies are known as	agglutinins
7.13	Agglutinins, like other humoral antibodies (page 346), are macromolecular substances (proteins) which are among the .... of the blood.	isoagglutinins
7.14	A patient whose blood serum contains antibodies as a result of a blood transfusion is .... against the blood-group antigen.	gamma globulins
7.15	Immunization creates a risk, for a second transfusion of blood containing the same antigen may cause the patient to experience a	immunized
		hemolytic transfusion reaction (possibly shock)

The ABO system. In the ABO system there are two antigens, A and B, and four blood groups: O, A, B, and AB. The group designation, such as **group A**, indicates that the person's red cells carry the A antigen but not B antigen. Group AB red cells carry both antigens, group O red cells carry neither antigen. If one or both of the A and B antigens is not present on a person's blood cells, he will naturally produce antibodies in his plasma against the missing antigens. Therefore the following red cell antigen-plasma antibody combinations are found.

Blood group	*Red cell antigen*	*Plasma antibodies*
O	neither A nor B	anti-A and anti-B
A	A only	anti-B only
B	B only	anti-A only
AB	A and B	neither antibody

The first requirement for a successful blood or red cell transfusion is that the donor's red cells must not be attacked by antibodies in the recipient's plasma. Since anti-A and anti-B antibodies are regularly present, in almost all cases a donor is selected who is of the same ABO group as the recipient. In emergency situations, when there is not enough time to determine the patient's ABO group, or if blood of the right group is not available, group O donor blood (which carries neither A nor B antigen) may be transfused (Fig. 7.1). In this case, the plasma of the donor blood is removed to prevent a reaction between the anti-A and anti-B antibodies in the donor plasma with the patient's red blood cells.

Universal donor

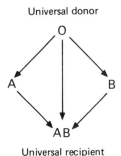

Universal recipient

Figure 7.1 The ABO blood system. Type A blood can receive from A (normally) or O (in an emergency) and donate to A (normally) or AB (in an emergency).

The Rh system. This blood group system was first identified in the Rhesus monkey. There are more than 25 antigens that belong to the Rh system, but in routine practice it is only necessary to consider one of them. If a person's red cells carry this particular Rh antigen, he is called Rh positive; if his cells lack this antigen, he is called Rh negative. The Rh negative individual does not usually have anti-Rh antibodies in his plasma which is in contrast with the ABO system. However, the Rh negative person can make the anti-Rh antibodies if he is transfused with blood from an Rh positive donor. If subsequent transfusions of Rh positive blood are given, a hemolytic transfusion reaction results. Therefore the standard procedure is to determine the patient's Rh type before transfusion. If he is Rh positive, he receives blood from an Rh positive donor. If he is Rh negative, Rh negative donor blood is used for the transfusion.

Rh immunization can also occur as a result of pregnancy. At the time the baby is born and the placenta separates from the inside of the uterus, some of the baby's red cells enter the mother's circulation. If the mother is Rh negative and the baby Rh positive, the mother may make antibodies against the Rh factor. This occurs in about 10 percent of cases. During a later pregnancy with an Rh positive fetus, the mother's anti-Rh antibodies cross the placenta and react with the fetus' red cells.

The injury to the fetus is the result of a breakdown of the red cells and the hemoglobin. The damaged red cells have a shorter than normal life span, and the fetus gets anemia. After birth, the baby becomes sick because of accumulation in the tissues of bilirubin, a breakdown product of hemoglobin (page 277). In particular, the brain will be damaged. The condition is fatal in severe cases. If the child survives, he may have paralysis, deafness and impaired muscle coordination unless treated.

The purpose of the treatment is to remove the damaged red cells and replace them with normal red cells in order to stop the production of bilirubin. An exchange transfusion immediately after birth protects the child from further brain damage.

Immunization of an Rh negative woman who has given birth to an Rh positive child can be prevented. This is done by injecting her with a small quantity of Rh antibodies after delivery. These antibodies will react with any fetal red cells (Rh positive) which may be present and rapidly destroy them before they are able to provoke antibody formation in the mother (Fig. 7.2).

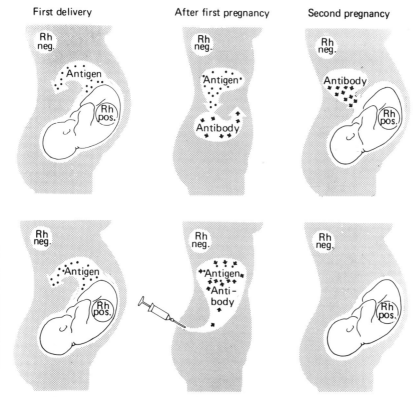

Figure 7.2 In Rh immunization of an Rh negative mother by an Rh positive fetus, antigen is transferred from the fetus to the mother. In a later pregnancy, antibodies formed in the mother can be transferred to the new fetus and cause injury to it.

7.16	In a blood transfusion, the . . . . (plasma, red cells) of the donor must under all circumstances be compatible with the . . . . (plasma, red cells) of the recipient.	
7.17	O blood has blood-cell antigen of the type . . . . (A + B, A, B, none).	red cells plasma
7.18	A person with O blood is therefore a . . . . (universal recipient, universal donor) with respect to the ABO system.	none
7.19	To reduce the risks of transfusion complications with regards to the Rh system, a universal donor must also be . . . . (Rh positive, Rh negative).	universal donor
7.20	A newborn infant's mother is Rh immunized, and he is born with jaundice. His blood group is . . . . (Rh positive, Rh negative); during the exchange transfusion he is given Rh negative blood.	Rh negative
7.21	Rh immunization of an Rh negative mother who has had an Rh positive child can be prevented by giving . . . . immediately after the delivery.	Rh positive
7.22	The child with a ruptured spleen in questions 2.45, 2.70 and 2.72 was taken to the hospital in a state of shock with signs of blood loss. As no blood typing could be performed, blood of group . . . . was given.	Rh antibodies
7.23	Before the transfusion was begun, a blood specimen was taken, so that a blood typing could be performed later on. A knowledge of the child's blood group was necessary in order to give blood . . . . at any subsequent transfusion.	O Rh negative
7.24	The percentage distribution of blood groups varies in different populations. In the USA, the distribution is: O, 45 percent; A, 40 percent; B, 10 percent; AB, 5 percent; Rh positive, 84 percent; Rh negative, 15 percent (weak Rh, 1 percent, not a separate group but an intermediate state). The most common blood group combination is thus O Rh positive, which occurs in . . . . percent.	of the same group

7.25	The rarest combination is . . . . which occurs in . . . . percent.	38 percent (45 · 84)
7.26	The consumption of blood of different groups is largely in proportion to the relative distribution in the population, though somewhat more O Rh negative blood is used because this is	AB Rh negative one
7.27	The percentage occurrence of universal donor blood is . . . . percent.	universal donor blood
		seven

Blood typing

Blood typing is one of the few laboratory tests in which a single error, such as incorrect ABO group, can lead to fatal consequences for the patient. It is therefore extremely important that procedures used should eliminate the possibilities of both technical errors and clerical errors, such as the confusion of two patient's names.

Manual blood typing procedures. These are used prior to blood transfusion to determine the patient's ABO group and Rh type. To a small drop of testing serum, containing known antibodies, is added a drop of the blood (red cells) to be typed (Fig. 7.3). If the corresponding antigen is present on the red cells, agglutination

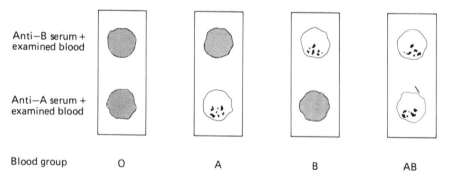

Anti—B serum + examined blood

Anti—A serum + examined blood

Blood group   O   A   B   AB

Figure 7.3 Determination of ABO group using the microscope slide method. Drops of saline suspension of the red cells to be typed are mixed with test sera. At the top of the slides are anti-B sera, that is, serum containing antibodies to the B antigen and no other antibodies, and at the bottom anti-A sera. The slide is rocked back and forth and observed for the appearance of agglutination, which usually begins within 30 seconds. (See also table on page 363.)

will occur. For example, to determine the ABO group, the red cells are tested first with serum containing anti-A antibodies and secondly with serum containing anti-B antibodies. To determine the Rh type, the red cells are tested with serum containing only anti-Rh antibodies.

The procedure is very simple in principle, but the tests must be carried out under the proper conditions of pH, temperature, protein concentration in the red cell suspension, etc. to get reliable results. The test sera must contain high levels of antibody and must be stored properly to maintain the antibody activity.

Automated blood typing instruments   are used primarily by large donor centers. A large number of samples can be tested but there should be no time constraint (i.e. no need for a very rapid result).

The AutoAnalyzer (page 313) is the instrument most commonly used. A suspension of red cells to be tested is sucked into the tubing of the instrument and various antisera are added. The mixture of cells and antiserum passes through a mixing coil. If necessary, it may also pass through an incubation coil where the temperature is raised to 37°C (body temperature). If a positive reaction occurs, the red cells will agglutinate. The cell suspension then flows across a **decantation tee** (Fig. 7.4). Agglutinated red cells have a greater tendency to fall out of the

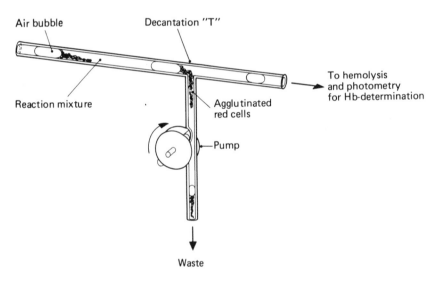

Figure 7.4 Decantation tee. Agglutinated red cells have a greater tendency to fall out of the vertical stem of the tee.

vertical stem of the tee, while unagglutinated cells will pass out through the horizontal limb of the tee. The unreacted cells move on to hemolysis, and by photometric assay of liberated hemoglobin an objective indication is obtained on the degree of agglutination.

BLOOD TRANSFUSIONS

Blood transfusions were originally performed by connecting the vein of the donor via a tube and a pumping device to the vein of the recipient. This method may be dangerous for the donor in that it is difficult to assess the amount of blood removed, and pumping may occur in the wrong direction. The donor must also be physically present during the transfusion, which makes transfusion during surgery very difficult.

At present, the transfusion of blood is divided into the following operations: **withdrawal** of blood from a donor; possibly **separation** of the whole blood into various components; **storage** of the blood; **pretransfusion** laboratory testing to select the best available donor blood for a given patient; and the actual **infusion** of the blood into the patient.

Blood withdrawal. The preferred blood donor is a healthy volunteer. The probability of transmission of infectious diseases such as hepatitis B from the donor to the patient is higher among those donors motivated to sell their blood for a profit because of needle-transmitted disease caused by drug abuse.

Before blood is taken from the donor, a short medical history is taken to determine that he is healthy and can donate blood without danger to himself. Additional assessment of his state of health is made by measuring his pulse rate, blood pressure, temperature, and hemoglobin level. He is also questioned about diseases which could be transmitted by his blood; these include hepatitis B, syphilis, and malaria.

A needle is inserted into a vein in the donor's arm and 450 ml, one "unit", of whole blood is withdrawn. It is collected in a sterilized plastic bag attached by a length of tubing to the needle. The bag contains a preservative-anticoagulant solution. The purpose of this solution is to maintain red cell viability by providing glucose for red cell metabolism, and prevent the forming of blood clots in the container by binding the ionized calcium in the blood with citrate ion to form un-ionized calcium citrate. (Ionized calcium is necessary for blood clotting to occur, see page 292.)

Separation. Only about half of the transfusions are given in the form of **whole blood**. The remainder of the patients receive **red cells**, **platelets**, **plasma**, or a **plasma protein concentrate**. The red cells are separated from the plasma of the donor blood by centrifugation and the plasma is transferred to another container. Platelets, which are lighter than red cells, will remain suspended in the plasma if the centrifugation time and speed are correct. The platelet-rich plasma can be converted to a platelet concentrate by removing more of the plasma. Thus the platelets from the entire 450 ml of blood can be concentrated in 50 ml of plasma. These platelet concentrates are used primarily in patients with leukemia who have a platelet deficiency and a consequent bleeding tendency.

Storage. To keep red blood cells alive, they must be stored at 1–6°C to slow the metabolic rate. Under these conditions about 1 percent of the red cells in the container die each day—the same rate at which they die in the body. The shelf-life of whole blood or red cells stored at this temperature is 3 weeks.

The shelf-life can be extended to five years if the red cells are frozen. To prevent the formation of ice crystals inside the cells, which would cause them to rupture, glycerine is added before freezing. The red cells may be stored in a mechanical freezer at −85°C or in liquid nitrogen at −196°C. Before transfusion the red cells are thawed and the glycerine removed by sequential washing with saline solutions. Several instruments are available for this purpose.

Pretransfusion testing. The risk of hemolytic transfusion reaction is least when the patient and donor blood are of the same ABO group and Rh type. Therefore the first step in the laboratory testing is to obtain a sample of the patient's blood and determine his ABO group and Rh type. Then appropriate donor blood is selected from the inventory in the blood bank refrigerator. Additional testing by a serological compatibility test, also called **crossmatching**, is performed to be sure that there are no unusual antibodies in the patient's serum which are capable of destroying the red blood cells of the donor. This involves mixing several drops of the patient's serum with a sample of the donor red cells in a test tube. Conditions such as temperature and protein concentration are then manipulated to assure that agglutination will occur if in fact there are such antibodies in the patient's serum. In addition, the donor's serum may be checked for compatibility with the patient's cells. The particular unit of donor blood is transfused only if this testing indicates that there is no incompatibility present.

Infusion of blood. A length of tubing with an in-line drip chamber is inserted into the plastic bag. A needle on the other end of the tubing is inserted into the patient's vein. The flow rate is adjusted by means of a pinch-clamp on the tubing. A blood filter prevents any clots from passing into the patient's venous system, where they would produce emboli (page 29). 450 ml of whole blood is usually infused over a period of 2–3 hours. The patient must be observed carefully during this period for signs of a hemolytic transfusion reaction (Fig. 7.5).

If the pretransfusion testing has been properly performed, there is less than one death in 10,000 transfusions due to hemolytic transfusion reaction. Those reactions that do occur are more often due to clerical mix-ups than to actual errors in the performance or.interpretation of the laboratory tests.

About 2,000 deaths occur in the United States each year that are due to blood transfusion. About half of them are due to transmission of hepatitis B from the donor to the patient, and half are due to hemolytic transfusion reactions.

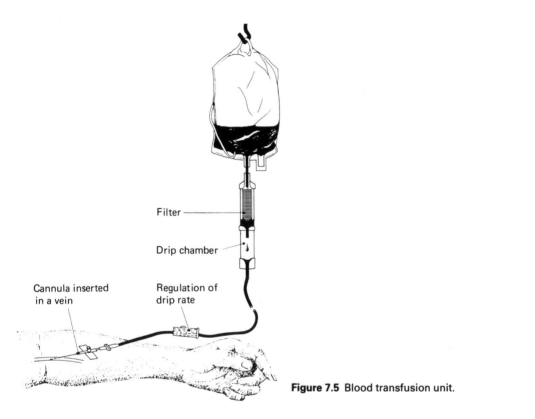

Filter

Drip chamber

Cannula inserted
in a vein

Regulation of
drip rate

Figure 7.5 Blood transfusion unit.

7.28	Blood typing is performed by adding the .... (blood, test sera with known antibodies) to the .... (blood, test sera).	
7.29	The presence of blood-cell antigen can be demonstrated by noting any .... after a certain time.	blood test sera
7.30	The transfusion of blood takes place in five stages: ...., ..., ..., ..., and	agglutination

7.31	When blood is withdrawn it is mixed with a preservative-anticoagulant solution which prevents .... and increases the .... of the blood cells.	blood withdrawal blood separation blood storage pretransfusion blood infusion
7.32	Blood to which preservative-anticoagulant solution has been added and which has been stored at 1–6°C can be stored for .... (time).	clotting length of life
7.33	Transfusions may be given in the form of whole blood, ..., ..., ..., or a	3 weeks
7.34	In a serological sensitivity test, a check is made that there is a match between the donor's .... and the recipient's	red cells platelets plasma plasma protein concentrate
7.35	Such a pretransfusion test is also called	blood cells serum
7.36	During infusion of blood, the patient is .... after a small amount of blood has been given.	crossmatching
7.37	During a blood infusion, a patient has chills and pain in the lumbar region. The infusion is discontinued immediately because symptoms indicate that .... blood has been given.	observed
7.38	The reason for this is most probably that a .... error has been made.	incompatible
		clerical mixup

TRANSPLANTATION

In order for the cells of a transplanted tissue to continue to function in the organism of the host, extremely good immunological similarity between donor and recipient is necessary. Thus, provided that the surgical technique is correct, transplantations between two sites in the same subject—that is, **autografts**—and between identical twins, which are genetically identical—**isogenic grafts**—are always successful, whereas those between genetically different individuals—**allografts**—are usually unsuccessful.

In the case of genetic dissimilarity, a graft begins to take at first, but then, after a week or so, an inflammatory reaction appears which gradually leads to necrosis (tissue death) of the graft, which is then rejected. This is because the recipient has developed cell-mediated immunity (page 346) to the transplanted tissue. In this case the donor tissue contains cell-bound antigens, which stimulate the recipient to produce specific cellular antibodies (page 346).

The organism's ability to develop such cell-mediated immunity probably normally serves to protect the organism against tumor growth. In transplantations, the cellular immune reaction is a great disadvantage. How to combat this is the major problem, and the level of success achieved determines the outcome of the transplantations.

To find a donor who corresponds closely immunologically with the recipient, a careful **tissue typing** is always performed before the transplantation. This takes some time, during which the organ must be kept alive by **tissue preservation**, if the donor is a deceased person. Tissue preservation is also needed during the transport of an organ to the recipient.

7.39	Provided that the surgical technique is correct, an autograft—that is, transfer of an organ from one site to another in the .... subject—and an isogenic graft—that is, transfer between .... identical individuals are always successful.	
7.40	In an allograft—that is between genetically .... individuals—the transplanted organ is generally rejected.	same genetically
7.41	Rejection of the organ is preceded by an .... reaction in the organ, after which it undergoes	different
7.42	The rejection is due to the fact that after a time the recipient develops cell-mediated .... to the transplanted tissue.	inflammatory necrosis (tissue death)
7.43	To find a donor that closely corresponds immunologically with the recipient, careful .... is performed.	immunity
		tissue typing

TISSUE TYPING

Transplantation antigens occur on most of the body's cells. These antigens can be divided into a number of different transplantation antigen systems. The different systems have different importance from the aspect of transplantation: there must be close agreement between the strong transplantation antigens if the grafted organ is to survive for long, while the weak transplantation antigen systems are of less importance.

One of the transplantation antigen systems is identical with the ABO antigen system that occurs in blood group serology. For transplantation, the donor must have the same blood group as the recipient.

Another transplantation antigen system is the HL-A system (human lymphocyte antigens). 25 different antigens have been identified in this system. Each individual inherits only two of these antigens from each parent—an individual thus cannot have more than four antigens in the HL-A system. The number of possible combinations, however, is large. Therefore it is usually difficult to find a suitable donor for a particular recipient.

To select a donor and recipient with a small immunological difference—that is, good **compatibility**—tissue typing is used. Two kinds of tests are used: **serological** methods and **cellular** or **biological** methods. With the cellular methods, only the summated effect of transplantation antigens present can be measured. With the serological methods, individual antigen differences can be observed.

Serological tests. The serological methods for typing are similar to those used in blood group serology. Antisera are obtained from volunteers that have been actively immunized or from women that have been immunized against transplantation antigens by repeated pregnancies with immunologically incompatible fetuses (cf, page 365). With the serological methods major incompatibilities can now be avoided with a high level of probability.

Cellular tests. Lymphocytes from individuals with different transplantation antigens react with each other, and this provides the basis for the cellular or biological methods of tissue typing.

The mixed lymphocyte culture is the most important test. It is based on the fact that in a tissue culture, lymphocytes from two individuals are more powerfully stimulated to undergo cell division, the greater the differences in the antigens are. The donor is chosen whose lymphocytes produce the weakest stimulation when mixed with the recipient's.

7.44	Tissue typing is performed to find for a particular recipient a donor who has a small immunological difference—that is, one who displays a good . . . .

7.45	Tissue typing can be performed using two different types of test: .... methods and .... methods.	compatibility
7.46	One of the strong transplantation antigen systems is identical with the .... antigen system in blood group serology.	serological cellular (biological)
7.47	Another transplantation antigen system is the .... system.	ABO
		HL-A

TISSUE STORAGE AND PRESERVATION

Tissues survive for a limited time after being removed from the donor's body. At room temperature and without a supply of oxygen given by artificial circulation, most organs die within an hour or so. This is too short a time to enable tissue typing to be performed and for the organ to be transported to the recipient.

The survival time can be increased by three measures: **hypothermia**, lowering the temperature, **perfusion**, flushing, and **hyperbaric oxygenation**, oxygenation under pressure.

Using just hypothermia at about 5°C, the organ's metabolism can be reduced to about 5 percent; this increases the survival time to about 12 hours. By perfusion with cooled oxygenated plasma, the survival time can be increased to about 24 hours. Some further improvement is attainable if the organ is also stored in oxygen under pressure, 5–15 atm.

The organs for transplantation must be stored in special chambers. The actual organ lies in an organ container, which forms an inner part of the storage chamber, the organ's arteries are connected to tubes which conduct sterile, oxygenated plasma to the organ. Plasma leaves the organ via the veins, which are not connected—it drains into the storage chamber. The plasma is oxygenated, and recirculated through the organ again. The organ container is surrounded by a pressure vessel, which enables an elevated oxygen pressure to be maintained; the oxygen is obtained from a bottle after reducing the pressure. The organ container is also thermostated with the aid of a cooling unit.

The oxygenation of plasma can be performed in different ways (page 566)—for example, by means of a membrane oxygenator. In this, the plasma passes on one side of an oxygen-permeable membrane while oxygen flows past on the other side. In the bubble oxygenation system, oxygen is bubbled through the plasma or this is oxygenated by allowing it to flow as a thin layer in an oxygen atmosphere. For the latter types, a bubble trap must be placed in the circulation to eliminate bubbles from the plasma so that gas emboli (page 29) cannot arise.

7.48	At room temperature and without artificial circulation, most organs die within . . . . (period).	
7.49	The survival time can be increased by three measures: . . . . , ... and	1 hour
7.50	With these measures the survival time can be increased to . . . . (period).	hypothermia (lowered temperature) perfusion (flushing) hyperbaric oxygenation (oxygenation under pressure)
		about 24 hours

REFERENCES

HUESTIS, D. W., BOVE, JR. and BUSCH, S. *Practical Blood Transfusion*. Boston (Little, Brown) 1969. 383 pages.

WEED, R. I. (ed.). *Hematology for Internists*. Boston (Little, Brown) 1971. 467 pages.

ZMIJEWSKI, C. M. and FLETCHER, J. L. *Immunohematology*. New York (Appleton-Century-Crofts) 1972. 334 pages.

chapter 8

Diagnostic Radiology

Medical radiology includes both diagnostic and therapeutic methods, which utilize ionizing radiation. In this chapter only the diagnostic methods are described; the therapeutic methods are dealt with in Chapter 13. In addition to the procedures which use ionizing radiation—of which x-ray diagnosis is by far the most important—a number of visualizing systems based on the use of other types of radiation (infrared radiation and ultrasound) are treated, although, strictly speaking, they do not fall within the field of radiology.

X-RAY DIAGNOSIS

In the investigation of most diseases when the diagnosis is not immediately evident, a radiological examination is one of the most important diagnostic aids. The examination technique varies according to the clinical problems. In the simplest cases, such as in suspected fracture, only a few radiographs are taken, or else fluoroscopy is performed, whereas in a complicated examination, such as examination of the heart or brain, more complex techniques and special training are required.

A radiograph is a shadow picture produced by x-rays emanating from a point source (Fig. 8.1). The image so obtained has a large depth of field; at the same time the divergence of the rays results in a geometric enlargement and causes distortion of the image, because the parts of the object located closer to the focus are enlarged more than the parts closer to the image plane.

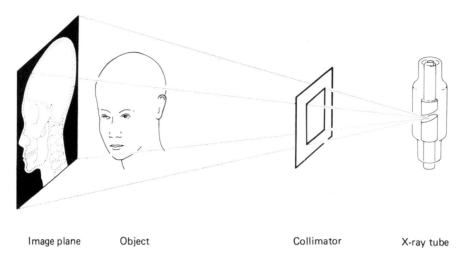

Image plane   Object   Collimator   X-ray tube

Figure 8.1 The x-ray image is a shadow picture produced by x-rays emitted from a point source.

Radiography and Fluoroscopy

There are two procedures of x-ray diagnosis that differ in principle, namely, **radiography** and **fluoroscopy**.

In radiography, an x-ray picture called a **radiograph** is produced for subsequent interpretation. The picture is usually obtained on photographic film placed in the image plane. (By more sophisticated techniques, which are described below, the picture can also be obtained in miniature photo format by photofluorography, by cinefluorography or by videotape recording.) In **fluoroscopy**, the patient's condition is examined by viewing the shadow image directly. This can be viewed on a fluorescent screen which converts x-rays to visible light. (Fluoroscopy is now often performed with an electronic image intensifier, which is usually combined with a television system.) The two methods are complementary.

Using x-ray film, radiographic images with a high geometric resolution can be obtained because the technique can be optimized. A wide range of contrast can be observed by choosing the best level of illumination in the subsequent inspection. There is ample time for a detailed inspection without concern for the patient's condition. Because of the short exposure times, the patient dose is usually comparatively low, while the examiner can move completely out of range during the exposure. Finally, an objective documentation of the patient's condition at the time of examination is obtained. This is of medical significance because comparisons can be made in the case of later examinations. The objective documentation is also of medicolegal value.

With direct fluoroscopy, it is possible to carry out a rapid survey from which an immediate diagnosis can be made. Moreover, the patient can be positioned during the procedure in order to obtain the most suitable radiation direction and the best field size of the x-ray beam, and the appropriate radiation quality can be chosen. In addition, movements of organs can be observed—for example, pulsations of the heart and the larger vessels, movements of the diaphragm during breathing, displacements of the larynx during swallowing and peristaltic movements in the gastrointestinal tract. Foreign bodies can be observed and removed under direct fluoroscopic control and fractures can be reduced (fractured bones correctly repositioned).

An x-ray examination consists of visualization of the organ under examination by means of a suitable technique, and of demonstrating its anatomic relationships so clearly that the patient's state can be determined. The primary purpose is thus not the production of pictures. The purpose is to reach a diagnosis, whether normal or in what way pathologically altered. The x-ray examination thus includes both anatomy and pathology and also much physiology.

Question		*Answer*
8.1	A radiograph is a .... produced by rays emitted from a point source.	
8.2	In this way the x-ray image has a large .... but at the same time there is a geometric .... because of the thickness of the object.	shadow picture
8.3	There are two x-ray diagnostic procedures, which differ in principle: ...., in which a photographic image is obtained for subsequent inspection, and ...., in which the patient's shadow image is viewed directly.	depth of field image distortion

8.4	The radiographic procedure, in which a picture is produced for subsequent inspection, has the following advantages: (1) a high geometric . . . . (2) wide range of . . . . (3) possibility of a detailed inspection with ample . . . . (4) relatively low . . . . because of the short exposure time (5) objective . . . . of the patient's condition.	radiography fluoroscopy
8.5	The value of the radiograph, as a document for preserving information, lies mainly in the fact that it enables a . . . . to be made in the case of later examinations; it also can be used as objective evidence in . . . . contexts.	(1) resolution (2) contrast (3) time (4) x-ray dose (5) documentation
8.6	Direct fluoroscopic examination of a patient has the advantage that: (1) the patient's condition can be . . . . surveyed (2) the most suitable ray direction and field size of the x-ray beam can be chosen because the patient can . . . . (3) the . . . . of the organs can be viewed directly (4) . . . . can be removed under direct observation, and . . . . can be reduced.	comparison medicolegal
		(1) rapidly (2) be positioned (3) movements (4) foreign bodies fractures

Contrast

Contrast provides the information content of the x-ray image. The appropriate technical parameters are chosen for each examination, so that the contrast is optimal for that diagnostic procedure.

A different contrast is obtained from a particular part of the body by changing the x-ray tube voltage: low-energy radiation, generated at 50–70 kV, produces high contrast for the skeleton and also for soft tissues, while higher energies give successively lower contrast. The higher energies are used for visualizing differences between lung and soft-tissue structures, which are reproduced better if obscuring skeletal components are imaged with low contrast.

Image contrast is a result of differential attenuation of the x-rays by the tissues. The attenuation is determined by Lambert-Beer's law: $I = I_o e^{-\mu \rho s}$, where I_o is the intensity of the incident radiation and I the intensity of the emergent radiation after passing through a distance, s, in a medium of density, ρ, and mass attenuation coefficient, μ. The mass attenuation coefficient differs from one element to another and varies with the radiation energy (Fig. 8.2). The attenuation can also be defined by the expression $I = I_o e^{-\mu x}$, where x is the mass of substance per unit area of the object, in g/cm^2 (kg/m^2).

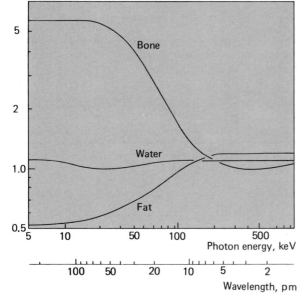

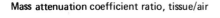

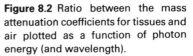

Figure 8.2 Ratio between the mass attenuation coefficients for tissues and air plotted as a function of photon energy (and wavelength).

Image contrast results when rays pass through two adjacent parts of the object with different mass attenuation coefficient, μ, different density, ρ, or different thickness, s. An example of contrast due mainly to a difference in mass attenuation coefficient is that obtained when visualizing the skeleton with low x-ray energies: bone is rich in calcium and phosphorus, which have higher atomic numbers and hence higher mass attenuation coefficients than the surrounding soft tissues, which consist mainly of oxygen, carbon, nitrogen and hydrogen. The higher density of bone further increases the contrast. Contrast due mainly to a difference in density is sometimes obtained when visualizing the fatty tissues, surrounded by other soft tissues of higher density (water and proteins). Differences in contrast due to differences in thickness may be so great that they complicate the evaluation of the x-ray findings.

In practice, we do not always distinguish between the three possible causes of contrast. Instead, the term **radiopacity** has been introduced. A structure in the body with a higher x-ray attenuation than the surrounding soft tissues—with an attenuation corresponding to that of water—is "radiopaque"; a structure that has the same attenuation is not radiopaque.

To visualize soft tissues it is often necessary to administer a **contrast medium**. There are **positive** and **negative** contrast media. If gas is administered (carbon dioxide, air or oxygen), a negative contrast results because of the higher density of the surrounding tissues. If contrast media consisting of elements with high atomic numbers are administered—usually barium or iodine—positive contrast is obtained because of the higher mass attenuation coefficient and higher density of these elements.

8.7	The technical parameters for a particular x-ray examination are chosen to give optimal	
8.8	Contrast provides the . . . . of the x-ray image.	contrast
8.9	Image contrast results when rays pass through two adjacent parts of the object with different . . . ., different . . . . or different	information content
8.10	The contrast varies with the energy of the x-rays because the . . . . is dependent on the energy.	mass attenuation coefficients densities thicknesses
8.11	Contrast media used to visualize the soft tissues are of two different types, producing . . . . and . . . . contrast.	mass attenuation coefficient
8.12	Negative contrast is obtained by using substances having a . . . . density than the surrounding tissues. For this purpose . . . . are administered.	positive negative
8.13	Positive contrast is obtained by using elements with a higher . . . . , and hence a higher . . . . than the surrounding soft tissues.	lower gases

8.14	Substances with a lower density than the surrounding soft tissues give .... contrast, while substances with higher mass attenuation coefficients give .... contrast.	atomic number mass attenuation coefficient (and also higher density)
8.15	Common negative contrast media are ...., ... and	negative positive
8.16	Contrast media which result in positive contrast usually contain the elements .... or	carbon dioxide air oxygen
8.17	A structure that absorbs x-rays more than the surrounding tissues is said to be	barium iodine
		radiopaque

X-RAY EXAMINATION OF THE ORGANS

The radiographic techniques used for imaging different organs vary considerably. Examples of common types of examination are given below, with illustrations.

Skeleton

The skeletal structures are easy to visualize, since there is no need to administer a contrast medium into the body. Even the untrained eye can sometimes observe fractures (Fig. 8.3); in other cases carefully chosen techniques, such as the adjustment of ray direction, are required in addition to great experience in interpreting fracture films. The position of the bones may also be radiographically checked after reduction or repair (Fig. 8.4). An example of pelvic film showing a fracture of the left femur is given in Fig. 8.5.

In all fracture examinations at least two exposures taken in perpendicular directions are required for reliable determination of the position of the fracture.

Infection of the bone, osteitis, can be diagnosed on the basis of resulting changes in the degree of mineralization—both decalcification and formation of new bone can occur. The same changes are seen in rheumatoid arthritis (Fig. 8.6).

Bone deformities have many causes: hereditary skeletal disorders, vitamin D deficiency, hormonal disturbances and many different kinds of bone tumors.

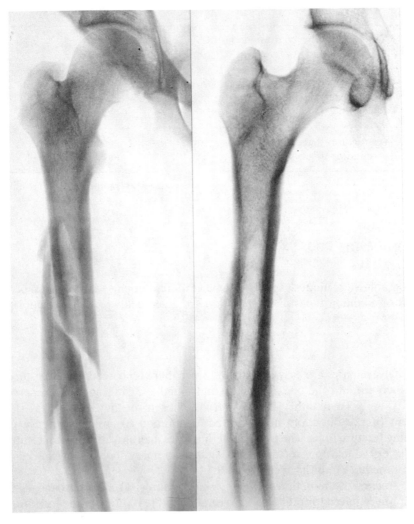

Figure 8.3 Fracture of the femur. Left—new fracture. Right—healed after 9 months.

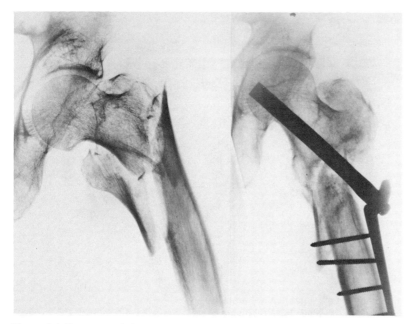

Figure 8.4 Fracture of femoral neck. Left—new fracture. Right—after nailing.

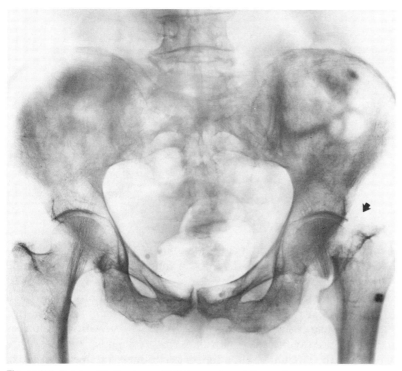

Figure 8.5 Pelvis with fracture of left femoral neck (arrow).

385

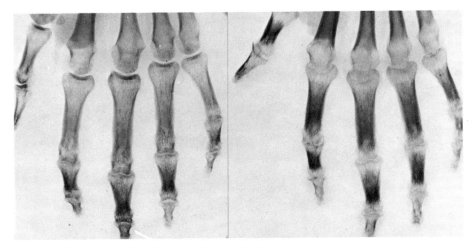

Figure 8.6 Bones of the hand. Left—practically normal. Right—decalcification at the joints as a result of rheumatoid arthritis. The films are from the same patient at an interval of one year.

8.18	To determine the position of a fracture, at least two radiographs must be taken in two directions	
8.19	In infections of bone, ... and in rheumatoid arthritis, there are changes in the degree of mineralization; both . . . . and . . . . can occur.	at right angles
		osteitis decalcification formation of new bone

Respiratory organs

Chest radiographs are taken mainly for examination of the lungs and heart. In order to reduce interfering skeletal shadows in lung examinations, high tube voltages, 150 kV, are chosen (Fig. 8.7).

Because of the air enclosed in the respiratory tract, the larger bronchi are seen as negative contrast, and the pulmonary vessels are seen as positive contrast against the air-filled lung tissue. Pneumothorax (page 57), in which the lung is collapsed and the pleural cavity is filled with air, is easy to diagnose: the vessels are not visualized. When the amount of air in the lungs is reduced (atelectasis), and in

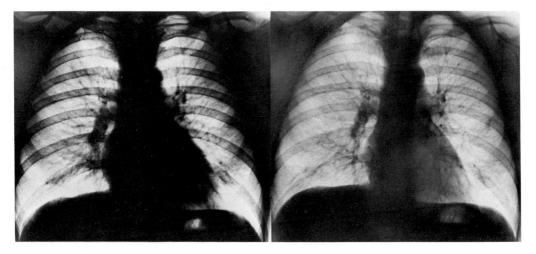

Figure 8.7 Lung radiographs taken with different tube voltages (left, 70 kV; right, 150 kV), thus producing different contrast. Note that whereas the vascular pattern is more clearly visualized at the higher voltage, the skeleton is reproduced more distinctly at the lower voltage.

pneumonia, there is an increased x-ray attenuation relative to the surrounding field. Different types of lung infections are accompanied by characteristic changes, which often enable a diagnosis to be made from the location, size and extent of the shadow.

Lung tumors may be primary or secondary in type (page 33). Bronchial carcinoma, which occurs as a primary growth in the lungs, is difficult to diagnose at an early stage. A special method of examination used in cases of suspected tumor is **bronchography**. A viscous, water-soluble contrast medium containing iodine is injected into the bronchi of one lung. The contrast medium is injected with a tube via the larynx after anesthetizing the mucous membrane—much is coughed up after the examination and the rest is absorbed. A tumor produces a filling defect in the contrast medium, which fills the rest of the bronchial tree.

If there is secondary spread of a tumor to the lungs, with growth of lung metastases, they displace the air-containing lung tissues, thus producing a local positive contrast.

8.20   In lung radiography, a . . . . (low, high) tube voltage is often chosen to eliminate interfering . . . . shadows.

8.21	The bronchi are seen as .... contrast because of the enclosed air.	high skeletal
8.22	When the amount of air in the lungs is reduced as in atelectasis or in pneumonia, there is an increase in the x-ray absorption relative to the surroundings, and a .... is seen.	negative
8.23	Bronchial carcinoma in an early stage is .... (easy, difficult) to diagnose by radiography.	shadow
		difficult

Circulatory organs

Heart examinations are performed by taking frontal and lateral films (Fig. 8.8). The evaluation is performed partly by calculating the total heart volume and partly on the basis of any changes in shape.

The heart volume is calculated by assuming that the heart is an ellipsoid of length, L, breadth, B, and depth, D, measured from the two x-ray projections (Fig. 8.8). The focus-film distance is standardized at 1.5 m, and the enlargement is therefore moderate. The enlargement—which is much the same for different patients—is compensated for by suitable choice of the constant in the formula for the volume of an ellipsoid:

$$\text{heart volume} = 0.42\, LBD$$

The heart volume normally varies within quite wide limits for different persons. It is dependent not only on body size but also on physical condition and occupation. To eliminate normal individual variations and to afford a better basis for the determination, the heart volume is normalized. The best correlation factor is the blood volume (page 184), but as the value for this is seldom available the heart volume per square meter of body surface area is used for normalization; this can be obtained from the Du Bois formula:

$$\text{body surface area} = W^{0.425}\, H^{0.725}\, 0.007184\ \text{m}^2$$

or from a simpler formula that is often used:

$$\text{body surface area} = (W + H - 60)/100\ \text{m}^2$$

where W is the body weight in kilograms and H is the body height in centimeters. The correlation to body weight alone is poorer and is not used. The normal upper

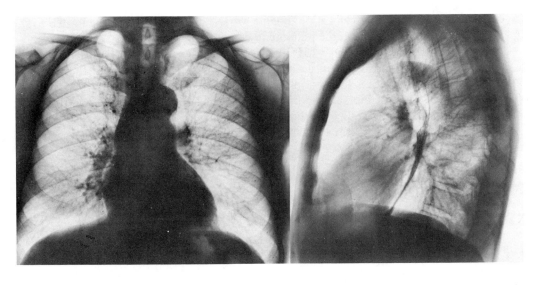

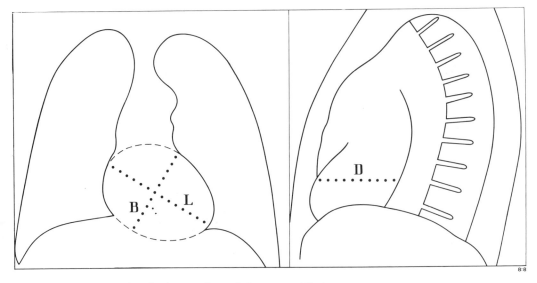

Figure 8.8 In determining the heart volume, it is assumed that the organ has an ellipsoidal shape.

limit for men is 500 ml/m² of body surface area and for women 450 ml/m² of body surface area. Most normal heart volumes are considerably lower.

Valvular defects and congenital deformations of the heart often produce characteristic changes in the shape of the organ. The first symptom of mitral stenosis (page 131) is widening of the left atrium—early in the disease, the right ventricle and the central pulmonary vessels also become enlarged—due to the increased pressure in the pulmonary circulation.

Aortic stenosis (page 131) likewise produces enlargement of the left ventricle. In aortic stenosis, calcification can often be seen in and around the valves—a feature that serves to confirm the diagnosis.

Because of the surrounding air-containing tissues, the heart and the major vessels can be visualized without administering a contrast medium. The examination is easy to perform and usually yields enough information for an assessment of the patient's condition.

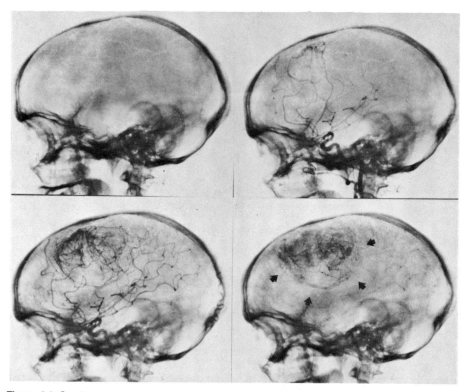

Figure 8.9 Cerebral angiography (visualization of the brain vessels with the aid of a contrast medium). Taken at intervals of 1 second, the films show clearly how the contrast medium is transmitted through the vascular system and fills out a hypervascularized tumor (arrows).

For visualization of the rest of the circulatory system and for special examinations of the heart, use is made of injectable, water-soluble organic compounds of iodine, which are readily excreted by the body. All the larger organs of the body can be examined by visualizing the associated vessels, **angiography**. Contrast medium is injected into an artery or vein, usually through a catheter placed in the vessel. The examination is designated according to the organ examined—for example, **angiocardiography**—the heart, **coronary angiography**—the coronary vessels of the heart, **nephroangiography**—the kidneys and **cerebral angiography**—the brain (Fig. 8.9).

When the actual vessels are studied to demonstrate constriction, vascular tumors or collaterals (page 186), the method is called **arteriography** in the case of arteries, and **phlebography** in the case of veins.

8.24	A radiographic examination of the heart includes calculation of the .... and note of any	
8.25	The heart and the major vessels are readily visualized against the surrounding air-containing ...., without requiring a contrast medium.	heart volume change in shape
8.26	The heart volume is calculated by assuming that the heart is an ...., and the volume is obtained as the product of a constant and the ...., ... and	lung tissue
8.27	The absolute heart volume is of minor interest; the relative heart volume is calculated per	ellipsoid length breadth depth
8.28	The body surface area in square meters can be estimated from the formula: ...., where W is the body weight in kilograms and H is the height in centimeters.	square meter of body surface area
8.29	The normal upper limit for the heart volume is .... for men and .... for women.	$(W + H - 60)/100$
8.30	Valvular defects and congenital deformities often cause	500 ml/m^2 of body surface area 450 ml/m^2 of body surface area
8.31	For examinations of the heart and vessels, a water-soluble contrast medium containing .... is injected. The method is called	changes in heart shape
8.32	In angiocardiography, the .... is examined.	iodine angiography

8.33	In cerebral angiography, the .... is examined.	heart
8.34	In arteriography, the .... are examined.	brain
8.35	In phlebography, the .... are examined.	arteries
8.36	A patient troubled with shortness of breath when walking up-hill, passage of large quantities of urine at night, and swollen legs has a heart with the dimensions $L = 20$, $B = 13$ and $D = 12$ cm and a body surface area of 2.2 m². The heart volume is ...., which is .... (a moderate size, enlarged).	veins
		600 ml/m² enlarged

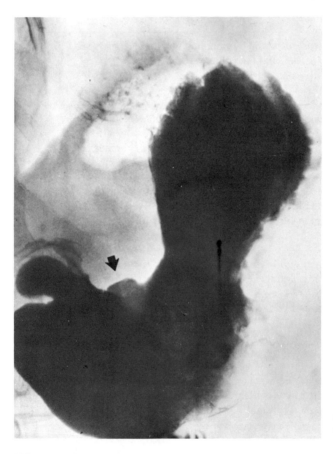

Figure 8.10 Radiography of a stomach with a large ulcer—seen as a niche at the arrow.

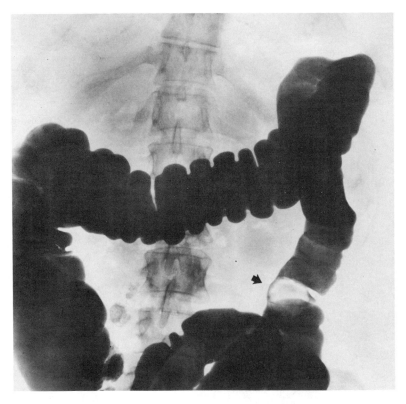

Figure 8.11 Colon radiography (examination of the large intestine with a contrast medium). Note that there is a filling defect in the contrast medium caused by an internal object, indicated by the arrow. The findings prompted a more detailed examination (see Fig. 8.12).

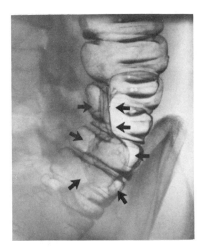

Figure 8.12 The patient shown in Fig. 8.11 was examined using the double contrast procedure. The origin of the filling defect was determined to be a polyp.

Digestive organs

The whole gastrointestinal tract can be imaged by using an emulsion of barium sulphate as a contrast medium. Barium sulphate is non-toxic, due to its low solubility product; otherwise barium ions are highly toxic. The contrast medium is swallowed or administered by means of an enema, depending on which part of the tract is to be examined (Figs. 8.10 and 8.11 on pages 392 and 393).

Sometimes a double-contrast procedure is used: a small amount of barium sulphate is introduced, and then air or carbon dioxide is blown in. Thus, a thin layer of contrast medium adheres to the mucosa, which is distended by the gas.

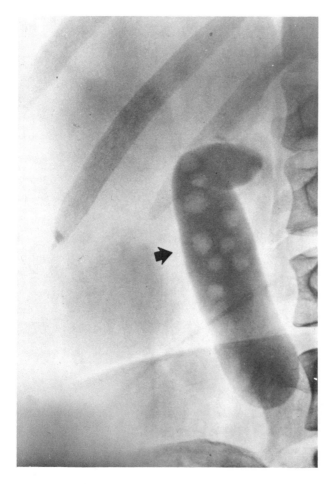

Figure 8.13 Gallbladder with a dozen stones. Note that the stones give a filling defect in the contrast medium in the gallbladder. One stone is indicated by the arrow.

Any structures that bulge into the intestine will be covered with the medium and a clear contour results (Fig. 8.12 on page 393).

Common pathological conditions of the gastrointestinal tract which are diagnosed by means of an x-ray examination are ulcers, tumors, swallowed foreign bodies, inflammatory conditions and varicose veins. An x-ray examination is by far the most important diagnostic procedure in diseases of the gastrointestinal tract.

Some organs can be visualized, since they selectively absorb certain organic compounds of iodine. The gallbladder can be seen with a contrast medium, which is given orally on the day before the examination and which is excreted via the liver; this technique is called **cholecystography**. The bile ducts can be visualized in the same way after intravenous injection of an opacifying medium, **intravenous cholangiography**. The size of the gallbladder and the width of the bile ducts can be observed, as can the degree of filling of the gallbladder and the flow of bile through the bile ducts to the duodenum. Gallstones show up as filling defects in the contrast medium (Fig. 8.13).

In connection with operations, contrast medium is often injected into the bile ducts, **operative cholangiography**, to detect the presence of any remaining stones and to show anatomic differences that may be important to the surgeon.

8.37	In an examination of the gastrointestinal tract, an emulsion of . . . . is used as the contrast medium.	
8.38	In the double contrast technique, ... is used as well as barium sulphate.	barium sulphate
8.39	Common pathological conditions of the gastrointestinal tract that can be diagnosed by means of x-rays are . . . . , ... , ... bodies, ... and	gas (air or carbon dioxide)
8.40	In cholecystography, the . . . . is examined, and in intravenous cholangiography, the . . . . ; the contrast medium used is an organic compound of iodine, which is selectively excreted by the	ulcers tumors foreign inflammatory conditions varicose veins
8.41	The bile ducts are examined after direct injection of a contrast medium during an operation or by means of a percutaneous (page 73) puncture in . . . . (name of x-ray examination).	gallbladder bile ducts liver

8.42	A somewhat obese middle-aged woman consults her physician after the Christmas holiday for pain in the right costal arch, especially after eating. Gallstones are suspected and the patient is given a contrast medium orally the day before . . . . (name of x-ray examination) is to be performed.	operative cholangiography
		cholecystography

Excretory organs

The urinary tract is examined by means of different contrast media, which are administered either via the urethral ostium or via the blood stream, when the contrast medium is excreted through the kidneys.

In **intravenous pyelography** (urography), the kidneys are visualized with an intravenous contrast medium containing iodine (Fig. 8.14). The fact that the medium is strongly concentrated by the kidneys ensures good radiopacity. It is possible to study the anatomy of the urinary tract and examine for kidney stones, tumors, inflammation and dilation of the urinary tract resulting from urinary obstruction (due, for example, to a kidney stone). An impression of renal function can also be obtained by observing the time for the excretion of the contrast medium and the accumulation of contrast medium in the renal tissue that occurs in pathological conditions involving obstruction of urinary flow in the ureter.

In **retrograde filling**, the contrast medium is injected via the urethral ostium or hrough a catheter placed in the urethra. The urethra and the urinary bladder can be visualized, **urethrocystography**, or simply, **cystography**. The renal pelvis and ureters can be examined if a contrast medium is injected via a urethral catheter introduced with the aid of a cystoscope, **retrograde pyelography**. The method is now used only in special cases, since the above described urographical method is simpler and can be carried out with less risk.

8.43	In intravenous pyelography, the . . . . are examined by intravenous injection of	
8.44	In urethrocystography the urethra and the urinary bladder are examined by . . . . injection of contrast medium via the	kidneys contrast medium
		retrograde urethral ostium

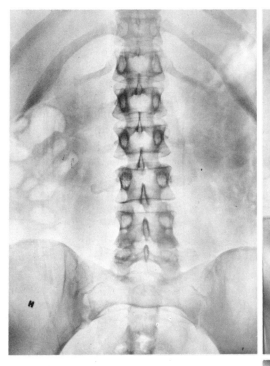

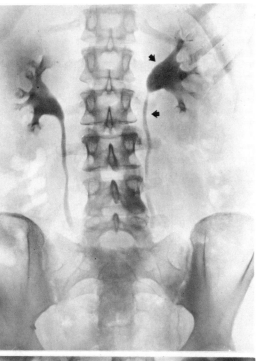

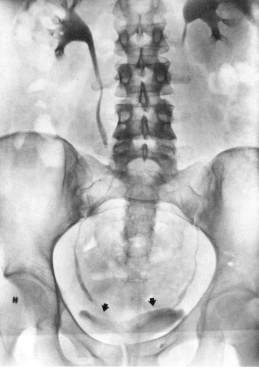

Figure 8.14 Urographic examination. Upper left—before injection of contrast medium. Upper right—20 minutes after intravenous injection of contrast medium. The renal pelvis and upper parts of the ureters are clearly visualized. Lower—partial visualization of urinary bladder.

Nervous system

The central nervous system is usually examined by **pneumography**—that is, filling the body cavities with air. The ventricles of the brain can be visualized by draining the cerebrospinal fluid and replacing it with air, **ventriculography**. In **encephalography**, air is injected into the subarachnoid space (a space below the middle meningeal membrane, the arachnoid mater, page 82), after puncturing the spinal canal (lumbar puncture) or the subarachnoid space around the brain (cisternal puncture). By encephalography, the whole cerebrospinal fluid system can be examined—not only the ventricles but also the cranial fossae and the cisternae.

The angiographic method is described above (page 390); this is of great neuroradiological importance both for diagnosis of vascular anomalies and in suspected tumors and hemorrhage.

Negative and positive contrast media are used for visualizing the spinal canal—in both cases the examination is known as **myelography**. It is performed in discal herniation and suspected tumor.

The introduction of computerized axial tomography (page 447) has reduced the need for some of these invasive neuroradiological methods, which involve discomfort and a certain risk for the patient.

8.45	In pneumography, organs are examined by injecting .... as the contrast medium.	
8.46	Ventriculography is pneumography of the cavities of the	air
8.47	In myelography, the .... is examined.	brain
8.48	A patient who in recent months has had increasingly severe headache, with neurological symptoms pointing to intracranial tumor, is referred for examination; the vessels of the brain are filled with contrast medium by injection into the carotid arteries—a technique known as .... The cavities of the brain are also filled by using air as a contrast medium; this technique is called	spinal canal
		cerebral angiography (also carotid angiography) ventriculography

X-RAY TECHNIQUES

Diagnostic radiology requires techniques adapted to the relevant medical problem. This section describes the most common physical technical principles, while a subsequent section summarizes the aspects of information theory concerning the technical components used and the applied physical procedures. Here, we examine the effect that the type of object has on the choice of technique, the way in which x-rays are generated and filtered and how the transmitted x-rays are converted to an image.

The X-ray Object

Physical properties of the x-ray object

The objects submitted to x-ray examination have different physical properties. One important factor is the thickness: in an x-ray examination of a tooth, a tissue layer of up to a few millimeters thickness is examined, while in the examination of a vertebral column in lateral projection, the x-rays must penetrate a tissue layer more than a hundred times as thick. The thickness of the object may also vary for a particular exposure, and different sections will be under- or overexposed unless special measures are taken to even out the exposure.

The elements making up the composition of the x-ray object vary. Radiography of the skeleton often requires softer x-radiation (lower energy) than soft-tissue radiography (page 380).

When x-rays pass through the object a considerable portion is scattered, as light is in frosted glass. The **scattered radiation** does not form a shadow image but has the opposite effect, causing fogging of the film and thus lowering the contrast. To reduce this effect, the x-ray field size should be made as narrow as possible, the x-ray object should be compressed to the smallest possible thickness and a grid (page 408) may be used.

The demands on resolution vary with the object. In skeletal radiography, a high resolution is often needed, and this calls for special technical procedures. In an examination of the abdominal organs—for example, the stomach or colon—the detail is not so fine as to require a special technique for high resolution. Instead, methods are required that minimize the patient dose—which would otherwise be high because of the great thickness of the object—and that minimize the required exposure time—among other things, to reduce the unsharpness due to movement of the organs during the exposure.

Short exposure times are particularly important in an examination of the lungs and heart, because of the powerful pulsations of these organs. For the same reason short exposure times must be used in x-ray examinations of children, who cannot be relied on to hold their breath.

In diagnostic radiology, a tube potential of 50–150 kV and exposure times of a few milliseconds to a few seconds are used. Because of the varying properties of x-ray objects and medical requirements, it is necessary to compromise in the choice of technical methods.

8.49	Part of the x-rays passing through the object are .... radiation, and this lowers the	
8.50	To reduce scattered radiation, the field size of the x-ray beam should be .... and the object	scattered contrast
8.51	Short exposure times are desirable in order to eliminate unsharpness due to	reduced compressed
8.52	In medical radiology, x-ray tube potentials in the range .... are used, and exposure times of between a few .... and a few	movement
		50–150 kV milliseconds seconds

Radiosensitivity of the x-ray object

X-rays, like other ionizing radiation, affect living cells. The lethal power increases with the dose (page 619), and with large doses, the cells are killed, although not all cells die at once. At lower doses the biological effect consists mainly of changes in the cell metabolism and structure. The effect appears only after a certain latency time, which is shorter for higher radiation doses. The latency time ranges from a few days to a few weeks or more; any genetic damage does not appear until the next generation.

Different tissues have different levels of sensitivity. The most sensitive ones are lymph-node tissue and bone marrow. Early signs of radiation damage are therefore anemia and changes in the blood picture, that is, in the number and appearance of the blood cells. The number of white cells decreases, and immature forms appear. Fetal tissues, sex glands and other glands, the skin and mucous membranes are also sensitive. The effect of radiation is cumulative; small doses received at long intervals are added to one another.

Exposure of the patient to radiation must be minimized. It is impossible to stipulate a general maximum permissible dose for diagnostic work because it depends on the urgency of the examination. It is inadvisable to follow fetal development in the mother by x-ray examinations, because of the sensitivity of the fetus to radiation, even if the dose to the mother and fetus does not exceed one rad

(10 mGy, page 617) or so. For example, in the case of a potentially fatal gastric disease, the use of a 10 times greater dose is justifiable if it means a more reliable diagnosis and more rapid treatment. The planning of an x-ray examination includes an assessment of risk, as is so often the case in medicine.

The dose must be the lowest that will yield an acceptable amount of information. In order to reduce the dose, high energy radiation (short wavelength, high kilovoltage) is used, which has a greater penetrating power. This may cause a reduction in the desired image contrast (cf, page 380), which constitutes the required information. In order to remove the low energy (longest wavelength, low kilovoltage) radiation, which would be absorbed in first few centimeters of the patient, filters—often 2 or 3 mm of aluminum—are placed in the beam before it strikes the patient, to reduce the dose.

The examination technique must be designed to protect the examining personnel. The maximum permissible whole-body irradiation dose for radiological staff is 0.1 rad (1 mGy) per week. The recommended upper limit of the accumulated dose for radiological personnel is $5(n - 18)$ rad (in SI units 0.05 $(n - 18)$ Gy), where n is the age. These limits do not, however, mean that there is no effect; there probably is, but compared with the other risks to which the individual is exposed, this one is too small to require a reduction of the dose.

8.53	A number of small radiation doses at long intervals are .... to each other, that is, the radiation effect is	
8.54	The tissues of the body with the highest sensitivity to radiation are the .... and	added cumulative
8.55	The earliest signs of radiation damage are .... and a change in the	lymph node tissues bone marrow
8.56	In an altered blood picture, there is a .... number of white cells, and forms of blood cells appear in the blood that are	anemia blood picture
8.57	Fetal tissue, sex glands and other glands, the skin and mucous membranes have a .... (high, moderate, low) sensitivity to radiation.	reduced immature
8.58	The permitted dose in x-ray examinations is dependent on the .... of the examination and is determined for the different types of examination by making an	high

8.59	The dose is reduced by using . . . . radiation.	urgency assessment of the risk
8.60	When high energy radiation is used, the contrast is generally . . . . (reduced, increased) and hence also the amount of information.	high energy
8.61	To eliminate the low energy radiation, the x-rays are passed through . . . . filters before they reach the patient.	reduced
8.62	For persons in radiological work, the maximum permissible dose for irradiation of the whole body is . . . . (dose per unit time).	aluminum (metal)
8.63	For a student nurse 23 years of age, the maximum cumulative dose is	0.1 rad/week (1 mGy/week)
8.64	For a retired radiologist aged 68 years, the maximum cumulative dose is	$5(23 - 18) = 25$ rad (0.25 Gy)
		250 rad (2.5 Gy)

X-ray Generators

X-rays are generated in high-vacuum tubes which are energized at a high voltage. Radiation of desired quality and quantity is obtained by varying the high voltage and current and the time that the high voltage is applied. The radiation is filtered and spatially limited to produce optimal contrast. The contrast should be optimized relative to the dose to which the patient is exposed.

X-ray tubes

X-ray quanta are liberated when electrons having a high enough energy penetrate a material. In an x-ray tube, the electrons are emitted by a hot filament cathode which is heated by a current. The cathode is designed to focus the electrons so that they impinge on a restricted area of the anode—the focal spot (Fig. 8.15). The x-ray output, Q, is proportional to the product of the current, I, and the time, t, expressed in milliampere-seconds, abbreviated to **mAs**—and also proportional to the square of the tube voltage, V:

Thus

$$Q = \text{constant } It\, V^2$$

This formula applies to the radiation emitted by the anode. The voltage dependence will actually be greater than this because of the inherent filtration of the tube and the extra filtration due to the tube housing, aluminum filters, and patient. With 15 mm Al filtration, Q is proportional to V^4, and with 20 mm Al, corresponding to about 200 mm of water, to V^5.

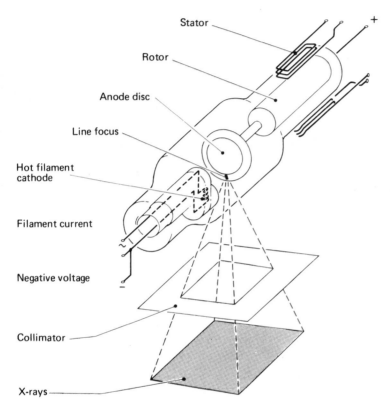

Stator

Rotor

Anode disc

Line focus

Hot filament cathode

Filament current

Negative voltage

Collimator

X-rays

Figure 8.15 X-ray tube with rotating anode, driven by a rotating magnetic field.

Tube load. It is technically difficult to simultaneously obtain a small focal spot (which is desirable from the aspect of image resolution) and a high current, exposure time and tube voltage (which are desirable from other aspects, as indicated above, page 399) without the anode melting.

The x-ray generation efficiency is low:

$$\eta = \text{x-ray energy/cathode beam energy} = 1.4 \cdot 10^{-9} ZV$$

where Z is the atomic number of the anode material and V the tube voltage.

In diagnostic radiology, tungsten is commonly used as the anode material because of its high melting point (3 370°C) and high atomic number, $Z = 74$. At 100 kV the efficiency $\eta \approx 0.01$. The rest of the energy, 99 percent, must be dissipated as heat from the anode, and this is usually accomplished by thermal radiation.

To increase the permissible load while retaining a small focal spot, a rectangular focus—known as a line focus—and a rotating anode are used. With the rectangular focus—measuring, for example, 1×5 mm—the thermal energy is distributed over a fivefold greater area; from the aspect of image formation the projected focal spot is small, about 1×1 mm, because the angle between the anode surface and the emerging central ray is small ($\approx 20°$) (Fig. 8.15). Rotation of the anode disc distributes the heat over its whole periphery. The ratio between the size of the thermal focus and that of the x-ray focus is equal to the ratio between the perimeter of the conical anode area and the width of the focal spot.

The x-ray output is also dependent on the type of high-voltage rectification. This is due to the fact that the output is dependent on the square of the voltage. Half-wave rectification yields one half the x-ray output of that obtained from a full-wave rectifier; a much better output is provided by three-phase rectifiers, in which the voltage does not drop between the half cycles (Fig. 8.16).

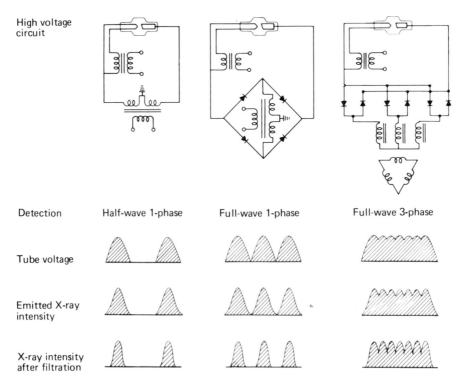

High voltage circuit

| Detection | Half-wave 1-phase | Full-wave 1-phase | Full-wave 3-phase |

Tube voltage

Emitted X-ray intensity

X-ray intensity after filtration

Figure 8.16 The x-ray output from an x-ray generator depends on the type of circuit used in the high-voltage rectifier.

To make an exposure, the cathode filament is heated. Then the line voltage is turned on to the primary winding of the high-voltage transformer during the desired exposure time.

Radiation energy distribution. The radiation quality, or the wavelength, is directly dependent on the kinetic energy of the electrons when they strike the anode. The emitted radiation is, however, not mono-energetic. There are two types of emission: **bremsstrahlung** (braking radiation) or white radiation, and **characteristic radiation**.

Bremsstrahlung has a wide energy distribution (Fig. 8.17). The distribution that is incident on the patient at a certain voltage is determined by the filtration (Fig. 8.18). The radiation of the lowest energy, that with the longest wavelength, is

Relative intensity

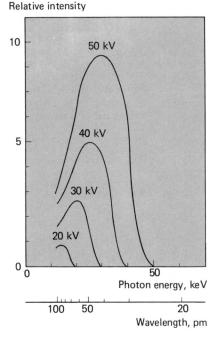

Figure 8.17 Bremsstrahlung spectra from an x-ray tube with a tungsten anode, emitted at the indicated tube voltages. The photon energies are always lower than the respective tube voltages.

absorbed in the primary filter, which is always used to protect the patient. The absorbed portion is so "soft" that it would not appreciably penetrate the patient and contribute noticeably to the image contrast; it would only result in an unnecessary skin dose. The energy distribution is also changed when the x-rays pass through the patient (Fig. 8.18). The high energy limit of the bremsstrahlung, the shortest wavelength, λ_0 (pm), is determined by the voltage, V, (kilovolts): $\lambda_0 = 1240/V$. The maximum intensity occurs at a higher wavelength ($\lambda_{max} \approx 1.5 \cdot \lambda_0$), representing softer radiation.

Relative intensity

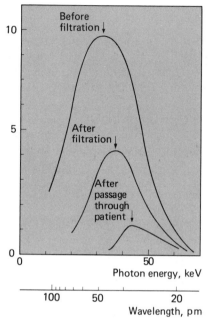

Figure 8.18 The spectral distribution of x-radiation is altered by filtration and by passage through the patient.

Relative intensity

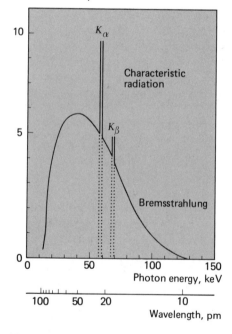

Figure 8.19 X-ray spectrum emitted by tungsten anode at 130 kV. The characteristic radiation is superimposed on a bremsstrahlung spectrum.

The characteristic radiation is excited in the atom's K shell; the x-rays that arise from the L shell have such a low energy that they do not penetrate the tube wall. The characteristic radiation for tungsten lies at $K_{\alpha 1} = 59.3$ keV, $K_{\alpha 2} = 57.9$ keV, $K_{\beta 1} = 67.4$ keV, $K_{\beta 2} = 69.3$ keV, corresponding to wavelengths of 17.9–21.4 pm. The intensity of the characteristic radiation increases rapidly with the voltage. As the voltage rises, K photons from tungsten constitute an increasing proportion of the total number of photons emitted, and at 100 kV are about 10 percent.

8.65	The quality and quantity of the radiation generated in an x-ray tube are adjusted by varying the ...., ... and	
8.66	The output from an x-ray tube is proportional to .... (combine the terms listed in the previous question into a formula).	current, *I*, exposure time, *t*, high voltage, *V*,
8.67	The permissible load on an x-ray tube is limited by the size of the anode's .... (x-ray, thermal) focal spot.	ItV^2
8.68	An attempt is therefore made to obtain a large ratio between the thermal and the x-ray focal spot by designing the latter as a .... and by .... the anode.	thermal
8.69	An x-ray technician accustomed to a full-wave 1-phase apparatus moves to another department with a 3-phase unit. She uses the same kV and mAs setting. The first picture will be .... (underexposed, normally exposed, overexposed).	line focus rotating
8.70	The shortest wavelength obtained in a bremsstrahlung spectrum at 124 kV is	overexposed
8.71	The x-rays passing through the patient have a .... (higher, equal, lower) photon energy distribution than the incident x-rays.	10 pm
8.72	To reduce the skin dose, which is caused by the low energy part of the bremsstrahlung spectrum, an .... is used.	higher
		aluminum filter

Collimators and grids

The x-ray beam is limited in order to increase the image contrast and to reduce the dose to the patient. The devices for this purpose fall into two groups: **collimators** and **grids**.

A **collimator** is an aperture diaphragm which restricts the beam. It is placed between the x-ray tube and the patient (Fig. 8.20). It may consist of a sheet of lead

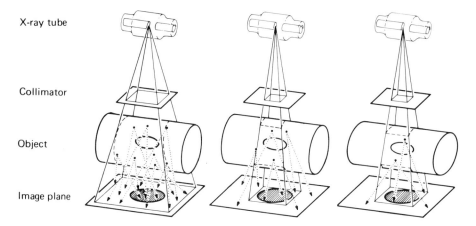

X-ray tube

Collimator

Object

Image plane

Figure 8.20 By choosing the smallest possible field size and collimator, the loss of contrast due to scattered radiation is decreased. By compressing the object, the scattered radiation from it can be further reduced.

with a rectangular or circular hole of suitable size, or of four adjustable lead strips which can be moved relative to each other. Collimators are usually furnished with an optical device, by which the x-ray field is simulated by a light field. This can be projected on the patient and permits positioning of the apparatus.

In a particular examination, the smallest possible field size is used. The patient dose is then low and less scattered radiation reaches the image plane—this increases the image contrast because scattered radiation produces diffuse illumination and fogging of the image without increasing its information content.

In order to reduce the scattered radiation, it is also important to compress the region of the patient being examined (Fig. 8.20).

Grids are inserted between the patient and the image plane (film cassette) to reduce the loss of contrast due to scattered radiation. A grid consists of thin lead strips separated by spacers of a low-attenuation material. The lead strips are usually angled and directed toward the x-ray focus so that the primary radiation from the focus, which carries the information, can pass between them, while the scattered radiation from the object is largely attenuated (Fig. 8.21).

X-ray tube

Collimator

Object

Grid

Film

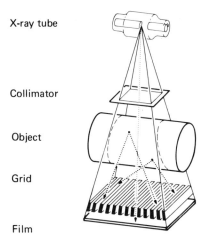

Figure 8.21 The principle of the grid. The focal radiation from the x-ray tube can pass between the lead strips, whereas much of the scattered radiation from the object is cut off because of its direction.

Because of the shadow cast by the lead strips, the image will be striped. These grid lines do not often interfere with the interpretation of the image, since the observer learns to disregard them. Fine details in the image may, however, be concealed. To avoid this, the grid can be displaced during the exposure so that the lead strips are not reproduced. Such moving grids are known as Bucky grids.

8.73	Collimators are used to increase the image .... and to reduce the patient	
8.74	A collimator is placed between the .... and the	contrast dose
8.75	A grid is placed between the .... and the	x-ray tube patient
8.76	In fluoroscopy of the stomach of a patient with gastric ulcer, the physician first cannot detect any typical "niche" (cf, Fig. 8.10). When the field size and collimator are reduced to a fraction of their original area and the body is compressed, the ulcer is visualized. This improvement in contrast is achieved by reducing the	patient image plane
8.77	A grid consists of parallel .... directed towards the	scattered radiation

8.78	A grid produces an improvement in contrast, because the scattered radiation from the object has a different .... from the primary radiation from the focus, and is therefore .... by the lead strips.	lead strips tube focus
8.79	A Bucky grid is a .... grid.	direction absorbed
		moving

Image Detection

Similar methods are used in both fluoroscopy and radiography (page 378) for obtaining the image information transmitted from the patient. The purpose is different, however. With fluoroscopy, a survey of the object is performed, while the apparatus is finely adjusted preparatory to radiography. The demands on resolution in fluoroscopy are not so great; because of the time required for fluoroscopy, it is more important to minimize the x-ray dose per unit of time. In radiography, greater demands are placed on the resolution; here too, the dose should also be kept low by ensuring that the maximum amount of the image information carried by the x-ray beam is actually utilized in the conversion to a visible image.

Imaging techniques in fluoroscopy

In fluoroscopy, the image may be viewed on a screen, where the x-ray photons are converted to visible light (Fig. 8.22). The active component in the screen

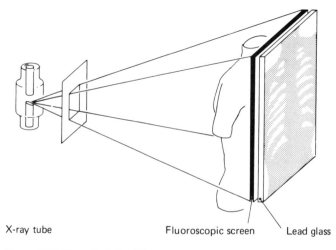

X-ray tube   Fluoroscopic screen   Lead glass

Figure 8.22 The principle of fluoroscopy.

fluoresces when the photons strike it. Zinc cadmium sulphide is generally used; the yellowish-green light emitted corresponds to the maximum sensitivity of the eye. Between the screen and the viewer, a sheet of lead glass is placed to protect against direct exposure to x-rays, but some scattered radiation cannot be completely avoided.

The efficiency of the fluoroscopic screen is low; only 7 percent of the photon energy is converted to visible light. The screen therefore emits only a weak light, 1–15 mcd/m^2 (millicandela/m^2). When using this simple fluoroscopic technique, the examining physician must adapt his eyes to the dark for about 20 min before the examination, and this is a major disadvantage. Another shortcoming is the fact that with the low brightness levels obtainable with the method, the resolution and contrast discrimination of the eye is poor. There is a considerable loss of information. Due to these disadvantages, fluoroscopy is no longer used.

In order to increase the brightness to a level suitable for the human eye, **x-ray image intensifiers** have been designed (Fig. 8.23). The input fluorescent screen

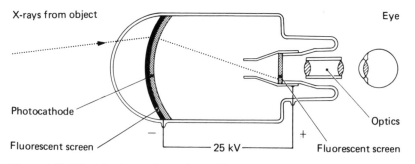

Figure 8.23 Principle of x-ray image intensifier.

converts the x-ray photons into light photons. When these strike a photocathode which is incorporated in the screen, photoelectrons are emitted. These are accelerated and focused by means of an electrostatic lens on a small output fluorescent screen. This can be viewed with a simple optical enlarging system, giving an amplification of about 5000 over that using the input screen alone.

To further increase the brightness and to permit electronic contrast enhancement of the image, and to enable several persons to view the image at the same time, a **television system** is often connected to the image intensifier (Fig. 8.24). By using an image intensifier combined, if required, with television, it is possible to reduce the radiation dose to which the patient and the investigator are exposed to several tenths of that obtained with the ordinary fluoroscopic technique.

The fluoroscopic system—whether it consists of a screen, an image intensifier or an image intensifier combined with a television system—is usually connected mechanically to the x-ray tube so that the two units move together during the patient examination. In order to decrease the dose to the patient and the

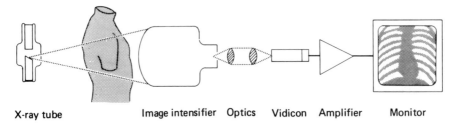

X-ray tube   Image intensifier   Optics   Vidicon   Amplifier   Monitor

Figure 8.24 An x-ray image intensifier is often combined with a television system.

investigator and to improve the image contrast, the image is constantly reduced to the smallest possible area with an adjustable collimator. In fluoroscopy without an image intensifier, a tube current of about 3 mA was used, while with the image intensifier a current of a few tenths of this value is enough. The voltage is adjusted to the patient thickness in order to obtain the required penetration.

In fluoroscopy, much information is lost because the viewer cannot fix his gaze on more than a small part of the image at any particular moment. By recording the fluoroscopic image on a videotape or videodisc, the information is preserved and the dose to the patient reduced.

8.80	A fluoroscopic screen fluoresces with a . . . . color, which corresponds to the . . . . of the human eye.	
8.81	Between the screen and the viewer a plate of . . . . is placed to protect against the x-radiation.	yellowish-green maximum sensitivity
8.82	Disadvantages of using a simple fluoroscopic technique with a screen are that the physician must . . . . before the examination, and that much information is lost because, at the low screen brightness level, both the . . . . and . . . . of the eyes are poor.	lead glass
8.83	An image intensifier permits a light intensification of about . . . . and a patient dose reduction to . . . . of that using a fluoroscopic screen.	adapt his eyes to the dark resolution contrast discrimination
8.84	The active components of an image intensifier, in order from the x-ray tube, are . . . . , ... , ... and	5000 a few tenths

8.85	The image intensifier is often combined with a television system to further increase the .... and to permit electronic .... enhancement of the image.	fluorescent screen photocathode electrostatic lens fluorescent screen
		brightness contrast

Methods for recording the radiographic image

Different methods are used for capturing the radiographic image. A photographic film combined with an intensifying screen is generally used, and sometimes just the film. Other procedures include photography of a fluoroscopic image on film of reduced format, photography of the image intensifier tube and videotape recording of the image.

X-rays exert a photographic effect. The efficiency of the process is extremely low for two reasons. First, the **film** absorbs only a small part of the x-rays, because it contains only small amounts of substances with high atomic numbers, even though it has an emulsion layer on both sides of the film base. Second, each absorbed x-ray photon represents a much greater amount of energy than is required to render a silver bromide grain developable. There is some small compensation from the fact that each photon, at least at fairly high energies, renders several silver bromide grains developable. For these reasons, film alone is used only for special purposes—for example, in skeletal radiographs of small areas, where high resolution is required. For such applications, special film with a high silver bromide content and relatively high x-ray attenuation is used.

To increase the efficiency and to reduce the information loss, one **intensifying screen** is placed on each side of the film (Fig. 8.25). The screens generate visible

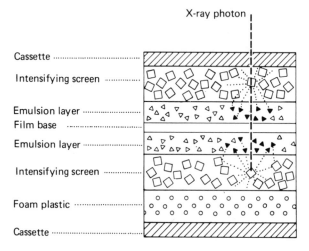

X-ray photon

Cassette ....

Intensifying screen ....

Emulsion layer ....
Film base ....

Emulsion layer ....

Intensifying screen ....

Foam plastic ....

Cassette ....

Figure 8.25 By placing intensifying screens in contact with the emulsion layer of the film, each x-ray photon causes a large number of silver bromide grains to become developable.

light and increase the efficiency for two reasons. First, the x-ray absorption is greater for the screens than for the film: 20–130 times greater depending on the x-ray photon energy. Secondly, light energy has 60 times greater power to blacken film, since each x-ray photon generates many light photons, each of which renders one silver bromide grain developable. The improvement obtained by using intensifying screens for a particular film is thus 10^2–10^3; in practice, however, the gain is by no means so great because different types of film are used with and without screens.

The gain in sensitivity is obtained at the cost of poorer resolution. As light is generated throughout the thickness of the intensifying screen, there is considerable light scatter and a loss of image detail (Fig. 8.25). It is necessary to compromise between high sensitivity and acceptable resolution—different types of screens are used for different purposes. Fine-grain screens, which have small fluorescent grains and thin layers, have a low sensitivity but high resolution. Screens with a high sensitivity, which have large grains and a thick layer, have a poor resolution. Universal screens are a third type with properties intermediate between the two types mentioned. The active substance in intensifying screens for low and moderately high energies is calcium tungstate. This fluoresces with a blue light, which corresponds closely to the maximum sensitivity of film.

The film should provide high contrast. This is the case if a large change in the degree of blackening results from a given change in exposure. The measure of film blackening is the photographic density: $D = \log_{10}(L_0/L)$, where L_0 and L are the incident and transmitted light intensities, respectively for the blackened, developed film. If the density is plotted against the logarithm of exposure to light, characteristic curves of the type shown in Fig. 8.26 left, are obtained; by exposure

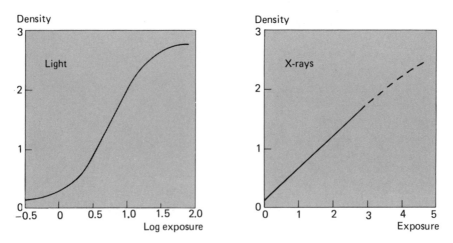

Figure 8.26 Left: the film density after exposure to light is a linear function of the logarithm of the exposure, only within a certain range. Right: the film density after direct exposure to x-rays is a linear function of the exposure.

to x-rays, the film density is a linear function of the exposure, Fig 8.26 right. In diagnostic radiology, the logarithmic relationship shown in Fig. 8.26 left, usually applies, since the x-radiation is generally converted to light via intensifying screens. The linear part of the curve is used in practice. The slope of this part of the curve (the tangent of the angle it makes with the abscissa) is known as the **gamma** (γ) of the film. Films used in diagnostic radiology have a film gamma value of about 3. Higher gamma values limit the working range (exposure latitude) of the film.

In order to reduce film costs, the images are often recorded on film of reduced format. In **photofluorography** (fluorography), the image of a fluorescent screen is photographed on small film, usually 70 or 100 mm roll film. However, there is a typical increase in patient dose of 5–10 times. Using the same format, it is possible to photograph the image obtained with an image intensifier tube; this procedure, **photospot filming**, not only lowers costs but also reduces the patient dose. There is some loss of quality compared to the ordinary procedure with full-scale display, but 70 or 100 mm fluorography is still a useful technique for examining several organs—for example, the stomach and colon. It is also possible to photograph the television monitor, but the image quality is then still poorer. Recording on **videotape** is also used in connection with the television system.

8.86	X-rays blacken photographic film, but the efficiency of the process is low because of the low . . . . and low degree of utilization of each . . . . Each represents a much greater amount of energy than is required to render a silver bromide grain	
8.87	In order to improve the efficiency, ... are used; one is placed on each side of the film, which has an emulsion layer on each side of the film base.	absorption x-ray photon developable
8.88	The gain in sensitivity, when screens are used, is obtained at the cost of a poorer	intensifying screens
8.89	In order to obtain high contrast, a film with a high . . . . is used. The value is about	resolution
8.90	The film gamma is defined as the slope of the linear part of the characteristic curve of density versus	gamma value 3
8.91	For an exposed and developed film the relationship between the density, D, the incident light, L_0, and the transmitted light, L, is given by the formula	$\log_{10}$ exposure

8.92	In photofluorography, a .... is photographed using a film of reduced format in order to lower	$D = \log_{10}(L_0/L)$
8.93	In photospot filming, the image from an .... is photographed.	fluorescent screen film costs
		image intensifier tube

INFORMATION CONTENT OF RADIOGRAPHS

The visual information obtained from a radiograph is determined, from the physical aspect, by two factors. First, the resolution is of importance because it determines the number of image elements that can be reproduced in the image. The second factor is the contrast, which is dependent on the precision with which the density of each image element can be reproduced and observed by the eye.

The resolution can be improved by using an x-ray tube with a finer focus, screens with finer fluorescent grain size or short exposure times for reducing the movement unsharpness (Fig. 8.27). In practice, the perception of fine detail is governed not by the properties of the human eye, but rather by the physical and technical conditions under which the exposure is taken.

The ways in which the contrast can be increased are more complex, and the possibilities are limited not only by technical factors—such as statistical fluctuations in the number of x-ray quanta that make up the image—but also by the limited ability of the human eye to perceive small differences in brightness.

Studies have been made of the different parts of the information chain—from the x-ray focus to the way in which the viewer perceives the image that is projected on the retina—but we still lack a comprehensive theory that will serve as a basis for choosing the optimal technical conditions for reproducing different types of x-ray objects. When such a theory has been worked out, the technical procedures in diagnostic radiology will probably be modified.

Here only four points are dealt with. Modulation transfer functions are being increasingly used to characterize the reproducing system, and are also being applied to describe the technical characteristics of the x-ray system. An important factor is the number of x-ray quanta available for building up the image, since limitations in this number often prevent transmission of the desired amount of information. Some examples are given of how unwanted image information can be selectively suppressed in order to enhance wanted information and hence facilitate the diagnosis. The section ends with a description of the nature of the visual process and the manner in which it limits utilization of the information present in the image.

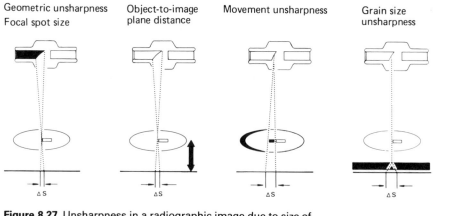

Geometric unsharpness
Focal spot size

Object-to-image
plane distance

Movement unsharpness

Grain size
unsharpness

ΔS   ΔS   ΔS   ΔS

Figure 8.27 Unsharpness in a radiographic image due to size of
focal spot, distance between object and image plane, movement
of object and grain size in intensifying screens and film emulsion.

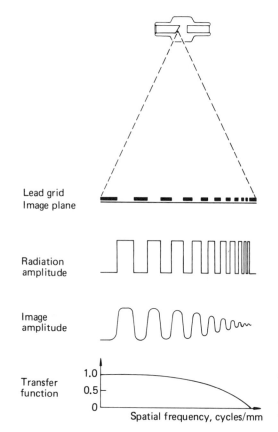

Lead grid
Image plane

Radiation
amplitude

Image
amplitude

Transfer
function

1.0
0.5
0

Spatial frequency, cycles/mm

Figure 8.28 In x-ray systems, the modulation transfer functions are determined experimentally by measuring
the reproduced contrast when a lead
grid is reproduced. (The transfer function is simplified in the figure; in fact, it
has a periodic character at higher spatial frequencies but this is irrelevant to
the following discussion.)

Modulation transfer functions

Resolution, which may be defined as the reciprocal of the distance between two points that can just be discriminated, is of limited value in diagnostic radiology. It does not include the image contrast, which is one factor determining the eye's ability to perceive detail. To obtain a more complete description of the properties of an imaging system, the concept of the modulation transfer function, MTF, has been adopted.

MTF is determined experimentally by measuring the image contrast obtained when a line grid with varying line widths is reproduced (Fig. 8.28). Thus, the contrast is studied as a function of the spatial frequency, expressed in cycles per millimeter.

Provided that each component of the system has a linear response, the MTF's can be combined by simple multiplication if they are plotted linearly (or by addition if they are plotted logarithmically).

Examples of MTF's for a typical radiographic system are shown in Fig. 8.29.

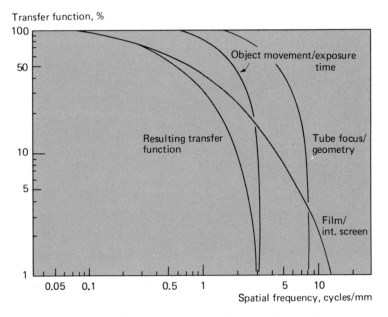

Figure 8.29 Example of modulation transfer functions in a typical radiographic imaging system.

Since there must be some geometric enlargement, the x-ray focus causes an absolute limit of 8 cycles/mm. It is true that the screen-film combination can reproduce somewhat higher spatial frequencies, but this is of no practical importance, since the contrast is then poor. (Even at a frequency of 1 cycle/mm the contrast is only 40 percent; this is due to the light scatter arising from the thickness of the screen.) Movement unsharpness eliminates all frequencies over 3 cycles/mm; because this problem is common in diagnostic radiology, there is no point in using systems capable of extremely high frequency reproduction.

An image intensifier tube cannot reproduce high contrasts, even at low spatial frequencies (Fig. 8.30). This is due to light generated on the image intensifier tube

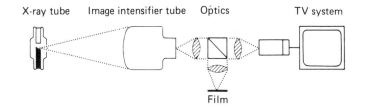

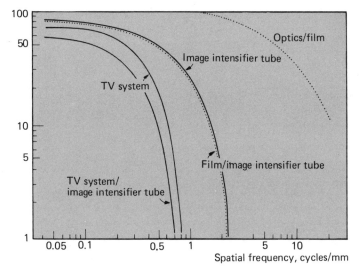

Figure 8.30 Example of modulation transfer functions in x-ray television systems.

screen, even though x-rays may not fall on the corresponding part of the image. Further deterioration is due to the properties of the television system. Clearly, for maximum utilization of the information in fluorography, the image on the intensifier tube screen should be recorded directly on a film by means of a mirror system as shown in Fig. 8.30, rather than by photography of the television monitor. Only if it is desired to perform electronic modification of the information—for example, dodging (page 430) or contrast enhancement—should the image be taken from the monitor, and then it will be at the cost of a general loss of information.

The MTF's of the described systems should be related to the spatial frequency content of the x-ray objects. These vary greatly. As has been stated above, some skeletal films require extremely high resolution and it is hardly surprising that these contain high frequencies—as shown for foot bones in Fig. 8.31. An

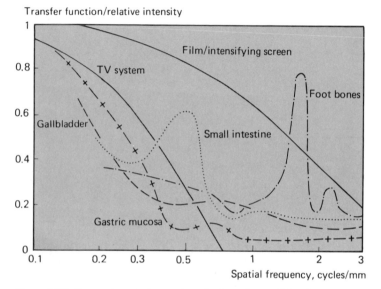

Figure 8.31 Comparison between transfer functions of imaging x-ray systems and spatial frequency content of some common x-ray objects. (Redrawn from M. Pfeiler, K. H. Reiss & O. Schott, Die Intensitäts-verteilung im Strahlenrelief als Eingangsgrösse beim Röntgenfernsehen, in Elektromedizin, Band 12/1967, by permission.)

examination of a gastric mucosa requires considerably higher frequencies than does one of a gallbladder, where the search is for a relatively large object; the contrast is, however, often lower for gallbladder examinations because of the difficulty of supplying large enough amounts of contrast medium. (This is excreted via the liver, whereas the intestines are filled directly by swallowing a barium meal.) The value of knowing the expected spatial frequency range of the x-ray object should not be exaggerated. Any diagnostic interpretation of an image is a complex mental process, where experience often compensates for any short-comings in the reproduced image.

8.94	In a determination of the MTF of an imaging system, the .... is measured as a function of	
8.95	The spatial frequency is measured in	contrast spatial frequency
8.96	Provided that each component of a system has a linear response, the MTF's of an image system can be combined by simple .... to obtain the overall MTF.	cycles per millimeter
8.97	In practice, the MTF of an x-ray image is often degraded considerably by .... of the organ.	multiplication
8.98	The largest spatial bandwidths are required to reproduce	movements
8.99	For visualization of the stomach (Fig. 8.10), colon (Fig. 8.11) and gallbladder (Fig. 8.13), ... (high, moderate, low) spatial frequencies are required.	skeletal structures
		low

Limitations imposed by the number of available quanta

The main technical problem in diagnostic radiology is to obtain the desired image information with the smallest possible patient dose. It is therefore important to determine the theoretical maximum possible ratio between information and dose for different x-ray systems. The information limit is set by the number of photons composing the image. It is thus necessary to know the number of quanta in different parts of the x-ray system. It is also important to know the eye's fundamental limits in perceiving contrast in the presence of image noise. It is then possible to determine the discrimination of detail that is theoretically possible for different systems.

An important factor in determining the noise content of the image is the integration time for the formation of the image. In radiography, the integration time is equal to the exposure time. In fluoroscopy, the integration time is taken as 0.2 s, the interval over which the eye integrates information. Events covering a shorter time merge into a single visual impression at the low light intensities of ordinary fluoroscopy (at higher light intensities the integration time is shorter, about 0.1 s). When an image intensifier tube is used in combination with a vidicon, the integration time can also be taken as 0.2 s because of the lag of the vidicon.

Number of quanta in different methods of diagnostic radiology.   Between each
stage in a diagnostic radiology system, the information is transmitted as quanta.
These quanta differ in their nature in the different stages. Thus, when they leave
the patient, quanta consist of x-ray photons. In an image intensifier tube, they
consist of electrons, and in a film, they are the blackened photographic grains. In
the transmission of information to the retina, quanta consist of light photons.

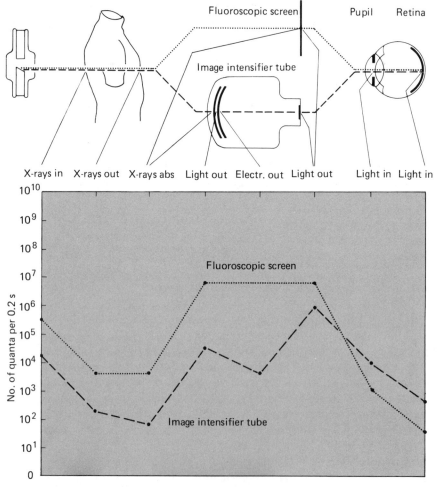

Figure 8.32 Number of quanta in fluoroscopy, with and without
image intensifier tube. Note the low degree of utilization of the
light leaving the fluoroscopic screen. When an image intensifier
tube is used, the smallest number of quanta is represented by the
x-ray photons absorbed in the image intensifier tube, but with the
usual fluoroscopic technique by the number of light photons
incident on the retina.

The strength of a chain is that of its weakest link. In an information chain of the type comprised by a diagnostic radiology system, the transmission capacity is thus determined by the part of the system where the number of quanta is lowest. Even if, at a later stage, quanta can be multiplied—for example, by making several grains developable for each absorbed x-ray photon—the amount of information is not increased. It is important to determine the number of quanta in the different stages for alternative systems.

Fluoroscopic techniques using fluorescent screens and image intensifier tubes differ considerably, as shown in Fig. 8.32. When an ordinary fluoroscopic screen is used, the transmission of information is limited by the fact that only a small part of the light emitted in all directions by the screen can be captured by the pupil of the eye—about 0.02 percent. Of the light photons that enter the pupil, only a fraction, less than 5 percent, can stimulate the retina. When a fluoroscopic screen is used, the information in the image is therefore determined by the number of light photons absorbed by the retina.

When an image intensifier tube is used in fluoroscopy, the amount of information is determined by the number of x-ray photons absorbed by the image intensifier. This number is smaller than the number of light photons absorbed by the retina. An improvement in the system can thus be achieved only by increasing the x-ray photon absorption. Any further increase in fluoroscopic screen brightness, unaccompanied by an increase in the x-ray photon absorption, does not augment the amount of information.

Comparison of the two fluoroscopic methods at the same retinal noise level shows that an image intensifier tube requires a dose that is one twenty-fifth of that used with ordinary fluoroscopic screens. The noise in the fluoroscopic screen is thus $\sqrt{25} = 5$ times as great as in the image intensifier tube for the same patient dose (page 400). This gain is often exploited by using a lower radiation intensity so as to reduce the patient dose.

In Fig. 8.33, conventional full-scale radiography, using film with screens, is compared with the use of image intensifier tubes (photospot filming). The weakest link in radiography is the number of absorbed photons by the intensifying screen-film combination; it is, however, only slightly lower than the number of quanta transmitted through the patient. There is thus little reason for further improvement of the system. In the case of an image intensifier tube, its low absorption of x-ray photons is the deciding factor. Figure 8.33 shows that the noise in the fluoroscopic image is about $\sqrt{100} = 10$ times as great as for the conventional radiographic image. The lower patient dose has been obtained at the cost of greater noise.

Perception of contrast in the presence of image noise. The eye has a limited ability to perceive contrast in the presence of noise—that is, fluctuations in the brightness of adjacent image elements. Examples of images with different noise levels are shown in Fig. 8.34.

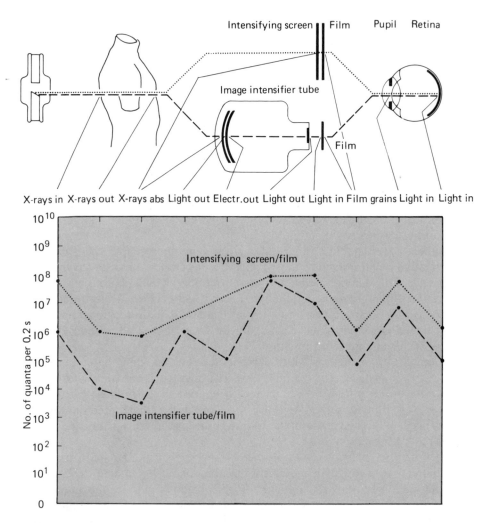

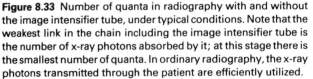

Figure 8.33 Number of quanta in radiography with and without the image intensifier tube, under typical conditions. Note that the weakest link in the chain including the image intensifier tube is the number of x-ray photons absorbed by it; at this stage there is the smallest number of quanta. In ordinary radiography, the x-ray photons transmitted through the patient are efficiently utilized.

Since the number of x-ray photons transmitted through the object per unit time varies statistically about a mean, the brightness of the image elements fluctuates correspondingly. It is therefore obvious that the ability of the eye to detect a particular detail is lowered if the brightness of adjacent image elements fluctuates.

Figure 8.34 Noise in the image interferes with the eye's ability to perceive differences in contrast.

The image contrast, C, in two adjacent areas with light intensities, I_1 and I_2, can be defined as $C = (I_1 - I_2)/I_1$. If I consists of n quanta per unit time, the standard deviation of the fluctuation will be $\sqrt{n}$ quanta. This gives a contrast fluctuation of $C_f = 1/\sqrt{n}$ for a small area compared with the surrounding background.

It has been found empirically that the eye can just perceive a minimum image contrast C_{min}, that is approximately 3 times C_f (minimum contrast-to-fluctuation ratio of 3); thus, $C_{min} \approx 3/\sqrt{n}$. If n is known, it is thus possible to calculate the smallest perceivable contrast.

Size of image elements for different x-ray diagnostic techniques. The lower limit for the size of the structures that can be perceived is determined by the image noise; the greater this is, the larger will be the image elements that the eye can just perceive.

By knowing the required ratio between contrast and noise, $C_{min} = 3/\sqrt{n}$, the size of the structures that can just be perceived can be determined. Figure 8.35 shows that the resolution is best for conventional radiography—the quantum noise does not appreciably limit the information content of the image; it should be pointed out, however, that the data in the figure relate to a low tube voltage and that the quantum noise increases considerably with the x-ray photon energy.

The fluorographic image has a somewhat greater noise level. Comparison between the fluoroscopic techniques with an ordinary screen and with an image intensifier tube shows that the latter is superior, since details having a lower contrast and a smaller area can be perceived.

Under ideal conditions, the eye is not able to distinguish differences in contrast of less than about 1 percent. This lower limit cannot always be achieved in diagnostic radiology because of the image noise and the small dimensions of the

Contrast, %

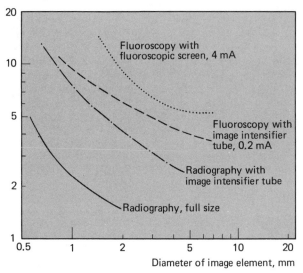

Figure 8.35 Resolution for different radiographic systems. The contrast of the image element is shown as a function of the smallest observable image element. Typical values at 70 kV tube voltage.

image structures. If fine details are to be observed—for example, objects a millimeter across—a contrast of at least 10 percent is necessary. If the contrast is low, the image elements must be of the order of one centimeter.

8.100	The information transmission capacity in an x-ray imaging system is limited by the smallest number of . . . . in any part of the system.	
8.101	Statistical fluctuations in the number of quanta give rise to . . . . in the image.	quanta
8.102	In calculating image noise from the number of quanta, the integration time in fluoroscopy is taken as . . . . and in radiography as the	noise
8.103	Quanta are of different types in the different stages of a diagnostic radiology system; for example, in the radiation leaving the patient they consist of . . . . , in a radiographic image of . . . . , and in the eye, of	0.2 s exposure time

8.104	The weakest link in a diagnostic radiology system—that stage of the system with the lowest number of quanta—differs according to the system. For example, in fluoroscopy without an image intensifier tube, the weakest link is the . . . ., in fluoroscopy with an image intensifier tube, it is the . . . ., in radiography, the . . . . and in photospot filming it is the	x-ray photons silver bromide grains light photons
8.105	Under favorable conditions, in the absence of noise, the eye cannot perceive contrasts smaller than about	retina input fluorescent screen of image intensifier tube intensifying screen input fluorescent screen of image intensifier tube
8.106	If the image contrast is low, about 1 percent, the object in a high-noise radiographic image must be of the order of . . . . across.	1 percent
8.107	If the contrast is high, more than 10 percent, it is possible under favorable conditions to perceive structures of the order of . . . . across.	1 centimeter
		1 millimeter

Information selection in diagnostic radiology

The radiographic image generally contains much more information than can be utilized in the clinical examination of the patient. In the inspection of the radiograph, therefore, a selection of information is made, those details being chosen that are of significance in the individual case. For example, shadows produced by the ribs are disregarded when the lungs or heart are being examined.

Normally, the conditions of the examination are optimized to reduce unnecessary details, so that the image of the organs under reexamination is free of interfering shadows as far as possible. Undesirable image structures can be further suppressed by using special procedures such as **tomography**, **subtraction**, and **dodging**.

Tomography. In the ordinary x-ray image, all the tissue layers traversed by the x-ray beam are visualized. When it is desired to eliminate all image shadows except those originating from a particular plane in the patient, tomography can be applied. (Synonymous terms to tomography are body section radiography, planigraphy, laminagraphy and stratigraphy.)

The principle of tomography is to produce intentional movement unsharpness in all planes except the one to be visualized. This is accomplished by moving the x-ray tube and film during the exposure about an axis located in that particular plane (Fig. 8.36). Linear, circular or helical motion can be chosen. The greater the

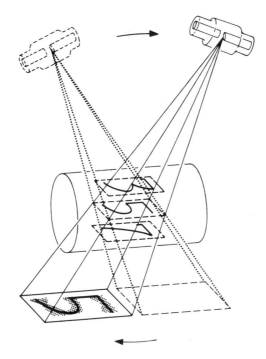

Figure 8.36 In tomography, an intentional movement unsharpness is produced for all the image planes that are not to be visualized.

distance of tube travel, the greater the movement unsharpness produced for undesired structures, and the thinner the layer that can be observed.

Subtraction. Information can be selected by subtracting unwanted details from the original x-ray image. For this to be possible, there must be two images, the difference between which constitutes the desired information. This is often the case in examinations in which a contrast medium is used—for example, angiography (page 390) in which several films are exposed as the contrast medium passes through the vascular system.

With the photographic technique, the subtraction procedure is as follows. A negative copy is made of one of the radiographs. This copy is placed exactly on the other radiograph. The two films consequently have reversed contrasts, and details common to the two films are then eliminated, while the differences remain—the shadow of the contrast medium (Fig. 8.37). Because of technical defects, certain common details in the radiographs generally persist, and these are used to locate

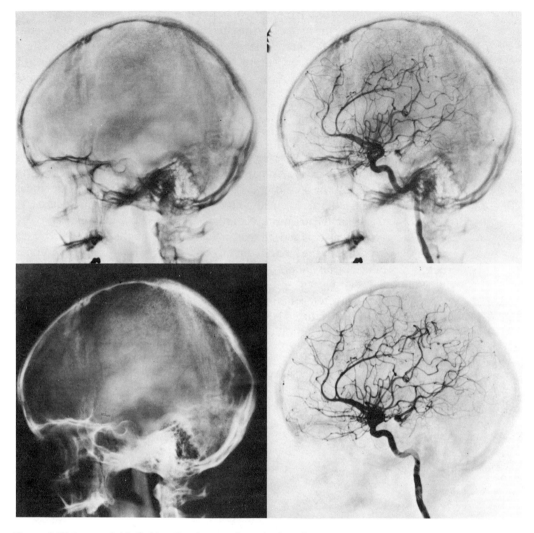

Figure 8.37 Lower right: Subtraction image of cerebral angiography. Upper left and right: The two original films. Lower left: Image with reversed contrast used in the subtraction process.

the difference shadow, relative to the surrounding anatomical structures. The photographic subtraction procedure is time consuming and requires experience in order to obtain a correctly exposed film with reversed contrast. For this reason the method is not widely used.

The subtraction procedure can be simplified by using television. The two films are converted to two video signals by two identical television channels and the subtraction is performed electronically. The images can also be easily processed by electronic means—for example, by making the difference picture positive or negative and adjusting the image contrast and brightness until optimal subtraction is obtained. For storing, the image on the television monitor can be photographed. The advantages of electronic subtraction—rapidity, simplicity and controllability—are obtained at the cost of poorer resolution; the highest spatial frequencies cannot be reproduced by the television system.

Dodging. Radiographs are often so unevenly exposed that large areas of the images are either under- or overexposed. This is mainly due to large differences in attenuation in different areas arising primarily from variations in thickness. In a lateral projection of the skull, the tissue thickness is large and the mean attenuation is high in the areas enclosed by the braincase, whereas in the areas of the face enclosing air the tissues are thinner and the mean attenuation lower. Thus, if the x-ray intensity is chosen to reproduce details in the braincase, there is marked overexposure of the face. If, on the other hand, low intensity is chosen in order to reproduce facial details—for example, the nasal cavities—the braincase will be underexposed.

Radiographs thus often contain unwanted spatial frequencies—the extremely low frequencies are reproduced with too high amplitude. These can be eliminated by dodging. There are two kinds of dodging used, primary and secondary.

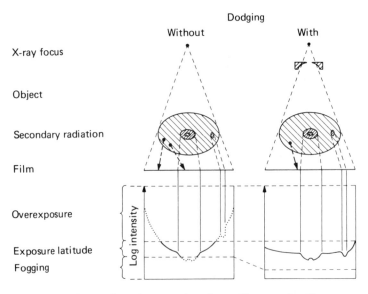

Figure 8.38 Comparison between imaging without and with dodging. The improvement in image quality is due to better utilization of the film's exposure latitude and reduction in secondary radiation from the object, thereby reducing the fogging.

In primary dodging, filters are placed in the beam between the x-ray tube and the patient in order to compensate for the varying mean attenuation (Figs. 8.38 and 8.39). The images are improved for two reasons: the working range (exposure latitude) of the film is better utilized, and the scattered radiation from the object is decreased, thus reducing the background fogging.

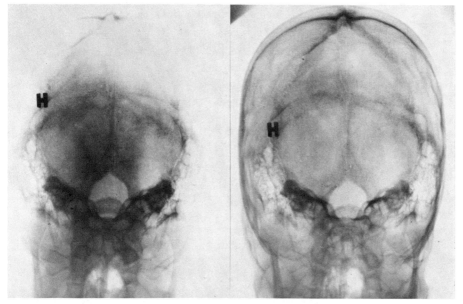

Figure 8.39 Radiographs of a skull taken without (left) and with dodging (right). (*Courtesy* S. Hirzel Verlag, Stuttgart.)

In secondary dodging, the information processing is performed after the radiation has passed through the patient—for example, by means of photographic techniques on the developed radiograph or by electronic methods in a television system.

The primary dodging technique has the great advantage of reducing the dose to the patient to about half the value of that needed with a conventional x-ray exposure.

8.108	Information selection in diagnostic radiology can be performed in three ways: . . . ., ... and . . . .

8.109	In tomography, unwanted image information is suppressed by producing .... for unwanted objects.	tomography subtraction dodging
8.110	The motion unsharpness is produced by moving the .... and the .... in opposite directions during the exposure.	motion unsharpness
8.111	A subtraction procedure for eliminating unwanted details can be utilized when there are two radiographs with a difference consisting of the	x-ray tube film
8.112	In photographic subtraction, the first step is to make a new negative film with .... contrast by copying the original film.	desired information
8.113	In dodging, the .... of the very low spatial frequencies is reduced.	reversed
8.114	To avoid over- or underexposure in different areas of an x-ray film, ... is used.	amplitude
8.115	A 2½-year-old girl develops acute coughing, respiratory distress and pain in the chest, and after a day or so, fever. Repeated radiographic and fluoroscopic examinations disclosed nothing abnormal Bronchoscopy (page 118) was performed to search for a possible foreign body in the windpipe, since the patient had been eating peanuts at the time she fell ill. No peanuts were found; a diagnosis of asthma was made and the patient was sent home. Three months later her condition deteriorated in connection with upper respiratory tract infection. For short periods ventilation ceased completely. A new radiological examination showed that both lungs were distended and the chest dilated. A foreign body was still suspected, and to visualize the bronchi without interfering contrast shadows an examination known as .... was performed. A peanut was then discovered. It was located and removed under bronchoscopic control.	primary dodging
		tomography

The visual process and contrast discrimination

The perception of an anatomic detail in a radiograph is a visual process. Sophisticated signal processing in the retina and central nervous system greatly improves our ability to observe the environment; in radiological work, however, it results in subjective impressions of the image that cannot be correctly interpreted unless the nature of this nervous signal processing is known. The eye has developed so that it performs best in detecting objects in our environment—game moving in the field, enemies hiding in the bushes; the eye is not well adapted for interpreting radiographs.

The rods of the retina react to changes in illumination; they adapt rapidly to constant illumination. The discharge frequencies for the action potentials from the rods in the retina are a logarithmic function of the change in illumination. To produce changes in illumination on the retinal receptors when the gaze is fixed on a stationary image, the eye is in constant motion—a state known as fixation nystagmus. These small eye movements can only be observed with the aid of instruments. As a result of nystagmus, in the presence of contrast, the retinal receptors are exposed to a stimulus that varies in time, and whose magnitude is determined by the illumination gradient, but is independent of the level of illumination (Fig. 8.40).

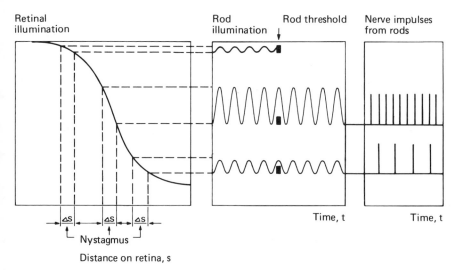

Figure 8.40 By means of small eye movements—fixation nystagmus—spatial illumination gradients on the retina are converted to time-variable changes in illumination on the rods. If the temporal changes of illumination exceed the threshold value for stimulus of the rods, nervous impulses are generated, whose frequency is a function of the temporal changes of illumination.

Nystagmus is essential for vision. This is evident from the fact that if the effect of eye movements is eliminated by means of an optical technique (a mirror device mounted on a contact lens that follows the eye movements) so that the image is constantly projected on the same place on the retina, the subjective image fades and disappears after a few seconds. Only by moving the image or replacing it with a new one can a subjective image be produced, which will again last for a few seconds. The perception of an image is thus dependent on the spatial illumination gradient on the retina.

With sight we thus first perceive only boundaries between areas in the image of different levels of illumination—that is, contrasts. In the retina and central nervous system there is further signal processing in which the negative second derivative of the illumination is added to the signal. This is easily perceived when two uniformly gray areas of different illumination are observed side by side: the lighter area appears lighter and the darker one darker near the boundary, although both are in fact of uniform illumination. The increase in contrast at the boundaries, which is a useful optical illusion, is known as the **Mach effect**, after its discoverer. Visual processing thus has a similarity to a Xerox copying machine: on the copy most of the ink powder is attracted in proportion to the negative second derivative of the electric field distribution, which represents the image. Large black areas on the original are thus reproduced as an outline, rather than as a filled-in area.

The situation is further complicated by the fact that in the central nervous system, the areas outlined by gradients in the image are filled in, so that subjective images are obtained also of the included areas, and these areas have a certain subjective brightness. We are unconscious of the filling-in of the image between intensity gradients. The blind spot, which is due to the absence of receptors in the retina at the place where the optic nerve leaves the eye fundus, should actually give a constant black spot in the visual field; it does not do so because the brain fills in gaps in the image.

Vision is thus a complex phenomenon which is dependent on the retinal illumination and its first and second derivatives. Figure 8.41 gives a diagrammatic representation of how we perceive the radiographic image of two different x-ray objects. An object with a diffuse boundary of the type shown on the left gives an inflection point in the curve of intensity versus distance. The point of inflection corresponds to the boundary we perceive subjectively. In the case of a blurred object—that is, one with a low spatial intensity gradient—the second derivative d^2E/ds^2 contributes little to the subjective image. Note also that no subjective image results when the spatial illumination gradient on the retina falls below the threshold for evoking action potentials from the rods. Nor does the eye see large differences in illumination if these are distributed over a large distance.

In practice, it is easy to increase the value of the spatial illumination gradient on the retina by viewing the image with an optical reducing system so that gradients present in the image are amplified on the retina. Another approach is to view the image at a greater distance, as the radiologist often does. One low

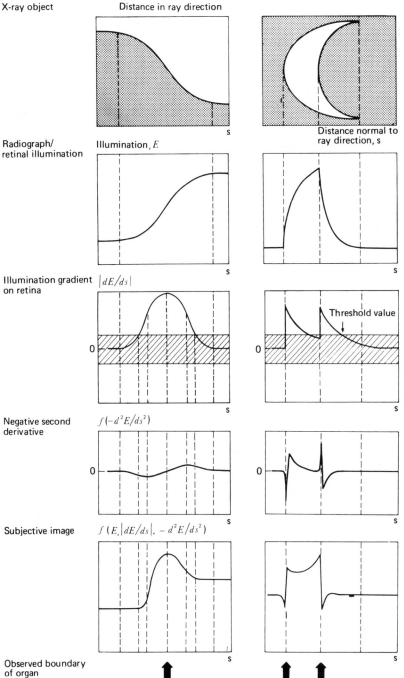

X-ray object

Distance in ray direction

Distance normal to ray direction, s

Radiograph/
retinal illumination

Illumination, E

Illumination gradient
on retina

$|dE/ds|$

0

0

Threshold value

Negative second
derivative

$f(-d^2E/ds^2)$

0

0

Subjective image

$f(E, |dE/ds|, -d^2E/ds^2)$

Observed boundary
of organ

Figure 8.41 The subjective image is a compound function of the
retinal illumination and its first derivative and negative second
derivative. The figure shows only a qualitative indication of the
subjective effect.

435

gradient may be suppressed in order to better observe a higher gradient, by enlarging the image or viewing it at a shorter distance.

An object of the type shown on the right in Fig. 8.41—for example, pneumothorax (page 126)—cannot be correctly perceived with the projection shown. The eye places the boundaries of the air-filled cavity where the negative second derivative of the retinal illumination (absolute quantity) is a maximum. The slit-shaped areas of the crescent-shaped object are overlooked because they produce an illumination gradient on the retina below the threshold for evoking action potentials.

8.116	In order to perceive a subjective image when the gaze is fixed on a stationary image, the image must contain a difference in light intensity—that is, a . . . .—and this must be converted in the individual retinal receptors to a stimulus that varies in . . . . (time, space).	
8.117	This conversion occurs through fixation nystagmus—that is, small	contrast time
8.118	The perception of an image is thus dependent on the spatial	eye movements
8.119	Low contrast cannot be perceived because the movement-induced retinal rod stimulation does not exceed the	·illumination gradient
8.120	To increase the stimulus—that is, the value of the spatial illumination gradient—the image may be viewed with an optical . . . . (reducing, enlarging) system.	stimulus threshold
8.121	A simple way of increasing a low contrast illumination gradient is to view the image at a	reducing
8.122	The visual sense places a blurred boundary at the point of . . . . of the curve of retinal illumination versus distance.	greater distance
8.123	In the retina a term is added to the image that is a function of the . . . . of the retinal illumination.	inflection
8.124	The mechanism described in the previous question produces a(n) . . . . (increase, decrease) in the perceived contrast.	second derivative

8.125   A step-shaped distribution of retinal illumination of   increase
         the type shown in the figure below gives perception
         of the type (indicate as a curve):

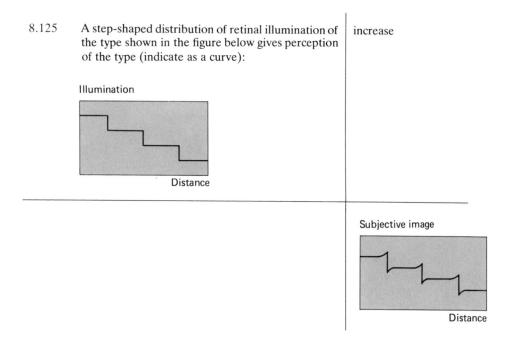

DATA ANALYSIS IN DIAGNOSTIC RADIOLOGY

The diagnostic procedure consists of collecting the facts relating to the position of pathological changes in the body or an organ, and the number, size and severity of the changes. Any changes occurring since previous examinations are also noted. These descriptive facts are usually supplemented with a tentative diagnosis and an estimate of the probability that this is correct. The report may also contain suggestions for further examinations.

The examining physician converts the image information in the radiograph to visual information, then to verbal information in the report. For the conversion from image information to verbal information, computer techniques have only rarely been used. It is, however, possible to systematize the verbal information so that all evaluations of radiological examinations adhere to a standardized format.

The mental process leading up to the report consists of a stepwise climb in a tree of diagnostic information, where the trunk consists of the x-ray diagnosis as a whole, and the finest branches consist of the detailed description of the available findings and the possible diagnoses. The ideal information tree consists of the accumulated, generally accepted knowledge in the whole field of diagnostic radiology. The information tree of a particular physician is modified by his level of training, experience, forgetfulness, and personal interest which lead to the incorporation of knowledge that is not generally accepted. Because of these individual differences, reports based on the same primary examination data can differ to a greater or lesser extent.

This difficulty can be minimized by using special computer terminals when issuing the report. The investigator chooses the route in a defined information tree represented by image frames. These are stored on a film strip and projected in turn on an image screen. Each display permits a choice of alternative branches, for example, 48. The choice is made by pressing buttons placed in rows beside the image display. The first frame provides a choice of organ system—for example, the circulatory system, respiratory system, gastrointestinal system, etc. In the next frame, organs are chosen—for example, the esophagus, stomach, etc. In the next frame, the choice is made between, for example, ulcer, benign and malignant tumors, etc. Further series of frames relate to descriptions of findings, the position and size of pathological changes, changes in the findings since earlier examinations, etc. Verbal information can also be inserted with an ordinary typewriter; this must be used when the findings cannot be adequately described by the frames. The terminal is linked to a computer which constantly records the results.

Advantages of such methods are that all the reports are prepared in the standardized format and can be made short and concise, information can be directly stored, and the stored information on the patient can be rapidly retrieved and subjected to statistical analysis. Disadvantages are that the physician must adapt himself to the machine and cannot report findings so descriptively and exhaustively as in a direct verbal description.

8.126	The mental process leading up to a report of a radiographic examination can be described as a stepwise climb in a	
8.127	The cumulated, generally accepted knowledge in the field of diagnostic radiology represents the . . . . information tree.	tree of information
8.128	Physicians have different levels of training, experience, personal interest and forgetfulness. Because of this, their verbally described x-ray diagnostic interpretations vary due to . . . . in the information tree utilized.	ideal
8.129	Advantages of the application of the ideal information tree stored in a computer system are that the report can be prepared in a . . . . format, the information can be directly . . . . , and rapidly . . . . , and that the information can easily be submitted to . . . . analysis.	individual differences

8.130	Disadvantages of the above described computer system for preparing a report are that the physician must .... himself to the computer, and that the findings cannot be reported in such great .... as in a direct verbal description.	standardized stored retrieved statistical
		adapt detail

QUANTITATIVE RADIOLOGICAL MEASUREMENTS

The x-radiation transmitted through the patient contains information about the amount of substances in the body. The information is contained in the difference between the energy distribution for the transmitted and incident radiation. The attenuation of low-energy x-ray quanta increases with the amount of elements of relatively high atomic numbers (Figs. 8.2 and 8.18).

The information relating to the quantitative composition is used to only a small extent in ordinary radiography. It is true that in the case of extremely low bone mineral levels in the skeleton—less than 50 percent of normal—it is possible to observe this on radiographs because the skeleton gives an abnormally weak contrast shadow. In most cases, however, the reduction in the bone mineral content is too small for such a subjective evaluation to be of clinical value. Quantitative methods have therefore been developed for determining the composition in the body: **film densitometry** and **x-ray spectrophotometry**. These methods are mainly used for determining the degree of mineralization of the skeleton.

Computerized axial tomography is another unique method for quantitative estimation and discrimination of small contrast differences in selected planes of the object.

Film densitometry

The amounts of certain substances in the body can be approximately determined by measuring the degree of x-ray film blackening, a technique known as film densitometry. The fact is used that the film blackening increases with x-ray exposure. For exact, quantitative measurements to be possible, however, there must be a known relationship between the level of blackening and the quantities of the substances in the body; but, as described below, there is no such well-defined relationship, and the method is therefore only approximate.

The procedure for exposing x-ray film in the measurement of the bone mineral content of the skeleton (calcium hydroxyapatite—calcium phosphate) is as follows. The part of the body involved is surrounded by a medium, usually water, having about the same mass attenuation coefficient and density as the soft tissues of the body. This smooths out the variations in the degree of film blackening that would arise if the thickness of soft tissues were distributed less uniformly over the image. Near the object is placed a reference step-wedge, consisting of a material having attenuation properties corresponding to those of the bone mineral. The increase in attenuation as the step-wedge gets thicker produces a reference shadow with decreasing blackening, which is determined photoelectrically with a film densitometer. This provides a calibration curve for the relationship between the bone mineral content and the degree of film blackening. The calibration curve is used for estimating the bone mineral content in the skeletal structures reproduced on the same film (Fig. 8.42).

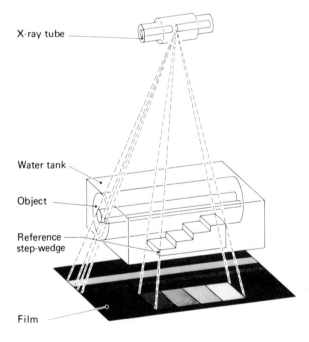

X-ray tube

Water tank

Object

Reference step-wedge

Film

Figure 8.42 Principle for measuring the bone mineral content of an object by simultaneous imaging of a reference step-wedge.

There are a number of measurement errors in the method that cannot be compensated for. The thickness of the film emulsion layer varies to some extent and in an unknown manner, and this produces an error that cannot be measured. Scattered radiation from the object—and from the reference step-wedge—is not uniformly distributed but results in a variation in background blackening. More serious is the fact that x-radiation from an ordinary x-ray tube is not mono-energetic and that the energy distribution as well as the intensity varies for different solid angles. Moreover, the energy distribution is modified to a different extent during passage of the beam through different parts of the object. These factors produce unknown variations in film blackening.

Differences in energy distribution and intensity at different solid angles from the x-ray tube are due to the so-called heel effect of the anode (Fig. 8.43). The

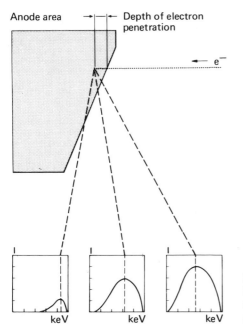

Figure 8.43 Because of the anode's heel effect, the radiation intensity and energy distribution vary with the solid angle.

electrons penetrate the surface of the anode a certain distance and x-ray photons are therefore liberated at a certain depth. The photons passing out at an extremely small angle relative to the surface of the anode undergo greater attenuation because of their longer path in the anode material; as a result of filtration, this radiation has a lower intensity and a higher energy distribution than the radiation that passes out at larger angles.

8.131 The radiation transmitted through the patient contains information relating to the amount of .... in the body.

8.132	This information is represented as a difference in the .... of the incident and transmitted x-radiation.	substances

8.133	The errors in x-ray film densitometry that cannot be eliminated are due to: (1) differences in the .... and .... of the x-radiation at different solid angles (2) .... emitted by all parts of the object (3) varying thickness of the film's	energy distribution

(1) energy distribution
intensity
(2) scattered radiation
(3) emulsion layer

X-ray spectrophotometry

Quantitative measurements of some of the body's substances can be performed by attenuation measurements using either radiation from an x-ray tube or from certain radionuclides. One advantage over film densitometry is that the radiation can be made more homogenous—that is, almost monoenergetic, and this reduces the measurement errors that arise due to changes in energy distribution during passage through the object. In addition, by restricting the measured radiation to a narrow beam, 1–20 mm in diameter, the measurement errors arising from scattered radiation from the object are eliminated. As a further advantage, the procedure usually includes counting and recording each photon, which enables digital circuit techniques to be used, and this results in greater accuracy in signal analysis.

X-ray spectrophotometry involves making enough experimental measurements to solve an equation system of the type:

$$I_{\lambda 1} = I_{0,\lambda 1} \exp - (\mu_{1,\lambda 1} x_1 + \mu_{2,\lambda 1} x_2 + \ldots + \mu_{n,\lambda 1} x_n) \tag{1}$$

$$I_{\lambda 2} = I_{0,\lambda 2} \exp - (\mu_{1,\lambda 2} x_1 + \mu_{2,\lambda 2} x_2 + \ldots + \mu_{n,\lambda 2} x_n) \tag{2}$$

$$\vdots$$

$$I_{\lambda m} = I_{0,\lambda m} \exp - (\mu_{1,\lambda m} x_1 + \mu_{2,\lambda m} x_2 + \ldots + \mu_{n,\lambda m} x_n) \tag{m}$$

where $I_{\lambda j}$ and $I_{0,\lambda j}$ are the transmitted and incident intensities of energies, $\lambda_1 \ldots \lambda_m$, and where $\mu_{i,\lambda j}$ are the attenuation coefficients for the substances $1 \ldots n$ at the energies $\lambda_1 \ldots \lambda_m$, and x_i are the amounts of the substances per unit area for the substances $1 \ldots n$.

In practice, an x-ray object is considered to consist of a maximum of five substances: soft tissues consisting of water and proteins (but not fat), fat, bone mineral, endogenous heavy elements (iodine in the thyroid) and exogenous heavy elements (contrast media). Water and proteins have such similar physical properties and occur in such homogeneous mixtures that they can be regarded as a single substance. In order to solve the equation system, the number of equations must be equal to the number of groups of substances under examination—that is to say, it is necessary to use the same number of different energies, where there are sufficiently large differences in attenuation coefficients. In practice, this is often difficult to achieve, and it is then necessary either to use special technical procedures or to accept approximate solutions. A number of different types of instruments are available that permit different levels of measurement accuracy.

With all types, the measurement is performed by means of a narrow beam. Either point measurements are performed over the given part, or the organ is scanned in one or more linear sweeps. In point measurement, the amounts of the substances are obtained in mg/mm^2 of body surface area. Because of the irregular shape of the organ, it is usually impossible to calculate the amounts per unit of organ volume (mg/mm^3); an exception is the head of the humerus, which has a regular form that can be determined by radiography.

Scanning produces a concentration profile (Fig. 8.44). If the area of the profile is integrated while the beam sweeps over the object—or in a subsequent signal analysis—the amount of substance in a one-millimeter-long section of the organ is obtained, mg/mm. If several parallel sweeps over the whole organ are performed, the total and absolute amount of the substance in grams is obtained. Such scanning is usually time consuming and the determination is therefore unreliable because the part of the body under examination cannot be adequately immobilized.

Radiation sources. The radiation source for x-ray spectrophotometry can be either an x-ray tube or radionuclides.

The radionuclides must have an emission that is nearly monoenergetic and that lies within the x-ray range. Use has been made of ^{125}I, which emits mainly at 27.3 keV and ^{241}Am at 59.6 keV. One advantage of radionuclides is that the intensity is known and remains constant during each measurement; one disadvantage is that the attainable intensities and radiation qualities greatly limit the range of application of the apparatus. The number of photons is insufficient for examination of the thick parts of the body, which have high attenuation. The accuracy, which is determined by statistical fluctuations in the photons detected, is also limited. When the radiation is generated by an x-ray tube, the energy distribution is limited to a narrow band by filtration. One advantage of the x-ray tube as a radiation source is that it yields a greater number of quanta per unit time than do radionuclides, thus permitting more rapid measurement and a higher level of accuracy.

Detectors. Radiation intensity is measured using scintillation crystals, NaI(Tl), combined with a photomultiplier. Radiation of energies, different from that

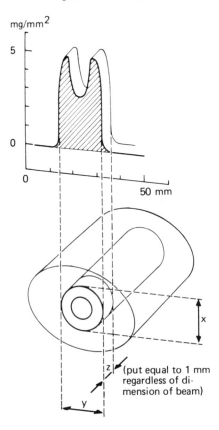

Figure 8.44 By integrating the concentration profile of an object, the amount of the substance under examination per centimeter of the organ can be determined.

desired are eliminated by amplitude discrimination of pulses from the photomultiplier. This allows only the wanted pulses to pass—for example, in the case of ^{125}I, those corresponding to 27.3 keV.

Examples of measuring systems.   There are systems of varying complexity, depending on the acceptance of approximate solutions of the equation system $(1)\ldots(m)$, page 442. Two examples of measuring systems are given below. In one of these, only one energy is used, and the object must then have a constant thickness of soft tissue. In the second system, three energies are used, which permit greater freedom in choosing the measuring object and greater accuracy.

For measuring the degree of mineralization of the peripheral skeleton (skeleton of the extremities), it is satisfactory to employ radiation of only one energy as long as certain systematic measuring errors are acceptable. A measuring system such as that shown in Fig. 8.45 is used. The part of the body in question is assumed to be of constant thickness. It is therefore surrounded by a material equivalent to soft tissue—that is, one having the same attenuation and density properties as the body's soft tissues. The radiation is obtained from a radionuclide.

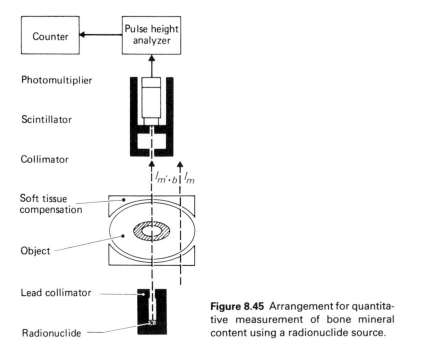

Figure 8.45 Arrangement for quantitative measurement of bone mineral content using a radionuclide source.

It is collimated—that is, restricted to provide a narrow beam—by means of lead collimators placed at the ray source and the detector. The bone mineral content, m_b (mg/mm^2), is given by the expression:

$$m_b = \rho_b \ln (I_t/I_{t+b})/(\mu_b\rho_b - \mu_t\rho_t)$$

where I_t and I_{t+b} are the respective intensities when the beam is passed through soft tissues alone and through both soft tissues and bone, μ_b and μ_t are the mass attenuation coefficients for bone mineral and soft tissues, and ρ_b and ρ_t are the corresponding densities. The greatest disadvantage of the method is the low radiation intensity. This means that measurements are limited to peripheral parts of the body, such as the forearm.

In the arrangement in Fig. 8.46, three energy bands are used, which are obtained from a special x-ray tube. The radiation is generated by intense x-ray bombardment of a conical secondary anode, divided into sectors, which are covered with substances that induce the emission of K lines. The anode is rotated so that the different energies are each produced in turn. A narrow x-ray beam is used in the measurements. The beam first passes through the servo-driven wedges, consisting of the substances in which measurements are to be made—for example, in the figure, soft tissues, bone mineral and iodine (used as a contrast medium). Then the beam passes through the measured object. (In the described system the presence of fat is disregarded, and this constitutes a minor source of

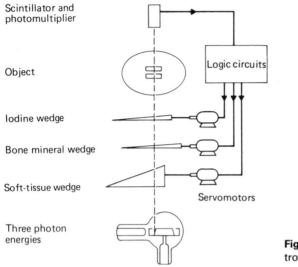

Scintillator and photomultiplier

Object

Logic circuits

Iodine wedge

Bone mineral wedge

Soft-tissue wedge

Servomotors

Three photon energies

Figure 8.46 Principle of the x-ray spectrophotometer.

error.) The intensities of the three energies are measured in the detector, which consists of a scintillator and a photomultiplier tube. The electronic system adjusts the position of the wedges so that the intensities of the three energies at the detector are always constant. When certain amounts of the three substances are inserted in the beam, the wedges are displaced a distance that is a direct measure of the amounts of the substances in the beam. In practice, on their path from the tube to the detector, the rays always pass through equal amounts of the three substances, irrespective of the composition and shape of the objects, and this enables measurements to be performed in different parts of the body. Because high radiation intensities can be obtained from the x-ray tube, relatively high scanning speeds can be used, which reduce errors due to movements of the measured part of the body.

8.134	In x-ray spectrophotometry, the x-ray sources can be .... or a(n)	
8.135	In point measurement at a site in the body, measurement values are expressed in .... (units).	radionuclides x-ray tube
8.136	By scanning a part of the body with a sweep, the quantity of the substance can be expressed in .... (units); this gives the amount present in a part of the organ that is .... in length.	mg/mm^2

8.137	By scanning with several parallel sweeps covering the whole organ, the .... amount of substance in the organ can be calculated, and then the amount is expressed in .... (unit).	mg/mm 1 mm
		total milligrams

Computerized axial tomography, CAT

It is possible to reconstruct the attenuation properties of the object in one particular plane by recording and processing a set of image projections. The technique is applicable in radiological and other imaging processes, such as gamma cameras; it is here described as applied to x-ray imaging.

A thin layer of the object is scanned with a pencil beam, Fig. 8.47. The attenuation is recorded with a scintillator in a group (i.e., 160) of parallel scans, and after each group the direction of the beam is slightly turned (i.e., 1°) for a

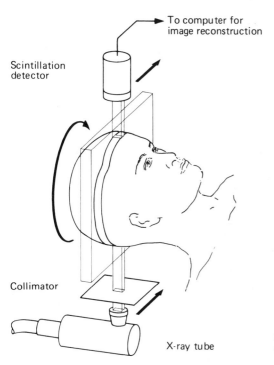

To computer for image reconstruction

Scintillation detector

Collimator

X-ray tube

Figure 8.47 Pencil beam arrangement for multiprojection scanning.

second group of scans. This process is repeated for 180 groups, so the apparatus completes the entire one-half turn in about five minutes. The attenuation values are digitized and stored in a computer memory.

The reconstruction of the image, after completed scanning, can be done in several ways. One main principle involves an iterative process. A matrix of the attenuation coefficients in the layer is built up stepwise. For each projection the matrix is adjusted so that it conforms to the values recorded for that particular scan. This process is continued until all projections have been used several times and no further improvement in the image of the layer is obtained.

Another principle for image reconstruction employs a convolution process, which can be described in the following way. Each projection is fourier transformed, filtered and retransformed into the spatial domain. The projections are then "back projected" on a matrix, and the sum of all is the reconstructed image.

An example of such a reconstructed image, called a data tomogram, obtained by an iterative process is shown in Fig. 8.48. The ventricular system of the brain is seen as dark areas even though no contrast medium has been introduced into the brain. It is possible to visualize directly several pathological processes that are

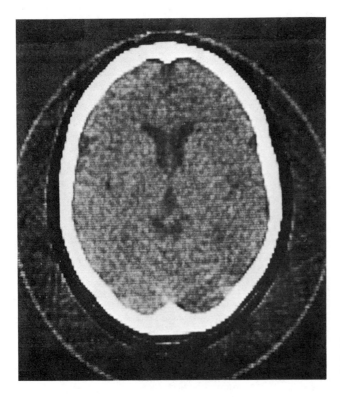

Figure 8.48 Data tomogram of the normal skull. The dark area in the center shows the ventricular system.

difficult or impossible to diagnose with other methods such as angiography. The scanning procedure for recording the necessary data for image reconstruction is performed without discomfort to the patient.

Several alternate techniques are possible to use when scanning the patient. Thus it is possible to have a fan beam geometry instead of a pencil beam. The scanning time is considerably shortened since the attenuation values for one projection can be obtained during the same time as one single value with the pencil beam. The projections can also be recorded with a photographic technique without using a scintillator detector; the image processing is then performed by incoherent optical methods.

Computerized transverse tomography, computer-assisted tomography, and 2-D reconstruction are other names applied to these image reconstruction processes which have dramatically improved the diagnostic capabilities in radiology. They are widely used in studying the brain, for evaluating abdominal organs and for similarly evaluating other parts of the body.

VISUALIZATION OF ORGANS CONTAINING RADIONUCLIDES

An organ can be visualized if it has selectively taken up a compound containing a radionuclide. Such a **labeled** compound may consist of a simple salt, for example $Na^{131}I$, or a complex organic compound, which incorporates the radionuclide. By appropriate choice of the labeled compound, it is possible to obtain an accumulation of the nuclide in the required organ or system of organs.

A large number of radionuclides are used for different organs. ^{131}I has been used not only in ionic form for examining the thyroid gland (cf, page 318) but also in a number of compounds because of the ease with which iodine is incorporated in different organic molecules. The liver can be visualized after injection of $^{99m}Tc_2 S_7$ in colloidal form or with ^{198}Au in colloidal form. For the kidneys, ^{99m}Tc-iron-ascorbic acid complex can be used. Tumors and metastases (daughter tumors) can be localized with many radionuclides such as ^{67}Ga and ^{99m}Tc administered in a form suitable for the particular type of tumor.

A radionuclide for selective organ uptake must have a comparatively short half-life in order to reduce the radiation dose. ^{131}I has a half-life of 8 days. For visualizing the thyroid gland, about $50 \mu Ci$ (≈ 2 MBq) of ^{131}I is injected which results in a dose of about 100 rad (1 Gy). Thus, the dose for organ visualization can be high and the method must be used with discretion.

With the introduction of ^{99m}Tc and other radionuclides, the dose has been considerably reduced. The half-life of ^{99m}Tc is only 6 hours. This radionuclide can easily be obtained immediately before use by elution with saline from a column containing ^{99}Mo, which is the parent isotope of ^{99m}Tc. In a thyroid examination with ^{99m}Tc, a dose of about 1 rad (10 mGy) is obtained; this is only one hundredth of the dose required when ^{131}I is used.

If the organ can be removed and sectioned, a very exact representation can be obtained by **autoradiography**. A photographic film is placed in contact with the sectioned plane of the organ. The film blackening so obtained after a period ranging from one hour to several weeks indicates directly the amount of radionuclide in different parts of the organ. Although it provides extremely high resolution, this technique is of interest only for research. For clinical use, the distribution of the radionuclide in the body must be determined from the intact organism; this can be accomplished by rectilinear scanning and gamma camera techniques.

Rectilinear scanning

An apparatus for recording the distribution of a radioactive substance in the body by scanning is generally known as a rectilinear scanner (Fig. 8.49). The radiation

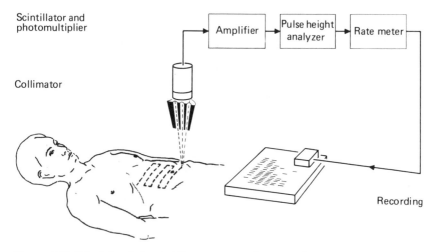

Figure 8.49 Principle of the rectilinear scanner for recording radionuclide distribution in the body.

from the object is restricted by a **collimator** so that the scintillation detector sees only a limited tissue volume (Fig. 8.50). Usually, multihole collimators are used; these gather radiation from a larger solid angle and therefore have a considerably higher sensitivity than single-hole collimators with the same resolution.

An absorbed gamma ray produces a scintillation (light burst) in a sodium iodide crystal. The light is detected by a photomultiplier tube, which produces electric pulses whose amplitude corresponds to the energy of the incoming quanta. Amplification is followed by pulse height discrimination, in which only pulses corresponding to quanta with the energy emitted by the radionuclide are

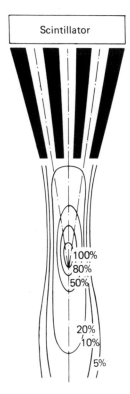

Scintillator

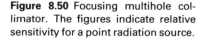

Figure 8.50 Focusing multihole collimator. The figures indicate relative sensitivity for a point radiation source.

passed on to the recording apparatus. Pulses due to scattered radiation, which have lower energy, are eliminated. This results in a more contrasty image, since scattered radiation is largely generated outside the visualized object, in the surrounding tissues.

Rectilinear scanning is often performed with a mechanical arrangement that records a mark on a sheet of paper for, say, every eighth incoming photon. The scanning process thus forms an image that represents the radionuclide distribution (Fig. 8.49). It is also possible to use a photographic procedure, in which a film is blackened with a flash of light for each incoming photon. The image so obtained is richer in half-tones than that produced by a mechanical printer, but the mechanical system has the advantage that the result can be viewed during scanning, which takes considerable time. The object is usually scanned with parallel straight sweep lines.

In rectilinear scanning, the emitted radiation is poorly utilized because the detector sees only one "image element" of the object at a time. The scanning times are long, ranging from tens of minutes to more than an hour. Therefore, movement unsharpness is a problem, and any dynamic study is impossible.

Gamma cameras

The drawbacks of the rectilinear scanning method have been largely eliminated in the gamma camera technique. A common feature of gamma cameras is that the image of the entire object is built up simultaneously.

In the method shown in Fig. 8.51, a number of photomultiplier tubes are used

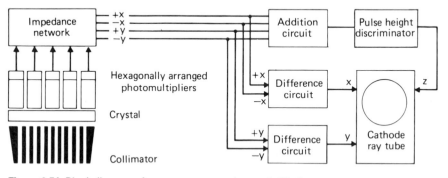

Figure 8.51 Block diagram of gamma camera using a scintillation crystal and nineteen hexagonally arranged photomultipliers. The pulse heights in the photomultipliers increase with the nearness of each scintillation; the X and Y coordinates of each scintillation can then be obtained from the impedance network.

which record scintillations in a large crystal. The radiation from the organ is focused on the crystal through a multihole collimator with a thousand or so holes; a light distribution corresponding to the shape of the organ is obtained in the crystal. Each scintillation in the crystal causes an electric pulse in all the photomultipliers; their amplitudes are, however, a function of the position in the crystal where the scintillation occurs. The closer the scintillation is to a particular photomultiplier, the higher the pulse amplitude in it. The information relating to the position of each scintillation in the crystal is thus coded as the ratio between the amplitudes of the electric pulses arising from the various photomultipliers.

The information is transmitted to a cathode ray tube, the beam deflection corresponding to the position of the scintillation. This is accomplished by summing the outgoing impulses of the photomultipliers in a network and presenting them as X and Y signals, corresponding to the position coordinates for each quantum absorbed in the crystal. Each scintillation produces a bright spot on a storage cathode ray tube screen. During a period of seconds to some minutes, depending on the individual examination, an image of the radionuclide distribution in the organ is thus built up.

With the gamma camera technique, studies can be made of the changes in the radionuclide distribution in an organ over comparatively short periods.

8.138	A substance in which a radionuclide has been incorporated to enable the substance to be traced in the body is called a .... compound.	
8.139	7 to 30 percent of ^{131}I in ionic form is normally taken up by the	labeled
8.140	Radionuclides such as ^{67}Ga and ^{99m}Tc in suitable pharmaceutical form can be used for localization of	thyroid gland
8.141	An apparatus for visualizing the distribution of a radioactive tracer substance in the body by a moving detector is called a	tumors
8.142	In rectilinear scanning, the radiation from the object is restricted with a .... so that the scintillation detector sees only a single ".........."	rectilinear scanner
8.143	In rectilinear scanning, pulse height discrimination is used to increase the	collimator image element
8.144	The scanning time in rectilinear scanners ranges from some tens of .... to a(n) .... or so.	image contrast (eliminate scattered radiation)
8.145	The exposure time for gamma cameras typically ranges from .... to some	minutes hour
		seconds minutes

PHOTOGRAPHY

Photography with visible light is used in a number of diagnostic applications. For the purpose of documenting findings to permit subsequent comparison, photography is obviously of value. Photography is also useful for following the course of healing—in the case of burns, for example.

Documentation of findings is also valuable when observation is difficult—for example, in gastroscopy (page 118). Where photography is not possible, it is necessary to perform an evaluation and make a diagnosis directly at the time of the examination. Color photography provides an opportunity for later and more leisurely assessment of the findings. With a miniature camera, color pictures with a negative diameter of 5 mm can be taken of selected areas of the gastric mucosa.

The camera is mounted in the tip of a gastroscope. It contains no shutter, the exposure being obtained with a flash. Photography with a gastrocamera is a useful complement to x-ray examinations in cases of superficial gastric ulcer in order to locate the site of bleeding in the stomach.

Infrared photography can be used to visualize superficial veins. These show up because the skin preferentially transmits certain wavelengths in the infrared region.

8.146	Photography is used in diagnosis for . . . . of findings of the examination.	
8.147	Photography with a gastrocamera is a complement to x-ray examinations in cases of gastric ulcer, to locate the site of	documentation
8.148	In infrared photography, the superficial . . . . in the skin can be visualized.	bleeding
		veins

VISUALIZATION WITH NONIONIZING RADIATION

Imaging with x-rays has certain limitations. Some organs do not provide sufficient contrast and cannot be filled with a radiopaque medium and therefore produce no shadow. In addition, the tissues are sensitive to radiation damage, especially the fetus, sex glands, eyes and thyroid gland, and therefore the number of x-ray examinations should be limited in which these tissues in particular are exposed to radiation. An x-ray examination always exposes the patient to some radiation.

There is a need for methods that do not rely on ionizing radiation; however, no method has yet been devised that provides more than a fraction of the information yielded by radiography. The **infrared** and **ultrasonic** methods have so far only supplemented the information provided by radiography; they have not replaced this technique.

THERMOGRAPHY

The body heat is dissipated mainly through the skin (cf, page 94), which is therefore usually at a higher temperature than the surroundings. But the skin temperature is not the same over the whole body; it is often lower for the protruding parts, such as the nose and ears, than for the more central parts of the body. The temperature distribution over the body surface normally has a known profile, but there are large individual differences.

In pathological conditions of the skin or the underlying organs, there may be disturbances of the normal temperature distribution, a fact that is exploited in the diagnostic technique known as thermography.

Physical Basis

The heat produced by metabolism leaves the body by radiation (about 45 percent), convection (30 percent), evaporation (20 percent) and conduction (5 percent). The ratio between these four processes varies greatly however, depending on the external temperature, humidity and clothing. The heat given off by an unclothed, normal, resting subject at different environmental temperatures is shown in Fig. 8.52. At room temperature, the main source of heat loss is radiation, and this constitutes the basis for medical thermography.

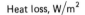

Heat loss, W/m²

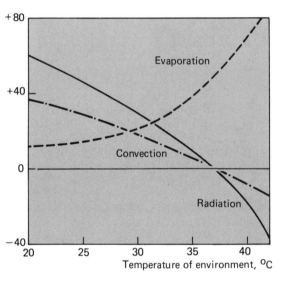

Figure 8.52 Heat loss from an unclothed subject versus temperature of the environment.

According to Wien's displacement law, objects at 37°C (98.6°F) have a radiation as shown in Fig. 8.53, with a maximum intensity at a wavelength of about 9.3 μm. The temperatures of different parts of the body surface normally vary between 25 and 36°C (77 and 97°F). The spectral distribution changes little between these temperature changes.

The radiation from the skin surface, as from all bodies, obeys Stefan-Boltzmann's law: $P = \sigma \varepsilon T^4$, where P is expressed in watts per square meter, $\sigma = 5.7 \cdot 10^{-8} \ \text{Wm}^{-2}\text{K}^{-4}$, ε is the emissivity and T the absolute temperature (K).

Photons/ $(m^2 \cdot s \cdot \mu m)$

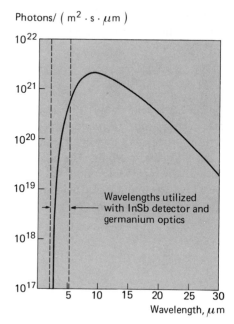

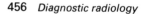

Figure 8.53 Spectral distribution for thermal radiation from the skin.

The emissivity is very close to 1 and in the wavelength range of interest, 2.0–20 μm, the body surface absorbs and radiates energy like an ideal black body; this enables skin temperature to be measured by thermography.

To obtain equilibrium, about 10 minutes before the examination the patient is placed in a draft-free room at about 20°C (68°F) with the relevant areas of the body uncovered. The parts of the body must be separated as far as possible in order to reduce the rise in temperature that occurs due to the mutual irradiation of skin surfaces facing each other. At equilibrium, the skin temperature distribution can be recorded and the skin temperature quantitatively measured by an infrared optical procedure.

8.149	At normal room temperature, 20–25°C (68–77°F), the body gives off heat mainly by	
8.150	The radiation has a wavelength range of interest of	radiation
8.151	The skin absorbs and radiates energy as an ideal . . . . body; the skin temperature can thus be quantitatively measured by	2.0–20 μm

8.152	Before the examination, the patient must be placed in a draft-free room with the relevant parts of the body bare in order to reach	black thermography
8.153	The temperature of the various parts of the body surface normally varies between about	equilibrium
		25 and 36°C (77 and 97°F)

Medical Applications of Thermography

The heat image recorded by thermography depends on the temperature distribution of the skin. The distribution mainly reflects the temperature of the underlying vessels; only a few organs, such as the liver, produce enough heat to appreciably raise the temperature of the covering skin.

Pathological processes that are accompanied by a change in the local circulation in the skin or underlying tissues can therefore be studied by thermography. In addition to primary circulatory disturbances, changes in skin temperature also occur in the case of inflammation, tumors and pregnancy—probably mostly due to increased blood flow or vascularization. A local increase in temperature may be due to a local increase in metabolism.

Circulatory disorders. Any kind of circulatory disturbance, if severe enough, can produce changes in skin temperature. For example, peripheral vascular spasm in the fingers (Raynaud's disease), producing trophic (page 9) disorders and gangrene (page 27), results in a characteristic lowering of the temperature, and this can serve as a valuable diagnostic aid.

It is sometimes useful to perform a quantitative recording of circulatory impairment when arterial emboli (pages 29 and 186) are suspected. This disorder occurs in elderly persons and often requires prompt diagnosis and vascular surgery within a few hours if amputation is to be avoided. Thermography can be performed to identify the patients that should be submitted to further examination by arteriography (page 391); the x-ray examination provides information on the exact position of circulatory obstruction, which is essential for the surgical treatment. By using the completely risk-free and relatively simple thermographic method in differential diagnosis of arterial emboli, fewer examinations would be required with the more complicated and risky arteriography; where arterial embolism is present, however, the thermographic examination would only delay the always necessary arteriography.

The circulation to the head passes through the common carotid artery. This vessel divides into the internal carotid artery, which runs to the brain and eyes, and the external carotid artery, which supplies other parts of the head. Impairment of the circulation in the internal carotid artery can be catastrophic, since of all the body tissues, the brain is most sensitive to oxygen deficiency. Such a circulatory disorder can often be diagnosed by thermographic demonstration of a reduced temperature over the temple on the affected side. The picture is complicated, however, by the development of collateral circulation (page 186) from the branches of the external carotid artery in the face via the nose into the cranium. This results in an elevated temperature in the nose, which is thus indirectly a sign of impaired circulation in a cranial vessel; this can be demonstrated by thermography.

Inflammation.   Since erythema and elevated tissue temperature are two of the four cardinal symptoms of inflammation (page 30), it is logical that this condition should be demonstrable by thermography. In arthritis (inflammation of the joints), the temperature of the skin over the joints is elevated. The thermographic image varies with the form of arthritis. Thermography provides a valuable quantitative method for following the effect of treatment of arthritis, which otherwise is appraised largely by the patient's subjective opinion.

Inflammation within the abdominal cavity is sometimes accompanied by an increase in skin temperature; this is found in, for example, about one half of all cases of appendicitis. Only patients with a thin abdominal wall—less than 1 cm of subcutaneous fat—yield diagnostically useful thermographic pictures; in more obese persons, thermal insulation rules out application of the method. The method cannot be used to diagnose cholecystitis (inflammation of the gallbladder, see Fig. 1.19) probably because of the normally elevated skin temperature in this region, due to the high metabolism in the liver.

Tumors.   Thermography is sometimes used in diagnosis of breast carcinoma. About 85 percent of palpable tumors of the breast that subsequently prove to be malignant are accompanied by a temperature rise of about 1°C (1.8°F), or more, of the skin over the tumor (Figs. 8.54 and 8.55). Although other morbid processes in the breast also produce a rise in temperature, the simple, harmless, comfortable thermographic method is used in some clinics for screening (selection of cases for refined diagnosis). The method is troubled with an excessive number of false positive and false negative diagnoses.

Pregnancy.   In the early stage of pregnancy, there is a rise in the temperature of the skin over the breasts, with a temperature distribution that is characteristic for this condition. Similar thermographic images are obtained when the patient uses pills for birth control.

Of greater practical importance is the fact that in some cases the placenta (page 596) can be located by thermography—the highly vascularized placental tissue produces an increase in skin temperature. The ability to locate the position of the placenta is important, since an abnormal position may complicate delivery. However, there is some debate about the value of thermography for this purpose.

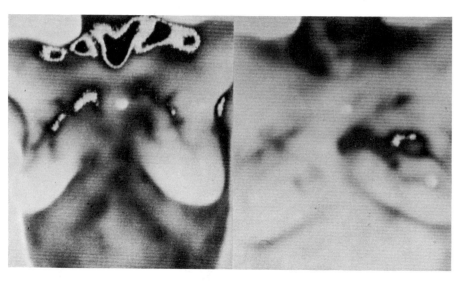

Figure 8.54 Thermogram of normal breasts. The image is reversed, the dark areas corresponding to higher temperatures. In addition, isotherms have been inserted as continuous white areas (AGA).

Figure 8.55 Thermogram of breasts with cancer on left side—the elevated skin temperature over the tumor represented by the dark area (AGA).

8.154	By means of thermography, the temperature distribution of the . . . . can be studied.	
8.155	The skin temperature is mainly due to the temperature of the underlying	skin
8.156	Only a few organs produce enough heat to raise the temperature of the overlying skin appreciably; one such organ is the	vessels
8.157	By means of thermography it is possible to examine pathological processes that cause an altered . . . . in the skin or underlying tissues.	liver
8.158	In addition to primary circulatory disturbances, the following three conditions produce alterations in skin temperature through their effect on the circulation: . . . . , ... and	circulation

8.159	A female patient has reduced circulation in her hands due to vascular spasm (Raynaud's disease); thermography can be used to demonstrate .... (elevated, lowered) skin temperature.	inflammation tumors pregnancy
8.160	When the circulation is impaired in the internal carotid artery, which runs to the brain, a compensatory circulation through collaterals from the external carotid artery can .... (raise, lower) the skin temperature in the nose.	lowered
8.161	In a patient with weakness and pain shifting from the epigastrium to the lower right quadrant, thermographic examination disclosed an elevated temperature in a palm-sized area of skin over the right iliac fossa (see Figs. 2.6 and 2.7). The patient in whom .... has been diagnosed probably has a subcutaneous (page 3) fat layer that is .... thick. (This is in itself an uninteresting result, since the diagnosis can be made with a simple physical examination, and the patient, whether lean or obese, should have an operation.)	raise
8.162	In a 40-year-old woman with a swelling in her breast, the physician finds an increase of 3°C (5.4°F) in the temperature of the corresponding skin area. The swelling is .... (certainly, possibly, certainly not) a malignant tumor.	appendicitis < 1 cm
		possibly

Thermographic Measurement Technique

Direct photography of the skin is impossible with available infrared sensitive films; only by infrared illumination of the skin can photographs be obtained with infrared sensitive film. Even with an infrared sensitive image converter it is necessary to use infrared illumination. With these methods, images of the reflected radiation are produced that, although possibly of some medical interest (page 453), do not contain information on the skin temperature distribution. This can only be obtained by the more complicated thermography.

Thermograms are produced by mechanico-optical scanning of the object, and electronic detection of the intensity distribution of the thermal image.

Radiation detection. Most thermography cameras employ a detector of indium antimonide, or mercury cadmium telluride, which is cooled to the temperature of liquid nitrogen, −196°C (−321°F). Thermistors have been used, but are no longer employed, due to low sensitivity. The sensitivity of the InSb detectors falls off rapidly at wavelengths above 5.4 μm, and HgCdTe falls off above 13 μm, while the body-heat radiation has an intensity maximum at about 9.3 μm (Figs. 8.52 and 8.53).

The mechanico-optical camera systems are complex and reminiscent of the earliest television cameras (Figs. 8.56 and 8.57). The lenses and prisms are made

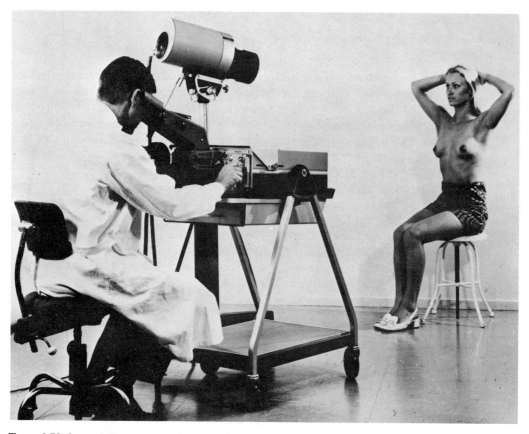

Figure 8.56 Arrangement for thermography of the breasts (AGA).

of germanium or silicon, which both have a good transmission throughout the relevant wavelength range for InSb. For HgCdTe, spherical mirrors are used throughout, to avoid absorption in the lenses.

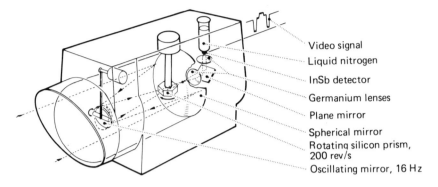

Figure 8.57 Principle of the thermography camera (AGA).

Image presentation. The electronically amplified video signal from the detector intensity modulates the electron beam of a cathode ray tube. Synchronizing pulses from the mechanico-optical scanning unit trigger the vertical and horizontal sweeps. Image frequencies used are between 16 frames per second and 1 frame in 3 minutes; the geometric and thermal resolution both decrease with an increase in the image frequency.

In a thermographic image, different light intensities correspond to different skin temperatures. Reversal of the polarity of the video signal can produce reversed images (Figs. 8.54 and 8.55). A gray scale can be used as the temperature reference. For more exact temperature measurement, isotherms can be inserted by using superimposed intensity modulation, so that they appear as saturated white areas—the skin surfaces of equal temperature appear as loops or connected areas (Fig. 8.54). By means of isotherms, skin temperature differences of 0.1–0.3°C (0.2–0.5°F) can be discriminated.

8.163	With infrared sensitive films and image converters, the skin can be imaged only if it is first .... with infrared light, and the image is then formed from the .... radiation.	
8.164	In thermography, an image is produced from the .... radiation from the actual skin.	illuminated reflected
8.165	The radiation detectors in thermography cameras are often ...., which must be cooled with	emitted

8.166	The lenses and prisms are made of .... or	InSb or HgCdTe detectors liquid nitrogen
8.167	A temperature reference may be placed on the thermograms by means of a .... or by inserting	germanium silicon
8.168	Skin temperature differences of .... can be discriminated.	gray scale isotherms
		0.1–0.3°C (0.2–0.5°F)

ULTRASONICS

Imaging with ultrasonic techniques has proved to be a valuable supplement to radiological examinations for certain purposes. The reason for this is that many different soft-tissue structures, such as muscle, connective tissue, nerve tissue, blood and, to some extent, fat, can be imaged by ultrasonic techniques although their mass attenuation coefficients and densities do not differ sufficiently to produce x-ray contrast. Ultrasonic imaging is safe, even for use during fetal examinations.

Ultrasonic diagnosis differs from radiological diagnosis in that no shadow images are normally obtained; in the majority of the more sophisticated ultrasonic methods, sectional images are obtained through parts of the body, which appear similar to a radar image.

Physical Principles

Sound is reflected when it meets an interface between two media with different acoustic impedances. Since tissues of the body have different impedances—this also applies to some extent to the different soft tissues of the body—many structures can be imaged by visualizing the way in which the sound is reflected from them.

The acoustic impedance is defined as the product of the velocity of sound, c, and the density, ρ. Table 8.1 shows that the acoustic impedance differs greatly for bone, air and the group that makes up the soft tissues. For the soft tissues, the differences are only slight.

Table 8.1. Velocity of sound, density and acoustic impedance
of the body tissues and ultrasonic transducers

Material	Velocity of sound m/s	Density kg/m^3	Acoustic impedance $kg/(m^2 s)$
Air	330	1.2	416
Fat	1,480	970	$1.36 \cdot 10^6$
Nervous tissue	1,520	1,040	$1.56 \cdot 10^6$
Muscle	1,570	1,060	$1.66 \cdot 10^6$
Bone (compact)	3,600	1,700	$6.12 \cdot 10^6$
Quartz	5,750	2.650	$15.2 \cdot 10^6$
Barium titanate	4,460	5,400	$24 \cdot 10^6$

When an incident ultrasonic wave is perpendicular to an interface between two media, which have impedances $c_1 \cdot \rho_1$ and $c_2 \cdot \rho_2$, there is partial reflection of the wave as given by the expression:

$$R = \left[\frac{c_1\rho_1 - c_2\rho_2}{c_1\rho_1 + c_2\rho_2} \right]^2$$

When the media differ greatly in impedance, as is the case for soft tissues and air, the coefficient of reflection, R, is close to 1; that is, practically all the energy is reflected. As a result, structures located behind an organ containing air cannot be observed. Between bone and soft tissues, $R \approx 0.3$; thus, most of the ultrasonic energy passes across the interface and the presence of bone only partially interferes with the observation of structures located behind; it will, however, produce a geometric distortion of the image (page 475). Between muscle and fat, $R \approx 0.01$, so a very sensitive detection system is needed in order to reproduce such a boundary—especially because a reflected wave is further attenuated by additional reflections at other tissue structures lying in the path to the detector, and by attenuation in the tissues.

For ultrasonic imaging, the procedure is essentially the same as that in radar technology. In the simplest design, the **A-scan**, the sound pulse reflection is recorded on an oscilloscope. The echo intensity deflects the Y-axis, while a linear sweep deflects the X-axis, which indicates the time for the echo to return (Fig. 8.58). If the sound velocity in the tissues is known, the distance between their interfaces can be determined from the time displacement of the echo.

In the **linear B-scan**, the ultrasonic transducer is moved laterally over the body surface so that the organ is scanned by repeated sound pulses, travelling along parallel paths (Fig. 8.59).

The successive echoes intensity modulate a cathode ray tube. The electron beam is deflected in the Y direction in proportion to the time delay of the echo,

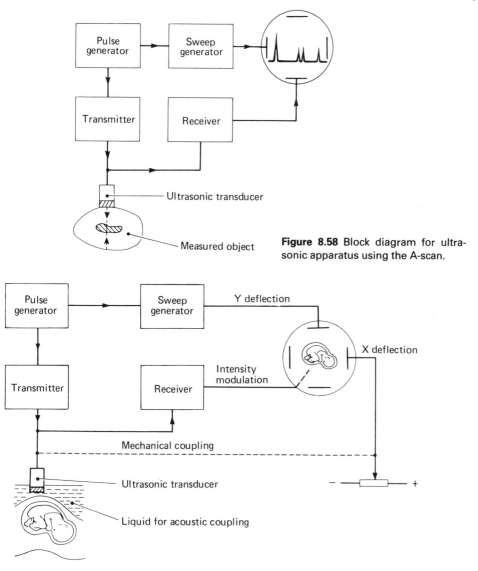

Figure 8.58 Block diagram for ultrasonic apparatus using the A-scan.

Figure 8.59 Block diagram for ultrasonic apparatus using the linear B-scan.

and in the X direction in proportion to the movement of the ultrasonic transducer. The sweeps combine to give an anatomic sectional image—known as an **ultrasonic tomogram**—of the plane in the body that is scanned.

In other designs, the ultrasonic transducer moves on a circle around the part of the body, which is sometimes immersed in water to obtain good acoustic coupling. It is also possible to have the transducer rotate about an axis similar to a radar antenna, in which case the transducer is inserted in a body cavity, such as a major blood vessel. In both cases images are obtained on a plan position indicator, PPI tube.

To obtain a more detailed anatomic structuring of the image, a more complicated scanning procedure is used—known as a **compound B-scan**. The ultrasonic transducer executes a rocking movement superimposed on a lateral displacement in a circular path (Fig 8.60). With this complex motion, it is possible

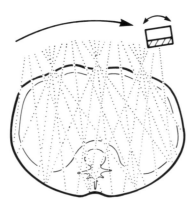

Figure 8.60 In the compound B-scan the organ is scanned with an ultrasonic beam from a transducer which executes a combined rocking and lateral, circular movement.

to minimize the problem that the incident sound beam in a regular B-scan is often not perpendicular to the tissue structures and thus is not reflected back towards the sensor, but is lost in many other directions.

8.169	Ultrasonic techniques can be used to visualize many of the .... (type of body structure) that do not produce contrast in a radiograph.	
8.170	In diagnostic radiology, a shadow image is obtained, and in ultrasonic diagnosis a	soft tissues
8.171	The acoustic reflectivity is determined by differences in the .... between two media.	sectional image
8.172	Acoustic impedance is defined as the product of .... and	acoustic impedance
8.173	When an ultrasonic transducer is directed towards the abdomen of a patient, the strongest echoes are obtained from the .... in the intestines.	density velocity of sound

8.174	On the screen of the simplest ultrasonic apparatus, the Y-axis carries the amplitude of the echoes and the X-axis the time delay of the echoes; this mode of presentation is known as	gas bubbles
8.175	In B-scanning, an anatomical sectional image is obtained by .... of the electron beam by the amplitude of the echoes.	A-scan
8.176	When the organ is scanned with repeated parallel sound pulses, this is called	intensity modulation
8.177	In compound B-scanning, the ultrasonic transmitter executes a .... movement, superimposed on a circular .... displacement.	linear B-scan
8.178	The sectional images thus obtained are known as	rocking lateral
		ultrasonic tomograms

Medical Applications of Ultrasonics

The different tissue structures of the body give echoes of different intensities. Organs rich in connective tissue give strong echoes, as do sharply defined interfaces between soft tissues and body liquids, and between soft tissues and bone. On the other hand, only weak echoes arise within muscles and bone.

With the A-scanning technique, numerous echoes are obtained from most places in the body—they can generally not be interpreted with this form of display. Only in some cases can the simple A-scanning procedure be used: in neurology for examining the midline of the brain, in ophthalmology for measuring the distance between the different parts of the eye, and in cardiology for studying the movements of the heart valves and for demonstrating the fluid effusion in pericarditis. When ultrasonics is used for examining other organs, and also the above mentioned organs for other purposes, more complicated scanning procedures are required.

Neurology. The two hemispheres of the cerebellum are separated by a thin, strong connective tissue membrane, the dura, which serves to support the softer brain tissue. Events may occur in the skull, which cause expansion—for example, bleeding on one side after external trauma, or a tumor in one half of the brain—and then the midline will be displaced. Immediate diagnosis of this condition can be a matter of life and death, since bleeding results in an increase in intracranial pressure. This must be relieved before interference with the circulation causes oxygen deficiency and resulting brain damage. Cerebral angiography (page 391) is a sophisticated operation which entails some risk. It certainly provides detailed information on the brain circulation, but should only be performed when it is obviously required. The ultrasonic method, **echo encephalography** is, however, risk-free and fairly easy to perform and rapidly discloses information on any displacement of the midline. An ultrasonic sensor is placed on the skull, using a thin layer of oil for acoustic coupling, and the echo received is recorded by an A-scan (Fig. 8.61). Normally, the midline lies within

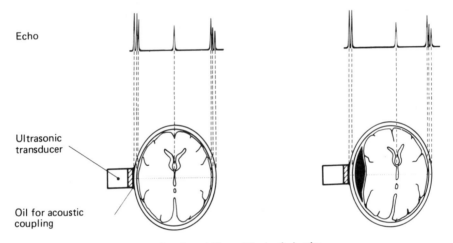

Echo

Ultrasonic transducer

Oil for acoustic coupling

Figure 8.61 Principle for locating the midline of the brain by the A-scan. Note that the midline is displaced to the right in the right picture.

±2 mm of the center of the skull. A displacement of more than 3 mm is pathological and calls for further examination, for example, trepanning (cutting a hole in the skull) to show the existence of a hemorrhage and to drain it.

Ophthalmology. By means of a simple A-scan, the distance between the different elements of the eye can be measured. The cornea, the anterior and posterior surfaces of the lens, and the retina give distinct echoes. The method has not been extensively applied because the measurement of distance is of minor diagnostic significance.

In cataract, when the lens is cloudy, it is sometimes desirable to examine the posterior parts of the eye to find whether the patient would benefit from surgical removal of the lens. Ultrasonic diagnosis using a linear or compound B-scan can then be used to demonstrate, among other things, detachment of the retina. In this case, the retina is displaced into the vitreous humor and produces distinct echoes. The same method can be used to locate foreign bodies in the eye.

Cardiology. The heart can be examined relatively easily by ultrasonic techniques. Practically no other organ in this part of the body produces an echo, since the heart is surrounded by the air-containing lungs. This facilitates interpretation of the echoes. Identification is further helped by the fact that the echoes, which are reflected by the heart wall and valves, move in a known manner. In fact, it is possible to measure directly, for example, the movements of the anterior mitral valve using a time motion, TM-scan in **echocardiography**. The displacement per unit time of the echo during diastole is a measure of the mobility of the mitral valve. In mitral stenosis, the mobility is reduced in relation to the severity of the condition, a fact that is helpful in deciding whether an operation should be carried out.

In certain forms of pericarditis (inflammation of the membrane enclosing the heart), there is an effusion of fluid. By means of ultrasonics, it is possible to demonstrate or exclude the presence of fluid in the pericardium. The possibility of a misinterpretation is present in, for example, the case of fluid in the pleural cavity (in the lung sac) or in pneumonia (inflammation of the lung), when ultrasonic waves are not totally reflected at the boundary between the pericardium and the lung. Linear and compound B-scanning can be applied in cardiology to determine the cross section of the heart chambers, but very high scanning speeds are required to prevent blur due to heart movements. Also, simultaneous recordings in 20 or 30 parallel stationary channels give good cross-sectional images of the heart, thus facilitating dynamic observations of heart function.

Obstetrics and gynecology. By means of ultrasonic diagnosis, the diameter of the fetal skull can be measured to determine the age of the fetus and to assess whether or not the fetus can be delivered through a narrow pelvis. In addition, the position of the fetus and placenta can be determined, which is of importance for delivery. It can also indicate the presence of twins.

In obstetric gynecological applications, the compound B-scan is a useful aid, see Fig. 8.62.

The anatomical structure of a pregnant uterus is ideal for ultrasonic tomography. It does not contain air, and the fetus is surrounded by a fluid giving an optimal acoustic coupling without causing echoes in itself. Ultrasonic images of a pregnant uterus are comparatively easy to interpret.

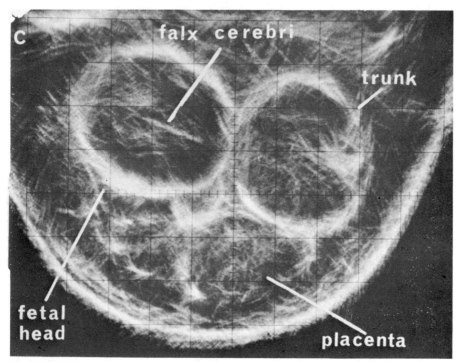

Figure 8.62 Ultrasonic image of pregnant uterus, with the fetal head at top left and the trunk on the right. (By permission of W. J. Garrett and G. Kossoff, Sydney, Australia.)

8.179	Strong ultrasonic echoes occur at the interfaces between . . . . and between	
8.180	The most powerful ultrasonic echoes from the soft tissues are obtained from organ structures that contain much . . . . tissue.	soft tissues and body fluids soft tissues and bone
8.181	The weakest echoes are obtained from tissue within . . . . and . . . . (tissues).	connective
8.182	The method of locating the midline of the brain by means of an A-scan is known as	muscle bone

8.183	A youth is involved in an accident on his motorcycle and is found unconscious, but recovers after a few minutes. The patient is taken to the hospital by ambulance. Paralysis of the left leg develops, he loses the power of speech and immediately becomes unconscious. The history is typical of extradural hematoma; an echo encephalographic examination discloses a 10 mm displacement to the .... (right, left) of the midline—(see page 80 and question 1.342). Trepanning is performed immediately at a number of places on the right side, and a bleeding vessel is located, which is sutured (page 523). The patient makes a full recovery.	echo encephalography
8.184	A man bumps his head on the roof of his car when he is getting out. Two weeks later he has a headache, which increases after a few days, and he goes into a coma. The history is typical of subdural hematoma, and the diagnosis is confirmed by displacement of the midline, which is detected by means of an ultrasonic examination using the ....- scanning procedure.	left
8.185	The method of measuring the movements of the heart valves by the ultrasonic technique is known as	A-
8.186	A patient consults a physician for shortness of breath, coughing, difficulty in climbing stairs, swollen legs and urination at night. Echocardiography discloses diminished mobility of the mitral valve. The history and the findings are typical of mitral	echocardiography
8.187	A pregnant woman in the seventh month of pregnancy has an abnormally large uterus, and twins are suspected, especially since there is a familial history of twins. The presence of two fetuses cannot be determined by palpation (page 122), but they are immediately visualized by ultrasonic tomography in which the ....-scan is applied.	stenosis (see page 131)
		compound B

Technical Aspects of Ultrasonic Diagnosis

When imaging with ultrasonics, there are several technical difficulties which limit the use of the method. Ultrasonic waves are attenuated by the tissues, especially the short wavelengths which give the best resolution. In addition, pictures obtained with the available imaging methods contain too few real and too many unreal image elements.

Resolution

Resolution is defined as the reciprocal of the distance between two points that can just be discriminated. Resolution is different in the axial direction, Z, of the ultrasonic beam and in the scanning direction perpendicular to this, X (Fig. 8.63).

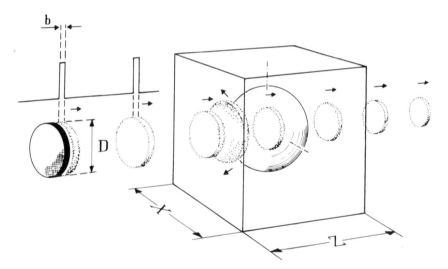

Figure 8.63 When imaging with ultrasound, the resolution is better in the direction of the beam, Z, than perpendicular to it, X. This is because the length of the impulse, *b*, is smaller than its diameter, *D*.

The resolution in the Z direction, A_z, is dependent on the duration of the impulse and thus, indirectly, on the wavelength. The resolution in the X direction, A_x, is largely dependent on the cross-sectional area of the beam.

Resolution in the axial direction of the beam. In order to discriminate two echoes reflected from adjacent boundary surfaces, the distance between them must be more than one half the length of the impulse; otherwise the trailing edge of the first echo will merge with the leading edge of the second. The impulse length *b* is limited by the wavelength λ since one cycle must consist of at least one period $A_z = 2/b < 2/\lambda$. As the impulse length changes with the velocity of sound, the resolution varies according to the type of tissue. For example, the impulse length in bone is 2.5 times that in fat (Table 8.1), and the resolution is thus 2.5 times poorer in bone than in fat. To obtain a high resolution in the Z direction, a short wavelength should thus be chosen.

The attenuation in the tissues increases, however, with frequency; for the required depth of penetration and a given sensitivity of the detector this results in an upper frequency limit—and a lower wavelength limit. The attenuation in a wave of intensity, I_0, decreases exponentially, so that after a distance, z, the intensity, $I_z = I_0 e^{-\alpha z}$, where α is the attenuation coefficient. This increases with frequency and varies according to the type of tissue. It can be represented by the half distance $Z_{1/2} = (\ln 2)/\alpha$, that is, the distance over which the intensity is halved. The half distance at 1 MHz is about 2 mm in bone, about 30 mm in muscle and about 70 mm in fat. In ultrasonic diagnosis, frequencies of 0.5–10 MHz are used, which correspond to a resolution A_z of between about 1 and 10 cycles per millimeter.

Resolution in the scanning direction. Two objects separated in the X direction by less than the diameter of the ultrasonic beam cannot be discriminated. The resolution in the X direction, A_x, is $1/D$, where D is the diameter of the beam. But no unique value of the diameter can be specified because the ultrasonic energy in the cross-sectional area of the beam decreases with the distance from the central ray.

The resolution in the scanning direction also decreases with increasing scanning speed. Thus, for two objects to be discriminated, their distance apart in the X direction must be greater than the distance between two consecutive sound pulses. However, normal impulse frequency is so high that scanning speed is not limited.

With available ultrasonic systems, a resolution in the direction of scanning, A_x, of about 0.3 to 0.03 cycles per millimeter can be obtained in practice.

8.188	In imaging with ultrasonic techniques, the resolution is defined as the .... of the .... between two points that can just be discriminated.	
8.189	The resolution is greater in the .... direction of the ultrasonic beam than in the direction perpendicular to this.	reciprocal distance
8.190	The resolution in the axial direction is dependent on the length of the ultrasonic	axial

8.191	Since an oscillation must consist of at least one cycle, the impulse length, b, is determined by the wavelength, λ, and its relation to the resolution is given by the expression: $A_z = \ldots\ldots\ldots\ldots$	impulse
8.192	The resolution A_z in bone is $\ldots\ldots\ldots\ldots$ (lower, higher) than in fat, since the sound velocity is $\ldots\ldots\ldots\ldots$ (lower, higher) in bone.	$2/b < 2/\lambda$
8.193	The resolution, A_z $\ldots\ldots\ldots\ldots$ (increases, decreases) with the ultrasonic frequency.	lower higher
8.194	The attenuation in the tissues $\ldots\ldots\ldots\ldots$ (increases, decreases) with the ultrasonic frequency.	increases
8.195	The intensity of a wave with an initial intensity I_0 decreases with the distance z and the attenuation coefficient α, as given by the expression: $I_z = \ldots\ldots\ldots\ldots$	increases
8.196	In ultrasonic diagnosis, frequencies of $\ldots\ldots\ldots\ldots$ are used, which correspond to a resolution A_z of the order $\ldots\ldots\ldots\ldots$	$I_0 e^{-\alpha z}$
8.197	The resolution in the scanning direction is largely determined by the $\ldots\ldots\ldots\ldots$ of the ultrasonic beam.	0.5–10 MHz 1–10 cycles/mm
8.198	An attempt is made to visualize two closely located tumors, separated by a lateral distance of 5 mm as seen from the ultrasonic transducer. The ultrasonic beam must have a diameter of $\ldots\ldots\ldots\ldots$	diameter
8.199	The ultrasonic beam in the previous question was, however, 10 mm in diameter, and no satisfactory image was obtained. By changing the position of the ultrasonic transducer and directing the beam to the tumors from a $\ldots\ldots\ldots\ldots$ direction, the better resolution in the $\ldots\ldots\ldots\ldots$ of the beam can be exploited.	<5 mm
		perpendicular axial direction

Image distortion

The ultrasonic image obtained on the oscilloscope does not correspond exactly to the cross-sectional area of the organ under examination. This may be due to distortion of the image geometry, to displacement of the relative positions of the image elements, to failure to reproduce some image elements or to generation of unreal image elements.

Because the sound velocity differs with the type of tissue, the propagation velocity for a sound impulse varies during its passage through the different tissue layers. But since the deflection speed in the cathode ray tube is constant, the image will be distorted. The image of structures with a high sound velocity, such as bone, will be diminished in the ray direction (Z direction) relative to the surrounding tissues. In the image, organ structures behind a tissue with a high sound velocity will be displaced towards the ultrasonic source. If only part of such a structure is shielded, its contour will be distorted (Fig. 8.64).

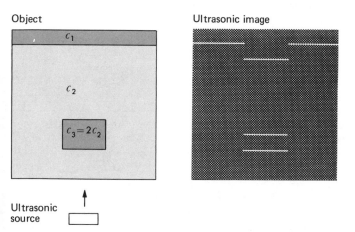

Object   Ultrasonic image

Ultrasonic source

Figure. 8.64 When the object contains structures with different sound velocities, objects located posteriorly will be reproduced with a distortion of contour.

Because the ultrasonic waves are strongly attenuated by the tissues, the intensity from deeper organ structures decreases or the echoes disappear completely. This effect is pronounced when the ray must pass through bone, which has a high attenuation. To compensate for this decrease, it is usual during the sweep cycle to increase the amplification of the ultrasonic apparatus exponentially with the sweep voltage. The amplification then increases with the depth of the structure. At the same time, however, the signal/noise ratio of the video signal decreases, and the deeper structures are therefore visualized with increasing noise.

Another image error can arise if the organ structure is completely shielded by a structure in front of it, whose surface is oriented at such an oblique angle relative to the ultrasonic beam, that total reflection occurs.

Geometrically correct visualization of biological tissues using ultrasound is thus in principle impossible. There are theoretical limits that cannot be overcome. For an organ consisting only of soft tissues, the image errors are small and usually negligible; in the case of bone, the errors may be large. Only through a subjective evaluation based on knowledge of the mechanism underlying image errors, and the anatomic structure of the organs under study, can a correct interpretation of the images be obtained.

8.200	An image error in the ultrasonic tomogram can arise through .... of the image geometry, the .... of certain image elements, or the generation of .... image elements.	
8.201	Geometric distortion arises because different tissues have different ...., while the electron beam on the oscilloscope tube is deflected at constant speed.	distortion absence unreal
8.202	Bone structures having a high sound velocity will be visualized with dimensions that are too .... (small, large) in the direction of the beam, relative to the surrounding soft tissues.	sound velocities
8.203	In the visualization of the brain's ventricle system with compound B-scanning, the ultrasonic beam passes through different cross-sections of the brain-case of varying thickness (because on the inside it follows to some extent the convolutions of the brain). Because the echoes are combined from a particular structure from different directions, these are visualized with certain .... relative to each other, and a .... image results.	small
8.204	The decrease in the intensity of the echoes from deeper organ structures, due to attenuation by the tissues, can be compensated for by using an .... change in amplification, synchronized with the oscilloscope sweep. However, deeper structures will be reproduced with a poorer	displacement blurred

8.205	In compound B-scanning, all the echoes sometimes disappear when shielded by more superficial tissue structures; this is due to the fact that rays are totally reflected by tissue structures that are oriented . . . . to the beam.	exponential signal/noise ratio
8.206	Geometrically correct visualization using ultrasonic tomography is in principle . . . . (possible, impossible).	obliquely
8.207	To be able to evaluate ultrasonic images, it is necessary to have a knowledge of the mechanism underlying the . . . . and of the . . . . structure of the organs.	impossible
		image errors anatomic

REFERENCES

BROOKS, R. A. and DI CHIRO, G. Theory of Image Reconstruction in Computed Tomography. *Radiology* Vol. 117 (1975) pp. 561–572.

GEBAUER, A., LISSNER, J. and SCHOTT, O. *Roentgen Television; Technical Bases and Clinico-roentgenologic Application.* New York (Grune & Stratton) 1967. 154 pages.

GERSHON-COHEN, J. Medical Thermography. *Sci. Amer.* Vol. 216 (1967) No. 2. pp. 94–102.

GORDON, R. et. al. Image Reconstruction from Projections. *Sci. Amer.* Vol. 233 (1975) No. 4. pp. 56–68.

HENDEE, W. R. *Medical Radiation Physics.* Chicago (Year Book) 1970. 599 pages.

JOHNS, H. E. and CUNNINGHAM, H. R. *Physics of Radiology.* Springfield, Illinois (Charles C. Thomas) 1969. 800 pages.

LEDLEY, R. S. et al. Computerized Transaxial X-ray Tomography of the Human Body. *Science,* Vol. 186 (1974). pp. 207–212.

McCULLOUGH, E. C. and BAKER, J. L. An Evaluation of the Quantitative and Radiation Features of a Scanning X-ray Transverse Axial Tomograph: The EMI Scanner. *Radiology.* Vol. 111 (1974). pp. 709–715.

SANDERS, R. C. (ed.) B-scan Ultrasound. *The Radiologic Clinics of North America.* Vol. 13 (1975).

SIEDBAND, M. P. Limitations of Exposure Reduction During Fluoroscopy by Image Storage. *Proc. Soc. Photo-optical Instrumentation Engineers,* Vol. 43 (1973). pp. 151–154.

TER-POGOSSIAN, M. M. *The Physical Aspects of Diagnostic Radiology.* New York (Harper & Row) 1967. 426 pages.

WELLS, P. N. T. *Physical Principles of Ultrasonic Diagnosis.* New York (Academic) 1969. 281 pages.

WELLS, P. N. T. *Ultrasonics in Clinical Diagnosis.* Edinburgh (Churchill Livingstone) 1972. 187 pages.

<table>
<tr><td>**chapter 9**</td><td># Internal Medicine

and General Principles

of Treatment</td></tr>
</table>

The word **medicine** has several meanings. In its broadest sense it includes the practice of preventive care, and the diagnosis and treatment of all diseases; it is in this sense that the word is used in the title of this book. In a more restricted sense, medicine deals with a large number of internal diseases which are treated mainly with drugs. To distinguish between these two meanings, the term **internal medicine** is used; in daily speech, however, this is often shortened to "medicine"; one may say that a patient is treated by a physician in the department of medicine. Finally, another important use of the word "medicine" is as a synonym for drugs, or, as they are also called, **pharmaceutical preparations**.

Medical care is divided into various specialties according to the kind of diseases dealt with and the type of treatment given.

A distinction is drawn between **somatic care**, that is, medical care of the body, and **psychiatric care**. The latter, which is subdivided into areas such as general psychiatry, child psychiatry and forensic psychiatry, are not dealt with here since they do not present particular engineering problems.

In medicine, taken in its broadest sense, two main groups may be distinguished, namely, **internal medicine** and **surgery** (Chapter 10). These may be further divided into a large number of subgroups (Table 9.1). It is, however, not always possible to observe a strict division, for a number of similar types of treatment may be used in different somatic specialties. Examples of such kinds of treatment are **intensive care** (Chapter 11), **radiotherapy** and **physical therapy** (Chapter 13).

Internal medicine is divided into a number of specialties, sometimes on an organizational basis and sometimes on the basis of theoretical knowledge, where similar diseases and ones difficult to diagnose are assigned to special groups. For example, it is inappropriate to treat patients with infectious diseases together with others; there are special hospitals or wards for infectious diseases where cases of **epidemic** diseases are isolated and given treatment. Because of the special problems associated with the care of children, the larger hospitals have special **pediatric** departments. Nervous diseases are particularly difficult to diagnose because of the complex structure and function of the central nervous system; patients with such diseases are often referred to **neurological** departments.

Table 9.1 Some specialties of internal medicine

Branch of medicine	*Dealing with:*
allergy	allergic diseases (allergy, hypersensitivity)
cardiology	heart diseases
dermatology	skin and its diseases
endocrinology	the glands of internal secretion, hormones and diseases of these glands
epidemiology	infectious diseases (also the spread of diseases in general, not only infectious ones, in various populations)
gastroenterology	diseases of the digestive system
geriatrics	care and diseases of the elderly
nephrology	diseases of the kidneys
neurology	diseases of the nervous system (excluding mental diseases)
pediatrics	diseases of children
rheumatology	rheumatic diseases (inflammation of the connective tissue in joints and muscles)
venerology	venereal diseases

The first part of this chapter deals with some general aspects of medical care and principles of treatment; the latter part of the chapter deals with the more specific problems of internal medicine.

Question	*Answer*
9.1 Medical care is divided into . . . . (of the body) and . . . . care.	

9.2	Somatic care is in turn divided into two main groups, namely . . . . and . . . . care.	somatic psychiatric
9.3	Special forms of care are . . . . , ... and	medical surgical
9.4	A sailor contracted syphilis in a port. A physician that he consulted did not consider himself compe-tent to treat the patient and referred him to a clinic for	intensive care radiotherapy physical therapy
9.5	A patient sought treatment at a medical clinic for severe eczema, which was due to hypersensitivity to a number of substances. Since he could not be cured there, he was referred to an . . . . clinic.	venereal diseases
9.6	A man of middle age noticed that his hands and feet had begun to grow and that his facial features had become coarser. At a medical clinic, the physician immediately recognized the patient's disease as **acromegaly**, which is due to an abnormal production of growth hormone in the pituitary. The disease is not very common and is difficult to treat, so the patient was referred to an . . . . clinic.	allergy
9.7	Relatives of a 50-year-old man noticed increasing rigidity in his body movements, and that the hands, especially the thumbs, had a fine tremor. The condi-tion, which is the first sign of **Parkinson's disease**, is due to an organic brain disorder. The patient was referred to a department of . . . . for exami-nation and treatment.	endocrinology
9.8	At the larger hospitals there are special departments of . . . . (for children's diseases).	neurology
		pediatrics

Types of care

For administrative purposes, medical care is divided according to type. This division is motivated mainly by economic reasons. The hospital resources must be used only for patients that are really in need of them; patients with minor complaints should not be admitted to the hospital. An important approach to improved economy in medicine is more efficient use of resources.

An early diagnosis is important to avoid long and expensive care for the individual—**medical checkups** and **screening** (mass examination for the detection of diseases) therefore form an important part of a health system. Because of the large number of patients examined, engineering methods will be used to an ever-increasing extent. The need for laboratory automation (page 312) and data processing in evaluating ECGs (page 214) has been dealt with above. Health checkups will increase in extent both with regard to the number of patients examined and the number and complexity of the methods of examination used. Computer techniques will be used to an increasing extent for storing and analyzing the large amounts of information (Chapter 14).

Medical checkups also have the disadvantage of possibly creating anxiety neurosis—a form of iatrogenic disease (page 486). Complications, even fatal ones, have arisen in the treatment of clinically healthy subjects.

Most patients receive **out-patient care**. The patient visits the hospital only for the time required for diagnosis and treatment. Out-patient care is provided at clinics and at hospital out-patient departments.

Another form of medical care provided by hospitals is **day-care**, in which the patient spends the day at the hospital but the night at home or in a hotel. The costs for the care of the patient at night are thus eliminated and the space can be used more rationally. The staff density in a day-care ward can also be relatively low. Day-care can often be utilized when the patient need not remain in bed.

The type of care used for most hospitalized patients with acute illnesses is known as normal **in-patient care**. Such patients are admitted for the time needed to make a diagnosis and to give treatment.

In the case of potentially fatal conditions, specially trained staff and sophisticated medical equipment are required. In facilities where access to such special resources is available, **intensive care** (Chapter 11) is given. There are various types of intensive care, depending on the training and apparatus required: **coronary care units**, **dialysis units** and **surgical intensive care units**.

When all therapeutic resources have been tried in vain, **chronic care** must be resorted to. A special form of this is **geriatric care**, the care of the elderly.

9.9	A patient suffering from weakness, loss of weight and mild fever consults his physician. At the .... clinic, he makes a preliminary examination and finds that a more detailed investigation is needed.	
9.10	The physician refers the patient to a local hospital, where he is admitted for a few days. Thorough radiographic and chemical examinations are carried out. The patient stays at a nearby hotel. The examination is thus performed using .... -care.	out-patient

9.11	The examination does not dismiss the suspicion that the patient is suffering from a serious disease. An operation is planned to confirm the suspected diagnosis and to try to give effective treatment. The patient is admitted to a surgical ward a few days before the operation. The ward is of the .... care type.	day
9.12	During the operation, the abdomen is opened and major surgery is performed. The patient's condition deteriorates and he is transferred to an .... care ward for a few days.	normal in-patient
9.13	After three days, the patient is transferred in a somewhat better state to a .... care ward.	intensive
9.14	The patient does not recover, because only supportive measures could be taken for the tumor disease from which he was found to be suffering. For social reasons, the patient could not be returned home, so he was moved to another, smaller, hospital for .... care.	normal in-patient
9.15	At this hospital there were also many elderly patients receiving .... care.	chronic
9.16	The outcome of the patient's disease might have been better and the costs for medical care lower if the disease had been diagnosed earlier by means of a	geriatric
		medical checkup or screening

Mortality, morbidity and lethality for different disease groups

The number of different pathological conditions is very great. There are more than a thousand that are by no means uncommon, and to these must be added a large number of rare conditions—estimated at some 35,000. The diseases may be grouped according to the organs and tissues involved: **circulatory organs, respiratory organs, digestive organs, kidneys and urinary tract, nervous system, endocrine, blood** and **connective tissue**. The diseases also may be classified according to a cause, which can attack several organs simultaneously. They fall into the following groups: **infectious diseases, tumor diseases, injuries** and **accidents, diseases of the newborn** and **congenital deformities**. These disease groups differ widely with regard to mortality, lethality and morbidity (page 10). Table 9.2 shows that the diseases of the circulatory organs are the most important group with regard to mortality; from the aspect of morbidity the infectious diseases are the most important.

Lethality is the number of deaths from a given disease relative to the number of persons contracting the disease, while mortality is the number of persons dying from the disease relative to the number of individuals in a population. A rare disease always leading to death has a high lethality but a low mortality.

The mode of treatment varies widely. For some groups, medical treatment is usual—for example, for diseases of the circulatory organs; for injuries and accidents, surgical and other methods are most common. Many diseases can be treated in a number of different ways.

Table 9.2 The mortality (death rate per annum and per million of the population of countries with a high living standard)

Diseases of the circulatory organs	4 300	Renal and urinary tract diseases	300
Tumor diseases	2 000	Endocrine diseases	200
Diseases of the nervous system	1 400	Infectious diseases	100
Injuries and accidents	700	Diseases of newborn, congenital deformities	80
Diseases of the respiratory organs	600	Blood diseases	40
Diseases of the digestive organs	500	Connective tissue diseases	—

9.17	Patients with a ruptured **cerebral aneurysm** (localized dilatation of a brain artery) have little chance of survival, since an operation is technically difficult to perform once a rupture has occurred. The condition is found in relatively young persons and differs entirely from the cerebral hemorrhage in older persons. Ruptured cerebral aneurysm has a high .... (mortality, morbidity, lethality) and a low .... and .... (mortality, morbidity, lethality).	
9.18	The three disease groups having the highest mortality are ...., ... and	lethality mortality morbidity (relatively uncommon disease)
		diseases of the circulatory organs tumor diseases diseases of the nervous system

GENERAL TREATMENT PRINCIPLES

The treatment objective depends on the state of the patient. Where possible, treatment seeks to bring about a full recovery. If this is not feasible, the physician must be content with a reduced objective, for example, alleviation of the patient's symptoms. The correct choice of treatment thus depends to a large extent on a correct diagnosis. The earliest chapters described the various diagnostic procedures—it should be evident that with the array of methods that are available, a high level of diagnostic precision is possible. With a patient that has had a thorough diagnostic examination, the choice of therapeutic methods usually presents no major problem; in other cases the physician is faced with a difficult choice. Based on his knowledge and experience, the physician chooses that form of therapy that he judges is best. He follows the patient's progress and observes whether the intended effect of the treatment is achieved; if not, he reevaluates the therapy and possibly chooses another method.

Forms of Treatment

The forms of treatment may be categorized according to the desired effect.

Preventive treatment or *prophylactic treatment.* The purpose of this is to prevent the patient from becoming ill—for example, an injection of gamma globulin (page 349) is given before a journey to countries where hepatitis A is common.

Causal treatment is a form of treatment in which the actual causes of the illness are attacked—for example, antibiotics against a bacterial infection or surgical removal of foreign bodies that have entered the body in an accident.

As a special form of causal treatment, it is usual to include **substitution therapy**—administration of a substance that is essential for the body, but that the body cannot produce because of a disease; an example is insulin in diabetes. In some cases, substitution therapy is not causal—for example, the administration of hormones in hypofunction of the adrenal glands, Addison's disease (page 272), when this is due to a tubercular infection of the adrenal glands.

Palliative treatment is a supportive treatment that is usually combined with another form; for example, giving the patient a general strengthening medicine in the case of an infectious disease. In malignant tumor diseases, an attempt is made to give a palliative treatment in order to delay the progress of the disease.

Symptomatic treatment is given to alleviate the patient's symptoms, for example, aspirin for headache in the case of a bacterial infection, or morphine to relieve pain due to injury inflicted in an accident.

Psychotherapy is treatment by means of conversation with the patient, during which the presence of unconscious internal conflicts is explained. The object of psychotherapy is resolving the conflicts in order to promote better functioning of the personality. A number of psychosomatic diseases respond to psychotherapy. These diseases are to some extent due to unconscious, emotional reactions that appear as bodily symptoms—the patient somatizes his feelings—for example, anxiety. Headache, gastric ulcer, heart disorders, giddiness, high blood pressure are examples of diseases that are not infrequently of a psychosomatic nature.

Suggestion therapy is a form of treatment that is used to give the patient a feeling of well-being, but the physician is aware that it is not a form of therapy according to any of the above principles.

Suggestion therapy is sometimes given as part of psychotherapy. Conversation therapy, aiming at building up the mental health of the patient, may well be concluded by pointing out the positive aspects of the patient's situation—there will always be some—and this can have a beneficial effect. The value of suggestion therapy should not be exaggerated or underrated. It is sometimes the best treatment in a therapeutic situation where all the physician can do is to rely on the body's own self-healing capacity. The correct application of suggestion therapy calls for a good psychological insight of the physician.

A drug that has no pharmacotherapeutic effect is called a **placebo**, and suggestion treatment performed with such a preparation is known as **placebo therapy**. Such treatment is used for examining the effect of new drugs: one group of patients is given the new medicine and another group only a placebo. Neither the treating physician nor the patients know which subjects received the placebo preparation and which the new drug. The difference in effect between the two groups represents the effectiveness of the new drug. With this procedure, the effects of suggestion can be eliminated from the effect of the pharmacotherapy. Ethical difficulties arise when the effect of new drugs must be evaluated by such **double blind tests**.

Iatrogenic damage

A treatment always creates a risk for the patient, just as is the case in many diagnostic examinations. For each patient the physician must assess what may be gained from a certain treatment and the risk of an undesirable effect. The physician is often obliged to give a treatment that only alleviates the symptoms of the disease and does not provide a complete cure, since the latter treatment might result in more serious injury than the disease from which the patient is suffering. An important doctrinal rule is that no treatment should cause injury to the patient. "Primum non nocere."

Despite every precaution, injury may still occur. Such a condition that arises as a result of therapeutic or diagnostic measures is known as an **iatrogenic** disease. There are a variety of iatrogenic injuries. For example, prescription of a sedative drug can lead to the patient becoming addicted to narcotics, or a patient given blood transfusions may contract hepatitis B, because the donors were asymptomatic carriers of infection. A common iatrogenic injury is cardiac neurosis—that is, symptoms including pains in the heart region, thumping heart and anxiety, with no objectively demonstrable changes in the circulatory organs.

An important reason that many medicines may only be obtained by prescription is to prevent patients, that are unaware of the risks, from causing themselves iatrogenic injuries, due to the effect of harmful medicines.

9.19	Treatment with an antibiotic is	
9.20	Treatment with gamma globulin is	causal
9.21	Palliative treatment	preventive
9.22	Children are regularly given vitamin D during growth to avoid contracting rickets. This treatment is	is supportive or it delays the progress of the disease
9.23	An elderly man has difficulty during urination because of prostatic hypertrophy (enlargement of the prostate gland). He must have his bladder drained daily, and this is done by inserting a catheter in the bladder. This measure is . . . . treatment.	preventive
9.24	The patient has an operation in which the prostate gland is removed. This is . . . . treatment.	palliative
9.25	The operation is performed at two sessions. Before the actual prostate is removed, a minor operation is performed in which the two spermatic ducts are cut. This is done to prevent infection from spreading down to the testes at the subsequent prostate operation. This minor operation is a . . . . measure.	causal
9.26	The patient is troubled with pain after the main operation. The administration of a sedative is a . . . . measure.	preventive
9.27	In homeopathic treatment, sugar pills are given which contain the supposed therapeutic substances in such dilution that they cannot have a pharmacological effect. That some patients still find homeopathic treatment beneficial is due to . . . . therapy.	symptomatic

9.28 A physician and an engineer discuss in the presence of a patient certain problems concerning the apparatus used in the treatment. Medical and technical terms are used that the patient does not understand. The patient is not informed of the gist of the conversation and he misconstrues the situation, believing that two physicians are concerned about his disease. Already apprehensive, he becomes still more disturbed and withdraws into himself. The situation is not clarified before he leaves the hospital. He does not follow the prescribed treatment as an outpatient and eventually dies. The patient has received an . . . . injury of a psychic nature with tragic consequences. It could have been avoided if the nature of the discussion had been explained briefly and if the engineer, who was previously unknown to the patient, had been introduced.	suggestion
	iatrogenic

Pharmacology

Pharmacology is the science of the effect of drugs on the organism and their use in the treatment and diagnosis of diseases. Drugs can be substances that normally occur in the body—for example, hormones. More commonly, they are substances that are foreign to the body.

In **pharmacotherapy**, treatment with drugs, it is necessary to choose a suitable form of administration, a suitable substance or combination of substances to obtain the required effect, and, finally, to observe any toxic effects of the drug—the unwanted side effects.

Administration of drugs

Drugs can be given in different ways. In choosing the method of administration, the physician must consider how soon the desired effect is required and the properties of the drug—how it is absorbed by the body and the damage it may cause at the site of application.

Peroral administration, intake by mouth, is used for drugs intended to act locally in the gastrointestinal tract and for drugs that are effective only after absorption—that is, after they have been taken up by the intestine and have become accessible to the body's cells via the blood stream. Examples of agents with a local action are those that are given to prevent a damage due to excessive production of acid in the stomach and that act by neutralizing the acid there. An example of a drug which acts after absorption is sulfa tablets, which are given for urinary tract infections—the active substance is absorbed by the intestines and excreted from the blood by the kidneys so that a high concentration is obtained in the urinary tract.

Rectal administration (also known as administration per rectum) through the rectum, is likewise used to obtain a local effect—for example, an enema—and to obtain an effect after absorption—for example, sedatives. Many drugs that cannot be taken orally because the patient is unconscious or has nausea—for example, seasickness—can be given rectally. The commonest form of preparation for such rectal administration is the suppository.

Administration via the skin and mucous membranes is used to obtain a local effect at the site of application. There are a number of different forms of preparation. A common one is drops for application in the ears, nose and eyes, and ointments for the skin and eyes. Gases and aerosols (liquids in droplet form) can be inhaled, and these exert an effect in the respiratory tract—for example, certain muscle relaxants that act on the smooth muscle of the bronchi in asthma.

Application via mucous membranes is sometimes used to obtain an effect after absorption—for example, **sublingually**, beneath the tongue. It is used when a relatively rapid effect is desired with a method of administration that the patient can manage himself. For example, nitroglycerine, a vasodilator, is used to treat spasm in the coronary vessels of the heart which manifests as angina pectoris, a substernal chest pain (page 107).

Parenteral administration is a general term for supplying drugs by injection (parenteral, other than via the gastrointestinal tract); the injection can be given in several different ways, usually **subcutaneously**, in the loose subcutaneous tissue, **intravenously**, into a vein (usually in the arm) and **intramuscularly**, in a muscle (almost always in the upper outer quadrant of the large muscle of the buttocks, which is the only place where damage to nerves can reliably be avoided).

Of these methods, intravenous injection has the most rapid therapeutic effect (ten seconds or so) because the drug is immediately conveyed out into the body by the blood stream. The subcutaneous injection is the slowest to take effect (some ten minutes or longer).

It is often desirable to obtain a **slow release** during parenteral administration. In subcutaneous injections, the effect of a drug can be greatly prolonged by mixing the active component with another substance in which this is insoluble. The drug diffuses slowly from the mixture so that a therapeutic effect is achieved over a period of days or several weeks. In diabetes, for example, insulin can be given in this way once a day instead of several times a day. Similarly, a delayed effect is obtained in intramuscular injections, if the active substance is emulsified in an oil. Tablets that are inserted surgically into the tissues can exert an effect over several months as a result of such a slow-release effect.

Parenteral injection causes some risks. At the injection site an infection can be introduced into the body. To avoid local tissue damage at the injection site, certain drugs can only be given intravenously, when they are immediately diluted. Others must under no circumstances be given intravenously, since they can damage the blood—for example, they may cause hemolysis, breakdown of the red blood cells (page 288).

9.29	Many drugs are given by injection into the subcutaneous tissue; this is a form of .... administration (other than via the gastrointestinal tract).	
9.30	Of the modes of parenteral administration, the most rapid therapeutic effect is obtained with .... injection and the slowest with .... injection.	parenteral
9.31	The therapeutic effect of a drug injected subcutaneously or intramuscularly can be prolonged considerably if it is mixed with another substance in which the drug is	intravenous subcutaneous
9.32	A four-year-old child is extremely anxious and is afraid of hospitals. The child must therefore be calmed before any treatment can be given. The child refuses to take medicine .... (by mouth) and it is decided not to frighten the child more with an injection. A suppository is given ...., and within half an hour the child has fallen into a peaceful sleep.	insoluble
		perorally rectally

Drug effects

Our knowledge of the effect of drugs in the body is based entirely on experience. The mechanisms are largely unknown. The biochemical processes are so complicated that we cannot say with confidence how a substance with a given chemical structure will act if it is introduced into the body. New drugs are therefore tested experimentally—first in animals and then in human subjects. Only some general principles of drug action are known.

One theoretically established mode of drug action is **substitution therapy**. Here, a substance is given that is identical with, or resembles closely, one that the normal organism can produce, but that is absent in the patient. Many endocrine disorders due to hypofunction or deficiency of hormones can thus be treated successfully. For example, thyroid hormones are given for hypothyroidism (page 74), insulin for diabetes (page 75) and sex hormones to women after menopause, when the natural production of these substances decreases.

A distinction is made between two opposing pharmacological effects, **stimulation** and **inhibition**. In stimulation, the activity of the cells is increased. For example, certain brain cells are stimulated by caffeine, with a consequent increase in the level of alertness. In the case of inhibition, the cell activity is reduced. An example of this is morphine, which decreases the activity of the respiratory and cough centers in the medulla oblongata.

The mechanisms of inhibition (and also stimulation) can be clarified by the concept of **substrate competition**. The biochemical pathways in the body consist of complicated chain reactions having many stages. Consider two successive reaction stages $A + B \rightarrow AB$ and $AB + C \rightarrow D$. If a substance B' is given that is very similar to but not identical with B, A may react with B', forming AB' instead of AB. If, however, $AB' + C$ cannot produce D, the reaction is arrested by substrate competition, and the reaction is inhibited. As body functions are often controlled by two opposing mechanisms (for example, by the parasympathetic and sympathetic nervous systems in the autonomic nervous system, page 87), inhibition of one reaction—which normally reduces a certain body function—may result in an ultimate increase in the organ function.

Activation of the parasympathetic system normally decreases the heart rate. When this system is inhibited, the heart rate increases.

To understand the effect of drugs it is important to know how they are metabolized in the body, **drug metabolism**. Most drugs undergo chemical conversion in the body and their therapeutic effect disappears. The detoxification occurs to a large extent in the liver. In this way, the body renders the foreign substance harmless, and it is excreted by the kidneys and intestines. Many drugs are excreted in unchanged form, mostly by the kidneys and intestines, but also by the liver via the bile. Volatile substances, such as gaseous anesthetics, are excreted through the lungs.

The effect of a given drug in a particular case is dependent on individual variations in sensitivity due to genetic factors, and on the type of disease (for example, renal and hepatic diseases), which can partly or completely change the metabolism of the drug. An important point is how the presence of one drug present in the body affects the metabolism of another drug—so-called **interaction**. A drug may be given at the same time as another only if it is known that it cannot produce a harmful interaction.

9.33	When a gallstone prevents bile from flowing to the intestines, the absorption of fat is disturbed. Since vitamin K, which is formed by the intestinal bacteria, is soluble in fat, vitamin K deficiency arises. This increases the tendency toward bleeding (page 292 and question 5.51). For this reason vitamin K is always given parenterally before gallbladder operations. This measure is a form of .... therapy.	
9.34	The hormone epinephrine, which is normally liberated from the adrenal glands (page 75), increases the heart rate, raises the blood pressure and increases the circulating blood volume. Epinephrine, and similar substances given as drugs, have a .... effect on the heart.	substitution
9.35	There are other groups of drugs known as **antiadrenergic substances**, that have the opposite effect to epinephrine, reducing the blood pressure. They are used in hypertension (page 66). Such substances have an .... effect.	stimulating
9.36	The antiadrenergic drugs act because they are chemically similar to, but not identical with, certain substances that are involved in the reaction of the sympathetic nervous system, and blocking therefore occurs. The drug acts through a mechanism called	inhibitory
9.37	The body eliminates the effects of foreign substances, including drugs, by two mechanisms, namely, chemical ...., which occurs largely in the liver, and ...., which takes place in the kidneys, liver and intestines.	substrate competition

9.38   A patient with a blood clot is given warfarin, a drug | conversion
that reduces the tendency of the blood to coagulate. | excretion
The proper dose must be determined individually by
following the prothrombin activity (page 292). If the
drug is introduced during a period when the patient
is taking phenobarbital as a tranquillizer, then a
relatively large dose must be given because
phenobarbital is known to reduce the action of
warfarin. If the patient stops taking phenobarbital
and instead takes aspirin, then he may die from
cerebral hemorrhage because aspirin increases the
effect of warfarin. The case provides two examples
of .... which the physician must warn the
patient about.

drug interaction

Toxic effects

Most drugs have side effects. The majority of them are trivial; others are so serious
that permanent damage can occur. The toxic effect—that is the poisonous
effect—is sometimes an extension of the desired therapeutic effect. Examples of
this are cerebral hemorrhage arising during medication with drugs that inhibit
clotting, in the case of a clotting disease. The risk of such damage can be reduced
by careful monitoring of the treatment.

Usually, the serious injuries are due to the fact that the patient is hypersensitive to the drug or that he develops such increased sensitivity during the course of
the treatment.

The toxic effect of a drug can show itself in many ways. **Hypersensitivity** can
result in a variety of symptoms such as fever, skin eruptions, vascular damage
(capillary hemorrhage), bone-marrow damage resulting in blood changes (for
example, agranulocytosis—a condition in which the white blood cells are
destroyed, leading to dangerous infections), liver disorders (different degrees of
severity up to death from hepatic coma) and irreversible renal damage (renal
failure, in some cases necrosis, tissue death, and death from uremia, urine
poisoning). Similar damage to the internal organs can arise without hypersensitivity, solely because the substance is concentrated at these sites and there is an
individual weakness of the organ.

Special care should be taken to avoid **teratogenic effects**—damage to a fetus
due to drugs taken by the mother. The risk of malformation is greatest during the
first weeks of pregnancy, when all the organs are forming in the fetus. Unnecessary medication should be avoided during pregnancy, especially at the beginning.
This is not a simple matter, because many women do not know when fertilization
occurs.

Finally, treatment with drugs entails a risk of **addiction**. This applies particularly to a large number of psychopharmacological drugs, which affect the mind. Hypnotics given over a long period lead to some addiction, but this rarely leads to serious damage. The major risks arise when the dose is increased, and when the drug is combined with others to obtain special intoxication effects. More powerful than the hypnotics are the **narcotics**, most of which are habit forming and readily lead to addiction.

9.39	Acetylsalicylic acid (Aspirin, Anacin, etc.) is used in liberal amounts for a wide variety of symptoms (on the average about 70 g per person per year; the therapeutic dose is 0.5 g). This is probably due to the fact that the agent reduces fever and alleviates pain. The drug is thus used for .... (causal, palliative, preventive, symptomatic) treatment.	
9.40	A child cries and seems to be tired. The mother is concerned and gives aspirin tablets. The child has a skin eruption. The physician suspects that the rash is due to the side effect of a drug and that the child is .... The diagnosis is confirmed by the fact that the rash disappears when the drug is withdrawn and returns when the drug is readministered.	symptomatic
9.41	A patient with a persistent dry cough is given cough medicine containing narcotics. Over a period of time the patient becomes	hypersensitive
9.42	A woman regularly takes headache tablets containing phenacetin. She dies from uremia because of an irreversible toxic effect on the .... (organ).	addicted
9.43	A woman begins using contraceptive pills. She has jaundice because of a side effect on the .... (organ). When she changes to another contraceptive method, she recovers immediately.	kidneys
		liver

EXAMPLES OF TREATMENT FOR INTERNAL MEDICAL DISEASES

When available, a form of treatment is used that directly eliminates the cause of the disease. But for most diseases there is no such therapy, and only palliative or symptomatic measures can be taken. The situation is illustrated by two examples of the treatment of internal diseases.

Infectious diseases

The **preventive treatment** of infectious diseases is often the most suitable measure. Because active immunization (page 349) can be provided for many infectious diseases—whether due to virus or bacteria—the mortality and morbidity have fallen in the last few decades. Passive immunization (page 348) is also of importance—for example, in preventing hepatitis A.

The most effective measure in cases of infectious diseases is treatment with **antibiotics** (penicillin, tetracycline, streptomycin, etc.) and **chemotherapeutic drugs** (sulfa preparations). The introduction of these drugs has completely altered the classical pathological pictures of a number of diseases. The course of the disease is interrupted at an early stage and recovery is achieved before the whole symptomatic picture has developed. Typical bacterial pneumonia (inflammation of the lungs) and syphilis are rarely seen today. The more effective treatments are an important reason for the reduced mortality of many infectious diseases (Table 9.3).

One problem in antibiotic treatment is that the bacteria often develop resistance (page 332). For example, in penicillin treatment, staphylococci can develop that are able to produce penicillinase, an enzyme capable of breaking down penicillin. The antibiotic therapy treatment then has no effect and it becomes necessary to use another antibiotic to which the microorganisms are sensitive. The development of resistant strains of microorganisms takes place more easily at low drug concentrations—treatment with antibiotics and chemotherapeutic drugs must be performed with a sufficiently large dose and for a long enough time, generally at least 5–7 days.

Table 9.3 Mortality for some infectious diseases per year and per million of the population during the period when chemotherapeutic agents and antibiotics were introduced in countries with a high living standard

Disease	1920	1940	1960
Pneumonia and influenza	2,000	700	400
Tuberculosis	1,000	500	60
Whooping cough	100	20	1
Bacterial meningitis	15	5	3

The sensitivity of microorganisms to different drugs varies considerably. Resistance should be determined before treatment is begun so that the most suitable drug can be chosen. For many infectious diseases there is no effective drug therapy.

The most commonly used modes of administration in antibiotic treatment and chemotherapy are by mouth and parenterally.

Local application to the skin and mucous membranes is often avoided because a high enough concentration cannot be achieved over the whole focus of infection—there is then a risk of developing resistant strains.

9.44	A mother is afraid of what she regards as "poison", and avoids all treatment with drugs. She objects to triple vaccination (against whooping cough, tetanus and diphtheria) for her newborn baby. When 6 years old, the child contracts whooping cough and becomes critically ill, but survives. The child develops bronchiectasis (dilatation of the bronchi), however, which results in invalidizing symptoms throughout his life in the form of constant bronchitis. Because of her attitude, the mother objected to .... (causal, palliative, preventive, symptomatic) treatment, which would have been effective.	
9.45	The treatment of syphilis formerly consisted of giving preparations containing arsenic, iodine, bismuth or mercury compounds, which were specifically effective against spirochetes (page 324). The treatment took several years. Today a single dose of penicillin given in slow-release form cures the disease. Both treatment methods constitute .... (causal, palliative, preventive, symptomatic) treatment.	preventive
9.46	A child has a "cold"—that is, a viral infection of the upper respiratory tract. (The viral infection may be later accompanied by a secondary bacterial infection, the purulent stage.) The father had previously discontinued taking penicillin for a different illness and gave his leftover pills to the child. The child does not recover and the treatment is discontinued on the second day when there are no more pills left. After a week the child's condition worsens. The physician, knowing nothing about the earlier treatment, gives penicillin for 7 days. The child's condition becomes still worse, however, and he is admitted to hospital where he subsequently dies from purulent meningitis. As a result of the first inadequate treatment, bacteria developed that were .... to penicillin.	causal
		resistant

Circulatory diseases

The reason that diseases of the circulatory organs result in such a high mortality and morbidity is that effective causal treatment is either not available or cannot be carried out for administrative or financial reasons.

Two diseases, valvular heart failure and arteriosclerosis, will be discussed to illustrate the situation.

Valvular heart disease is due to valvular defects which arise in different ways (page 130), and can result from rheumatic fever. This is usually due to an infection of the throat by hemolytic streptococci (page 324) 1–4 weeks earlier. (Infections due to such bacteria should therefore be treated with antibiotics; once rheumatic fever has appeared antibiotic therapy is ineffective except to prevent further valvular damage. Unfortunately, many cases of infections with hemolytic strep-tococci are not diagnosed.) Rheumatic heart failure is becoming increasingly rare. Syphilis in late stages can cause valvular defect, and early antibiotic therapy is therefore important.

The treatment of valvular defect is determined by the extent of the impairment of the pumping action. In mild heart failure, the symptoms are limited to poor work capacity and no actual treatment is necessary. It is enough to advise the patient to avoid extreme physical effort. Measures are required only if **congestive heart failure** develops—that is, if troublesome symptoms appear because the heart is unable to maintain an adequate circulation. Most symptoms are due to stasis, with stagnation of blood in the lungs (left ventricular failure) or large veins (right ventricular failure). Since in pulmonary stasis, the blood is inadequately oxygenated, the patient suffers from respiratory distress. The patient becomes cyanotic (page 28) and edema develops (page 28). In severe pulmonary stasis, coughing develops. In more advanced cases of left ventricular failure, **pulmonary edema** develops, and blood plasma enters the lung alveoli and interferes with gaseous exchange. Pulmonary edema is a dangerous condition.

The most important drug in the treatment of congestive heart failure is **digitalis**. This herbal drug, which has been in use since the eighteenth century, has a specific effect on the heart. The heart's power of contraction increases and the heart rate is lowered. In mitral valve stenosis, for example, the reduced heart rate makes increased filling of the ventricles possible, and this, together with the improved power of contraction, increases the cardiac output (page 160). Finally, the conduction time (page 195) is prolonged, and this lowers the number of heart contractions in certain arrhythmias (page 196)—these often occur in organic heart failure.

A patient with severe congestive heart failure is best cared for in the **sitting position**, with the foot-end lowered. The edema then collects in the legs thus reducing the pulmonary edema, and this helps respiration. In severe respiratory distress, pure **oxygen** is breathed through a mask so that the oxygenation of the blood in the lungs is improved. The patient's anxiety is diminished with **sedatives**.

In pulmonary edema, which is a very severe form of congestive heart failure and which constitutes an immediate threat to life, methods are applied to produce a rapid drop in the blood volume. This can be done with rapid-acting diuretic drugs or by venesection, in which a vein is punctured with a syringe with a large caliber needle and 300–500 ml of blood is allowed to flow out. Pulmonary edema can also preferably be treated with a ventilator (page 545) when there is one available.

Arteriosclerosis is a disease where the arterial walls become thickened and lose elasticity. Usually, the disease develops slowly over a period of 20–30 years. It begins with deposits of fat-like substances in the vessel walls. The deposits slowly increase and are finally calcified, and the narrower vessel lumen restricts circulation—**occlusive disease**. It is especially serious when the changes affect the coronary arteries that supply the actual heart muscle with blood. The disease is then called **coronary arteriosclerosis**. If a piece of calcified tissue is detached from the vessel wall or if a blood clot forms on the calcified inner side of the vessel, the blood circulation suddenly decreases (coronary occlusion) and part of the heart muscle dies—a **myocardial infarction** occurs.

Arteriosclerosis is probably due to several concurrent causes. From statistical studies on large groups of patients with myocardial infarction, it has been found that the cause is probably a combination of **heredity**, **overweight**, **diet** (too much fat in the food), **stress**, **smoking** and **insufficient physical activity**. Just one of these factors is probably not enough to cause arteriosclerosis to develop. All of these factors can be controlled, except for heredity. Therefore, most physicians recommend prevention to high-risk patients, by eliminating the causal factors.

There is still no causal treatment by which arteriosclerosis can be cured. This is also true in the early stages before the fat is calcified. One difficulty is detecting the presence of the disease; another difficulty is observing the effects of treatment in the individual case. Therefore, treatment is begun after the appearance of symptoms, such as angina pectoris—that is, pain in the heart region (page 107 and Fig. 2.2). The diagnosis of **coronary insufficiency** can be confirmed with the ECG (ST depression, page 199). Such attacks can be arrested with vasodilators, for example, nitroglycerine, if the vascular changes are not too severe.

Myocardial infarction should be treated with a special form of intensive care (page 560), because of the risk of cardiac arrest during the days immediately following the onset of the symptoms.

9.47   Antibiotic treatment for a patient with hemolytic streptococci is a .... (causal, palliative, preventive, symptomatic, suggestion) treatment of throat infections and a .... treatment for rheumatic fever which can result in, among other things, heart damage.

9.48	Digitalis treatment for congestive heart failure with valvular defect is a .... treatment.	causal preventive
9.49	To place a patient with congestive heart failure in the sitting position is a .... measure.	palliative
9.50	To give an anxious patient with congestive heart failure a sedative is a .... measure.	palliative
9.51	A patient with angina pectoris with ST depression is given a vasodilating agent. The treatment is	symptomatic
		palliative

REFERENCES

ALLYN, R. A Library for Internists II. *Ann. Intern. Med.* Vol. 84 (1976) pp. 346–373.

CHATTON, M. J. *Handbook of Medical Treatment.* Los Altos (Lange) 1974. 640 pages.

CLUFF, L. and JOHNSON, J. (eds.). *Clinical Concepts of Infectious Diseases.* Baltimore (Williams & Wilkins) 1972. 431 pages.

GOODMAN, L. S. and GILMAN, A. *The Pharmacological Basis of Therapeutics.* New York (Macmillan) 1968. 1,785 pages.

MEYERS, F. H. et al: *Review of Medical Pharmacology.* Los Altos (Lange) 1974. 721 pages.

SPIVAK, J. L. and BARNES, H. V. *Manual of Clinical Problems in Internal Medicine.* Boston (Little, Brown) 1974. 496 pages.

chapter 10 | Surgery

Surgical methods of treatment consist mainly of **operations**. These methods also include **reductions**—that is, the restoration of organs to the correct position in case of fractures and sprains. In addition, purely pharmacological treatment principles are used to a varying extent, for example, antibiotics to control infection. Surgical methods are used in **general surgery**, and also in some independent disciplines, examples of which are given in Table 10.1.

Table 10.1

Branch of surgery	*Dealing with:*
anesthesiology	anesthetic methods
gynecology	diseases of the genital tract of women
neurosurgery	surgical diseases of the nervous system
obstetrics	the art of managing pregnancy and childbirth
ophthalmology	diseases of the eye
orthopedics	disorders involving locomotor structures, especially bones and joints
otolaryngology	diseases of the ear, nose and throat
plastic surgery	reconstructive surgery
thoracic surgery	surgical diseases of the chest organs
urology	diseases of the urinary organs

Question		Answer
10.1	A patient who is a smoker has been increasingly troubled during the last year with sudden attacks of coughing. He consulted a physician on several occasions without the cause being found. Lung cancer is suspected so the patient is admitted for a specialized examination in the department of .... surgery.	
10.2	A patient with increasingly severe headache, vomiting and epileptic fits over the previous month is found to have a brain tumor. He is referred to the department of .... -surgery.	thoracic
10.3	A woman in the third month of pregnancy has hemorrhages. She is admitted to the department of .... because of threatened miscarriage.	neuro
10.4	A 12-year-old boy has made a bomb, which accidentally explodes. Metal splinters enter one of his eyes. Treatment is performed in the department of	gynecology
10.5	A woman gives birth to a child in the department of	ophthalmology
10.6	A patient with **sinusitis**, inflammation in the sinuses, is referred for treatment to the department of	obstetrics
10.7	A patient with repeated attacks of renal colic must undergo an operation. It is performed in the department of	otolaryngology
		urology

PRINCIPLES OF SURGICAL TREATMENT

An operation is the central feature of surgical treatment. The practical technique of operations is determined to a large extent by three factors: the risk of **infection**, the occurrence of **pain** and the body's **bleeding tendency**. Because of the risk of infection **antiseptic** routines must be followed—that is, the operation is performed in the absence of infection-producing microorganisms. Some form of **anesthesia**, general or local, is used to alleviate pain, and to give the surgeon better working conditions. The bleeding tendency to some extent determines the **surgical technique** to be used in the operation.

ANTISEPSIS

An operation is performed under antiseptic conditions. These are obtained by using sterile (page 336) instruments, material and protective clothing, by disinfecting (page 338) all the parts of the patient's skin and mucous membranes where the operation is to be performed, and by consistently applying strict **working routines**. For this to be possible, all but minor operations must be carried out in specially equipped **operating suites**.

The antiseptic technique thus aims at preventing infection of the operative area by pathogenic microorganisms from both the environment and from the patient's skin and mucous membranes and from the body cavities, where such microorganisms are normally found.

The operating suite

From a functional aspect, the operating suite can be divided into **three zones**, with increasingly strict hygienic requirements in order to achieve antiseptic conditions. The outermost zone consists of rooms and corridors outside the actual operating room. To this outermost zone, nobody has access except those having a need to be there. Before anyone enters the outermost zone, shoes should be changed or special footwear added to prevent microorganisms from being introduced from the other hospital departments; a pair of shoes may be reserved for use in the operating department. It is also usual to change into clean protective clothing.

The middle zone consists of the parts of the operating room that are not included in the area where strict sterility is required. This zone is called the **unsterile area**. Working in this zone are the anesthetists, assisting nurses, orderlies, and any technicians. All of them wear a clean protective gown with a cap to prevent contamination with hair and particles from the skin, and a mask over the nose and mouth to prevent droplet infection during speech and breathing.

The innermost zone, the **sterile area**, consists of that part of the actual operating room where strict sterility is required. The surgeon, surgeon's assistants and surgical nurses work in this area. All wear sterile surgical gowns and gloves. All instruments and linen in this zone are sterile. All objects that happen to become unsterile are immediately placed in a bin located in the unsterile area. To make it easier to distinguish between unsterile and sterile cloths, these are often of different colors: sterile ones are usually green, a color chosen to avoid glare in the strong illumination on the operating table. No efforts are spared to maintain antiseptic conditions in this zone.

Modern operating rooms have a special ventilating system, which supplies sterile, filtered air under a slight, positive pressure relative to that of the rest of the hospital. This prevents microorganisms from being carried in by air currents. Floors and walls are of materials that are easy to keep clean.

Some operating rooms are planned according to the two-corridor system. One corridor and the door between this and the operating room are used for the patient and staff working in the unsterile area. Another corridor and door, located on the opposite side, are reserved for staff in sterile clothing.

Working routines

An operation requires preparation and coordination, so that all technical resources and all information that may be required are at hand. An operation is therefore a matter of teamwork, to a greater degree than any other medical activity. The surgeon is dependent on one or more surgical assistants for manual assistance in the actual operating area, and a surgical nurse is responsible for keeping sterile instruments, drapes, sponges and drugs at hand. Another nurse works in the unsterile area and assists the surgical nurse. Hospital orderlies are responsible for cleaning, etc. In the case of major operations, the general anesthesia is managed by a physician who may be assisted by an anesthetic nurse. Sometimes a radiologist is required for examinations during the actual operation. In some major operations, engineers are needed for operating monitoring apparatus, heart-lung machines and other sophisticated technical equipment. All the staff follow a working routine that enables antisepsis to be maintained in the operation area.

The patient is brought into the surgical suite after being bathed and in clean clothes. The day before, the patient has been shaved at the places on the body where the operation is to be performed. The patient is moved to the operating table in an induction area so that the bed need not be brought into the operating room. The anesthesia is begun in this induction area, which is thus located in the outermost zone of the operation suite.

At the same time, the surgical nurses, with the assistance of another nurse or hospital orderly, put on sterile gowns, and place the necessary instruments, surgical drapes, drugs, etc. on tables. A so-called Mayo stand is draped. The second nurse mounts the radiographs, connects the suction unit and prepares other technical equipment in the unsterile area.

When the patient has been anesthetized, the operating table is rolled into the operating room. The surgical nurse or assistant prepares the operative field and adjacent parts of the patient's skin with an antiseptic solution. She then creates a sterile field by covering the patient's body with sterile surgical drapes so that only the area where the incision is to be made is exposed. The Mayo stand is placed so that its surface is above the patient; it is used for some basic surgical instruments to be accessible close to the operating field. Prior to this, the surgeon, in cap and mask, has cleaned fingernails and washed hands and forearms for 10 minutes so that they are antiseptic—a precaution against the rupture of a surgical glove during the operation. The surgeon enters the operating room where the surgical nurse assists in putting on sterile gown and gloves. The operation can now begin.

Throughout the operation, a strict distinction is made between what is sterile and what is unsterile. If an unsterile body cavity is opened, such as the intestine, special sterile sponges are placed around it so that they can be removed or changed in case any unsterile intestinal contents find their way to the operative area. All instruments and sponges used during the unsterile stage of such operations are immediately placed in receptacles and then are not used again during the operation.

After the operation has been completed, the operating room is cleaned; among other things, the floor is washed. Only then can a new operation be performed. To prevent spread of infection it is also important to plan the operation schedule so that all operations on patients without infection are performed before those on any that may be infected.

10.8	An object that is free from all microorganisms is	
10.9	An object that is treated so that the number of pathogenic bacteria is reduced is	sterile
10.10	The technique that aims to prevent infection of the operative area by pathogenic bacteria is called	disinfected
10.11	An operating suite has three zones. When a person enters the outermost from elsewhere in the hospital, he should change his .... and put on a	antisepsis
10.12	When passing into the middle zone he should wear a .... and	shoes protective gown
10.13	This second zone is called the	cap mask
10.14	In the third zone, called the ...., all persons wear .... and	unsterile area
10.15	A patient is to have a hernia operation. The day before, the patient is .... and the skin round the groin is	sterile area surgical gowns gloves

10.16	When the patient is brought to the surgical suite, he is moved from the bed to the operating table in an .... area, where the anesthesia is also begun.	bathed shaved
10.17	When the patient, who is lying on the operating table, is brought into the operating room, the surgical nurse cleans the skin of the abdomen, groin, thigh, penis and scrotum with a .... detergent.	induction
10.18	The surgical nurse then covers all parts of the patient except the groin with .... drapes.	disinfecting
		sterile

ANESTHESIA

Anesthesia serves two purposes. First it must ensure that the patient does not feel pain; this is of importance not only to prevent patient discomfort but also to have the patient in a physically better state; pain itself can cause a state of shock (page 557), which can endanger life. Second, the anesthesia must provide the surgeon with favorable conditions for the work, by removing the need to hasten the operation to avoid pain, and by providing a muscle relaxation, which is necessary in abdominal operations and reduction of fractures (broken bones).

Anesthesia can be given in two ways: as **regional anesthesia** or as **general anesthesia**. In the case of regional anesthesia, part of the body ennervated by specific nerves is rendered insensitive; in general anesthesia, there is a gradual blunting of protective reflexes and the patient usually loses consciousness.

Regional Anesthesia

Regional or **local** anesthesia can be produced by two procedures: **topical** anesthesia and **conduction** anesthesia; the latter type can be divided into **infiltration**, **field block**, and **nerve block** anesthesia.

Topical anesthesia

By spraying, brushing, instilling or dropping an anesthetic on mucous membranes these can be rendered insensitive. The anesthetic diffuses inwards and acts on the end-organs of the nerves so that these cannot emit nerve impulses. No deep tissue effects are obtained; hence the terms **permeation anesthesia** and **surface anesthesia** are also used (Fig. 10.1). Such anesthesia is used in minor operations in the nose, throat, eyes, urethra and urinary bladder and also in diagnostic examinations—for example, in endoscopy (page 116).

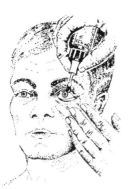

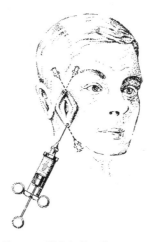

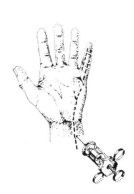

Figure 10.1 Topical anesthesia prior to operation on the eye.

Figure 10.2 Infiltration anesthesia prior to suturing a wound in the face.

Figure 10.3 Nerve block anesthesia of ulnar nerve before suturing a wound on the little finger side of the hand.

Infiltration and field block anesthesia

In both methods, the tissues are diffusely flooded by the anesthetic so that nerve endings and fine nerve fibers are anesthetized. In **infiltration anesthesia**, the injection is made in the tissues at the site of the wound or damage, for example, a fracture (not to be recommended because of infection risk). In **field block anesthesia**, the injection is made into the tissues surrounding the area to be made insensitive without infiltrating the area itself. The methods are commonly used in treatment of wounds and for skin incisions, for example, when removing superficial skin tumors. The methods are also used as an adjunct in general anesthesia when a more superficial anesthesia is sufficient (Fig. 10.2).

Nerve block anesthesia

The impulses in a nerve leading from an operative site can be blocked if somewhere around this nerve an anesthetic fluid is injected—this is called **nerve block anesthesia** (Fig. 10.3). It is important to deposit the anesthetic as close to the nerve as possible. Exact knowledge of the anatomy of the nerve tracts in the body is required. Nerve block anesthesia can be used for anesthesia of all the peripheral nerves in the body. For example, in operations on the hand or forearm, different areas can be anesthetized by inducing nerve block anesthesia of the radial nerve, the median nerve or the ulnar nerve (Fig. 1.35).

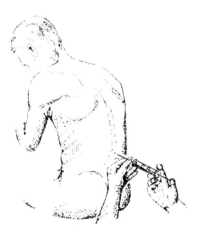

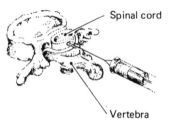

Spinal cord

Vertebra

Figure 10.4 In spinal anesthesia, the anesthetic is injected into the fluid bathing the spinal cord.

A special form of nerve block anesthesia is **spinal anesthesia** (Fig. 10.4). By means of a lumbar puncture between two vertebrae, the anesthetic is injected in order to obtain conduction anesthesia of the nerves leaving the spinal cord. Spinal anesthesia produces excellent relaxation of the muscles, which greatly facilitates the surgeon's work in operations on the lower part of the abdominal cavity. The method is used also in urological and gynecological operations and for operations on the legs.

10.19	Loss of feeling or sensation is called	
10.20	Topical, infiltration, field block and nerve block anesthesia are different forms of	anesthesia
10.21	When anesthesia is given, so that the patient loses consciousness, this is called	regional anesthesia
10.22	A male patient is suspected of having a tumor of the urinary bladder. Cystoscopy (page 118) must be performed—a painful method of examination unless an anesthetic is given. A viscous anesthetic is injected into the aperture of the penis so that it ascends in the urethra. By light compression, the agent is prevented from flowing out. Five minutes later, the cystoscope can be inserted without discomfort thanks to the .... (type of local anesthesia) given.	general anesthesia

10.23	A man has cut himself in the lower leg. The wound is cleaned and before it is sewn up, an anesthetic is given by injecting the anesthetic solution subcutaneously around the wound opening. Loss of feeling is obtained with	topical anesthesia
10.24	A patient is to be operated on for hemorrhoids. Anesthesia is induced by injecting the anesthetic agent in the sacral canal where the nerves to the pelvis floor run. This sacral anesthesia is a form of	infiltration anesthesia
10.25	A muscular, obese man is to have an operation for an abdominal complaint. Since it is known from experience that patients with this constitution are difficult to manage under general anesthesia, loss of feeling is obtained by injecting an anesthetic agent between the third and fourth lumbar vertebrae, around the nerves that leave the spinal cord. The method is known as	regional anesthesia (nerve block anesthesia, conduction anesthesia)
		spinal anesthesia

General Anesthesia

To induce unconsciousness by general anesthesia, the agent is administered to the body so that it reaches the brain via the blood stream. This can be performed in different ways.

In **inhalation anesthesia**, gaseous anesthetic agents are introduced via the lungs. Examples of such agents are diethyl ether, chloroform, cyclopropane, halothane ($CF_3CHClBr$), methoxyflurane and nitrous oxide (N_2O, laughing gas).

In **intravenous anesthesia**, the agent is injected into the blood. The most commonly used agents are barbiturates, which act as adjuncts to other anesthetics and have a very short duration effect; they are of the same group as the common hypnotics, nembutal or seconal. Intravenous anesthesia rapidly induces deep unconsciousness, and thus there is a risk involved. It is therefore often combined with some form of inhalation anesthesia to reduce the required amount of intravenously injected anesthetic.

A third way of inducing general anesthesia is to place a general anesthetic in the rectum; it is then absorbed by the mucous membrane of the intestine—**rectal anesthesia**.

Before the operation begins certain measures are taken to prepare the patient for general anesthesia. The stomach, urinary bladder and rectum must be emptied before the operation. The patient must not eat or drink for twelve hours preceding the operation. The patient is also given premedication. The purposes of this are to reduce the patient's awareness of his situation and to raise the threshold for evoking a number of reflexes (page 138). For example, the secretion of saliva and gastric juice should be reduced in order to prevent these from being breathed in during anesthesia—this breathing in is known as **aspiration**; associated with this aspiration is increased risk of postoperative complications, in particular, pneumonia. One common form of **premedication** is to administer a combination of morphine and scopolamine. Premedication is performed in the ward about an hour before the patient is taken into the operating suite.

The patient under general anesthesia must be carefully watched. It is important to keep the patient at the right **depth of anesthesia** by adjusting the administration of anesthetic. The **respiratory tract** must be free so that there is adequate oxygenation of the blood in the lungs while carbon dioxide is ventilated.

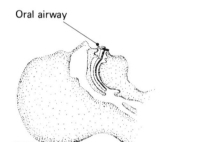

Oral airway

Figure 10.5 An oral airway inserted to produce a free airway.

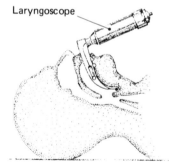

Laryngoscope

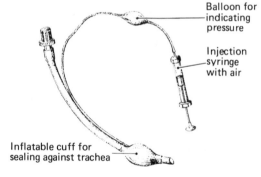

Balloon for indicating pressure

Injection syringe with air

Inflatable cuff for sealing against trachea

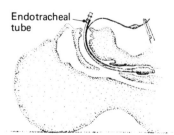

Endotracheal tube

Figure 10.6 In general anesthesia, tracheal intubation is often performed. When the endotracheal tube is inserted, a laryngoscope is used.

A satisfactory **blood circulation** must be maintained; the heart action is monitored by measuring the blood pressure and pulse. It is often possible to follow the electrocardiogram on a cardioscope, which is a simple form of cathode ray oscillograph with a long-persistence fluorescent screen or with a built-in electronic memory.

The respiratory tract can be kept free by inserting an **oral airway** (Fig. 10.5). If controlled (artificial) ventilation is to be given, **intubation** of the patient is almost invariably necessary; that is, a plastic or rubber tube—a so-called **endotracheal tube**—must be inserted in the trachea (Fig. 10.6). This is done by means of a laryngoscope.

10.26	The form of anesthesia in which gaseous anesthetic is administered via the lungs is known as	
10.27	When water-soluble anesthetics are injected directly into the blood, the form of anesthesia is called	inhalation anesthesia
10.28	An hour before being transferred to the operating suite, a patient receives an intramuscular injection of morphine-scopolamine. That is, the patient is given	intravenous anesthesia
10.29	Premedication serves a number of purposes including reduction of the patient's	premedication
10.30	Another use of premedication is to increase the .... so as to reduce the secretion of saliva and gastric juice during anesthesia.	awareness of his situation
10.31	To prevent the stomach contents from being breathed in by the unconscious patient—known as .... —three measures are taken, namely, preparation of the patient so that the stomach is ...., ... of the patient and, during anesthesia, insertion of an endotracheal tube in the windpipe—known as	threshold of reflexes
10.32	In the operation on the patient the anesthetist and the anesthetist nurse keep a constant watch on three fundamental conditions, namely, ..., ... and	aspiration empty premedication intubation
		depth of anesthesia respiration blood circulation

Stages of anesthesia

When increasing amounts of an anesthetic are administered, the depth of anesthesia steadily increases. This is carefully followed by observing a number of reflexes, which weaken and disappear at different depths of anesthesia. In particular, the blink reflex, eye movements, pupil size and respiration are noted (Fig. 10.7). In classical ether anesthesia done without premedication, four different stages of anesthesia are distinguished.

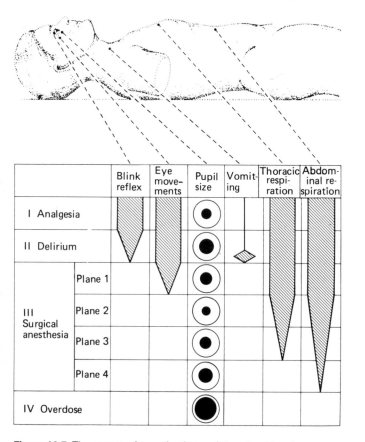

		Blink reflex	Eye movements	Pupil size	Vomiting	Thoracic respiration	Abdominal respiration
I Analgesia							
II Delirium							
III Surgical anesthesia	Plane 1						
	Plane 2						
	Plane 3						
	Plane 4						
IV Overdose							

Figure 10.7 The stages of anesthesia are determined by observing whether certain natural reflexes are abolished. The stages indicated here are typical of anesthesia induced with diethyl ether.

1. **Analgesia stage.** Consciousness is retained but there is alleviation of pain—that is, analgesia. The respiration is unchanged and the reflexes are slightly hyperactive. Anesthesia in this stage can be used in obstetrics, when the patient herself controls the supply of, for example, nitrous oxide.

Unfortunately this type of self-administration does not give complete relief from pain.

2. **Delirium stage.**   Loss of consciousness begins, but at the same time a number of motor reflexes are elicited so that involuntary muscular movements and jerking movements appear. There is a risk of vomiting and laryngospasm (closure of the glottis). The pupils are relatively wide. No operations are performed in the delirium stage.

3. **Stage of surgical anesthesia.**   As the depth of anesthesia gradually increases, the reflexes weaken and are abolished and the eye movements cease. The pupils first diminish in size and then, at a greater depth of anesthesia, they widen again. Respiration involves first both chest and abdomen—thoracic and abdominal respiration—in very deep anesthesia, only abdominal respiration is present.

   In the third stage of anesthesia, four planes are distinguished. The four planes represent different depths of anesthesia. On each occasion that anesthesia is induced a suitable plane is chosen according to the type of surgical operation. An attempt is made to keep the depth of anesthesia as shallow as possible.

4. **Overdose stage.**   If the dose of anesthetic is excessive, total respiratory paralysis results and all vital reflex mechanisms that are important for maintaining life are depressed. Unless resuscitation is performed with controlled (artificial) ventilation, death follows from asphyxia (suffocation and circulatory collapse).

   When emerging from the anesthetic, the patient passes through all the stages in the reverse order. The patient is carefully watched until reflexes are normal and consciousness returns.

10.33	A woman takes sleeping pills in an attempt to commit suicide. In the ambulance on the way to the hospital the pupils are dilated, respiration ceases and the skin becomes cyanotic (blue in color). The patient is in . . . . (depth of anesthesia).	
10.34	A woman is to give birth to a child. Alleviation of pain, which is called . . . ., is obtained by administration of nitrous oxide. She enters the . . . . stage. (This method is used in Europe, but not in the U.S.)	overdose stage (Stage 4)

10.35	A man is to have an operation for a tumor in the abdomen. An intravenous general anesthetic is first given so that he falls asleep, and this is followed by inhalation anesthesia. The pupils are small, the eye movements have ceased and the blink reflex is abolished. The patient is in the stage of	analgesia analgesia (Stage 1)
10.36	At a small hospital with no anesthetist a man is to have an operation for appendicitis (inflammation of the appendix). The anesthetic nurse gives general anesthesia with ether using an open mask. The method is easy to perform alone and requires little technical equipment. After the patient has lost consciousness he becomes disturbed for a few minutes and tries to free himself from the operating table with his arms, tosses his head about and talks incoherently. The patient is in the . . . . (stage of anesthesia).	surgical anesthesia (Stage 3)
		delirium (Stage 2)

Methods for inhalation anesthesia

During anesthesia not only is the **anesthetic** administered in the required amount, but also **oxygen**. Any excess **carbon dioxide** is also dispersed.

In the superficial stages of anesthesia the patient must breathe for himself—**spontaneous ventilation**. At a greater depth of anesthesia, it is often necessary to give artificial ventilation—known as **controlled ventilation**.

A number of different anesthesia machines are in use. They are all furnished with **flowmeters** for oxygen and gaseous anesthetics, so that gaseous mixtures with the required partial pressures can be obtained. In addition, there is some form of **vaporizer** for liquid anesthetics. These are designed to supply a known volume percentage of the anesthetic.

Most anesthesia machines are provided with a **gas reservoir**, which usually consists of a rubber bag. This serves to take up volume changes in the system that arise when the patient breathes—the gas reservoir serves as the source of gas when the patient breathes in. In most systems it takes up most, or all, of the change in volume that occurs in the system during exhalation. The gas reservoir can also be used for controlled ventilation. This is accomplished by compressing the bag with the hand. The anesthesia machine is connected to the patient by means of tubing and a mask, which is pressed over the mouth and nose, or else it is connected to an endotracheal tube in an intubated patient.

There are in principle two systems: rebreathing and nonrebreathing systems. Intermediate forms with partial rebreathing are the commonest.

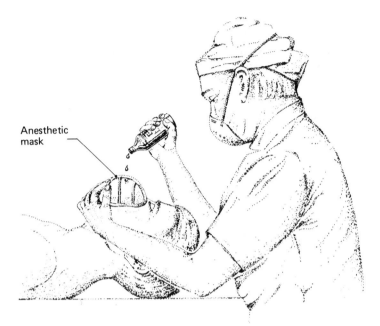

Anesthetic
mask

Figure 10.8 Dropping ether on a mask is a nonrebreathing
system. Ether is no longer in common use.

In a **nonrebreathing system**, the patient constantly breathes a fresh gaseous
mixture, and on exhalation none of the gas is rebreathed. An example of this
system is that in which ether is dropped on a mask, through which the patient
breathes (Fig. 10.8). With this system there is a loss of gas and an increased risk of
explosion when certain anesthetic agents are used. In order to control ventilation,
one way valves and reservoirs are available. The method has the advantage of
simplicity of design, but involves more work for the anesthetist.

In a **rebreathing system**, the patient rebreathes the same gaseous mixture.
Carbon dioxide is eliminated with an absorber, and oxygen is supplied to replace
what the patient consumes. In this system, there is thus complete rebreathing.
Such a system is usually connected in a **circle** whereby a gaseous mixture that is
freed of carbon dioxide and enriched with oxygen is conducted to the patient
through a tube, and the exhaled gaseous mixture is led away through another tube
(Fig. 10.9). A breathing valve is placed on the mask or endotracheal tube so that
the correct direction of flow is obtained in the circuit. The circle system has the
advantages that the gases breathed are cooler (the carbon dioxide absorber
develops heat), there is no risk of breathing in dust from the absorber, and the
dead space (page 145) is small.

A rebreathing system can also be designed as a **to-and-fro system**. The carbon
dioxide absorber is then directly connected to the mask or endotracheal tube and

REBREATHING SYSTEM

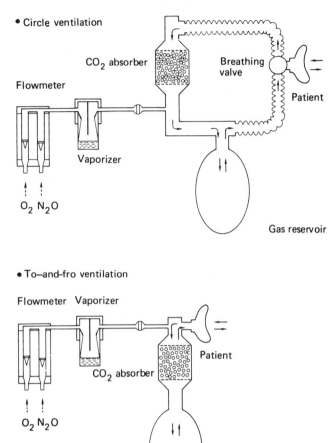

• Circle ventilation

CO$_2$ absorber

Breathing valve

Flowmeter

Patient

Vaporizer

O$_2$ N$_2$O

Gas reservoir

• To–and–fro ventilation

Flowmeter Vaporizer

Patient

CO$_2$ absorber

O$_2$ N$_2$O

Gas reservoir

Figure 10.9 Systems with complete rebreathing are entirely closed. Exhaled CO$_2$ is absorbed and consumed oxygen is replaced.

the patient breathes through it in both directions. Advantages of the to-and-fro system over the circle system are a lower respiratory resistance and a simpler cleaning procedure.

A theoretical advantage of a system with complete rebreathing is that the depth of anesthesia can be kept constant without supplying further anesthetic when the desired depth of anesthesia and equilibrium have been attained. This situation is seldom achieved in practice since leaks develop and change the concentration of the anesthetic agent. Moreover, it takes a long time to reach equilibrium. Another disadvantage is the difficulty of ensuring that the exact amount of oxygen is constantly supplied.

The systems with only **partial rebreathing** are easier to manage (Fig. 10.10). A given amount of new gaseous mixture is constantly supplied. During exhalation, a corresponding portion of the gas is lost through discharge while the rest is returned to the patient after absorption of the carbon dioxide.

PARTIAL REBREATHING

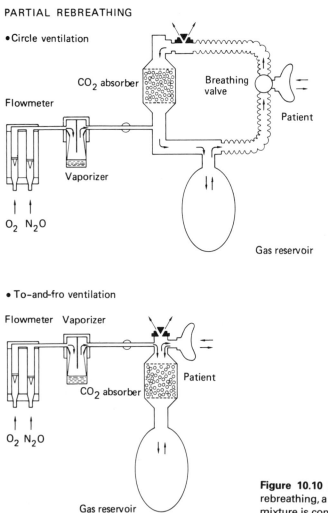

Figure 10.10 In systems with partial rebreathing, a fresh volume of gaseous mixture is constantly added.

To make the anesthetist's work easier in the case of controlled ventilation an anesthesia machine can be designed as a ventilator. Ventilators are described in the section on intensive care (page 545).

10.37	In anesthesia, the .... and .... are supplied and .... is eliminated.	
10.38	To be able to supply a gaseous mixture with the required partial pressures in general anesthesia the anesthesia machine is furnished with a..........	anesthetic oxygen carbon dioxide
10.39	For supplying volatile liquid anesthetics there is usually a	flowmeter
10.40	To take up the change in volume due to breathing, the anesthesia machine is usually provided with a .... consisting of a	vaporizer
10.41	A patient is anesthetized by a nurse dropping ether on a mask placed over the patient's nose and mouth. This anesthesia system is of the .... type. The patient has .... (spontaneous, controlled) ventilation.	gas reservoir rubber bag
10.42	A man is to have an operation for a gastric ulcer. Since the surgeon is dependent on good muscular relaxation, **curare** is given; this drug induces total muscle paralysis in the body. The patient is therefore unable to breathe unaided. The anesthetist must constantly perform .... ventilation. He uses an anesthesia system of the .... type.	nonrebreathing spontaneous
10.43	A patient is to have an operation for cancer of the mouth. The operation is expected to take a long time. A system with partial rebreathing is used. To avoid having too warm ventilatory gases during the long operation and because the anesthetist has limited room in front of the patient's face (the carbon dioxide absorber takes up room) where the surgeon is working, a .... (type of system) is used.	controlled (artificial) partial rebreathing
		circle system

Risks in anesthesia

In anesthesia, there is always a risk for the patient even though it is a very small one. Complications can affect, among other things, the respiration and blood circulation. The treatment of these complications is the same as that applied in intensive care, and is described in Chapter 11. In addition, technical mishaps can occur—for example, explosions and confusion of gas pipes.

Risk of explosion. Some anesthetics are highly flammable and sparks must be avoided. Electrosurgical units (page 520) must not be used in forms of anesthesia where there is a risk of explosion. More difficult to control are the sparks that can occur due to static electricity. Electrically conducting floors in operating rooms reduce, but do not entirely eliminate, the possibility of static charges building up.

Many substances that are not inflammable in air, such as steel, or that burn only with difficulty can cause an explosive fire in the presence of pure oxygen.

Risk of confusion. It is difficult to establish that the right gaseous mixture is being given. Thus with each induction of anesthesia, there is a risk of error. This may be due to interchange of tubes when the hospital's central gas unit is being repaired, flow of anesthetic gas into the oxygen lines due to absence of valves in the anesthetic unit, or to defective valves. A number of deaths have resulted from such technical mishaps.

- Because of a wrong choice of material for a gas pipe line, oxygen leaked from a combined gas and electricity outlet box in the ceiling of the operating room. Through a production error, the electric insulation gap had been made too small. During an operation a nurse stumbled over an electric cable to an ECG unit. The tugging of the cable slightly displaced the electric socket, causing a spark across the small insulation gap. In the oxygen atmosphere, the sheet steel from which the box was made, ignited and an explosive fire broke out. The patient died—not from burns, but because the anesthesia was not properly administered due to the distraction of the anesthetist.

- Rubber gas pipes in an operating room had worn out. A repairer changed them and the operating room was brought back into use. When, some weeks later, a patient was anesthetized, his condition rapidly deteriorated even though the anesthetist set the flow meter at 100 percent oxygen. The patient died because pure nitrous oxide had been given due to accidental interchange of the rubber pipes. The next patient was anesthetized in the same way and also died.

SURGICAL TECHNIQUES

In an operation, different technical procedures are used. The skin and organs are opened by an **incision**. Sometimes there is an organ defect—that is, deficiency or alteration of some tissue components or function. It is then necessary to **transplant** such organs or implant (**im-**, not in-) prostheses to replace these. It is also necessary to **suture**—that is, sew up the organ. Finally a **dressing** is applied to protect the wound.

Incisional Methods and Similar Procedures

Different techniques are used for exposing the operative area and performing incisions and operations in the organs. In principle, we distinguish between **sharp** and **blunt surgical techniques**, **electrosurgery** and special procedures such as **cryotechniques** and **laser techniques**.

Sharp and blunt surgical techniques

The common surgical knife, the **scalpel**, is available in many different sizes, from the largest, which are used for major skin incisions, to the smallest, which are used in eye operations (Fig. 10.11). **Scissors** are used to some extent—for cutting tissues with the sharp edges and for blunt dissection between two tissue layers. In

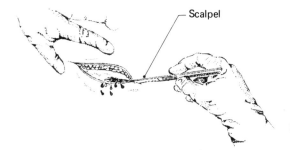

Scalpel

Figure 10.11 The surgical knife is known as a scalpel.

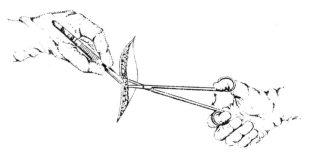

Figure 10.12 Blunt dissection with scissors.

blunt dissection, the scissors are operated in the direction opposite to the normal one, the blades being separated after inserting them between the tissue layers (Fig. 10.12). An advantage of blunt dissection is that the anatomical structures can be followed, so that little damage is caused and there is little if any bleeding. It is also possible to perform blunt dissection with a finger or tweezers.

Operations on bone are performed with saws, drills or trephines (cylindrical saws for cutting holes). They can be hand-driven, electric or pneumatic.

Electrosurgery

Electrosurgery (in Europe, **surgical diathermy**) can be employed for making incisions in tissues (Fig. 10.13). Use is made of a high-frequency alternating

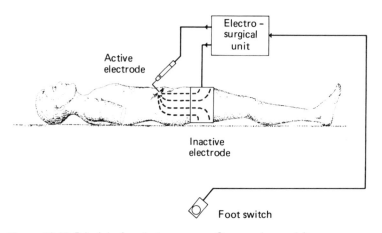

Figure 10.13 Principle for electrosurgery. Commonly used for cutting through layers of tissue.

current, 0.4–3 MHz, often 1.75 MHz. There is a large difference in area between the two electrodes, so that at one of them there is a greater current density and strong local heating, while at the other electrode there is no appreciable heating. The "active" electrode is small, usually with a cross-sectional area of a few square millimeters. The inactive electrode consists of a large conductive plate, at least 100 cm² in area. It may be placed at any arbitrary place on the body, but is usually located under the buttocks or thigh.

The heating at the active electrode can be so intense that the tissues boil and an arc forms between the tissues and the electrode.

Occasionally bipolar electrodes are used in electrosurgery where the current density is the same at both electrodes.

The principle of electrosurgery is as follows. The total current through the body is determined by the voltage (set on the electrosurgical unit) and the total impedance between the electrodes. The generation of heat per unit volume of tissue, $P/V\,(\text{W/m}^3)$, is given by the expression

$$P/V = \rho i^2$$

where ρ is the resistivity (Ωm) including the dielectric losses, and i is the current density (A/m^2). Note that the current density is not the same for all sections of the body, for the current tends to follow the path of minimum impedance. These current pathways are complex because the body is composed of tissues having very different resistivities and dielectric constants.

As a means of incising tissues, electrosurgery has the advantage that bleeding is diminished due to the coagulation of the vessels. In addition, some microorganisms are killed by heat.

Damage may result from incorrect use of electrosurgery. To understand the mechanism involved, note that the current follows a path of minimum impedance; the greatest heat is generated where the current density is greatest and the impedance highest. When the technique is properly applied this is the point of application of the active electrode, where because of its small dimensions, the current density is highest. If there is poor electrical contact between the inactive electrode and the skin there is intense generation of heat as a result of the high contact impedance. This may occur if a piece of cloth happens to be placed between the electrode and the skin, and burns then result.

Burns are thus not produced by electrosurgery, unless the current has passed through the part of the body in question. Lesions detected after an operation and ascribed to the use of electrosurgery, are often due to **chemical corrosion** or **pressure necrosis**, or a combination of the two. The chemical damage may be due to detergent which has been used to disinfect the skin and has run down between the inactive electrode and the table and remained in contact with the skin for a long time. Necrosis (tissue death) may be due to excessive and prolonged pressure on an area of the body, with resulting impairment of the blood circulation.

Cryotechnique and lasers

Tissues can be killed when desired by freezing to temperatures below $-20°\text{C}$. The cryoprobe consists of two concentric tubes, the inner one of which conducts liquid nitrogen to the tip. When applied to the required site, ice crystals form in the tissue and there is also an increase in the salt concentration within the cells; necrosis of the tissue results. The dead tissue can be left in place after the operation, and is then sloughed or reabsorbed. It may also be removed by the sharp or blunt technique.

One field in which laser beams can be used is in operations on the eye—for example, retinal detachment. By utilizing the optical properties of the eye, bursts of energy are transmitted into the interior of the eye. Thus the retina can be tacked in place by points of thermal coagulation.

10.44	A surgical knife is called a	
10.45	Scissors or a finger can be used to separate two loosely connected layers of tissue, this is known as .... dissection.	scalpel
10.46	In electrosurgery, the current passes through the body, following the path of lowest	blunt
10.47	In the electric circuit so formed, the greatest generation of heat occurs where the resistivity is .... (highest, lowest) and where the current density is	impedance
10.48	After a brain operation in which the patient lay for 4 hours with the facial bones bearing on a rubber cushioned support on the operating table, two large necrotic areas were observed at the sites of support. Electrosurgery had been used during the operation and the inactive electrode was under the buttocks. The neurosurgeon suspected that the injury was due to the electrosurgery; he was .... (right, wrong).	highest highest
10.49	A patient was operated on for a bladder tumor. The bladder was filled with isotonic saline. The inactive electrosurgery electrode was placed around the patient's forearm, although it was difficult to obtain good contact. An electrode was inserted through the cystoscope towards the tumor and the current was switched on. As there was no effect, the current was increased. After the operation a large burn lesion was found on the forearm. It was caused by the incorrect use of isotonic saline (0.9 percent) for filling the bladder. Because of the low electrical resistivity of the salt solution, good electric contact was obtained with the small active electrode, so that its area was in effect increased to cover the whole of the bladder contents. As a result, the highest impedance appeared at the .... electrode. The bladder should have been filled with a liquid having a higher resistivity, such as distilled water, and a better place than the forearm should have been chosen for the inactive electrode.	wrong (pressure necrosis)

10.50   A patient was operated on for an injury to the knee.   inactive
The nurse connected the electrosurgical unit by
placing the inactive electrode under the buttocks.
During the operation, the electrosurgical unit was
not used, but by mistake someone stood on the foot
contact. The patient, who had been given a spinal
anesthetic, complained repeatedly of an intensely
warm feeling. He said that he literally fried on the
operating table. After the operation, two large
burns were found on the buttocks corresponding to
the place where the inactive electrode had been
applied. There were also burns on the side of the
little fingers, which had been touching the metal
edge of the operating table. From a reconstruction
of the accident, it was decided that the active
electrode must have slipped down and come into
contact with metal parts of the operating table. The
burns arose through the coincidence of two unfortu-
nate circumstances, as a result of which burns were
obtained at the places on the body where the
. . . . was greatest.

resistivity

Suturing

For suturing—that is, sewing up tissues—different materials are used. Catgut
(twisted sheep-gut), synthetic materials, silk, nylon and stainless steel are
common suture materials. The choice depends on the required strength, on the
time that the suture must last and on whether it will be possible to remove the
suture after the operation.

Catgut is absorbed in the body because it consists of foreign proteins, which
can be readily broken down by proteolytic enzymes. This is an advantage, since it
is possible to suture the intestines and the peritoneal membrane, knowing that the
suture will disappear in some days, weeks or months, the actual time depending on
the thickness of the thread and on the type of pretreatment. One disadvantage of
catgut is that an inflammatory tissue reaction is set up around the suture because it
consists of foreign protein (page 346). The synthetic absorbable materials do not
produce a tissue reaction. Stainless steel is never absorbed, nor does it produce a
tissue reaction.

There are various suturing techniques. Usually a curved needle is used, which
is gripped with a holder (Fig. 10.14). Either an **interrupted** or a **continuous suture**
is made. To prevent the wound margins from rolling up, **mattress sutures** are often
used (Fig. 10.14). It is important not to knot the sutures too tightly. If this happens
the tissues adjacent to the sutures necrotize—that is, they die—because of impaired blood circulation.

Interrupted suture Continuous suture Mattress suture

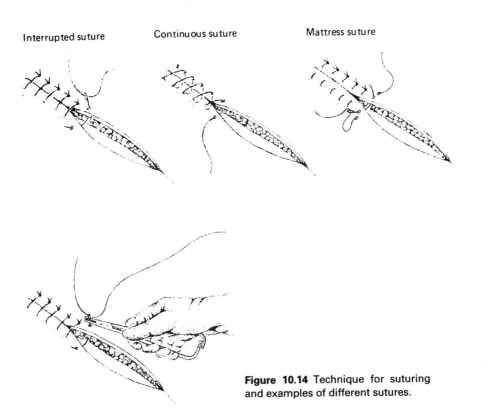

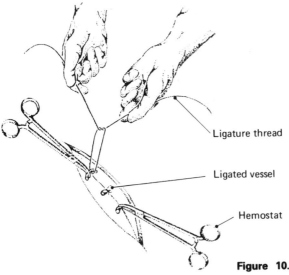

Figure 10.14 Technique for suturing and examples of different sutures.

Hemostasis

The bleeding that occurs during an operation must be stopped. The severed arteries and veins are **ligated**, or tied (noun, **ligature**). This is done by first attaching **hemostats** (lockable forceps) to all bleeding vessels (Fig. 10.15). A

Ligature thread

Ligated vessel

Hemostat

Figure 10.15 Stopping bleeding by ligating vessels.

catgut thread is then knotted around each vessel and the hemostats are removed. Bleeding from minor vessels can be controlled by coagulation with electrosurgery (page 520). Larger vessels are ligated by suturing—that is, the thread is first anchored to the vessel wall using a needle before it is knotted, thereby preventing the thread from slipping off the vessel.

Bleeding from capillaries stops spontaneously if the clotting time is normal (page 292); if not, it must be normalized by transfusing fresh blood. Pieces of specially prepared resorbable gelatin sponge, called gelfoam or surgicel, are often applied to an area of diffuse bleeding.

10.51	Intestines heal rapidly. They are therefore sewn with . . . ., which is absorbed the most rapidly of all suture materials.	
10.52	The strongest suture material and the one that is not absorbed at all is	catgut
10.53	Occupying a position between these suture materials are . . . . and	stainless steel
10.54	For healing to be possible it is important that the suture threads are not drawn so tight that they interfere with the	silk nylon
10.55	The procedure of binding a vessel with a thread—for example, catgut—is known as . . . . (verb); we say that a . . . . (noun) is made.	blood circulation
		ligating ligature

Transplantation Techniques

There are two main conditions for transferring living tissues; first the transplant must be anatomically connected to the host in a satisfactory way; second, the immunological rejection reaction must be prevented (page 373).

Surgical technique

The greatest practical problem when a transplant is to be surgically inserted in the host is the difficulty of connecting the minor vessels. The technique is, however, highly developed and consists of sewing the vessels together end-to-end or end-to-side. Ordinary permanent suture materials that are nonabsorbable, such as silk or nylon, are used.

The rejoining of nerves in the adult so that their function is restored is technically very difficult; in children this can more often be accomplished successfully, probably because the nerve tissues are in a state of growth. A totally detached organ, for example, a hand, can indeed be surgically reattached in the adult, and nerve function can sometimes be restored. This used to be considered impossible and a hand prosthesis assumed to be functionally superior. Reattachment operations require prolonged hospital care.

Small pieces of tissue, such as skin and fascia (connective tissue membranes), can be grafted (transplanted) without connecting the vessels, since the grafts can be oxygenated and can obtain nutrition via surrounding lymph. It is also possible to transfer relatively large bone transplants, probably because of the low metabolism of bones.

Transplantation immunology

The chief difficulty in transplanting organs between genetically different individuals is presented by immunological reactions.

Transplantation from one place to another of the same individual—autograft (page 372)—or between identical twins—isograft—presents no immunological problems. Tissues are often transferred from one site to another on the same individual, for example, skin after burns, and bone after skeletal injuries. Less commonly, an identical twin is available as the donor.

Problems arise in allograft (page 372). The transplant then has antigenic properties—to a varying extent depending on the immunological difference between donor and host, and on the degree of contact between the transplant and the antibody-forming organs of the host.

The immune reaction can be suppressed in several ways. Of the many methods that have been tested, treatment with certain drugs—so-called **antimetabolites** and **antilymphocytic globulin, ALG,**—are the two most common.

The antimetabolites attack the metabolism of the cells, with the result that the cells either die or they are weakened. Such substances were first tested in cancer treatment, but they have also proved to be of use in suppressing the immune response. The method has the disadvantage that there is a detrimental effect on the whole organism.

An adjunctive immunosuppressive agent is antilymphocytic globulin. These globulins which are prepared in animals, usually horses, by injecting human lymphocytes, consist of antibodies that have a specific effect against the lymphocytes. Since these lymphocytes are responsible for cell-mediated immunity, treatment with antilymphocytes leads to a reduction in the number of lymphocytes and hence also to a suppression of the immune reaction.

Some organs are less exposed to immunological rejection than others. This is due to the degree of contact between the transplant and the host's reticuloendothelial system, RES (page 343). All organs with a direct blood supply thus present difficulties—for example, kidneys, liver, heart, lungs and skin. The eye's cornea, on the other hand, is not supplied with vessels, and there is thus no spread of the antigen substances in the host. It has long been possible to transplant corneas successfully without a knowledge of the immunological factors involved.

10.56	A patient is suffering from high blood pressure, which is found to be due to narrowing of an artery to a kidney. The kidney therefore receives too little blood and tends to compensate for this by providing substances to the blood that raise the blood pressure. The causal treatment consists of surgical removal of the constriction, and this is done by replacing part of the artery with a graft consisting of a vein from the thigh, a dacron tube, or other replacement. The technical problem is one of .... (suturing the vessel, immunological rejection of the graft).	
10.57	In a patient with severe burns, the wound is covered with skin from a cadaver. The skin becomes attached, but after a few weeks rejection begins due to an .... (With this palliative operation it has, however, been possible to tide the patient over a critical stage.)	suturing the vessel
10.58	Kidney transplantations are relatively successful, with more than one half of the hosts surviving for at least three years. If the patients are divided into those receiving kidneys from closely related donors and from unrelated donors, it is found that two thirds survive in the former group but only one third in the latter. This would be expected because there is a closer .... similarity between donors and hosts.	immune reaction
10.59	When signs of rejection appear, persons with renal transplants must be treated with immunosuppressive drugs, including corticosteroids, antimetabolites and ...., ALG.	immunological
		antilymphocytic globulin

Implantation of Prostheses

When lost tissue or an organ cannot be replaced by means of transplantation, a **prosthesis** must be provided. Prostheses are thus all those parts made of nonliving materials that replace living organs and tissues. Examples of organs that can be replaced with prostheses are legs, joints, cartilage, vessels, heart valves and corneas.

The choice of the material is the greatest technical problem in the design of a prosthesis. The material must provide satisfactory mechanical function of the prosthesis, it must not have a harmful effect on the body and not be destroyed by the body fluids. Many materials cannot be implanted because they are absorbed to some extent. This is the case for many plastics, such as polyethylene. Nor must the material irritate the tissues so that inflammation results. Some materials are carcinogenic—that is, they give rise to cancer during prolonged implantation. The choice of material is thus dependent on the desired mechanical and biochemical properties.

Bone can be replaced with parts manufactured from special stainless alloys, usually Vitallium, which consists of cobalt and chromium. Thus, in the hip joint, the joint that is most often destroyed, the femoral head can be replaced with a Vitallium prosthesis. Bone can also be replaced with so-called inorganic bone, a material produced from calf bone by extracting all the organic components, leaving only the inorganic hydroxyapatite.

Cartilage is replaced with a silicone rubber known as Silastic. This material is very inert and is not absorbed; many other types of rubber are destroyed in the body and become brittle or cause inflammation of the tissues.

Vessels are replaced with tubes of a knitted or woven fabric produced from Dacron or Teflon. The tube is sutured to the vessel. The fabric is then saturated with blood, which clots, producing a tube consisting of a blood clot reinforced with the mesh. The clot is converted to connective tissue in the body so that the vascular prosthesis is accepted.

Heart valve prostheses of many different designs are available. A common one is the disc valve (which opens and closes like a lid). They are produced from stainless material, plastic and synthetic fabric. After the old valve is removed, the prosthesis is sutured into place at the same site. The area of contact is through the fabric-covered surfaces where ingrowth of fibrous tissue occurs.

10.60	A child is born without one outer ear. A plastic operation is performed and skin from the thigh is used. Cartilage, however, cannot be obtained in large enough pieces. A prosthesis is made of	
10.61	A man undergoes an operation for a thigh tumor, which has grown in and involved the femoral artery. To avoid amputating the leg, a vascular prosthesis of . . . . is sutured in.	Silastic (silicone rubber)
10.62	A woman has had a pain in the hip over many years due to destruction of the joint. A hip-joint prosthesis made of . . . . (an alloy of chromium and cobalt) is inserted.	Dacron or Teflon fabric
		Vitallium

Dressing Techniques

After an operation or an injury, the wound is covered with a dressing. The dressing has four functions:

Protection against microorganisms to hinder invasion of pathogens during the first couple of days of wound healing.

Mechanical support so that the wound margins are stabilized, thereby promoting healing. In the case of limb fractures, the dressing is shaped using a plaster cast or splint so that it removes some mechanical load from the limb. A plaster dressing and splint are also used for treating infected wounds; any movement aids the microorganisms in their attempt to invade the tissues, while immobility supports the body's defenses against infection.

Compression of the wound so that bleeding is stopped and the wound margins heal more evenly.

Absorption of tissue fluid, which can seep from the damaged tissues.

10.63	A patient with elevated blood pressure undergoes an operation in the abdomen. Careful hemostasis is performed, and after suturing the abdominal wall there is no bleeding. When the patient awakens from the anesthesia and is taken back to the ward, there is a rise in the blood pressure, which had been lower than normal under anesthesia. Small hemorrhages from the wound margins develop. In one place the wound dressing becomes saturated and must be changed immediately, since it no longer serves as a	
10.64	When the new dressing is applied, attempts are made to stop the bleeding by	protection against microorganisms
10.65	A patient injured his finger on a nail so that infection developed. After cleaning the skin, a dressing with a plastic splint is applied to immobilize the whole finger. The purpose of the dressing is to provide . . . ., an important measure in treating infection.	compression
		mechanical support

EXAMPLES OF TREATMENT OF SURGICAL DISEASES

The methods of surgical treatment are usually causal—an attempt is made to remove the cause of the disease. Sometimes it is necessary to be content with palliative (p. 485) measures.

Surgical treatment is designated according to a simple nomenclature. A cut is called an **incision**. For example, a boil is incised so that the pus can drain out. An incision is made in the abdominal wall to perform an operation on the gallbladder.

The removal of a piece of tissue or a foreign body by cutting is called **excision**. A birthmark on the skin is excised. The removal of part of an organ is called **resection**. Removal of an organ, completely or partially, is called **ectomy**. Appendectomy is performed in appendicitis—that is, the appendix is removed when it is inflamed. Removal of a tumor, usually completely, is called **extirpation**; the term is also used synonymously with ectomy in removal of an organ.

Performance of an incision in, and opening of, a cavity is indicated by the suffix **-tomy**—for example, herniotomy, when a hernia is opened and sewn up again to make its diameter smaller. Formation of an opening is indicated by the suffix **-stomy**—for example, tracheostomy, when a passage is created between the trachea and the skin in the case of airway obstruction of the larynx. The actual operation is called tracheotomy.

A communication created between two blood vessels, intestines or nerves is called an **anastomosis**.

Local transfer of tissue is made by **plastic operations**; the opposite is **transplantation**, when it is moved from one site to another. In a burn with scarring, a skin graft, or dermatoplasty, is performed—that is, the scar is excised and the surrounding skin is separated from the underlying tissues and drawn over the skinless area.

anastomosis	a communication, for example, between two blood vessels, intestines or nerves
ectomy	surgical removal of a whole organ or a part of it by cutting
excision	cutting out, cutting away
extirpation	complete removal of a tumor or an organ
incision	cutting or opening with a knife
plastic operation **-plasty**	an operation performed to restore shape and function by local transfer of tissue after injury, disease or deformity
resection	surgical removal of a part of an organ by cutting
-stomy	a suffix meaning to form an opening, mouth, or outlet
-tomy	a suffix meaning cutting, surgical opening
transplantation	moving of body substance, for example, skin, nerves and bone (graft) from one place on the body to another or from one individual to another

10.66	A patient is to have an operation for gastric ulcer. The first step is to make an .... in the abdominal wall.	
10.67	It is possible to choose between several methods of treatment for gastric ulcer. In one of these, part of the stomach that produces hydrochloric acid is removed; we say that a .... is performed.	incision
10.68	It is also possible to create a new outlet between the remaining part of the stomach and the small intestine—known as a gastroentero-	resection
10.69	Another possibility is to cut the parasympathetic nerves that conduct hydrochloric-acid stimulating impulses to the glands in the stomach. The parasympathetic nerve is the vagus nerve; a vago- .... is performed.	stomy
10.70	To compensate for a reduction in motor action that occurs in the stomach in vagotomy, an operation to promote emptying must be performed at the same time—that is, a better flow from the stomach is created. This is done by making an incision in, and moving the muscles in, the pylorus, the lower orifice of the stomach; a pyloro- .... is performed.	tomy
		plasty

Infectious diseases

Infections often result in an **abscess**, an accumulation of pus. This occurs due to decomposition of tissues. The abscess contains white blood cells, tissue fluid, fragments of decomposed tissue and bacteria. Abscesses can form anywhere in the body. In the skin they can arise after injury, when microorganisms have penetrated deeply, or through infection of different structures in the skin—for example, enlarged sebaceous glands. A pimple that contains yellowish white pus is a small abscess in an ordinary sebaceous or sweat gland. An appendicitis abscess, an accumulation of pus around a burst appendix, is a complication that can arise if the operation is not performed in time. After a successful appendectomy, an abscess can form in the abdominal wall some days after the operation. Such an abscess differs radically in its symptoms and treatment from appendicitis abscesses.

An abscess often calls for surgical treatment. The principle is to create free flow for the pus, which is called **drainage**. An incision or a blunt dissection is made to the abscess and the channel is then widened so that the pus cannot stagnate. It may be desirable to insert a rubber tube or the like in the wound channel to keep it open for some days, so that healing can take place from the bottom.

Infections that do not lead to abscess formation, but that are diffusely spread in the tissues are treated by **immobilization**—for example, with plaster casts. Immobilization treatment is particularly important in infections near joints, since otherwise the tissue layers are constantly exposed to displacement during movements.

10.71	An accumulation of pus that has arisen through decomposition of tissues is called an	
10.72	A woman that has had an illegal abortion in which the uterus was perforated by error has fever, abdominal pain and the urge to defecate. On palpation (page 122) via the vagina, an abscess is discovered in the lower part of the abdominal cavity. It is clearly demarcated and is located between the rectum and the uterus. To prevent spread into the abdomen, an incision in the vagina is made, and 10 ml of pus flows out. A rubber tube is inserted for	abscess
10.73	A patient with an injury to the hand has purulent infection of a tendon sheath. This is opened with an incision and the cavity is flushed with penicillin solution. Penicillin is also given parenterally (page 489). The further surgical treatment, which is important in this case, consists of .... with a splint.	drainage
		immobilization

Tumor diseases

Some tumor diseases are treated surgically, some by radiotherapy (Chapter 13) and some by means of drugs. A combination of these methods is common. Surgical treatment alone is chosen for cancer of the gastrointestinal tract and for lung cancer. Combined surgical and radiological therapy are relevant for mammary and ovarian cancer. Early diagnosis and treatment are important—one person in five in a country with a high living standard dies from carcinoma. The prognosis is dependent to a large extent on how soon the treatment is started. The type of tumor is also of importance; some forms of cancer cannot be cured even if diagnosed early.

The prime object of surgical treatment is to **extirpate** the tumor—that is, remove it completely by surgery. A **radical operation** is often performed, by which it is meant that not only the actual tumor is removed but also the surrounding tissues with the lymphatic vessels and lymph nodes. The reason for this is that tumors spread via the lymphatic vessels to the lymph nodes. In a radical **mastectomy** for mammary carcinoma, the whole breast is removed, and also the underlying muscle, fatty tissue and lymph glands in the axillae. If the tumor is confined to the breast, a simple mastectomy, or even a wide local incision, may be effective in eradicating the malignancy.

Another surgical treatment method is based on an endocrine mechanism. It is known that hormonal factors are important in the growth of many kinds of tumors. Thus, female sex hormones stimulate the growth of breast tumors and tumors of the female genitalia—cancer of the uterus. Similarly, male sex hormones stimulate the development of prostatic cancer. (One form of drug therapy for such tumors is therefore to give contrasexual hormones—that is, female sex hormones to men and vice versa.) The surgical treatment aims at eliminating the patient's production of his or her own sex hormones. The ovaries are therefore surgically removed in women and the testicles in men. This treatment in itself is insufficient for definitive elimination of the tumor but it alleviates the symptoms and prolongs the survival time.

10.74	A woman has noticed a walnut-sized swelling in the breast located in the upper outer quadrant. A needle puncture is performed for a biopsy and it is found that the patient has a malignant tumor. A . . . . operation is therefore performed.	
10.75	In the radical operation, not only the tumor but also much of the surrounding tissues, especially the . . . . and the . . . . , are removed.	radical
10.76	One year after the operation, swellings are noticed in the area of the operation, which prove to be metastases. Radiotherapy is performed as is also surgical endocrine treatment, which consists of	lymph nodes lymphatic vessels
		removal of the ovaries

Example of an abdominal operation

To summarize the surgical measures, a case of cholelithiasis (gallstones) will be described.

The patient is a woman aged 40 years, inclined to stoutness, who during Christmas has repeated attacks of pain in the stomach, brought on by fatty food. The patient occasionally had jaundice (page 278), and the urine had been port-colored. Radiography—cholecystography (page 395) disclosed a number of fairly large and small stones in the gallbladder.

The risk associated with cholecystectomy (removal of the gallbladder), that is, of not surviving the operation, is about 1 percent, when considering the patient's age, illness and her state of health. Technically, the operation is not of the simplest kind, for the physician must be sure that no stones remain in the common bile duct (page 52). The risk must be considered relative to the prognosis (page 102) if no measures are taken at all.

If the patient is given no treatment, there is a constant risk of a stone lodging in the bile ducts, especially at the opening into the duodenum where the pancreatic duct also emerges. If a stone obstructs flow, pancreatitis (inflammation of the pancreas) a feared, life-threatening condition, may develop. The liver may also be damaged. There is, in addition, a risk of acute cholecystitis (inflammation of the gallbladder), which can develop if the flow from the gallbladder is obstructed by a stone. Finally, the patient will certainly have further attacks of pain (biliary colic) as stones leave the gallbladder and pass through the bile ducts.

The physician concludes that, all things considered, the patient's situation might be decidedly worse if no operation is done, and accordingly he therefore strongly recommends one. Because of the episodes of pain, the patient readily agrees to the operation (a factor that is, however, not of critical importance in the appraisal of the risk—it only makes it easier for the patient to make up her mind).

The patient is admitted to a hospital ward some days before the operation. A number of chemical tests are carried out, including ones showing the state of the blood (page 285), the liver (page 277) and the electrolytes (page 272). The patient's blood group is determined in case a blood transfusion should prove necessary (page 359). An electrocardiogram, ECG, (page 198) is recorded to check that the heart is normal and to serve as a basis for comparison, should the patient have heart trouble during the course of her illness.

The day before the operation, certain preparatory measures are taken. An injection of vitamin K may be given to normalize the bleeding time (if prothrombin production by the liver is low, page 292). The patient is required to take a bath and is given an enema in the evening in order to empty the bowels. In order to obtain a peaceful night's sleep, a powerful sedative is given.

On the morning of the day the operation is to be performed, the patient waits in the ward; food and drink are withheld in order to eliminate the risk of aspirating vomited stomach contents (page 509). One hour before the patient is due in the operating suite, the ward is informed of the required premedication (page 509). The patient is given an injection and becomes calm and sleepy, and more or less indifferent to events.

The patient is taken to the operating suite in her own bed and transferred there to the operating table in the induction room. Her arms are restrained to arm rests fixed to the operating table, the right one above her face and the left one at right angles to the body. In the right arm, the blood pressure is measured with a cuff (page 133) and in the left, a hypodermic needle is inserted in a vein for intravenous general anesthesia and for any blood transfusion. To facilitate the induction of general anesthesia, an atmosphere of quiet and calm is maintained in the induction room; essential conversation is conducted in a lowered voice.

General anesthesia is initiated with an intravenous injection of a barbiturate and the patient falls asleep in a minute or so with no stage of delirium (page 512). Intubation is then performed (page 510). This is accomplished by bending the head strongly backwards by lowering the head-rest, and then inserting the endotracheal tube with the aid of a laryngoscope. The tracheal tube is connected to an anesthesia machine for inhalation anesthesia. To obtain good muscular relaxation in order to ease the surgeon's work, a curare preparation is adminis- tered. This produces complete muscular paralysis throughout the body, even in the respiratory muscles. Controlled ventilation (page 513) is therefore main- tained throughout the operation. The blood circulation, ventilation and depth of anesthesia are constantly monitored throughout the operation; all the values and any measures taken are recorded on a special anesthesia record sheet.

When the patient has been brought into the operating room, preparations for the operation are conducted under the guidance of the surgical nurse, who is dressed in sterile gown and gloves. The entire anterior and right sides of the patient's trunk are cleaned with disinfecting solution to obtain an antiseptic field. This is done with a cotton compress, which is held with sterile forceps. In this way the surgical nurse remains sterile. After this washing stage, sterile surgical drapes are laid over the patient leaving only the area of skin exposed where the incision is to be made.

The operation can now be started. The surgeon first decides exactly where the skin incision is to be made; this calls for good judgement, for it must provide easy access to the relevant organs. Where the diagnosis is reliable, as in this case, the incision is made just below the right costal arch; if it is uncertain whether the patient's illness is due to pathological changes in the stomach, the incision is made instead in the midline. First of all a skin incision is made and bleeding from severed vessels is stopped by ligating them (page 524). Likewise, bleeding produced when incising the muscle layer in the abdominal wall is stopped. Beneath the muscle layer, the bluish white peritoneum appears and it is opened with scissors, care being taken to avoid damage to the viscera; the scissors work between two fingers inserted in the abdominal cavity to raise the peritoneum.

The abdomen opened, the surgeon is in a position to appraise the situation. When palpating the gallbladder, he finds that it is filled with stones, thus confirming the diagnosis; it is highly improbable that a positive radiological diagnosis will be wrong. The surgeon makes a careful check of the anatomy and decides on the surgical procedure. Surgical sponges, all provided with radiopaque markers, are placed in the abdomen in order to hold the intestines aside. This ensures a clear surgical field, and also serves as a protection in case there should be leakage of bile during the operation; this would then be absorbed by the sponges which would be changed.

The cholecystectomy—removal of the gallbladder—presents the following problem. The anatomy is not always regular, and it is important to avoid damage to the hepatic artery or to the common bile duct, which runs from the liver to the duodenum. It is therefore necessary to locate these structures accurately before the operation is completed. The artery from the gallbladder is carefully dissected free and a check is made that there is no confusion with the hepatic artery. The bile duct artery is then encircled with two ligatures and cut between them. The bile duct is then ligated and cut between the gallbladder and the common duct. The gallbladder, which lies with one half bearing against the liver and the other half against the peritoneal membrane, is then separated from the liver by blunt dissection, using scissors. Any bleeding is arrested by ligating the severed arteries.

To ensure that there are no stones left in the common bile duct, an incision is made in it—an operation known as choledochotomy. Two suture threads are attached in the duct so that it can be stretched, and an 8 mm long incision is made in the wall. A flexible probe is inserted in the bile duct and passed through into the duodenum. By palpating around the probe with the fingers a search is made to find any residual stones. They are removed with a special scoop or flushed out. Cholangiography (page 395) is then performed—a radiographic examination of the bile ducts after contrast medium has been injected through a rubber tube. If this does not demonstrate more stones, the bile duct is closed by suturing around a T-shaped rubber tube, the free end of which passes out through the wound in the abdomen. For a week or so after the operation, this tube allows bile to drain away during the course of healing.

The abdomen is then closed. Another rubber tube is first inserted so that its end is located deep in the abdomen. This enables any blood to drain away, and also discloses any hemorrhage, which may necessitate immediate reoperation. With the tube in position, the peritoneum is first sewn up so carefully that any subsequent infection of the abdominal wall will be unable to spread into the abdomen but instead be able to drain outwards. Next the muscle layer is sutured. Finally, the abdomen is closed with mattress sutures (page 523). A sterile dressing is then applied.

The operation is now completed and the patient may be allowed to waken from the general anesthesia. She is transferred to the surgical intensive care unit for constant supervision. Here facilities are available for any required emergency measures.

After a few days there is no longer any risk of hemorrhage, so the rubber tube leading from the operative region is removed. The T-tube is withdrawn some days later, when it is considered that the bile can flow freely to the duodenum; the aperture left in the common duct then heals.

During the period after the operation the temperature is checked to see that there is no infection. Similarly, the legs are checked to ensure that no blood clots form, since they may become detached and form pulmonary emboli (page 63).

The risk of blood clots is reduced by encouraging the patient to get up as soon as possible. The patient is usually discharged 14 days after the operation and may stay at a convalescent home for another 14 days before returning home to her normal workload.

REFERENCES

DAVIS, L. E. *Davis–Christopher Textbook of Surgery; The Biological Basis of Modern Surgical Practice*. Philadelphia (Saunders) 1973. 2135 pages.

DRIPPS, R. D. *Introduction to Anesthesia*. Philadelphia (Saunders) 1972. 456 pages.

DUNPHY, J. E. *Wound Healing*. New York (Medcom Press) 1974. 82 pages.

HILL, D. W. *Electronic Techniques in Anaesthesia and Surgery*. Second edition. London (Butterworths) 1973. 421 pages.

SCHWARTZ, S. I. *Principles of Surgery*. New York (Blakiston) 1974. 1982 pages.

WILSON, J. L. *Handbook of Surgery*. Los Altos (Lange) 1973. 877 pages.

chapter 11

Intensive Care

When the body is temporarily unable to maintain vital functions, it requires intensive care. There are various causes, but since the therapeutic measures are often similar, hospitals have established special areas for intensive care.

Intensive care should only be given if the patient's basic disease is treatable.

In internal medicine there is often a need for intensive care. This is the case, for example, in **poisoning** with sleeping pills in connection with attempted suicide. One of the problems in this case is that the respiratory center in the medulla oblongata is temporarily paralyzed. The same condition occurs in **diseases of the central nervous system**, in which vital centers may be affected. **Lung diseases**, like asthma, can require intensive care because of difficulty in breathing. The same is true of several severe infections, such as general blood poisoning, pneumonia and meningitis, in which case the risk of infection is a special problem. Close observation is required for **myocardial infarction** during the days immediately following the infarct, when there is a risk of cardiac arrest. In **renal damage**, which can result in uremia (poisoning by retention of urinary constituents in the blood) due to reduced excretion, dialysis treatment is required.

In surgery, regular intensive care is needed during the days following major **operations** to prevent shock and to restore the "internal environment"; intensive care directly follows anesthesia. Many **cases of accidents** with damage to the central nervous system must be closely observed for the first few days. **Burns** require special intensive care because of the great loss of fluids by exudation from large wound areas, proneness to infection and the damaging effects on the heart and kidneys due to extensive tissue breakdown.

Intensive care requires rapid diagnosis and treatment. In the case of **respiratory** and **circulatory** failure, effective treatment must be started within a few minutes. In the somewhat longer term, the **internal environment**—the fluid balance, electrolyte balance and the acid-base balance—must be restored, and also **nutrition**. Within a few days steps must be taken to ensure **dialysis**, the excretion of waste products from the body.

Intensive care can be divided into **intensive observation** and **intensive treatment**—the former is a prerequisite of the latter. In intensive observation many of the diagnostic methods described in earlier chapters are used. Four vital functions are monitored: breathing, blood circulation, internal environment and level of consciousness. For intensive treatment special methods have been developed, often with advanced techniques. Some of these are described in the following.

Question		*Answer*
11.1	Intensive care is used to maintain vital functions . . . . (temporarily, permanently).	
11.2	A man in his fifties, previously in good health, is admitted to the hospital with myocardial infarction. As there is a risk of cardiac arrest, for the next few days the patient is placed in an . . . . unit.	temporarily
11.3	A patient, who has been smoking for some years, and who has lung cancer in an advanced stage with metastases (daughter tumors) in the brain, has been suffering from headaches, vomiting and epileptic attacks for the last six months. During the last few days the circulation has greatly deteriorated. The following intensive care is given:	intensive care
11.4	Intensive care is divided into . . . . and	none (not treatable)

11.5	In intensive observation, four vital functions are monitored, namely ...., ..., ... and	intensive observation intensive treatment
		breathing blood circulation internal environment level of consciousness

RESPIRATION

Reduced breathing, or **respiratory failure (insufficiency)**, can have different causes. Over one half of such cases are due to airway **obstruction**. This may be caused by mucus and blood which cannot be coughed up. Inflammation of various kinds can also produce airway obstruction due to accumulation of pus and due to swelling of the mucous membranes of the airways. In asthma, impaired breathing is due to bronchospasm, which is a special form of airway obstruction.

Another important cause of respiratory failure is due to factors which influence the **respiratory center** in the medulla oblongata. The activity of this center can be reduced or paralyzed by intracranial bleeding, which produces an increase in pressure in the skull. Such bleeding occurs, for instance, after trauma or in tumors. Paralysis of the respiratory center can also occur in infections, for example, polio. Respiratory paralysis frequently occurs because of a toxic effect, as in poisoning with sleeping pills.

The treatment of respiratory failure depends on its cause. When there is an obstruction, it must be eliminated. Usually it is possible to obtain an adequate airway by means of **intubation** (page 510) or by **tracheotomy** (page 530). Constant and careful bronchial hygiene is then important—that is, aspiration of mucus with a catheter consisting of a soft plastic or rubber tube connected to a suction device. An attempt to relieve bronchospasm is first made with drugs. Sometimes these measures are not enough and the patient is unable to maintain adequate breathing. In order to lower the patient's breathing work load, **ventilator treatment** is introduced. In paralysis of the respiratory center the most important measure is thus to connect the patient to a ventilator. A very special procedure with quite a different field of use from the above is **hyperbaric oxygen therapy.**

In an acute condition with depressed or arrested breathing, **artificial ventilation** is given immediately. This must be accomplished by all available aids—blowing in air using mouth-to-mouth resuscitation or a hand-squeezed bag or ventilator—until the patient can breathe on his own.

Artificial Ventilation and Free Airway

The procedure to restore satisfactory breathing depends on the level of unconsciousness. In the case of a mildly unconscious patient with respiratory movements, but where breathing is prevented because the tongue has fallen back into the throat, the body should be immediately placed in a stooping position (Fig. 11.1). This results in a free airway and the patient only needs to be watched.

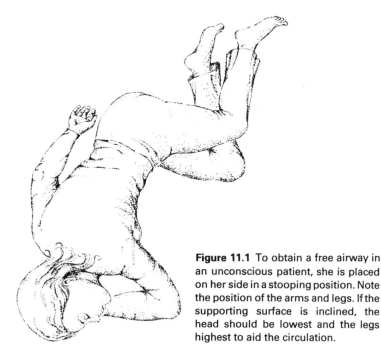

Figure 11.1 To obtain a free airway in an unconscious patient, she is placed on her side in a stooping position. Note the position of the arms and legs. If the supporting surface is inclined, the head should be lowest and the legs highest to aid the circulation.

Manual methods for artificial ventilation

Injured or very ill patients with severe forms of respiratory failure must be given artificial ventilation without delay. The measures are taken in a definite order:

1. **Supine position.** Place the patient on his back in the supine position with the head at a low level.
2. **Foreign bodies in the mouth are removed.** Remove dentures, dislodged teeth, etc.
3. **Free airway.** In the supine position the tongue falls back and blocks the airway (Fig. 11.2). Open the airway by bending the head back as far as possible (Fig. 11.3) and pull the chin forwards (Fig. 11.4).
4. **Blowing in air.** If there are no mechanical aids, use the mouth-to-mouth method (Fig. 11.5). If the patient has jaw spasm, blow air in through the nose. In the case of children, blow in through both mouth and nose.

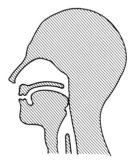

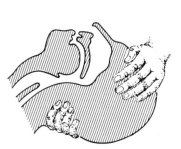

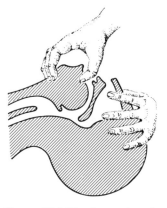

Figure 11.2 In the supine position the throat is blocked by the tongue which falls back.

Figure 11.3 The head is bent fully to obtain a free airway.

Figure 11.4 The lower jaw is drawn forwards to obtain a free airway.

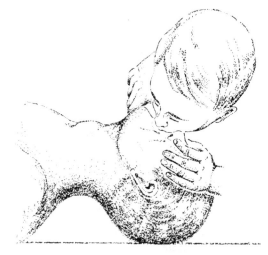

Figure 11.5 Blowing air through the mouth. Air can also be blown in through the nose. During the inflation check that the chest rises.

Mechanical aids for manual artificial ventilation usually consist of a mask, breathing valve and self-filling bag (Fig. 11.6). The mask, which is of soft rubber or plastic, is held firmly over the patient's mouth and nose so that it fits tightly. The breathing valve serves to guide the air so that fresh air or air enriched with oxygen is supplied to the patient and the expired air is conducted away. Squeezed with one hand, the bag functions as a pump. It is self-expanding and fills automatically with fresh air or oxygen when the patient breathes out.

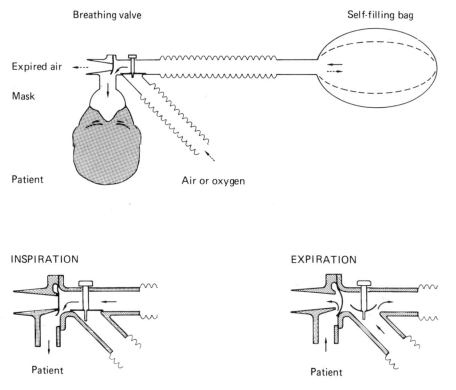

Figure 11.6 Mask, breathing valve and self-filling bag for artificial ventilation.

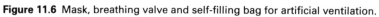

11.6	While visiting a family with a cat, a person that is allergic to this animal has an attack of asthma. He has difficulty in breathing, in spite of vigorous respiratory movements. The smooth muscles in the airways contract so that these are constricted. The difficulty is due to an .... (the commonest cause of respiratory failure).	
11.7	A woman takes an overdose of sleeping pills. The ambulance personnel find her deeply unconscious with disturbed respiration due to a paralysis of the	obstruction of the airways

11.8	A patient that has had a major chest operation does not recover satisfactory breathing after the anesthesia has worn off. Shallow general anesthesia is induced again for .... (insertion of a tube in the windpipe), and much mucus is sucked out. A .... (incision in the windpipe in the front of the neck) is performed to effect a .... (external connection with the windpipe).	respiratory center
11.9	After the operation, the mucus is sucked out of the windpipe—this action is known as	intubation tracheotomy tracheostomy (page 530)
11.10	Despite this, breathing is still difficult. The patient is connected to a	bronchial hygiene
11.11	You arrive on the scene of a traffic accident just after a collision. One of the drivers who was wearing a safety belt and received only minor injuries is in heated argument with an onlooker about the cause of the accident. You find three persons unconscious in the car. A child is sitting in the back seat of the car with his head resting on his chest, which is being spasmodically drawn in while the epigastrium and the abdomen are pressed downwards and outwards—so-called **paradoxical respiratory movements**. You carefully lift the child and place him on the roadside in a .... (position) with the head .... (high, low) and the legs .... (high, low). In this way a .... is immediately obtained and the child can breathe spontaneously.	ventilator
11.12	While doing this you have ordered the onlookers and the injured driver to help the two other injured persons—the driver in the other car and his passenger in the front seat, who was not using a safety belt. You find them unconscious on the ground. You and an onlooker place the victims .... (body position), after which you check that there are no .... in the mouth. You then obtain a .... by bending the head fully .... and drawing the chin forwards, after which you give artificial ventilation by the .... One of the injured persons rapidly resumes spontaneous breathing.	stooping position low high free airway

11.13	An injured person remains unconscious, with pallid skin color, in spite of attempts at resuscitation. You change to heart massage (page 555) while an assistant gives .... until the ambulance arrives.	supine foreign objects free airway back mouth-to-mouth method
11.14	The ambulance brings simple mechanical aids for artificial ventilation which consist of a .... and .... and an automatically filling ...., which considerably eases the rescue work.	artificial ventilation
		mask breathing valve bag

Ventilators

When artificial ventilation must be maintained for a long time, a ventilator is used. The ventilator patient requires more careful observation than some other patients in an intensive care unit.

Ventilator treatment is today always performed by the insufflation method. (The so-called iron lung used earlier, in which all the body but the head was enclosed in a steel cylinder has been abandoned.) For ventilator treatment, an airtight connection with the windpipe is required, via either a tracheal tube (page 510) or a tracheal cannula inserted through an incision in the windpipe (tracheotomy, page 530). The airtight connection is obtained for both the tube and the cannula by means of an inflatable cuff (Fig. 10.6).

Ventilators can operate in different modes: **controlled** breathing and **assisted** breathing. In assisted breathing, the patient's own spontaneous attempt to breathe in causes the ventilator to cycle on during inspiration. In the other mode, controlled breathing, most ventilators take over all the breathing work. If the patient has any spontaneous breathing, it must then be eliminated either by slight hyperventilation or by drugs; many patients that are awake and have some spontaneous breathing rapidly learn to follow the frequency of the ventilator in controlled breathing—that is, to synchronize. Certain servo-controlled ventilators switch automatically to an assisted mode so that the ventilator instead synchronizes to the patient.

The effects obtained with ventilator treatment are threefold:

Adequate ventilation. The ventilation is adjusted so that enough oxygen is supplied and the right amount of carbon dioxide is eliminated. It is necessary to avoid hyperventilation, which causes respiratory alkalosis, and hypoventilation which produces respiratory acidosis (pages 157 and 575).

Elimination of respiratory work. The ventilator takes over the respiratory work, which is due partly to the **resistance**, $\Delta P/\dot{V}$, consisting mainly of the airway resistance, and partly to the **compliance**, dV/dP, the elastic component in movements of the chest and lungs (page 151).

Increased intrathoracic pressure. Ventilator treatment produces abnormal pressure conditions in the thoracic cavity. The pressure is normally negative for a large part of the breathing cycle, because of the expansion of the thoracic cavity and the diaphragm, and this negative pressure helps to return the blood to the heart. Artificial ventilation with intermittent positive pressure interferes with the return flow, and this reduces the cardiac output. The increase in pressure is, however, beneficial in several pathological conditions; it prevents atelectasis, that is, collapse of portions of the lung, and counteracts edema of the lung (pages 28 and 497).

The gaseous mixture supplied must have a high enough moisture content to prevent dehydration of the mucous membranes. It must be heated to insure close to 100 percent relative humidity at body temperature.

With certain ventilators it is possible to withdraw air during expiration by applying a negative pressure. This can increase the circulation due to improved return of the blood, but there is a risk of collapse of the bronchi and uneven air distribution.

Every ventilator operates cyclically. During **insufflation** (blowing in), air or some other gaseous mixture is pumped into the lungs. During **expiration** the pressure ceases. This cycle is regulated by a mechanical, pneumatic or electronic circuit. The regulation can be accomplished using different principles; there are **pressure-limited**, **volume-limited** and **servo-controlled** systems.

Pressure-limited ventilators work on the principle that insufflation is terminated when the gaseous mixture pumped into the patient's lungs reaches a pre-set pressure. The pressure operates a diaphragm-controlled cut-off valve. The pressure at which the insufflation is terminated is varied by spring loading the diaphragm with different forces. The length of the expiratory phase can be varied by adjusting the recovery speed of the cut-off valve's diaphragm.

A number of pressure-limited ventilators can also be **flow-limited**, the insufflation being stopped only when the gas flow has ceased. This occurs when the insufflated volume is consistent with the chest wall compliance and the pressure set on the ventilator. Such flow-limited systems have the advantage that the inspiratory phase is not stopped in the case of sudden random increases in pressure.

All pressure-limited ventilator systems have the disadvantage that the ventilation volume is unknown. If the airway resistance is altered during the treatment the ventilation will also change. Pressure-limited ventilators can be used when the resistance and compliance do not vary or deviate too much from the normal—for example, in patients with respiratory paralysis but no lung complications.

Pressure-limited ventilators are driven by the compressed gaseous mixture used for ventilation. They are thus simple in design and reliable in operation.

Volume-limited ventilators. For this type of ventilator, the design aims at delivering a constant volume for each breath. This is accomplished by having a rubber bag fill to the required delivery volume. During insufflation the bag is emptied by applying external pressure to a chamber containing the bag. The power system is thus separated from the patient system by the walls of the bag (Fig. 11.7).

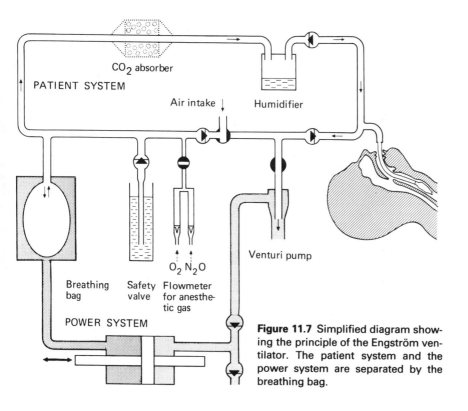

Figure 11.7 Simplified diagram showing the principle of the Engström ventilator. The patient system and the power system are separated by the breathing bag.

The maximum pressure developed in the patient system must be limited to prevent rupturing the lungs. A simple pressure-sensitive safety valve—a water lock or a spring-loaded valve—is provided. Volume-limited ventilators do not give the desired ventilation in cases where the pre-set maximum pressure cannot completely empty the bag.

Resistance to expiration should be as low as possible. However, in treatment of pulmonary edema an increased expiration pressure by loading the valve is useful. This causes a positive pressure in the alveoli to force the fluid back into the blood vessels.

A negative pressure in the lungs during expiration can be produced with a special electrically driven fan, or with a venturi pump placed in the expiration circuit (Fig. 11.7).

Servo-controlled ventilators. The use of modern electronic control techniques has made it possible to design ventilators with properties that could not be attained with mechanical ventilators (Fig. 11.8).

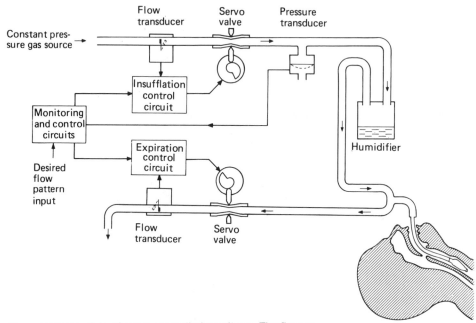

Figure 11.8 Principle of servo-controlled ventilator. The flow to and from the patient is controlled by feedback circuits.

The principle is simple. The flow to and from the patient is controlled by feedback circuits. The instantaneous flows are sensed by paddle-shaped transducers in the tubes connected to the patient, and electrical signals proportional to the flows are generated. The actual flow signals are compared to the desired flow signals, and any errors are amplified and used to control the flow valves. These servo valves, inserted in the tubes, ensure that the desired ventilation is maintained, independent of the airway resistance and compliance.

The electronic unit contains amplifiers and logic circuits that control the ventilation. It also monitors pressures, activates alarms, and computes mechanical lung parameters.

Varying flow patterns can be easily achieved. This is of importance in order to provide optimal ventilation for different types of pathological disorders. The insufflation may be performed with constant flow, accelerated flow, or decelerated flow. The insufflation time may be set to any desired fraction of the breathing cycle. A pause may be held at the end of the insufflation, during which a constant pressure is maintained in the lungs, and this equalizes the pressures and improves gas exchange. If there is enough spontaneous breathing, the ventilation may be triggered by the patient, for assisted ventilation.

A special sigh function is also included. The tidal volume supplied to the patient is then doubled or tripled every hundredth breath. This causes more natural breathing. Sighing opens up closed airways and alveoli, thereby counteracting atelectasis.

Examples of mechanical lung parameters that can be continuously calculated during ventilation are: compliance, airway resistance during expiration or insufflation, expired minute volume (to check for leaks), tidal volumes, and pause pressure.

Finally, servo-ventilators are smaller, weigh less and consume less power than high performance mechanical ventilators. The noise level is also very low, which makes ventilator treatment less irritating for the patient.

When reliable PCO_2 transducers become available for in vivo use, the patient can be included in the servo loop. Then the ventilation can be automatically adjusted to produce the desired blood gas concentration.

General considerations for ventilator use. One difficulty in determining the exact magnitude of the ventilation in liters per minute is presented by the so-called **compression losses**. As the pressure in the lungs and tubing increases during insufflation, the gaseous mixture in them is compressed. In this way the patient only receives part of the volume variation, and the ventilation is smaller than expected. To ensure low compression losses, the patient system of the ventilator must have a small volume. The compression losses are particularly great in the case of young children. The compression losses in the ventilator can be determined from the pressures and volumes in it.

It must be possible to clean, disinfect and, if necessary, sterilize the various parts of a ventilator after use.

A ventilator is used in inhalation anesthesia, when controlled breathing is necessary (page 513). Different gaseous mixtures are supplied to the patient system. The ventilators can also be used for administering anesthesia using the principles of re-breathing (pages 514 and 516).

11.15	The purpose of ventilator treatment is to provide adequate ...., eliminate the patient's .... and sometimes increase the intrathoracic	
11.16	Low ventilation results in accumulation of carbon dioxide in the body, which leads to .... (change in the "internal environment")	ventilation respiratory work pressure
11.17	Excessive ventilation leads to blowing off carbon dioxide, which results in	acidosis
11.18	Respiratory work is required to overcome .... in the airway and .... in the chest wall.	alkalosis
11.19	To prevent damage to the mucous membranes in the airway during ventilator treatment, the air or gaseous mixture used must have a sufficiently high .... and be	resistance $\Delta P/\dot{V}$ compliance dV/dP
11.20	The ventilator's operation cycle consists of two phases, ... (blowing in) and .... (air passing out).	moisture content heated
11.21	When the patient has insufficient spontaneous breathing, ... can be given, and then the insufflation is synchronized with the patient's	insufflation expiration
11.22	To control the ventilator's working cycle either the .... or the .... of the insufflated gas is used, or a combination of the two.	assisted ventilation inspiration
11.23	Pressure-limited systems have the disadvantage that the .... is not known.	pressure volume
11.24	A pressure-limited ventilator has, however, the advantage that the design is .... and	ventilation volume
11.25	Volume-limited ventilators have the advantage that the .... can be determined.	simple reliable in operation
11.26	The ventilation is expressed in .... (units).	ventilation

11.27	In calculating the ventilation for a volume-limited ventilator, particularly in .... (type of patient), a correction must be made for compression losses in the gas present in the	liters/minute
11.28	Two patients with respiratory failure, one that has taken an overdose of sleeping pills and the other with grave asthma, are admitted to a hospital where there are only two ventilators. One is an early pressure-limited type and the other a more recent servo-controlled type. The patient suffering from poisoning from the sleeping pills is given the ....-limited one in this case because the .... and .... are probably more or less normal and constant.	children ventilator
11.29	During treatment of the asthmatic patient the airway resistance changes. The servo-controlled ventilator then gives .... (increased, unchanged, reduced), ventilation.	pressure resistance compliance
		unchanged

Hyperbaric Treatment with Oxygen

The conveyance of oxygen from the air to the cells occurs in four phases: ventilation, diffusion, circulation and cell respiration (page 142). By means of artificial ventilation, with or without a ventilator, only the ventilation is directly affected. Deficiencies in the other stages can also be remedied by giving **hyperbaric oxygen treatment**, in which oxygen is given at increased atmospheric pressure.

Physiological principles

When air is breathed at normal barometric pressure, the oxygen in the blood is carried mainly by chemical binding with hemoglobin; only a small part of the transported oxygen is physically dissolved in plasma (Table 11.1). In arterial blood the hemoglobin is about 97 percent saturated, although the partial pressure of the oxygen is only about 100 mm Hg (13.3 kPa) (page 153). The arterial blood thus contains 200 ml of oxygen/liter of arterial blood, 3 ml of which is physically dissolved on the average. The tissues take up about 60 ml/liter during the passage of the blood through the capillaries (a–v O_2 difference). The venous blood contains about 140 ml/liter.

If the oxygen pressure is increased, for instance by breathing pure oxygen at 3 atm, the arterial PO_2 increases to about 2,000 mm Hg, and since the amount of physically dissolved oxygen increases linearly with PO_2 $(0.031 \text{ ml} \times 1^{-1} \times \text{mm Hg}^{-1})$, the physically dissolved oxygen increases to 60 ml/liter, and the entire oxygen needs of the tissues can be transported without the aid of the hemoglobin. Alternatively, an abnormally increased oxygen need or a reduced transport capacity can be compensated by hyperbaric oxygen treatment.

Table 11.1   Physiological principle for hyperbaric treatment

			Breathing of		
			Air 1 *atm*	100% O_2 1 *atm*	100% O_2 3 *atm*
Arterial blood	Oxygen content	ml/l	200	220	260
	Hb saturation	%	97	100	100
	PO_2	mm Hg	90	650	2,000
	Physically dissolved O_2	ml/l	3	20	60
Tissues	Extraction	ml/l	60	60	≈ 60
Venous blood	Oxygen content	ml/l	140	160	200
	Hb saturation	%	70	85	100
	PO_2	mm Hg	40	50	100
	Physically dissolved O_2	ml/l	(1.2)	(1.5)	(3.0)

In practice, the treatment is given in the following way. The patient is enclosed in a pressure chamber, which is filled with oxygen at the desired pressure; for safety the chamber can also be filled with air and the oxygen is then supplied via a special transport system. The pressure chambers are either just large enough to provide room for the patient lying or seated, or large enough to take four persons, so that surgical operations can be performed.

Hyperbaric oxygen treatment is attended by certain risks because oxygen is toxic and can cause explosive fires.

Oxygen poisoning produces spasms which begin as twitching in the face and develop into potentially fatal, epileptic-like attacks (page 241), and can lead to death. Treatment must therefore be limited in time—3 hours in pure oxygen at 3 atm is relatively safe; however, hypersensitive persons can develop symptoms after only 10 minutes at this pressure.

The risk of explosions in an atmosphere of pure oxygen should not be underestimated—many substances that do not burn in air burn explosively in pure oxygen—for example, sheet steel.

Clinical applications

Hyperbaric oxygen therapy is used in the treatment of certain diseases characterized by impaired utilization of oxygen or inadequate oxygen transport. Two
examples will be described below: anaerobic infections and carbon monoxide
poisoning. Hyperbaric oxygen therapy is also used in certain skin problems, such
as burns, and leg ulcers that are slow to heal.

Anaerobic infections. Anaerobic bacteria are characterized by the fact that they
can grow only at low oxygen tensions. Gas gangrene and tetanus are examples of
diseases caused by such anaerobic bacteria. Patients with gas gangrene can be
effectively and dramatically cured with hyperbaric oxygen treatment. The fever
falls from 40°C (104°F) to normal within 24 hours and the patient's general
condition is radically improved. In tetanus the treatment is less effective and
seldom used, because these patients also require other types of intensive care,
which are difficult to combine with the treatment in a pressure chamber.

Carbon monoxide poisoning is caused by blocking of the oxygen transport
capacity of hemoglobin. Carbon monoxide binds to hemoglobin 200 times more
readily than oxygen does. Hyperbaric oxygen treatment enables the cells to be
supplied with oxygen without requiring any transport by the hemoglobin. For
effective treatment the patient should be placed in a pressure chamber without
delay—within half an hour of poisoning.

11.30	Treatment with oxygen under positive pressure is called .... therapy.	
11.31	The treatment is based on the fact that the transport can be considerably increased because oxygen is .... in plasma.	hyperbaric oxygen
11.32	Hyperbaric oxygen treatment is performed at not more than .... (pressure).	physically dissolved
11.33	The risks associated with such treatment are due to the .... effect of the oxygen and to the fact that it can cause	3 atm
11.34	Hyperbaric oxygen therapy can be used for treating diseases where the .... of the body are increased or the .... is reduced.	toxic explosive fires

11.35	Examples of such disease; are .... and	oxygen needs oxygen transport
		anaerobic infections carbon monoxide poisoning

CIRCULATION

A reduced circulation, so-called **circulatory failure (insufficiency)**, can range from a moderate drop in blood pressure to complete arrest of the circulation. The pathological picture and the methods of treatment therefore vary widely; in grave forms of circulatory failure, intensive care is required in coronary care units.

In acute **cardiac arrest** unconsciousness follows within 6–10 seconds because the brain is deprived of oxygen. To prevent permanent damage to the brain, treatment must be started within 3 minutes. In **shock** the blood pressure is lowered and this decreases the oxygenation of the tissues. Prevention and treatment of shock are very common measures taken during operations, and the treatment is continued afterwards in the intensive care unit. A special form of intensive care is required in **myocardial infarction**, not always because of imminent circulatory failure but because of the risk of heart arrhythmia which can lead to cardiac arrest. Sometimes special methods are required to provide temporary **artificial circulation**—for example, heart-lung machines and equipment for assisting the circulation.

CARDIAC ARREST

Cardiac arrest is due either to ventricular fibrillation or to asystole—cardiac standstill (page 196). It is unnecessary to distinguish fibrillation from asystole immediately, since the initial treatment in either case is identical. The four clinical signs of cardiac arrest are:

- **unconsciousness**
- **absence of pulse**, for example in a neck artery
- **dilated pupils**, which do not react to light
- **respiratory arrest** (due to oxygen deficiency in the brain, and consequent paralysis of the respiratory center)

Treatment of cardiac arrest must be given immediately. It is of vital importance that the brain be given oxygen before the nerve cells are damaged. Treatment must be given in the right order:

1. **Artificial ventilation.** To maintain the blood circulation is meaningless unless the blood is oxygenated, and this can be accomplished only through the lungs. The first step is therefore to give artificial ventilation (page 540).

2. **External heart compression.** The chest is compressed 4–6 cm by pressing rapidly on the sternum about 60 times a minute (Fig. 11.9). By compressing

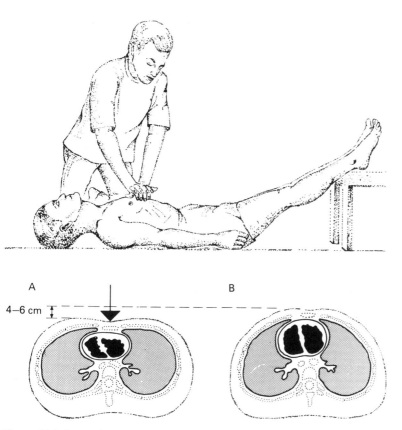

A   B

4–6 cm

Figure 11.9 External compression of the heart is accomplished by vertical compressions in the middle of the chest.

the heart the blood is forced out into the aorta and pulmonary arteries. It is important that the compression be performed with rapid compressions so that the blood is ejected into the circulation. Excessive force should be avoided on the chest, however, because of the danger of fracturing the ribs. Moreover, to avoid damage to the liver and other viscera, pressure should not be applied too far down on the sternum.

3. **Raise the legs.**   This eases the return of blood to the heart.

4. **Further treatment**   requires special equipment. An ECG is used to determine whether the circulatory arrest is due to asystole or ventricular fibrillation (page 196). In the latter case defibrillation is performed with a heart

defibrillator (page 217). The halted circulation rapidly produces metabolic acidosis, which must be treated (page 575). Drugs are also given to restore other changes in the internal environment.

It is easy to see when resuscitation has been successful: the dilated pupils contract, the pulse can be felt on the neck, the skin color improves and spontaneous respiratory movements return.

11.36	Reduced blood circulation is called circulatory .... or	
11.37	Ventricular fibrillation and asystole, paralysis of the heart, are the two causes of	failure insufficiency
11.38	A condition which includes low blood pressure and impaired oxygenation of the tissues is called	cardiac arrest
11.39	For some hours a patient has felt unusually tired, and has had slight pain in the middle of the chest. The symptoms are due to myocardial infarction. Complications in the form of ventricular fibrillation ensue. The four symptoms of cardiac arrest are: ...., ..., ... and	shock
11.40	Unconsciousness and respiratory arrest are due to	unconsciousness absence of pulse dilated pupils respiratory arrest
11.41	In cardiac arrest the first three measures to take are (1).........., (2).......... and (3)..........	oxygen deficiency in the brain
11.42	In heart compression the chest wall is compressed by applying pressure to the sternum .... (gradually, rapidly) with a force that is .... (weak, moderate, as much as the rescuer can manage) at a rate of about	(1) artificial ventilation (2) heart compression (3) raise the legs

11.43   Signs of successful resuscitation are that the pupils
        ...., that the return of the .... can
        be felt on the neck, that the patient's ....
        color has improved and that spontaneous
        .... have returned.

rapidly
moderate
(4–6 cm
  compression)
60 times/min

contract
pulse
skin
respiratory movements

SHOCK

Shock is a state that arises as a result of reduced blood circulation. The most important symptom is **low blood pressure**. The pulse may be rapid or slow, depending on the causes of the shock. There is **reduced oxygenation** of the tissues. The external signs in a shocked patient are pallor and cold and moist skin, which sometimes has a characteristic marbled appearance. The urine output is reduced by the low blood pressure. The low tissue oxygenation leads to incomplete glucose combustion, and hence the formation of organic acids. Because the pH is displaced in the acid direction, **hypoxic metabolic acidosis** rapidly develops.

Types of shock

Shock can occur in different ways. Although the symptoms are to a large extent similar, it is necessary to recognize the different types because they require different kinds of treatment.

Cardiogenic shock.   An inadequate pumping action due to damage to the heart gives rise to cardiogenic shock (*cardio*, heart—*gen*, cause). The reason may be myocardial infarction if so much of the heart muscle has been damaged that the heart can no longer maintain the blood pressure. The pumping efficiency can also be lowered by arrhythmia—for example, by a sudden block (page 196).

Hypovolemic shock is caused by reduction of the blood volume (*hypo*, too little—*vol*, volume—*emi*, blood). The most common cause is bleeding, for which reason the condition is also called **hemorrhagic shock**. Hypovolemic shock can also arise in the case of extensive burns, when there are large losses of plasma from the damaged skin area.

A rapid drop in blood volume of 10–15 percent—that is, 500–750 ml in an adult male—does not produce symptoms in a healthy person who is lying down. During effort, however, there is some reduction in functional capacity. A rapid loss of blood amounting to 15–30 percent produces hypovolemic shock. The body can sometimes correct the loss by contraction of the blood vessels. Losses exceeding 30 percent lead to shock with a high risk of immediate death.

In hypovolemic shock the pulse rate is high, for the body tries to compensate for the reduction in circulation by increasing the heart rate.

Neurogenic shock is the commonest cause of low blood circulation. It is also known as primary shock. It is caused by a disturbance of the nervous regulatory system which controls the degree of contraction of the vessels. Vasomotor centers (page 82) in the medulla oblongata are affected. The lack of vessel contraction results in a lower hydrodynamic resistance and blood pressure. The blood collects in the dilated vessels in the abdomen instead of returning to the heart. This lowers the heart's blood supply and aggravates the symptoms.

In this type of shock, unlike other types, the pulse rate is low. The body is unable to compensate for the circulatory failure caused by the lack of vessel contraction because the regulatory system is not functioning.

Neurogenic shock can occur as a result of a mental reaction to pain or frightening experiences (**psychic shock**), due to the effect of poisons (**toxic shock**), due to hypersensitivity to certain substances (**anaphylactic shock**), during operations and general anesthesia (**surgical shock**) and due to general exhaustion (**exhaustion shock**).

Cardiogenic or hypovolemic shock is often complicated by ensuing neurogenic shock. When the regulatory functions of the body are overloaded, **irreversible shock** can develop. For example, severe maximum vascular contraction of the intestines can prevent oxygenation and nutrition and hence lead to necrosis (tissue death) of the intestinal mucosa. Cause and effect are linked in a feedback loop and death can rapidly result.

Supervision and treatment of shock

Prevention of shock is an important measure. The patient is therefore watched carefully. The blood pressure, pulse, temperature and central venous pressure are followed. The measured values are recorded on the medical record so that any changes can be rapidly recognized. The patient's skin color and general condition are, of course, also observed.

The stages preceding shock are, nevertheless, not easily recognized. The body's regulatory system keeps the measured variables within the normal range until the capacity of the system is exceeded, and then shock develops.

The **central venous pressure**, **CVP**, is measured by means of a catheter inserted in the superior vena cava or subclavian vein and an attached water manometer. A falling CVP is a sign of impaired return of blood to the heart. A low CVP can be produced by hypovolemic shock.

If the CVP is high this indicates that the venous blood flowing back to the heart cannot be pumped on to the required extent. In cardiogenic shock the CVP is therefore high. Similarly, the CVP is elevated if too much fluid has been given intravenously. The CVP is normally 2–10 cm H_2O (0.2–1 kPa).

Causal therapy should be used in the treatment of shock. In hypovolemic shock the blood volume must be restored immediately. This is done by giving transfusions of blood or plasma. Blood transfusions are required in the case of major hemorrhages requiring replacement of red cells.

In neurogenic shock, too, the cause should be discovered when possible. If pain causes the shock, a pain-alleviating drug is given. If bacterial toxins cause the shock, steps are taken to combat the infection.

An important measure in shock is to **lower the head**. The blood pooled in the dilated abdominal vessels then flows back to the heart. A lowered head facilitates the blood flow from the heart to the brain. This simple method of treatment is used during operations; if the blood pressure falls, the head is lowered immediately.

11.44	In a patient with a large myocardial infarct, the pumping action of the heart is impaired. The patient becomes increasingly dazed and restless and cold sweat develops. The pulse rate is high, and the blood pressure falls. The symptoms point to	
11.45	The patient's CVP, ..., is .... (high, normal, low).	cardiogenic shock
11.46	A 4-year-old child falls from a fourth-floor window and is admitted to the hospital with pale skin, cold sweat, rapid pulse and low blood pressure. No signs of external bleeding. The abdomen is distended and tense. Diagnosis:	central venous pressure high
11.47	If the CVP had been measured (which, however, should not be done) a .... (low, normal, high) pressure would have been found.	hypovolemic shock
11.48	The patient is suspected of having a ruptured spleen, which causes bleeding into the abdomen, and is immediately given	low
11.49	In a medical course for engineers a film of an operation is shown. Several of the audience feel sick. They become pale and develop a cold sweat. One faints. Diagnosis:	blood transfusions
11.50	The CVP in this person is	neurogenic shock

11.51	The person beside the one that fainted presses his colleague's head between his knees. The dilated . . . . in the abdomen are thus compressed so that the . . . . flow to the heart and . . . . is improved. The treatment has a rapid effect. (It would have been still more effective to have placed the person on the floor and raised the legs.)	low
11.52	When the film is continued, the participants in the course who have recovered, perform self-therapy to eliminate the cause of the shock by	vessels blood brain
		closing their eyes

MYOCARDIAL INFARCTION

The mortality from myocardial infarction is high. More than one half of all deaths in a country with a high living standard are due to cardiovascular diseases, and of these about one half are due to myocardial infarction. The direct cause of death in about one half of the myocardial infarction cases is temporary disturbance of the heart rhythm, and in the other half a lowered pumping efficiency of the heart. If the arrhythmia is discovered in time and treatment is given, the mortality from myocardial infarction can be greatly reduced.

If a clot blocks the blood supply in a coronary vessel, this causes an infarct that lowers the pumping efficiency. If the infarct includes a large part of the heart muscle, the pumping efficiency of the heart is considerably reduced.

Cardiac arrhythmia in myocardial infarction

In most cases of myocardial infarction, rhythmic disturbances develop within three days. They are of different kinds (pages 194–96), often consisting of ventricular extrasystoles and various forms of block. The arrhythmias sometimes develop into ventricular fibrillation or asystole, with circulatory conditions that must be treated within a few minutes or death will follow. For this reason, the patient must be observed and provided with preventive care. Resuscitative equipment must be immediately available. Most patients who exhibit only arrhythmias, without excessive loss of pumping efficiency, survive with such intensive care.

The various arrhythmias have different **prognostic significance**. More than five ventricular extrasystoles per minute is a sign of threatening ventricular fibrillation. Similarly, a 3rd degree AV block is a serious condition, not only as a premonition of fibrillation or asystole but also because the patient often goes into shock. On the other hand, a 1st or 2nd degree block is in itself not associated with an excess mortality; however, a 2nd degree block often leads to a total block (3rd degree block), and prophylactic treatment must therefore be given. A bundle block does not cause any hemodynamic deterioration in the patient, but may precede total block.

In arrhythmia, drugs are used as the **preventive treatment**, to avoid the development of more life-threatening arrhythmias. Certain drugs, for example, the anesthetic lidocaine (xylocaine), reduces the risk of ventricular extrasystoles leading to fibrillation. These patients are therefore given drip infusion of lidocaine. Second degree block and bundle block are treated with pacemakers (page 219).

In circulatory arrest, **resuscitation** should be started within 30 seconds. Ventricular fibrillation can be treated successfully with electrical defibrillation (page 217). Asystole is treated with drugs—for example, epinephrine injected directly into the heart—or pacemakers; the results are, however, poor.

For **circulatory failure** due to myocardial infarction and other causes, the following supportive treatment is given, usually in a coronary care unit (page 497). The oxygenation of the blood is improved by giving oxygen. Digitalis is administered to increase the contractile force of the heart muscle. Morphine alleviates pain and is beneficial in lung edema. In addition, drugs are given to prevent the blood from clotting in the damaged part of the heart muscle or in the venous system; should this happen the clot could come loose and cause an embolism (page 29).

Observation of myocardial infarction

One problem in the treatment of myocardial infarction is the high initial mortality. Many persons die before they seek help or can be transported to a hospital. Even for those who enter a hospital, diagnosis often cannot be made for 12–24 hours. About one half of the patients with initial symptoms suggesting a heart attack have an infarction.

In a coronary care unit electronic instrumentation is widely used to monitor the patients. The most important measurement is the ECG, which gives direct information on any arrhythmia that has developed. Continuous monitoring of other physiological parameters, such as temperature and ventilation, are of less importance in a coronary care unit. Blood pressure can be measured automatically, but there are practical difficulties when the patient is awake, and it is not usually performed routinely. Further details of electronic monitoring techniques are given on pages 585–86.

ECG observation is performed by continuous monitoring of the electrical heart activity and by electronic analysis, whereby any dangerous change sets off an alarm signal. The chief purpose of the analysis is to detect extrasystoles and changes in heart rate. For each patient, individual limiting values for the alarm signal are set and there is no need for a constant watch of the monitors. In addition, the last few minutes of the ECG is stored on a short-time tape loop or solid state memory; in the case of an alarm it can then be played back and visualized, so that the events leading up to the alarm can be established.

11.53	A patient has myocardial infarction. It is highly probable that he will develop . . . . in the course of the next 24 hours.	
11.54	Cardiac arrhythmia may be benign or malignant. A warning of ventricular fibrillation is	cardiac arrhythmia
11.55	To reduce the excitability of the heart muscle and the risk of arrhythmia a drug can be given as an intravenous drip, namely	ventricular extrasystoles
11.56	In the case of a 2nd degree block and in fully developed 3rd degree block the patient can be provided with a	lidocaine (xylocaine)
11.57	In the case of ventricular fibrillation . . . . is performed.	pacemaker
		defibrillation

EXTRACORPOREAL CIRCULATION AND ASSISTED CIRCULATION

In major operations on the heart—for example, the installation of a valve prosthesis or correction of a congenital malformation—the heart cannot maintain the circulation. It is then necessary to provide **extracorporeal circulation** with a special machine.

Although it is technically possible to replace the function of only the right half of the heart (right bypass), the usual practice is to bypass the whole heart. At the same time an artificial lung is used so that the blood is oxygenated and carbon dioxide is removed; for it is difficult to maintain the pulmonary circulation when the heart is not functioning. A **heart-lung bypass** is created. The apparatus used is known as a **heart-lung machine**.

This technique is not presently used in intensive care units but only during operations. It is described in this section, however, because it fulfils the criterion of intensive treatment, namely, that it temporarily takes over vital functions.

There is a need for devices to provide **circulatory assistance** to support a faulty heart. Such devices have not been generally adopted but designs are being tested. Several **artificial hearts** are under development, and these may some day provide a permanent replacement.

Heart-Lung Machines

The technical problems presented by extracorporeal circulation are great. To empty the heart, the blood is led from the vena cava to the heart-lung machine. Here gaseous exchange is accomplished by an artificial lung, after which the blood is returned to the aorta by means of a blood pump (Fig. 11.10). Throughout the

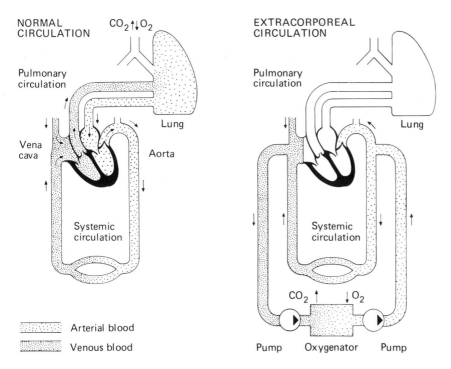

NORMAL CIRCULATION

EXTRACORPOREAL CIRCULATION

$CO_2 \uparrow\downarrow O_2$

Pulmonary circulation

Pulmonary circulation

Lung

Lung

Vena cava

Aorta

Systemic circulation

Systemic circulation

$CO_2 \uparrow$ $\downarrow O_2$

:::::: Arterial blood

▬▬ Venous blood

Pump Oxygenator Pump

Figure 11.10 In extracorporeal circulation the pulmonary circulation and the whole heart are bypassed.

procedure the amount of blood in the vascular system is kept more or less constant. The heart-lung machine operates under sterile conditions so as to prevent infection. It is designed to avoid damage to the blood cells; it is particularly important to avoid hemolysis—breakdown of the red blood cells. Clotting of the blood must be avoided. In addition, the anesthesia depresses the patient's own temperature regulating system, so the temperature is controlled. When the heart-lung machine is connected to the patient and later disconnected, interruption of the circulation must be kept to a minimum. No large fluctuation of the circulating blood volume should occur. The blood in the lungs and in the actual heart muscle must be returned to the circulating blood volume.

The time during which the heart can be bypassed is limited. The actual heart muscle itself can be deprived of its blood supply for at most 10 minutes at normal body temperature. To increase the time available for the operation, **hypothermia** is used—that is, cooling of the whole body, or still better only the heart; the metabolic rate is thus lowered and the time can be increased. At 30°C (86°F) the metabolic rate is reduced by 50 percent and the heart can then tolerate nearly 20 minutes without blood flow. Considerably lower temperatures, down to 15°C (59°F), are also used. This is possible in heart operations, but not in other operations under hypothermia; for at temperatures below about 28°C (82°F) ventricular fibrillation readily occurs. Fibrillation does not interfere with the heart operation and may even be an advantage, since pumping movements do not occur; but in operations on other organs, for example the kidneys, the risk of fibrillation sets a lower limit for the permissible cooling.

The total duration of the extracorporeal circulation with presently available apparatus is restricted to a few hours because of the hemolysis of the red cells.

11.58	To perform an operation on the heart, it must be emptied and an .... (outside the body) circulation must be used.	
11.59	The whole heart is bypassed, which stops the .... circulation. Thus it is necessary to use an artificial	extracorporeal
11.60	The apparatus used for such extracorporeal circulation is known as a	pulmonary lung (oxygenator)
11.61	When a heart-lung machine is connected blood is taken from the .... and after gaseous exchange it is pumped back to	heart-lung machine
11.62	At normal body temperature the heart can be without blood for a maximum of .... (time).	vena cava a large artery
11.63	The time can be increased by inducing	10 minutes
11.64	At 30°C (86°F) the metabolic rate is reduced by .... percent.	hypothermia (cooling of patient)
11.65	Under 28°C (82°F) .... (a condition in the heart) easily occurs (this does not interfere with the heart operation, and may even be an advantage).	50

11.66	The total time during which a heart-lung machine can be connected is limited by the . . . . that occurs, and must not exceed	ventricular fibrillation
		hemolysis a few hours

Oxygenators

The demands on an artificial lung are great. Every minute 5 liters of blood must be spread in a layer thin enough to ensure adequate gaseous exchange. Enough oxygen must be transported to saturate the hemoglobin. The right amount of

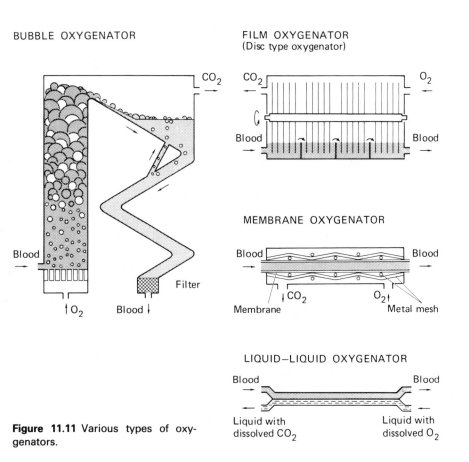

Figure 11.11 Various types of oxygenators.

carbon dioxide must be given off so that the acid-base balance is not disturbed. The oxygenated blood must have all bubbles removed, which would otherwise cause air emboli (page 29). Throughout the process the blood must be carefully handled to reduce the damage of the delicate blood cells; otherwise the body would be unable to dispose of all the decomposition products from the hemolyzed cells.

In oxygenators a mixture of oxygen and 2–5 percent carbon dioxide is usually employed. This sets a lower limit for the arterial carbon dioxide tension, and respiratory alkalosis is avoided (pages 157 and 575).

There are four types of artificial lungs: **bubble oxygenators**, **film oxygenators**, **membrane oxygenators** and **liquid-liquid oxygenators** (Fig. 11.11).

Bubble oxygenators consist of two main components: a column in which oxygen is bubbled through the blood in a finely dispersed form, and a gas-separating component that removes the bubbles and foam. To provide adequate oxygenation is easy; to rid the blood of carbon dioxide is more difficult. To provide adequate carbon dioxide transport it is necessary to have a larger volume of gas than the blood volume in the column. This leads to pronounced foaming and damage to the red cells. Bubble oxygenators are therefore suitable only for short operations. They are the least expensive and the most commonly used.

Film oxygenators are of several types. A feature common to them all is that the blood is spread out in a thin film. This is accomplished on plates, metal screens or rotating discs or spirals. An oxygen mixture flows over the thin layer of blood. These oxygenators are slightly less traumatic to the red cells. Film oxygenators have the disadvantage of being difficult to clean.

Membrane oxygenators have the advantage that the blood does not come into direct contact with the oxygen mixture; bubbles and foam therefore do not form. The blood flows on one side of a membrane permeable to gas and a stream of oxygen flows on the other. The membrane is made of microporous polyethylene, whose gas permeability is 10^4 times greater than that of ordinary polyethylene and 100 times greater than that of silicon rubber. In a membrane oxygenator the carbon dioxide transport is limited by the permeability of the membrane. The oxygen transport is limited by the thickness of the blood layer; that is, by the distribution of the blood at the membrane. Membrane oxygenators are not in common use because they are expensive.

Liquid-liquid oxygenators use fluoridized organic compounds as a working fluid. These readily dissolve oxygen and carbon dioxide which then diffuse to and from the blood. Although the blood is in direct contact with the liquid, it is chemically too different from the blood constituents to react with them. It therefore has no harmful effect on the blood. These oxygenators appear to have advantages.

Blood pumps

The central problem in the design of blood pumps is to avoid hemolysis—that is, disintegration of the fragile red cells. The cells must therefore not be exposed to turbulence or being squeezed between moving parts of the pumps. Many of the common techniques for pumping liquids are therefore unsuitable.

A blood pump must meet many other requirements. It must deliver up to 5 liters/min against a pressure of 180 mm Hg (≈ 24 kPa). The pump flow must be controllable and accurately known so that it can be kept constant.

This is usually accomplished by keeping the blood volume in the heart-lung machine constant after equilibrium has been reached. The pump flow is controlled by sensing the blood volume.

The pump must be easy to clean and sterilize. It should not contain dead space where blood can collect and clot. The ideal blood pump has yet to be designed.

The principle on which most blood pumps operate is that one or more tubes are subjected to peristaltic compression. The commonest is a roller pump in which two or more eccentrically mounted and rotating rollers compress the tube which is placed in a semicircular loop on the inside of a cylindrical wall (Fig. 11.12).

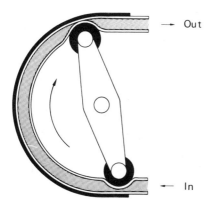

Out

In

Figure 11.12 A roller pump, which has been carefully adjusted so that the rollers just compress the tube, is fairly nontraumatic to the blood cells; however, the maximum time that extracorporeal circulation can be permitted is limited by the hemolysis that occurs.

11.67   The gaseous exchange in a heart-lung machine takes place in an . . . .

11.68	In this, the hemoglobin in the blood is .... with oxygen and its carbon dioxide content is .... so that the acid-base balance is not altered.	oxygenator
11.69	If too much carbon dioxide is blown off .... (type of disturbance of the internal environment) arises.	saturated reduced
11.70	To avoid this, use is made in oxygenators of oxygen to which .... (vol percent) of .... has been added. This sets a lower limit for the arterial	respiratory alkalosis
11.71	Oxygenators are of four types: ...., ..., ... and	2–5 carbon dioxide carbon dioxide tension
11.72	To reduce hemolysis, the blood pump design should provide a flow that minimizes .... Also, the blood cells should not be subjected to unnecessary	bubble oxygenators film oxygenators membrane oxygenators liquid-liquid oxygenators
11.73	Most blood pumps use the principle of .... compression.	turbulence mechanical stress
		peristaltic

Apparatus for Assisting the Circulation

Devices are needed to assist a heart in temporary failure. A balloon is inserted in the aorta via the femoral artery in the groin. The balloon is filled during diastole (dilatation of the heart) and emptied during systole (the contraction) (Fig. 11.13).

Provided that the aortic valves are functioning normally the blood is then ejected into the tissues during diastole and the heart is relieved of the load during systole.

There is a possibility of assisting the circulation without an operation. This could be done by exploiting the fact that the arteries in the lower extremities contain a large volume of blood. The legs are placed in a pressure chamber, which closes tightly against the thighs. In a manner similar to the aortic pump, the chamber is pressurized in synchrony with the heart. The vessels act as a pump chamber, thus relieving the heart's pumping work load. There have been practical difficulties with the method and it is not generally used.

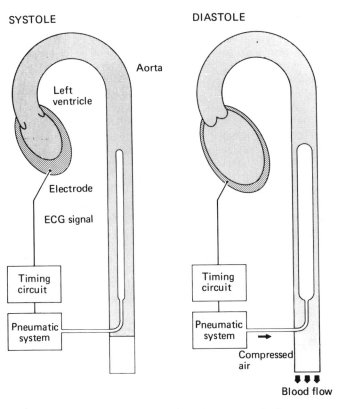

SYSTOLE   DIASTOLE

Aorta

Left
ventricle

Electrode

ECG signal

Timing
circuit

Timing
circuit

Pneumatic
system

Pneumatic
system

Compressed
air

Blood flow

Figure 11.13 Principle of the balloon pump inserted in the aorta
to assist the circulation.

Artificial Hearts

There are three fundamental difficulties in designing an artificial replacement for
the heart. First, any material that is in contact with the blood must not cause
hemolysis or blood clots. The material must be tough enough to withstand 10^5
cycles/24 hours (the heart rate). Second, the pump motor must be designed small,
light, reliable, and efficient enough to enable it to be inserted surgically into the
heart's cavity. Third, the energy supply must be sufficient. A power of 5–50 W is
required depending on the efficiency of the motor.

11.74	The technical procedure, temporarily relieving the load on a failing heart is called ....

11.75	Such aids are often based on the principle of raising the aortic pressure during . . . . and lowering it during	circulatory assistance
		diastole systole

INTERNAL ENVIRONMENT AND NUTRITION

Most problems in intensive care arise due to a disturbance of the body's internal environment. In the healthy individual a large number of regulatory systems ensure that **nutrition, fluid balance, electrolyte balance** and **acid-base balance** are maintained. When there is not enough water we become thirsty and drink, when hungry we eat, when the fluid supply is too great the urine output is increased, when the blood's pH deviates from normal, urine composition is altered and also the amount of expired carbon dioxide so that the acid-base balance is restored.

The critically ill patient cannot always regulate these functions unaided. If the patient cannot take food or drink by mouth, liquid and nutrients are infused, usually in the form of an intravenous drip. The composition is chosen to restore the internal environment. In partial or complete renal failure it is very important to follow the patient closely because the body is deprived of its most important mechanism for restoring the balance (page 293). The blood composition is monitored by chemical analysis and other methods.

Fluid treatment using intravenous drip **infusion** is given for three reasons: to provide **nutrition**, to treat a **disorder** in the internal environment (disturbance of the fluid, electrolyte and acid-base balances) and as a **prophylactic measure** before a major operation. As a basis for the treatment a record is kept on a special fluid-balance sheet of the calculated **needs**, measured and estimated **losses** and supplied **quantities** of various substances.

NUTRITION

The body requires carbohydrates, fats, proteins and certain salts. By intravenous feeding the required nutrients can be supplied so that normal metabolism is maintained over a long period. Carbohydrates are given as a solution of glucose and fructose. Fats are supplied as an emulsion of triglycerides of palmitic, stearic, oleic and linoleic acids; the emulsion contains soybean and cotton seed oils. The proteins can be given in the form of human serum albumin, but this is expensive and entails risk of hepatitis B. It is therefore better for the proteins to be supplied in the form of amino acids in solution from which the body can rapidly synthesize specific proteins. To these nutrient solutions are added minerals, mainly sodium and potassium chlorides; magnesium is also required in long-term intravenous

Table 11.2 Physiological daily needs of certain nutrients

	Water *ml*	*Calories* *kcal* *(kJ)*	*Carbo-* *hydrates* *g*	*Fats* *g*	*Protein* *(amino* *acids)* *g*	*Na+* *mEq* *(mmol)*	*K+* *mEq** *(mmol)*
Per kg body weight	25–35	25–30 (100–125)	2	2	1	≈1 (≈1)	≈0.7 (≈0.7)
For adult man, 70 kg	2,500	2,000 (8,500)	150 (≈600 kcal, ≈2,500 kJ)	150 (≈1,400 kcal, ≈6,000 kJ)	70	80 (80)	50 (50)

* For definition of mEq see page 274.

feeding. The amounts required of these substances are dependent on body size (Table 11.2).

The estimated daily requirement is corrected for any losses. These can occur in many ways. For example, vomiting can cause a large deficiency of electrolytes, mostly chloride and potassium ions—and also a decrease in the hydrogen ion concentration, with resulting alkalosis. In burns there are large fluid losses from the areas where the skin has been lost—the serous fluid is rich in proteins so the patient must be given compensatory amounts of proteins or amino acids.

11.76	During severe illnesses the body's regulatory systems have difficulties controlling ...., ... balance, ... balance and .... balance.	
11.77	The correct internal environment can be restored by	nutrition fluid electrolyte acid-base
11.78	The quantities of the nutrients given are determined by estimating the .... and correcting for any .... that have occurred.	intravenous feeding
11.79	The daily caloric requirement of an adult 70 kg man is about	needs losses
11.80	In intravenous feeding, 600 kcal (2,500 kJ) is usually given in the form of .... and 1,400 (6,000 kJ) in the form of	2,000 kcal (8,500 kJ)

11.81	The protein needs, 70 g/day for a 70 kg man are best supplied in the form of	carbohydrates fat emulsion
11.82	By using the supplied amino acids the body can rapidly .... proteins.	amino acid solutions
11.83	The electrolytes that are most needed in intensive care are .... and	synthesize
		Na$^+$ (sodium) K$^+$ (potassium)

FLUID BALANCE

For normal function the body must have water in the correct amount and in the correct distribution. The body water accounts for between two thirds and one half of the body weight; with variation due to the amount of fat. The body water is about two thirds intracellular and about one third extracellular fluid (page 26). The extracellular fluid includes the plasma volume in the blood; the plasma volume amounts to about 4 percent of the body weight.

When the blood volume varies beyond certain limits severe circulatory disorders arise. One common condition is reduced blood volume resulting in hypovolemic shock (page 557). It is essential to rapidly restore the proper volume of circulating liquid in the vascular system. If blood is not available, plasma is given. In this way the volume of circulating fluid is adjusted so that the heart works satisfactorily. This measure is one of the most important for preventing or treating hypovolemic shock.

The amount of interstitial fluid (fluid between the cells) may increase—a condition called edema. This has several causes. When the colloidal osmotic pressure in the plasma is lowered due to a decreased albumin content, the fluid leaks from the capillaries and cannot be adequately reabsorbed on the venous side (page 281). The patient develops edema, especially at the sites of loose connective tissue such as around the eyes. The correct measure is to raise the colloidal osmotic pressure of the blood.

Edema also occurs in impaired circulation. The excess interstitial liquid collects particularly at the lowest parts of the body: the patient develops edema in the legs. If the circulation cannot be improved, drugs are given to remove liquid by increasing the excretion by the kidneys. Since sodium chloride binds the liquid extracellularly, reduced intake of salt is therefore desirable in cases with impaired circulation.

In a state of too small an amount of body water, the interstitial volume is reduced in particular. The patient is **dehydrated**. The cheeks are sunken and the skin is dry and inelastic. If the skin on the back of the hand is pinched and released it does not recover immediately. The patient is given fluid in the form of isotonic saline (0.9 percent) often combined with other needed electrolytes and nutrients.

Too much fluid causes **hypervolemia**, which causes overloading of the heart. Signs of hypervolemia are elevation of the central venous pressure, CVP (page 558), and moist skin.

ELECTROLYTE BALANCE

The most important ions in the electrolyte balance are the positive ions Na^+ and K^+ and the negative ions Cl^- and HCO_3^-.

As pointed out earlier, most of the sodium ions are located extracellularly. They are thus responsible for a large part of the electrolyte osmotic pressure in the extracellular fluid space. The quantity of water in the body is thus dependent on the quantity of sodium ions.

Most of the potassium ions are located intracellularly. Potassium ion concentration greatly affects the excitability of the nerve and muscle cells (page 272). It is particularly important in intensive care to keep the potassium ion concentration in the plasma within such limits that heart muscle function is not impaired. The treatment of potassium disorders is performed with great care so that the heart rhythm is not disturbed.

The intra- and extracellular potassium ion concentrations are affected by the acid-base balance. In acidosis, potassium ions leave the cell and hyperkalemia results. In alkalosis, the potassium ions move into the cells with resulting hypokalemia. This must be borne in mind in the treatment of disturbances of acid-base balance.

Chloride is the most abundant negative ion in the extracellular fluid. The chloride ion concentration largely follows the sodium ion concentration. A chloride ion deficiency is compensated for by an increase in the quantity of bicarbonate ions and alkalosis develops. Bicarbonate ions are a major factor in determining the acid-base balance.

11.84   A child has severe diarrhea for some days, resulting in large fluid losses. The child is admitted to the hospital in poor condition with signs of dehydration; the skin is dry, cold and cyanotically pale, and the eyes are sunken. The first measure to restore the fluid balance consists of intravenous feeding of .... (blood, albumin solution, plasma, amino acid solution, glucose solution, fat emulsion, isotonic saline).

11.85	Immediately after this the child recovers and chemical analyses of the blood (hematocrit, page 287, electrolytes in the serum, page 272) show that the electrolyte balance is largely restored. The patient's caloric needs are then met by intravenous feeding of .... and	isotonic saline
11.86	A man uses an inflammable cleaning fluid, and a spark from static electricity in the clothes causes an explosion. He suffers extensive burns and is admitted to the hospital. He loses much plasma from the burns, which results in a loss of blood volume. The blood becomes concentrated, increasing the viscosity and further slowing the circulation. Edema develops in the areas of the burns due to a shift in the colloid osmotic balance. The first measure in shock due to burns is to give .... (the same alternatives listed for question 11.84).	carbohydrates fat emulsion (possibly amino acid solution)
11.87	Due to destruction of tissue in the burn, the intracellular .... ions leak out into the plasma, thus raising the concentration and risking .... The infusion solution must therefore not contain this ion.	plasma or albumin solution
		potassium cardiac arrest

ACID-BASE BALANCE

The human body can function only within a narrow pH range (pages 157–59). Normally the pH of the arterial blood is between 7.35 and 7.45. Shifts occur in many pathological conditions when the body's buffering capacity is reduced. This is evident, since the body's 24-hour production of hydrogen ions is equivalent to about 2.5 liters of concentrated hydrochloric acid. Hydrogen ions are eliminated by exhaling carbon dioxide and excreting various acids in the urine. If these functions are disturbed or if the hydrogen ion concentration increases as a result of pathological conditions, potentially fatal complications can rapidly develop. During intensive care it is very important to closely monitor acid-base balance.

In order to treat an acid-base disturbance, its cause must be determined. The patient's condition is checked by using a number of laboratory tests. The presence of an acid-base disturbance is checked by measuring the pH of the blood (page 158). Furthermore, it must be decided whether the changes are of respiratory or metabolic origin. The partial pressure of carbon dioxide in the arterial blood is measured, usually with a PCO$_2$-electrode (page 155). In acidosis of respiratory origin, the PCO$_2$ is over 40 mm Hg (5.3 kPa) and in respiratory alkalosis under 40 mm Hg (5.3 kPa).

To describe the patient's metabolic acid-base disturbance, three parameters are used, the **standard bicarbonate, buffer base** and the **base excess**.

The standard bicarbonate is the HCO$_3^-$ concentration that would exist in the whole blood at a standardized PCO$_2$ of 40 mm Hg (5.3 kPa). The **standard bicarbonate** value is thus the HCO$_3^-$ concentration when the influence of the respiration is eliminated. The standard bicarbonate is usually read from a nomogram based on the Henderson-Hasselbalch formula (page 157). In metabolic acidosis, the standard bicarbonate value is less than 24 mEq/l and in metabolic alkalosis it is more than 24 mEq/l (24 mmol/l).

The total buffer capacity of all buffers together, i.e., not only of the bicarbonate, is called the **buffer base**. The base excess is the change in the buffer base. Thus, the **base excess** is a quantitative measure of the amount of a strong acid or a strong base, expressed in mEq/l (mmol/l), that would be needed to restore the patient's buffer base to normal, i.e., the pH to 7.40 at a PCO$_2$ of 40 mm Hg (5.3 kPa) at 37°C. In metabolic alkalosis the base excess is positive, and in metabolic acidosis it may be called negative, that is, a base deficit prevails. When there is no metabolic acid-base disturbance the value is ± 0.

The situation is complicated by the fact that the organism tends to compensate for these shifts. For example, in metabolic acidosis the ventilation of carbon dioxide increases. Other laboratory tests may be required to completely determine the origin of the pathology.

Shifts in the acid-base balance due to respiratory problems are treated by changing the ventilation. To treat acidosis due to greatly reduced ventilation, a ventilator is used (page 545). Simpler measures, however, often suffice. If the resistance to air flow (page 150) is increased by bronchial spasm, as in asthma, drugs are given that dilate the airways. In mild forms of respiratory failure, breathing exercises may suffice.

If spontaneous hyperventilation leads to respiratory alkalosis—as is common in severe pain—the cause of the hyperventilation must be removed.

In metabolic acid-base shifts, attempts to discover the reason for the pH shift should also be made. For instance, acidosis due to shock (page 557) is corrected by treatment of shock. This form of acidosis, called hypoxic metabolic acidosis, is due to impaired oxygenation of the tissues because of reduced blood circulation, and consequent incomplete combustion of glucose. The result is that organic acids are produced instead of carbon dioxide and water. The acidosis often arises so rapidly, however, that it is necessary to compensate immediately for the pH displacement by giving an intravenous infusion of an alkaline solution. Sodium bicarbonate, sodium lactate and THAM (Tris, tris-hydroxymethyl-amino methane, an organic buffer) solution are used. Sodium bicarbonate produces a rapid correction because the blood's bicarbonate ion concentration is increased directly. One disadvantage is that sodium ions are given at the same time, and these bind water. Sodium lactate is effective only after combustion of the lactate ions in the liver, which results in the formation of bicarbonate ions. One advantage of THAM solution is that it does not increase the amount of sodium ions. Another is that it acts not only extracellularly but also intracellularly, since it diffuses through the cell membranes.

Metabolic alkalosis is a common complication of treatment with drugs that increase the urine output—so-called diuretics. It can also occur when the organism loses large amounts of acid gastric juice, and hence also chloride ions. A fall in the chloride ion concentration is compensated for by a rise in the bicarbonate ion level. Alkalosis can be treated by giving chloride ions (potassium, sodium or ammonium chloride).

11.88	The condition of a patient in an intensive care unit is deteriorating rapidly. Laboratory tests show the following values: pH 7.17 PCO_2 90 mm Hg (12 kPa) Standard bicarbonate 24 mEq/l (24 mmol/l) Base excess 0 mEq/l (0 mmol/l) Diagnosis . . . . Treatment . . . . (the most efficient one possible because the patient's condition is critical).	
11.89	A patient is admitted to the hospital unconscious. He smells of acetone, and diabetic coma is immediately confirmed. In addition to the treatment of the patient's diabetes with insulin, immediate measures must be taken to correct a disturbance of the acid-base balance. Laboratory values: pH 7.20 Standard bicarbonate 12 mEq/l (12 mmol/l) Base excess −18 mEq/l (−18 mmol/l) The patient thus has . . . . which is treated by . . . . (because there is no harm in giving sodium ions).	respiratory acidosis (respiratory failure) ventilator
11.90	The arterial carbon dioxide tension in the patient in the last question was 23 mm Hg (3.1 kPa). This does not mean that there is a respiratory pathological change but that the body is trying to . . . . the metabolic acidosis.	metabolic acidosis sodium bicarbonate infusion

11.91	A patient poisoned by an overdose of sleeping pills is admitted to the hospital with a temperature of 31°C (88°F). He is treated with a ventilator which is set at a normal value of 8 l/min. Blood gas analysis gives the following values: pH 7.60 PCO_2 18 mm Hg (2.4 kPa) Diagnosis . . . . The setting of the ventilator is changed to . . . . (increase, reduce) the ventilation.	compensate for
11.92	The patient in question 11.86 with burns and in a state of shock had the following values: pH 7.21 PCO_2 25 mm Hg (3.3 kPa) Standard bicarbonate 12 mEq/l (12 mmol/l) Base excess −17 mEq/l (−17 mmol/l) The acid-base disturbance is	respiratory alkalosis reduce (cooling reduces the body's metabolism)
11.93	A patient who has undergone a major abdominal operation vomits for several days afterwards, thereby losing large amounts of gastric juice. The patient becomes listless and the breathing is shallow. Laboratory values: pH 7.51 PCO_2 50 mm Hg (6.7 kPa) Standard bicarbonate 34 mEq/l (34 mmol/l) Base excess 11 mEq/l (11 mmol/l) Diagnosis . . . . Treatment	metabolic acidosis (partly respiratorily compensated)
		metabolic alkalosis (partly respiratorily compensated) infusion of NaCl and KCl

DIALYSIS

In the case of complete or advanced renal failure, **uremia** (literally urine in blood, physiologically—retention of urea and other nitrogenous metabolites) develops. Most of the metabolic breakdown products cannot be excreted and they collect in the body. The urea and creatinine levels in the blood rise. The concentrations of these substances are used as a measure of the degree of renal failure (page 297). The kidneys normally regulate the acid-base balance in the body by excreting non-volatile acids; in renal failure, acidosis develops (page 574). Because of the acidosis and the tissue breakdown, the amount of potassium in the extracellular fluid increases, and this may affect the heart function (page 272). The amount of body fluid also increases, since it cannot be excreted. The patient becomes weak and is nauseated. Partial renal damage is frequent. If there is some residual renal function, long survival is possible. If renal failure is complete, death occurs after a week or so. Renal failure can be chronic or acute. Chronic renal failure can be due to nephritis (inflammation of the kidneys), obstruction of the urine by stones or tumors, or disturbed renal circulation. Acute renal failure can be produced by a variety of causes including poisoning by organic and inorganic chemicals and circulatory insufficiency states secondary to trauma. Both acute and chronic renal failure can be treated by **dialysis**. In the presence of complete renal failure or advanced renal failure, dialysis is required two or three times a week.

Dialysis can be **extracorporeal** or **intracorporeal**. In extracorporeal dialysis **(hemodialysis)** blood is purified by an artificial kidney (a hemodialyzer) where waste products diffuse through a semipermeable membrane which is continuously rinsed by a dialyzing solution (dialysate).

In intracorporeal dialysis a membrane in the body is used for diffusion; in clinical application, the peritoneal cavity is employed. The method is known as **peritoneal dialysis**.

The two procedures are complementary. Hemodialysis is the more effective but it is technically more complex and presents some risk. For both the patient and the nursing staff there is a risk of, among other things, transmitting hepatitis B through handling the blood. Peritoneal dialysis is simple to perform but less effective. Hemodialysis is completed within 3–6 hours; peritoneal dialysis requires three times as long.

In dialysis three physical processes can be used: **diffusion**, **osmosis** and **ultrafiltration**.

Substances diffuse through the membrane in the direction from high to low concentration. Waste products are transferred to the dialysate until equilibrium is reached. Similarly, if the concentration is higher in the dialysate, low molecular weight substances diffuse from this into the blood. When equilibrium is reached, the internal environment is corrected to achieve the normal ion concentration. For example, the potassium concentration of the dialysate is adjusted so that the amount of this element in the extracellular fluid compartment is restored to normal. The concentrations of other ions in the dialysate are similarly controlled.

Fluid removal can be achieved by either osmosis or ultrafiltration. During peritoneal dialysis osmotic pressure can be adjusted by altering the glucose concentration of the peritoneal dialysis fluid. A 7 percent glucose concentration will remove large amounts of fluid with each exchange; a 1.5 percent glucose concentration will have a lesser effect.

An alternative way of removing fluid can be utilized in hemodialysis. The hydrostatic pressure of the blood is increased in relation to that of the dialysate in the artificial kidney. In this way the blood is ultrafiltrated and concentrated.

Hemodialysis

In hemodialysis, blood is routed or pumped into an extracorporeal dialyzer. For short term use a double lumen catheter is inserted into the femoral vein; for use over longer periods an **arteriovenous** shunt, a permanent connection between an artery and a vein, is used (Fig. 11.14). In dialysis, the shunt is opened and

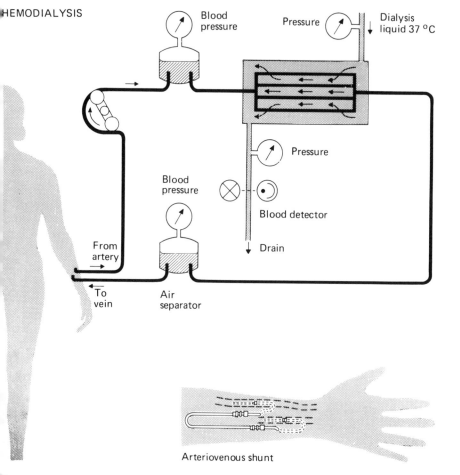

Figure 11.14 Principle of hemodialysis.

connected to the dialyzer. An arteriovenous shunt can function for up to two years if it is carefully managed. Rapid blood flow through the shunt, lowered clotting ability of the uremic blood and the non-thrombogenic properties of the shunt tubings prevent clotting. Careful hygiene is required to prevent infection from spreading into the body where the tube passes through the skin.

There are several types of hemodialyzers. A common feature of them all is that the blood flows on one side of a semipermeable membrane and the dialysate on the other (Fig. 11.14). The membrane is 1 m^2 or more in area.

In the Kolff kidney, also called the Travenol kidney (after one of the manufacturers), the membrane consists of cellophane tubing wound in a spiral on a loose polypropylene screen through which the dialysate is flushed. An advantage of this design is that it is easy to manufacture and use; a disadvantage is that a special pump is required to force the blood through.

In the Kiil kidney, dialysis occurs through a number of planar sheets of cellophane which are pressed together in a frame. Blood flows in alternate spaces, and the dialysate flows in the others. Since only small volumes of blood are required to fill the spaces between the dialysis membranes, this kidney need not be filled with transfusion blood before use. Moreover, as the hydrodynamic resistance is low, no blood pump is required. The arterial pressure is sufficient to maintain the flow. The design of the Kiil kidney is comparatively complex.

A hemodialysis apparatus requires several control circuits. Rupture of a membrane can lead to rapid loss of blood (alternatively the dialysate can enter the blood circulation if the pressure conditions permit). There is therefore a blood leak detector. The pressures in the inlet and outlet circuits are also usually measured. In addition it is wise to monitor the composition of the dialysate—for example, by measuring its electrical conductivity. Thermostatic control of the dialysate temperature at 37°C (98.6°F) is necessary.

Peritoneal Dialysis

In peritoneal dialysis the peritoneal membrane is used as a dialysis membrane. A catheter is inserted in the abdomen through a puncture just below the navel. A sterile dialysate fluid, 1.5–2 liters, is allowed to flow into the abdomen; diffusion takes place in 10–30 min, and the liquid is then removed by aspiration. The procedure is repeated 20–30 times. There is a risk of infection and sterile techniques must be used to avoid peritonitis—that is, inflammation of the peritoneum.

The method is thus simple. It can be performed manually with few technical aids but requires more work.

It is better to use an automatic procedure (Fig. 11.15). Here, sterile dialysate is pumped into the abdominal cavity with a volume-recording pump. The liquid is kept at 37°C (98.6°F) by replacing part of the tube with a stainless steel section, which is warmed by passing an electric current through it; to ensure the correct temperature of the liquid, the current is controlled by a feedback circuit.

The volume-recording pump is also used to empty the abdominal cavity. It is important that no liquid remains in the abdomen. The total amount of liquid per filling should not exceed about 2 liters. Otherwise, movement of the diaphragm is hindered, resulting in respiratory difficulties. A counter records the volume and a logic circuit triggers an alarm if the amount of liquid withdrawn is too small.

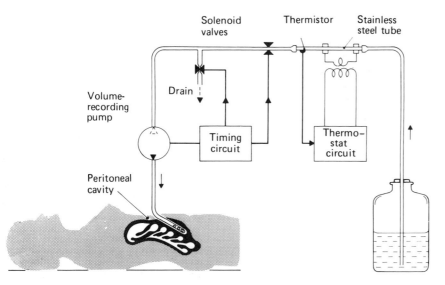

Figure 11.15 Peritoneal dialysis, the abdominal cavity is used as an artificial kidney.

11.94	A patient with chronic renal damage is waiting for a suitable donor for renal transplantation. He is dialyzed regularly twice a week at a special kidney clinic at a fairly large hospital. The patient, who is still able to work, wishes to have the most effective dialysis possible, which takes the least time. Therefore .... (type of dialysis) is chosen.	
11.95	A patient who has taken an overdose of sleeping pills is admitted to a small rural hospital which has limited technical and staff resources. The renal function is poor and it is considered important to eliminate the drug, which has caused respiratory paralysis. The patient is dialyzed for several days by .... (type of dialysis).	hemodialysis (extracorporeal dialysis)
11.96	In dialysis the waste products are transferred to the dialysate by .... (type of physical process).	peritoneal dialysis (intracorporeal dialysis)
11.97	The ions present in the dialysate are transferred to the patient's extracellular fluid so far as the ionic concentration permits by .... (physical process).	diffusion

11.98	In uremic poisoning the patient has excess body fluid. This can be eliminated in hemodialysis by .... and .... (physical principles), and in peritoneal dialysis by	diffusion
11.99	For efficient water removal in peritoneal dialysis a dialysate with a high .... content, usually .... percent, is used.	osmosis ultrafiltration osmosis (only because pressure difference cannot be produced)
		glucose 7

TECHNICAL ASPECTS OF INTENSIVE CARE

Intensive monitoring and intensive treatment present a complex problem of information analysis. The patient's condition is followed carefully by repeated measurement of many variables. Measurement artifacts are disregarded, while significant data are recorded, stored, and analyzed. The most important information analysis task is to reduce the volume of data—that is, to select from the amount of information available only that which is directly useful in the immediate care of the patient. When treatment is performed, the results are monitored and any indicated corrections are made to improve the therapy. Throughout this process technical devices may be heavily involved. These devices must, however, be reliable and simple to use; it is not beneficial to replace a nurse that watches the patient by a technician that watches the monitoring apparatus. The technical problems in intensive care are great.

PARAMETERS IN INTENSIVE MONITORING

In monitoring a seriously ill patient primary attention is devoted to the **respiration**, **blood circulation** and **level of consciousness**. Next in importance are the **temperature** and other body functions, such as **urine production**. A few of these monitored parameters are easy to record with technical devices, but most of them are difficult, mainly because of the lack of suitable sensors.

Some monitoring instruments are indispensible in intensive care. For example, in the heart patient continuous recording of the ECG is essential. The technical methods for recording many other parameters are still inferior to observation by hospital staff. It is true that the latter involves high wage costs, but this disadvantage is outweighed by the fact that the medical results are better; critical conditions are noticed sooner, false alarms seldom arise because artifacts can be discovered, and the patient benefits from the human contact. Thus, both technical aids and staff are needed.

Respiration

The respiratory function can be assessed by estimating the ventilation and by blood analyses.

Ventilation. In practice the possibilities of quantitatively monitoring the ventilation are limited. The patient must breathe through the apparatus to determine the ventilatory volume. This so disturbs the patient that obtaining these data may not be worthwhile.

Therefore usually only the breathing rate is monitored. One way in which this can be done is to place in the dorsal pharynx a thermistor from which a thin lead passes out through the nose. When breathing in through the mouth or nose the temperature falls, and when breathing out it rises. The variation is recorded by the thermistor.

The ventilation can also be followed qualitatively by impedance plethysmography (page 187). The electrodes are placed on each side of the chest at the level of the fifth or sixth intercostal space. The method is comfortable for the patient and the same electrodes can also be used for ECG monitoring. The method has been frequently used in the observation of newborn, when disturbances of respiration sometimes occur.

The ventilatory flow can be measured with a pneumotachygraph, which measures the pressure drop across a fine screen placed in the flow stream. The flow can be integrated to yield ventilation in liters per minute.

Blood gas analyses are best performed by means of arterial samples, which can easily be collected through an intra-arterial catheter. The pH of the blood could also be determined with a needle-shaped glass electrode, which is inserted in an artery. The method is usually not employed in intensive care because the artery might be damaged by the electrode. Sampling by arterial catheter is more comfortable and less risky.

Respiration may be indirectly estimated by measuring the partial pressure of the exhaled carbon dioxide since the alveolar PCO_2 is close to that in the arteries. Carbon dioxide analyzers have therefore been developed to continuously measure the expired PCO_2. These are based on the high absorption of carbon dioxide at certain infrared wavelengths. The method is occasionally used in intensive care.

Blood Circulation

Since the body can go into circulatory failure in a short time, automatic monitoring techniques are important. By measuring the arterial blood pressure, central venous pressure, and ECG, imminent circulatory failure can be detected and treatment, such as intravenous infusions, quickly begun.

Automatic blood pressure measurement is performed either directly or indirectly (see pages 133 and 170).

In direct measurement of the arterial blood pressure, a catheter is placed in an artery and connected to a pressure transducer; the radial artery in the forearm is often used. The detailed arterial pressure contour can also be obtained in addition to the systolic and diastolic values. Clotting of the blood at the catheter tip must be prevented. Therefore, a small amount of the infusion solution flows constantly through the catheter. The solution usually contains heparin, a substance that prevents clotting. An intra-arterial catheter could damage the artery, but with careful technique the risk is small.

Indirect methods for automatic blood pressure measurements (Fig. 11.16) are

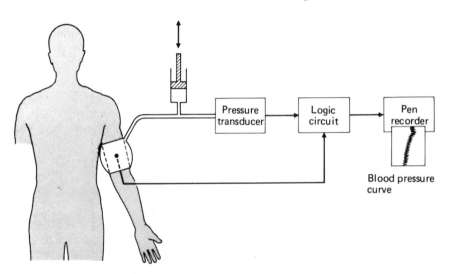

Figure 11.16 In automatic blood pressure measurement by the indirect method, different types of sensors may be used to record the systolic and diastolic pressures. The figure shows schematically a sensor placed under the blood pressure cuff. The sensor may consist of a microphone, an ultrasonic crystal directed towards the artery, or a device that senses pressure changes in the blood pressure cuff during pulsations of the heart.

based on a principle similar to the manual procedure using a blood pressure cuff (page 133). In the manual method, the pressure in the cuff is varied and the operator detects when the blood ceases to flow in the underlying artery. The auscultative method relies on the sound produced when the blood is forced through the compressed artery, and the palpatory method detects when the pulse cannot be felt in an artery peripheral to the compression. In the automatic methods, the pressure in the cuff produces changes in the blood stream, which are detected and recorded.

A number of methods have been developed for this purpose. All can be made to function satisfactorily in patients with normal blood pressure, but most of them fail on patients with shock, where monitoring is most needed. This does not, however, mean that they are not of great value in intensive care, since blood pressure measurements in patients without shock take up a large part of the working time of staff engaged in patient monitoring.

One of the best methods for recording the blood pressure under a cuff is to measure the volume changes that occur in the cuff when the blood pushes past the constriction formed by the cuff. A form of oscillometry is thus employed (page 186). If one cuff is used, only the systolic blood pressure can be measured. From the phase displacement of the volume changes in two cuffs, one of which is peripheral to the other, the diastolic pressure can also be measured.

For acoustic recording of blood pressure under the cuff a microphone is placed under it (see page 134). The position of the microphone is critical, however, and extraneous sounds make the method unreliable.

The blood pulsations can be observed by optical absorption measurements in tissues peripheral to the cuff—for example, in a finger. The method is sensitive to motion artifacts and is unreliable at low blood pressures.

By directing an ultrasonic beam at the artery, wall movements can be recorded. An ultrasonic crystal is placed under the cuff so that the beam is normal to the artery. This method uses the Doppler effect—the shift in frequency of the reflected sound is caused by wall motion. Accurate measurements of the movements of the artery wall can be made and both systolic and diastolic blood pressure can be recorded. The method has the disadvantages that it is somewhat sensitive to motion artifacts and that the orientation of the ultrasonic crystal is critical.

Impedance plethysmography—that is, the measurement of the tissues' electrical impedance—is also used for automatic indirect recording of the blood pressure by sensing arterial pulsations peripheral to the cuff.

The complexity of the problem is illustrated by the large number of indirect methods for automatic measurement of blood pressure that have been proposed.

Central venous pressure, CVP. The usual way of measuring the central venous pressure is by using a liquid manometer connected to a catheter inserted in a vein, so that its tip is located near the right atrium. Clotting is prevented by constantly infusing liquid through the catheter. A simple liquid manometer of this type is better than more advanced pressure transducers. Since the central venous pressure is only 2–10 cm H_2O (0.2–1 kPa) the value of the method is dependent on the accuracy with which the transducer or the liquid meniscus can be positioned in relation to the body (Fig. 3.15, page 170). Transducer measurement of the CVP provides no real advantage in practice, since the apparatus is more complex, difficult to manage and sensitive to motion.

Monitoring with ECG. An indispensible technical method in many intensive care cases is ECG monitoring. Only the ECG enables rhythm disturbances of the heart to be correctly diagnosed. Other heart disorders also can be detected rapidly by this means. The method is well suited for including an automatic alarm signal. The ECG also enables the heart rate to be measured; this is of great diagnostic importance—for example, for distinguishing between different kinds of shock (page 557). For monitoring, the ordinary ECG technique described above (pages 188–213) is used; there is, however, a great need for data reduction and some form of data storage.

In order to view the patient's ECG in real time and to reduce and store the resulting data, special intensive care equipment has been designed. **Cardioscopes**—cathode ray oscilloscopes with a long persistence screen or with digital memories—are located both at the bedside and at a central nursing station in the intensive care unit.

One special kind of cardioscope is the **contourograph**, on which a large number of ECG curves from the same patient are shown one above the other. In this way it is possible to examine the previous 5–10 minutes of the ECG. Disturbances in rhythm and rate are reflected as changes in the pattern of the ECG curves.

When the nurse is unable to keep a constant watch on the cardioscope, alarm signals are employed. Limiting value alarms are used for the heart rate—a signal is emitted if the heart rate exceeds or falls below certain preset values. Some cardioscopes contain arrhythmia detectors, which emit a signal if there is a disturbance in rhythm.

The heart rate meter contains a bandpass filter, which eliminates low and high frequency artifacts. The resulting R wave triggers a circuit that measures each R–R interval, then inverts it to form the heart rate. The beat-to-beat heart rate is continuously displayed on a meter that contains high and low limit alarms. These summon the nurse if the heart beats too rapidly or slowly for a period of more than, say, five seconds.

A small special purpose computer may be employed to search for ventricular extrasystoles. These can be recognized because they occur earlier than normal and are wider than normal. The computer declares an R wave **early** if its R–R interval is less than say 90 percent of that of a running average. The computer declares a QRS complex **wide** if its width exceeds more than say 120 percent of a previously stored normal value. If the wave is both early and wide, the computer signals a ventricular extrasystole. If more than, say, 3 occur per minute, an alarm summons the nurse. Computers may also be used to monitor other, more complex variables and to calculate and display data and data trends for a number of patients.

If an unusual event occurs on the ECG, the physician would like to examine the events that led up to it. Therefore, a permanently connected tape recorder records the ECG signal on a tape loop. If an event occurs, the signals stored on the loop are transferred to an ordinary ECG recorder. Thus, any time a decision is made, the recorder can reproduce events from one minute in the past to any time in the future. Since continuously operating tape recorders have high maintenance problems, electronic semiconductor memories are replacing the tape loops.

Level of Consciousness

Automatic observation of the level of consciousness is very difficult. The way in which EEG recording can in principle be used in this connection has been described above (page 244). The value of the method in intensive care is, however, restricted to special cases of deep unconsciousness. Simple observation of the patient yields considerably more refined information on the patient's condition, more rapidly and with less effort than does the EEG. With a glance and a brief question it is also possible to ascertain the patient's state of mind, physical activity, mental alertness, pupil size and the presence of spasms, etc. By direct observation of the patient such findings can be rapidly analyzed to give a diagnostic interpretation.

Temperature Measurement

Automatic temperature measurement is easy to perform. However, the sensor must be placed where the body temperature can be measured. The sensor is often a thermistor which can be placed in the rectum, the mouth or the esophagus. Since sensors and their cables are often disturbing to a conscious patient, automatic temperature measurement is more suitable in the case of the unconscious patient.

AUTOMATIC DATA ANALYSIS IN THE INTENSIVE CARE UNIT

In care of the critically ill patient large quantities of data are collected. For example, during a major heart operation and the following 24 hours, over a thousand observations, measurements and laboratory examinations are made. Without the aid of automatic data processing it is difficult to analyze this amount of information, and appropriate treatment is thus delayed. In addition, the choice of treatment could then be made only after simple, rough calculations. This results in only an estimate for the required therapy, followed by a remeasurement of the variable. Thus the therapy proceeds by trial and error.

With the aid of automatic data processing the collection of data, its storage, processing and presentation are more efficiently performed. Provided that reliable data sensors can be applied to the patient, some data can be collected on-line. This enables up-to-date judgments of the patient's condition to be made.

But the on-line technique is not always preferred, since with manual collection of data, artifacts are more easily discovered. Also, most data cannot be obtained on-line since they consist of laboratory results, therapeutic measures taken, etc.

With automatic data processing many calculations regarding the patient's condition can be performed continuously that would not otherwise be possible because of the time factor. The data can be presented much more rapidly and more effectively. The data are generally presented on a CRT screen in both graphic and alphanumeric form. Because of its high cost such equipment is used only in more advanced intensive care units.

Automatically Controlled Administration of Drugs

It is often desirable to select the dose of a medicine according to the patient's state at a particular time. For example, in neurogenic shock or in poisoning by sleeping pills, the centers controlling the blood pressure (page 93) in the medulla oblongata are paralyzed. Drugs are administered to raise the blood pressure, with the dose carefully adjusted according to the measured blood pressure. This is difficult to achieve by manual measurement. The problem is obviously one of control technique. Methods have therefore been developed for regulating the dose in cases where the body's own mechanism for regulating the blood pressure is not functioning.

One system is shown in Fig. 11.17. The feedback loop contains a sensor that

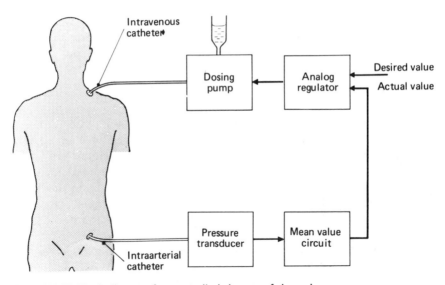

Figure 11.17 Block diagram for controlled dosage of drugs in automatic regulation of blood pressure in a patient in shock.

measures the pressure in the femoral artery. The pressure variations during the heart cycle are smoothed out in a mean value calculator, which gives a signal proportional to the "actual" value for the patient's blood pressure. A comparison is made with a "desired" value, which is determined for each case. The difference between these two values is the error signal, which actuates a PID regulator.

This regulator is set for optimal function of the control circuit by independent adjustment of the gain, integration time constant and differentiation time constant. The rate at which the drug is injected is chosen as a combination of a proportional, P, integrated, I, and differentiated, D, value of the error signal. In this way the blood pressure can be set in a short time with little overshoot.

Similar dosing systems have been developed for other types of drug therapy. For example, in diabetic coma, attempts have been made to control the supply of insulin on the basis of the instantaneous blood sugar level. Some time lag in the system is unavoidable because the chemical analysis takes a minute or so. This is not critical because the time constant of the body's blood sugar level control system is comparatively large. As has been mentioned above, attempts have been made to control general anesthesia by means of EEG signals (page 244).

11.100	In most intensive care units, the most important variable to monitor is the	
11.101	By measuring the following variables, it is possible to monitor the (1) circulation . . . . , ... and . . . . (2) respiration . . . . and . . . . (3) metabolism	ECG

11.102	The level of consciousness can be followed only in very special cases by means of the . . . . ; in practically all cases monitoring by the . . . . is required.	arterial blood pressure
		CVP
		ECG
		breathing rate
		blood gas
		  analysis
		temperature (cf. ques-
		  tion 11.91)

11.103	The purpose of automatic data processing in intensive care is to obtain better . . . . concerning the patient's condition, better . . . . which provides for quicker access, more effective . . . . and finally convenient . . . . for physicians and nurses.	EEG staff
11.104	Administration of drugs by using feedback control has been tested in the cases where the body's own . . . . have been paralyzed or disabled.	data collection data storage data analysis data presentation
		regulatory functions

REFERENCES

GOLDIN, M. D. (ed.). *Intensive Care of the Surgical Patient.* Chicago (Year Book) 1971. 500 pages.

GOTCH. F. A. *The Evaluation of Hemodialyzers.* (DHEW Publication NIH 72–103) Washington, D. C. (U.S. Government Printing Office) 1972. 84 pages.

LOWN, B. Intensive Heart Care. *Sci. Amer.* Vol. 219 (1968) No. 1. Pp. 19–27.

RAVIN, M. B. and MODELL, J. H. (eds.). *Introduction to Life Support.* Boston (Little, Brown) 1973. 183 pages.

RUBENSTEIN, E. *Intensive Medical Care.* New York (McGraw-Hill) 1971. 276 pages.

STEPHENSON, H. E. *Cardiac Arrest and Resuscitation.* 4 ed. Saint Louis (Mosby) 1974. 998 pages.

chapter 12	# Obstetrics

Pregnancy and delivery are natural processes, which usually run their course without complications. Nevertheless, modern medical care is still needed to reduce the risks for mother and child. The mother makes regular visits to her physician, who determines if the pregnancy is proceeding normally. This provides an opportunity to discover and treat any pathological conditions at an early stage.

During the delivery, both the mother and the fetus are closely monitored. The mother receives **obstetrical care**, which usually includes alleviation of pain. Complications may require rapid intervention. During delivery, certain technical equipment may be used for supervision and treatment. Anesthesia may also be required.

The branch of surgery concerned with pregnancy, labor and childbirth is called **obstetrics**.

Obstetric terminology

In both medical and legal contexts (inheritance decisions), it is important to know whether a woman has given birth to a living child, a dead child or has had a miscarriage. The following nomenclature has therefore been introduced.

A woman has had a **live birth** if the infant shows one of the three evidences of life (breathing, heart action, voluntary muscle movement). A birth certificate is filed with the local health department. Otherwise it is a **still birth**.

An **abortion** (miscarriage) occurs if a fetus is expelled before 20 weeks. The abortion can be spontaneous or induced. Most spontaneous abortions occur during the first trimester.

The number of pregnancies that a woman has had is denoted by the stem **gravida**—thus, Gravida I (primigravida), Gravida II, etc. (for more than one pregnancy, multigravida). The number of children delivered (beyond 20 weeks) is denoted by the stem **para**—thus, Para 0 (nullipara), Para I (primipara), etc. (for more than one child, multipara).

For denoting the stage of maturity of the child at birth the term **immature** is used for a child born with a gestation period between 20 and 28 weeks. Formerly the term **premature** was applied to birthweights less than 2500 g, but now a better indication is obtained from measurements on the amniotic fluid, and concentration of creatinine and **surfactant**—a surface tension-lowering substance secreted onto lung surfaces.

A distinction is made between the different periods of a pregnancy. **Natal** denotes the birth period, the time around delivery. **Prenatal** and **postnatal** are thus the times before and after birth, respectively. The **perinatal** period is the time from 20 weeks gestation to four weeks after delivery. The **neonatal** period is the first four weeks after birth.

Table 12.1 Obstetric terminology

abortion	expulsion of a fetus before 20 weeks or weighing less than 500 g
child	a newborn that after birth has breathed or shown other signs of life
gravida	the number of pregnancies
immature child	between 20 and 28 weeks gestation
mature child	formerly weight >2500 g, but now better defined by measurements on the amniotic fluid, and concentration of surfactant and creatinine
natal	period of birth
neonatal	first four weeks after birth
para	the number of children that a woman has carried and delivered after 20 weeks gestation
perinatal	from 20 weeks gestation to 4 weeks post delivery
postnatal	after birth
premature child	formerly weight <2500 g, but now better defined by measurements on the amniotic fluid, and concentration of surfactant and creatinine
prenatal	before birth

PREGNANCY

The sexual functions are governed by hormonal control systems. In the woman the pituitary (page 74), in combination with a number of other endocrine glands, controls the **sexual drive**, **menstrual cycle**, **pregnancy** and **lactation** (the secretion of milk).

Menstrual cycle

The woman's menstrual cycle exhibits a number of phases. Figure 12.1 applies only to a normal cycle of 28 days—for the sake of simplicity, the times are related to the first day of the cycle when bleeding occurs.

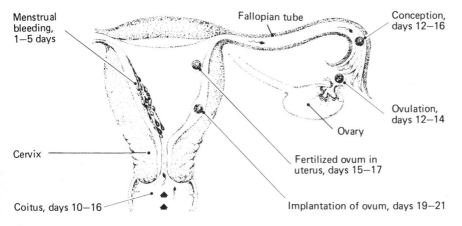

Figure 12.1 The menstrual cycle, fertilization and transport of the ovum. The times given are days of the cycle in a normal menstrual cycle of 28 days.

The menstrual cycle begins with bleeding, when the **endometrium**, the mucous membrane in the uterus, breaks down. After 3–5 days, the bleeding ceases and the mucous membrane proliferates, that is, the inner surface lining of the uterus is covered with new cells: the uterus prepares to receive the fertilized ovum. The ovum, which is normally released from one of the **ovaries** during the 12th–14th day of the cycle, emerges into the abdominal cavity and then enters the **fallopian tube**. It is slowly conveyed down through this to the **uterus**. If the ovum is not fertilized during its passage through the tube it does not become attached to the mucous membrane of the uterus but is lost. The mucous membrane is then broken down again and bleeding recurs.

The menstrual cycle is accompanied by rhythmic changes in metabolism, which can be followed objectively. Chemically determinable changes in the secretion of hormones in the urine reflect the conditions in the body. In addition, there is a rise in the body temperature of 0.3–0.5°C (0.5–1.0°F), after **ovulation**; by taking the temperature it is thus possible to obtain confirmation that this has occurred.

Conception

For **conception** (fertilization) to occur, there must be a close correspondence in time between **ovulation** and **coitus**, sexual intercourse. The survival time of the ovum after ovulation is short, about 8–12 hours, as is the survival time of the sperm in the female genital tract, about 3–4 days (Fig. 12.1).

During sexual intercourse, the seminal fluid is deposited around the cervix in the vagina. The sperm swim in the thin secretion with which the canal of the cervix is filled at this time in the menstrual cycle, and are aided by a rhythmic muscular activity in the uterus and fallopian tubes after coitus. The transport of the sperm from the vagina to the upper part of the fallopian tube, where fertilization of the ovum occurs, takes about one hour.

Fertilization is thus most likely to occur if sexual intercourse takes place between day 10 and day 16 of the cycle. There is also a possibility of fertilization at other times, presumably due to the rare occurrence of an **extra ovulation** or more commonly due to variations in the length of the menstrual cycle.

Only a few of the 100–150 million sperm deposited in the vagina reach the ovum. Most of them die in the vagina within an hour, because of the acid environment, and the rest die on their way up through the uterus and in the fallopian tube. As a result of this process, the most viable sperm are selected, so that only these reach the ovum, while the deformed sperm, which are probably bearers of abnormal genes, are eliminated. Only one sperm cell can fertilize a particular ovum.

The transport of the fertilized ovum through the fallopian tube takes three days. Only after four more days—that is, seven days after conception—is the ovum implanted in the mucous membrane of the uterus.

Under pathological conditions, the ovum may develop outside the uterus; **extrauterine pregnancy** then results. An extrauterine fetus cannot be born, but as a rule must be surgically removed after a few months when the diagnosis can be made.

Pregnancy diagnosis

Pregnancy is diagnosed by different methods. The diagnosis is difficult early in the pregnancy but the longer it continues, the more reliable are the signs that develop. A distinction is drawn between those subjective symptoms and objective signs that may point to pregnancy, and reliable signs of pregnancy.

The subjective symptoms that the woman experiences include absence of menstruation and a number of more or less diffuse signs such as nausea, loss of appetite, fatigue and sensations of tenderness in the breasts. About half way through the pregnancy, the woman feels fetal movements.

The objective signs consist of demonstrable enlargement of the uterus and a softening of its consistency, which is felt by palpation via the vagina. Typical skin changes, so-called striae, also often occur.

The reliable signs of pregnancy consist of positive pregnancy tests, fetal sounds—the beat of the fetal heart can be heard—and parts of the fetus that can be palpated. By means of radiography, ultrasonic diagnosis and recording of fetal ECG a thorough examination of the position and state of the fetus can be made.

Pregnancy tests. A pregnancy can be confirmed by different laboratory methods. The most reliable is the demonstration of pregnancy hormone, human chorionic gonadotropin, HCG, in the urine. The determination is based on an immunological reaction—HCG is a protein with antigenic properties (page 346).

The immunological pregnancy test requires the availability of HCG. The antibodies are obtained from rabbits that have been immunized by injecting HCG. The antibodies are found in the gamma globulin fraction of the blood serum. In addition, "carriers" of the antigen HCG must be available. Such carriers can be "sensitized" sheep blood cells—that is, ones to which HCG molecules have been attached. The carriers can also be polystyrene particles on which HCG molecules have been absorbed.

The pregnancy test is based on the fact that urine containing HCG inactivates antibodies in the serum. The inactivation occurs if urine from a pregnant woman is added to the rabbit serum. Inactivation is confirmed by observing that no agglutination (page 347) occurs when the sensitized sheep blood cells or polystyrene particles are added to the urine-serum mixture. If the urine does not contain HCG, the antibody serum remains active and the blood cells or particles agglutinate. The test becomes positive about 2 weeks after menstruation has failed to occur. The reliability of the reaction is about 99 percent.

Question		*Answer*
12.1	The menstrual cycle is counted from the . . . . of bleeding.	
12.2	Ovulation, ..., usually occurs on the . . . . day of the cycle.	first day
12.3	. . . . (fertilization) is most likely to occur after . . . . (sexual intercourse) on . . . . day of the cycle.	release of the ovum 12th–14th
12.4	Fusion of the sperm cell and the ovum occurs in the . . . . (organ).	Conception coitus 10th to 16th

12.5	The fertilized ovum migrates down through the fallopian tube over a period of	fallopian tube (oviduct)
12.6	The ovum is implanted in the uterus . . . . days after conception.	3 days
12.7	A woman having relatively regular periods has menstruation lasting 5 days, then has intercourse 2 days later without any form of contraceptive. Since the survival time of the sperm cells does not exceed . . . . days and since the release of the ovum probably does not occur earlier than on day . . . . of the cycle, she probably . . . . (became, did not become) pregnant.	7
12.8	The woman's menstruation did not occur, however; this may be due either to pregnancy because of unusually early . . . . or to . . . . ; or the menstruation can have been absent because of other factors, possibly anxiety.	4 12 did not become $(5+2+4=11<12)$
12.9	The woman consults a physician a little more than a week after menstruation has failed to occur. The physician performs an immunological test. He mixes rabbit antiserum with the patient's urine and then adds HCG sensitized sheep blood cells. The blood cells do not agglutinate. The patient . . . . (is, is not) pregnant.	ovulation an extra ovulation
		is

Fetal development

After the fertilized ovum has been implanted in the mucous membrane of the uterus, it grows rapidly. It is supplied via the **placenta**, where the fetus's blood vessels so closely contact the mother's that gaseous exchange and diffusion of nutrients to, and waste products from, the fetus can occur. The vascular systems are normally separated, and this enables the fetus and mother to have different blood groups (Chapter 7). The placenta is connected to the fetus by the **umbilical cord**.

The fetus is surrounded by **amniotic fluid**, fetal water, contained in a cavity formed by the **amniotic sac**, the fetal membranes. This membrane sac enclosing the fetus fills the uterine cavity (Fig. 12.2).

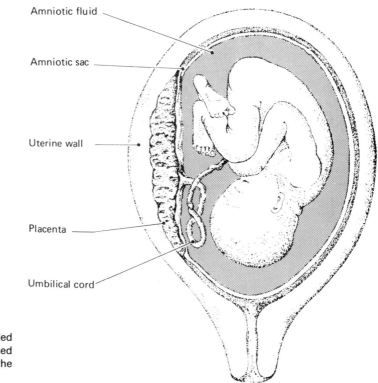

Amniotic fluid

Amniotic sac

Uterine wall

Placenta

Umbilical cord

Figure 12.2 The fetus lies surrounded by the amniotic fluid, which is enclosed in the amniotic sac formed from the fetal membranes.

The pregnancy lasts about 10 lunar (28 days) months, counting from the first day of the last menstrual period (MP). The date of delivery can be calculated according to the formula:

$$MP + 1 \text{ year} - 3 \text{ calendar months} + 7 \text{ days}$$

The duration of the pregnancy, however, varies; 50 percent of the deliveries occur at the expected time ±1 week; 80 percent of the deliveries occur at the calculated time ±2 weeks.

The approximate size of the fetus can be estimated according to the rule: fetal length in centimeters during the first five months of pregnancy is equal to the square of the respective number of months. For older fetuses, the number of months is multiplied by 5. A five-month fetus is thus about 25 cm long and a full-term fetus about 50 cm.

Table 12.2

Age Lunar Months	Fetal Length cm	Age Lunar Months	Fetal Length cm
1	1	6	30
2	4	7	35
3	9	8	40
4	16	9	45
5	25	10	50

The fetus begins to make movements in the third month of pregnancy, but the woman does not feel them until about the fifth month.

The fetal sounds—that is, the fetus's heartbeats—can be heard in the middle of pregnancy. Normally, the heart rate is 120–160 beats/minute.

The fetal heart can be examined during pregnancy by means of ultrasonic and ECG techniques (page 610).

As the fetus grows, so does the uterus. In the third or fourth month it can be palpated above the pubic bone in the median plane. At the end of the ninth month, the uterus reaches up to the costal arch. Finally, during the tenth month, the uterus drops slightly.

12.10	The fetus is supplied with nourishment, and gaseous exchange occurs, through the	
12.11	The placenta grows into the	placenta
12.12	The mother's blood vessels .... (continue, do not continue) into the fetus via the placenta.	uterine wall
12.13	The placenta covers only part of the uterine wall; between the uterus and the fetus there are also the .... and the	do not continue
12.14	The number of lunar months the pregnancy lasts after the first day of the last menstrual period is	amniotic sac (fetal membrane) amniotic fluid (fetal water)
12.15	A pregnant woman had her last menstrual period on New Year's Day. She calculated that the child would be born around .... (date).	10

12.16	In the third month of pregnancy, a woman has a hemorrhage and the fetus is expelled spontaneously. The woman has had an	October 7th
12.17	The woman, who had previously not given birth to a living child, but who had had a legal abortion performed earlier, is gravida .... and para	abortion (miscarriage)
12.18	Another woman who had given birth to three full-term children and one stillborn fetus is gravida .... and para	II 0
12.19	The stillborn child died in the .... (pre-natal, natal, postnatal) stage of pregnancy.	IV III
12.20	The highest infant mortality occurs within the first month of life, that is in the .... period.	prenatal
		neonatal

DELIVERY

Delivery (**parturition**) is due to contractions of the uterus. Its walls consist of smooth muscle which contracts rhythmically without voluntary control; this is **labor**. The process is controlled hormonally from the pituitary, which secretes a hormone, **oxytocin**, which stimulates the muscles of the uterus. Due to uterine contractions, the pressure rises uniformly throughout the uterine cavity and the fetus is pressed downwards toward the **cervix**, the neck of the uterus. The normal pressure during labor is about 25 mm Hg (3 kPa), which causes a gradual widening of the cervix.

The duration of labor is dependent on a number of factors, such as the size of the woman's pelvis, the size of the fetus and the strength of the contractions. Labor is divided into three stages: the first stage (**dilatation**), the second stage (**expulsion**), and the third stage (**placental**). During these stages the woman needs different forms of supervision and assistance.

The first stage lasts from the onset of uterine contractions until the cervix is dilated completely. The contractions increase in frequency and strength until in fully developed normal labor, there is one contraction every three to five minutes, each lasting one half to one minute. The woman experiences these contractions as pains in the back, groin and lower abdomen.

During the first stage, the cervix gradually widens. The first stage normally continues for about 15 hours for first births and about nine hours for subsequent births, but there are large individual differences.

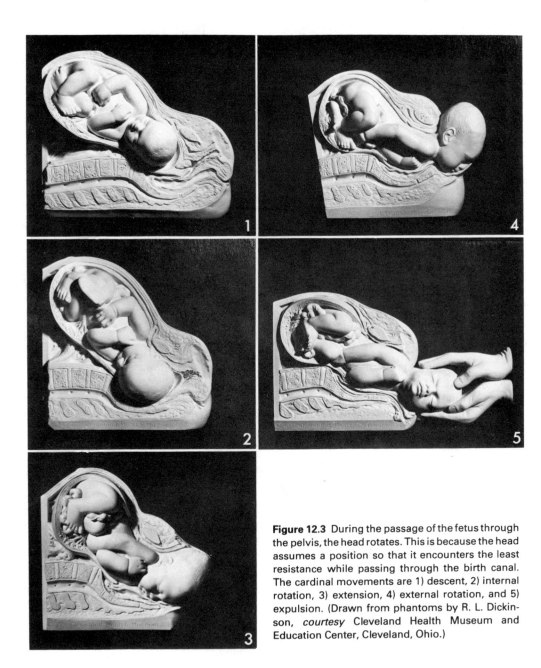

Figure 12.3 During the passage of the fetus through the pelvis, the head rotates. This is because the head assumes a position so that it encounters the least resistance while passing through the birth canal. The cardinal movements are 1) descent, 2) internal rotation, 3) extension, 4) external rotation, and 5) expulsion. (Drawn from phantoms by R. L. Dickinson, *courtesy* Cleveland Health Museum and Education Center, Cleveland, Ohio.)

The amniotic sac is normally intact during the greater part of the first stage. It is pressed down in front of the fetus with an intervening layer of amniotic fluid. It is thus the pressure transmitted via the amniotic sac that dilates the cervix.

During the first stage, the amniotic sac often ruptures and a portion of the amniotic fluid is discharged. If this does not happen spontaneously, the sac is ruptured with tweezers or forceps—the contractions then usually increase in intensity.

It is important to determine the exact position of the fetus. Normally the head of the fetus is the leading part, so-called **cephalic presentation**. The largest part of the fetus, which is the head, widens the birth canal and the subsequent parts easily pass through. The fetus may be born in the **face presentation** (when the face presents), in the **brow presentation** (when the brow presents), and in the **vertex presentation** (when the upper and back part of the head presents).

The fetus can also be born with the buttocks leading—so-called **breech presentation**, or with a foot or the feet leading—**footling presentation**. This is accompanied by an increased risk for the fetus, since the umbilical cord can be pinched by the head. Rarely, there is a **transverse presentation** (with the fetus lying crossways), which must be corrected to **longitudinal presentation** so that the delivery can develop normally.

During the first stage, the woman is watched carefully. By means of **palpation** of the abdomen and via the vagina it is possible to follow the dilatation of the cervix and the passage of the fetus down through the birth canal. It is possible to observe how the head rotates during its passage (Fig. 12.3). The sounds of the **fetal heartbeat** are listened to in order to monitor the state of the fetus. This provides information regarding **asphyxia**, lack of oxygen (page 604). It is sometimes necessary to take action to prevent the fetus from dying within the uterus.

The second stage lasts from the time the cervix is fully dilated until the expulsion of the fetus. During this stage, which lasts an hour or so for the primipara to half an hour for the multipara, the labor changes character. The fetus presses on the pelvic floor eliciting reflex mechanisms that cause the woman to bear down. The woman can and should collaborate by consciously bearing down with the abdominal muscles synchronously with the uterine contractions.

During the second stage, preparations for delivery are made. The woman's external genitalia are disinfected. The condition of the fetus is checked at frequent intervals. The obstetrician follows the events; they should proceed at the correct rate, so that the child is not in danger and the soft tissues in the pelvic floor are not **ruptured**, or torn. With his hands, the obstetrician guides the process to some extent (Fig. 12.3). At each contraction, the pelvic floor protrudes. Finally the leading part of the fetus, usually the head, appears, and the child can be helped out.

When the delivery is complete, mucus is aspirated from the child's mouth. The umbilical cord is tied and cut. The child usually breathes spontaneously and often emits a cry. The lungs are filled with air, and the blood circulation in the child undergoes a change so that the blood does not flow in the umbilical cord but through the lungs—a complex physiological process that takes place in a short period of time. A life is born.

The third stage begins when the child has been delivered. It lasts about a quarter of an hour. Uterine muscles begin to contract again so that the attachment for the placenta shrinks. This is detached and expelled. The placental contractions are painless.

During the third stage, the mother is monitored to see that there is no great loss of blood. By giving drugs that contract the uterus, the bleeding can be reduced.

12.21	During the tenth month of pregnancy, a woman occasionally feels pain in the sacral area. This indicates that .... (delivery) is imminent.	
12.22	Some days later, the contractions become regular—occurring first at intervals of 15 min and then more frequently. This is the beginning of the .... of delivery.	parturition
12.23	The woman, who is nullipara, goes to the hospital obstetrics department. It is estimated that the child will be born about .... hours after the beginning of the first stage.	first stage (dilatation)
12.24	The woman is examined; for example, the obstetrician feels the abdomen with his hands. By palpation he determines the	16 (15 + 1; large individual variation)
12.25	He also listens with a fetal stethoscope on the abdomen to judge the state of the fetus from the sounds of the .... They should normally have a frequency of	position of the fetus
12.26	After 12 hours, the woman notices a change in the contractions. She feels pressure and has a sensation which causes the urge to defecate. At each contraction, the pelvic floor protrudes: the woman has a type of contraction where she .... The mother is now in the .... of delivery.	fetal heartbeat 120–160 beats/min

12.27	The obstetrician supervises the second stage and to some extent regulates the rate at which it proceeds. In particular he tries to ensure that the child .... and that the pelvic floor of the woman does not	bears down second stage (expulsion)
12.28	After the delivery, mucus is aspirated from the	is not in danger rupture
12.29	The child usually begins to .... spontaneously.	child's mouth
12.30	The .... stage then begins, during which the .... is expelled.	breathe
		third (placental) placenta

Obstetric Anesthesia

To alleviate pain during delivery, different kinds of anesthesia are administered (page 505). Regional anesthesia, intravenous anesthesia and inhalation anesthesia are used.

In regional anesthesia (page 505), different locations of the nerve tracts that run from the uterus, vagina and pelvic floor are anesthetized. Regional anesthesia is commonly used in the United States.

In the United States barbiturate drugs, usually combined with scopolamine may be given intravenously to relieve pain during labor. The patient is frequently unable to bear down properly, which makes it necessary to deliver the child with forceps. Some children delivered this way do not breathe as spontaneously. Meperidine combined with scopolamine provide less risk to mother and child.

In the Scandinavian countries, barbiturate drugs may be given to stop labor in order to let the mother rest.

Inhalation anesthesia with nitrous oxide is commonly used in the Scandinavian countries. The gas is supplied intermittently at the beginning of the contractions, and preferably just before they begin. The woman is in the first stage of anesthesia, the so-called analgesia stage (page 511). Apparatus has been designed—so-called **analgesia inhaler**—with which the woman herself can manage the anesthesia without participation of the anesthetist or nurse. The apparatus provides a suitable mixture of nitrous oxide and oxygen—usually 50 percent of each.

The nitrous oxide anesthesia has some advantages. Relief of pain is rapid, producing patient comfort. Nitrous oxide has a low level of toxicity and does not have an irritant effect on the mucous membranes of the respiratory tract. The labor is not reduced, as is the case with many narcotic analgesics. Nitrous oxide is not explosive and does not interfere with the respiration or circulation. The disadvantage is that the pain relief is not complete.

12.31	In regional anesthesia, the nerve tracts that run from the . . . ., ... and . . . . are anesthetized.	
12.32	The preferable combinations of drugs for intravenous anesthesia are . . . . and	uterus vagina pelvic floor
12.33	In inhalation anesthesia using nitrous oxide, the gas is administered by an . . . . which the woman can manage	meperidine scopolamine
		analgesia inhaler herself

Obstetric Complications

Complications sometimes occur during pregnancy and delivery. Three examples are given below: **asphyxia**, where the fetus has oxygen deficiency, **placenta previa**, incorrect position of the placenta in the uterus, and **toxemia of pregnancy**, a pathological state of the pregnant woman that sometimes results in severe disturbances.

Asphyxia

The most common intrauterine injury to the fetus is due to **hypoxia**, oxygen deficiency, which leads to **fetal asphyxia**. Asphyxia not infrequently causes fetal death or brain damage. There are different causes of asphyxia.

In **placental insufficiency**, reduced function of the placenta, there is impaired gaseous exchange, which can lead to asphyxia. Placental insufficiency can, in its turn, have several causes, such as diabetes in the mother or toxemia of pregnancy. Lung and heart diseases in the mother can also produce fetal asphyxia. These conditions sometimes lead to fetal death long before the fetus has reached full term—**intrauterine fetal death**. This does not constitute a danger to the pregnant woman, though the knowledge that the fetus is dead will cause considerable mental stress, and the pregnancy should be interrupted as soon as the diagnosis has been made.

Another cause of asphyxia is **umbilical cord complications**. A knot in the umbilical cord can lead to death of the fetus at different stages of fetal development—the knot interferes with the blood circulation and the fetus is suffocated. If the amniotic fluid is discharged before the leading part of the fetus has entered the birth canal, the cord may **prolapse** (fall down). This constitutes a major risk of asphyxia due to clamping of the umbilical cord when the fetus is pushed down.

Asphyxia produces certain typical symptoms. The most important of these is a change in the fetal heart rate. Irregularity of fetal sounds is indicative of asphyxia. If the rate is below 120 beats/min, the condition is critical. If possible, the delivery must then be rapidly terminated.

Placenta previa

The placenta should normally not fuse with the part of the uterine wall around the cervix. If this happens the condition is known as **placenta previa**. It may be due to implantation of the ovum far down in the uterus or to excessive growth of the placenta. Placenta previa leads to intermittent bleeding during the last months of pregnancy. The bleeding is due to detachment of the placenta from the uterus. The bleeding is not accompanied by pain unless labor has begun. Placenta previa can be diagnosed by radionuclides or by ultrasonic scanning (page 469).

Placenta previa is both a fetal and a maternal problem; the maternal mortality is less than one percent. The delivery in these cases is performed by Cesarean section (page 607).

Toxemia of pregnancy

During pregnancy a serious pathological condition known as **toxemia of pregnancy** can develop in the woman. The cause of the disease is unknown. It is characterized by three cardinal symptoms: **edema**, interstitial accumulation of fluid (page 281), **hypertension**, elevated blood pressure (page 135), and **proteinuria**, protein in the urine (page 296). There are also a number of accompanying complications of the brain, eyes, liver and kidneys. Visual defects are relatively common. Severe toxemia produces an intense headache. In extreme cases, unconsciousness and convulsions—**eclampsia**—follow. The convulsions can lead to death.

Toxemia of pregnancy endangers both fetus and mother. The fetus can die **in utero** by asphyxia, due to placental malfunction, which accompanies the disease. Toxemia of pregnancy presents a direct threat to the mother's life during pregnancy and risk of permanent damage to different organs (brain, eyes, kidneys) after the pregnancy. After complications from hemorrhage, eclampsia attacks are the commonest cause of death of the mother.

As the cause of toxemia is unknown, no causal therapy can be given, and the treatment must be symptomatic. The edema and hypertension are treated with drugs. In addition, drugs to lower the blood pressure may be given if the hypertension becomes severe. Bed confinement is an important step to lower the blood pressure. Intense light and sound evoke attacks of eclampsia, so severe toxemia cases should be isolated in a quiet, dark room. Sedatives are given to prevent attacks of eclampsia.

12.34	A woman with a normal pregnancy and delivery is watched closely. Towards the end of the delivery, the fetal sounds become irregular and occasionally fall below 120 beats/min. Diagnosis	
12.35	The pregnancy is quickly terminated and the probable cause is found: the umbilical cord is wound several times around the neck of the fetus and is being pulled increasingly taut as the fetus is pushed down in the birth canal. The blood circulation through the umbilical cord is then impaired and the fetus is exposed to . . . . (cause of asphyxia).	asphyxia of the fetus
12.36	A woman is checked in the seventh month of pregnancy. Protein is found in the urine, a condition known as . . . . ; the blood pressure is 170/110 mm Hg (23/15 kPa), that is, ... ; and there is an increase in weight due to interstitial fluid, known as . . . . Diagnosis:	hypoxia (lack of oxygen)
12.37	During the next two months the condition gets worse, and the patient is admitted to hospital one month before delivery is expected. She is given special care to avoid any attacks of convulsions and unconsciousness—so-called . . . . , which would endanger her life.	proteinuria hypertension edema toxemia of pregnancy
12.38	An attack of eclampsia can be evoked by intense . . . . and	eclampsia
12.39	A woman has repeated intermittent hemorrhages during the last months of pregnancy. Possible diagnosis:	light sound
12.40	A woman has a hemorrhage in the third month of pregnancy. Probable diagnosis:	placenta previa
		abortion (spontaneous miscarriage)

Surgical Techniques in Obstetrics

Delivery sometimes leads to complications that necessitate an operation on the mother. A wrong position of the fetus, asphyxia, placenta previa, toxemia of pregnancy and many other conditions can require measures that are often of an urgent nature.

Rotation

Rotation is performed to correct the position of the fetus where normal delivery may be possible, and to terminate a complicated delivery without delay.

External rotation is performed to correct transverse or breech presentation. The fetus is then brought into a more normal position. To effect external rotation, the obstetrician places both hands on the woman's abdomen and tries to turn the fetus into the correct position. In external rotation it is important that the amniotic fluid has not passed out and that there is enough fluid present. The birth canal must be normal, with no narrowing, so that natural delivery is possible.

In an external rotation, which is performed 4–6 weeks before the time of delivery, there is some risk of umbilical cord complications. The advisability of instead performing a Cesarean section when the fetus is full term must be considered.

Internal rotation may be used when the fetal head is in an abnormal position that makes delivery difficult or impossible. The obstetrician inserts his hand into the birth canal and turns the fetal head to a more favorable position.

Cesarean section

In a Cesarean section (after Julius Caesar, who is said to have been delivered in this way) an abdominal incision is first made. The uterus is then opened and the fetus lifted out. A Cesarean section is performed when the risk to the mother and child are judged to be less than would be the case in vaginal delivery. For example, a Cesarean section is chosen in placenta previa when the life of both mother and child are endangered. Also in umbilical cord prolapse, when the risk to the fetus is great, this method is preferred.

The operation is performed under general anesthesia—that is, using a combination of intravenous and inhalation anesthesia (page 508). Regional anesthesia may also be used. Cesarean section causes a risk to the mother of 0.2–0.5 percent, depending on the pathological situation and the obstetric complications. The mortality associated with the operation itself is very small; risks arise from postoperative complications—for example, due to infection of the uterus. The mortality for the child in Cesarean section is between 3 and 10 percent.

Instrumental extraction

When the condition of the mother or the fetus calls for rapid termination of the delivery by the natural route—for reasons such as weak contractions, severe hemorrhage or fetal asphyxia—two technical methods can be used: **forceps** and **vacuum extraction**. With both of these, the fetal head can be **extracted**, drawn out, and **rotated** in the birth canal.

Forceps technique.   In a forceps delivery, the fetal head is gripped with the forceps and a combined tractive and rotary force is applied, Fig. 12.4. The forceps

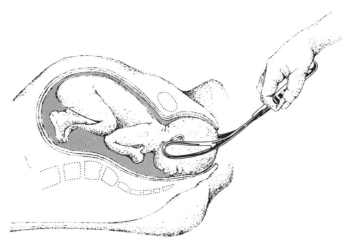

Figure 12.4 Forceps delivery.

can be separated into two branches. Each branch consists of a blade, shank, and handle. The branches are inserted separately so that the blades are applied to the head. The two branches are then connected with the locking device. By gripping the two connected handles, the fetal head can be maneuvered.

Vacuum extraction   is performed with a vacuum extractor, which is attached to the fetal crown (or buttocks in breech presentation), Fig. 12.5. The extractor is connected to a vacuum tank and a vacuum pump by a tube. By gradually reducing the pressure to a negative pressure of 0.6–0.8 atm (60–80 kPa), a firm adhesion between the vacuum extractor and the part of the fetus is obtained. By pulling on the tube, the desired traction can be applied to the fetus. The operation is performed with the patient under some form of anesthesia.

Vacuum extraction provides an opportunity for producing improved labor contractions. By pulling synchronously with the contractions, reflexes are evoked that reinforce the contractions.

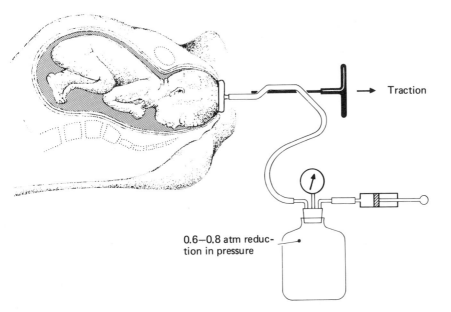

Figure 12.5 Vacuum extraction of the fetus.

0.6–0.8 atm reduction in pressure

Traction

In forceps delivery, injury can be caused to the mother and the child; in vacuum extraction the risk to the mother is minimal and to the child reduced. Vacuum extraction has replaced forceps techniques in many countries in Europe and the Far East; it is not used in the United States.

12.41	In the ninth month of pregnancy it is found that the fetus is in the transverse presentation. The obstetrician is faced with the choice of either immediately trying to perform an . . . . or of waiting until full term and performing a	
12.42	A woman is in her tenth month of pregnancy, when the amniotic fluid suddenly passes at home. Labor then begins. After arrival at the hospital, prolapse of the umbilical cord is found, which had occurred because the fetal head was not fixed in the birth canal when the amniotic fluid passed. The fetus shows signs of asphyxia. As the cervix is not dilated enough, there is only one way to save the fetus, namely by	external rotation Cesarean section

12.43	A primipara aged 35 years has a difficult labor. The delivery is prolonged even though contraction-stimulating drugs have been given. The cervix is dilated to 5 cm. To assist the mother (the fetus shows no signs of asphyxia) by accelerating the delivery, an .... is performed.	Cesarean section
		instrumental extraction (forceps delivery or vacuum extraction)

TECHNICAL ASPECTS OF OBSTETRIC DIAGNOSIS

Pregnancy and delivery present special diagnostic problems. It is important to determine the state of the fetus in order to select the proper treatment. The examination is not easy to perform, because the fetus is surrounded by the uterus and the abdominal wall of the woman. An x-ray examination of the fetus should be avoided (page 400). For this reason, a number of special diagnostic methods have been developed: **fetal electrocardiography**, **fetal phonocardiography** and **ultrasonic diagnosis**.

Fetal electrocardiography. The heart of the fetus, like that of the mother, emits electrical action potentials. There are technical problems involved, however, since the signals from the fetal heart, **f-ECG**, have a lower amplitude than those picked up at the same time from the mother, **m-ECG**. Moreover, the f-ECG recording contains interference not only from the m-ECG, but also from the muscles of the mother—electromyographic signals (page 253).

When the f-ECG is picked up, electrodes are placed on the mother's abdomen, and if possible also on the fetal scalp, in order to obtain a good signal-to-noise ratio (Fig. 12.6). After the amniotic fluid has been discharged and the fetal skull can be reached, an electrode is clipped on it.

To facilitate the diagnosis, the signals are processed to suppress the m-ECG and to enhance the f-ECG. This signal processing can be performed in different ways. Attempts have been made to subtract the m-ECG from the composite signal picked up from the abdomen. With this procedure, the positioning of the electrodes is very critical, since the subtraction potential must be of the right amplitude, phase and shape as the m-ECG in the recorded composite signal.

Frequency filtering can also improve the signal/noise ratio. Here, use is made of the fact that the mother's R wave has the greatest frequency content from 10–30 Hz, while that of the fetus is greatest from 15–40 Hz.

With the f-ECG, a pregnancy can be diagnosed from the 17th week of pregnancy. The chances are best in weeks 20–24 and 36–38; during weeks 28–32,

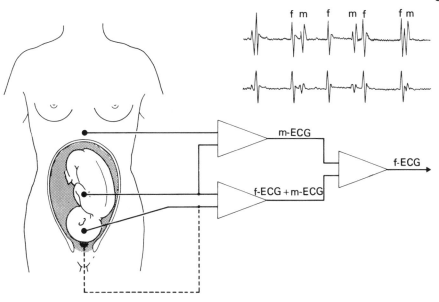

Figure 12.6 Example of electrode positions in recording of fetal ECG. By subtracting the mother's ECG signal from the signal picked up over the fetus, some improvement in the signal is obtained, as is shown in the lower curve.

the amplitude is lower, probably because the signals are attenuated by the relatively large amount of amniotic fluid. The f-ECG is used primarily to measure the fetal heart rate, from which it is possible to detect asphyxia.

Fetal phonocardiography can be recorded by placing a microphone on the mother's abdominal wall, over the site where the fetal sounds have maximum intensity. One of the biggest disadvantages is that the position of the microphone is critical, and artifacts due to extraneous sounds are easily recorded. The method does not represent any technical advance in fetal monitoring.

Ultrasonic diagnosis can be performed by the compound B-scanning technique (page 466) and by the Doppler ultrasonic method.

The fetal contours can be visualized by ultrasonic tomograms obtained by compound B-scanning. It is possible, for example, to detect the presence of twins.

The Doppler ultrasonic method provides diagnostic information about the blood circulation in the fetus. The required equipment consists of a transmitter, which emits a continuous ultrasonic wave towards the fetus, and a receiver, which picks up the reflected waves (Fig. 12.7). The emitting crystal is mounted together with the receiving crystal in a probe, which is held against the mother's abdominal wall. A frequency of about 2 MHz is used. A small amount of oil or gel is placed between the probe and the abdominal wall to obtain good acoustic coupling. The

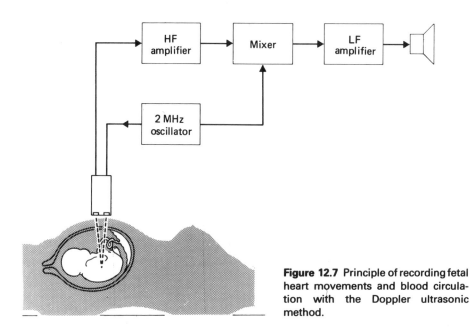

Figure 12.7 Principle of recording fetal heart movements and blood circulation with the Doppler ultrasonic method.

reflected signal is amplified and mixed with the emitted signal. The resulting beat frequency is proportional to the blood velocity in the fetus and mother. The beat frequency is amplified and can be heard with a loudspeaker.

With this method, the presence of a pulsating heart and blood flow in the fetus can be determined. The blood flow in the mother's blood vessels can be distinguished from that in the fetus due to the differences in the pulse rate. Different parts of the fetus can be identified and examined due to the variations in blood stream velocity in the different parts of the fetus.

The echo can be obtained from the fetal heart as early as the 10th–12th fetal week and from that time until delivery. The Doppler ultrasonic technique is thus superior to f-ECG. The method is, as far as is known, completely without danger.

The following sounds are obtained:

- Thump, Thump—low frequency note, rapid rhythm—fetal heart movement.
- Swish, Swish—high frequency note, rapid rhythm—umbilical cord sound.
- Thuummp, Thuummp—low frequency note, slow rhythm—mother's body movements due to vibrations transmitted from the heart.
- Woooch, Woooch—mid-frequency note, slow rhythm—mother's arteries.

Monitoring of the fetal condition is sometimes routinely done by a combination of fetal ECG and intrauterine pressure recordings, Fig. 12.8.

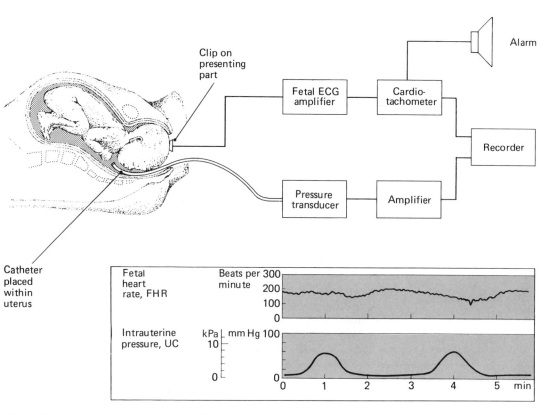

Figure 12.8 Simultaneous monitoring of the fetal heart rate and the intrauterine pressure.

When the cervix is dilated to about 2 cm or more, an electrode is clipped onto the presenting part, as described above. The resulting fetal ECG is large enough to provide a reliable signal for conversion to fetal heart rate. Alarms are actuated if the fetal heart rate goes outside preset limits.

To record the intrauterine pressure, a catheter is placed within the uterus and connected to a pressure transducer. Each contraction should produce a small slowing of the fetal heart rate, with a proper delay. If the resulting pressure during uterine contractions is too low, or does not drop to zero between contractions, drugs may be given to correct the condition. Intrauterine pressure recordings are associated with an increased risk of intrauterine infection that, however, can be treated by antibiotics.

Deviations from the typical recorded patterns shown in Fig. 12.8 provide an early indication of fetal distress, and, for example, provide the diagnostic information required to decide on termination of the delivery by Cesarean section. This reduces the number of cases of brain damage resulting from asphyxia.

12.44	The greatest difficulty in recording the .... (fetal electrocardiogram) is that the .... (mother's electrocardiogram) has a greater .... This disadvantage can be partially compensated for by using the fact that the former have somewhat higher .... than the latter.	
12.45	There are major difficulties in using the recording of fetal sounds, called ...., for monitoring purposes, among other things, because fetal movements cause the signal to disappear.	f-ECG m-ECG amplitude frequencies
12.46	A full-term fetus is examined by the Doppler ultrasonic method. By palpating the abdomen from outside, the head and neck can be located. The ultrasonic probe is directed towards both sides of the neck, and a large signal is received from both places. The umbilical cord is wound around the neck of the fetus. What is "heard" by the ultrasonic method is the .... in the umbilical cord.	fetal phonocardiography
		blood flow

REFERENCES

BENSON, R. C. Handbook of Obstetrics and Gynecology. Los Altos (Lange) 1974. 770 pages.

HELLMAN, L. M., PRITCHARD, J. A. and WYNN, R. M. *Williams Obstetrics.* New York (Appleton–Century–Crofts) 1971. 1242 pages.

HON, E. H. An Introduction to Fetal Heart Rate Monitoring. New Haven (Harty Press) 1969. 95 pages.

chapter 13

Radiotherapy
and Physical Therapy

In the treatment of a number of diseases, different kinds of radiation can be applied. The principles of treatment and the various fields of application vary widely depending upon the type of radiation used. In **radiotherapy**, or radiation therapy, ionizing radiation is employed. The treatment with some other forms of energy, such as ultrasound and high-frequency electromagnetic radiation in the radio frequency range is commonly referred to collectively by the term **physical therapy**. The term also includes a number of other methods such as massage, heat, hydrotherapy and exercise.

Radiotherapeutic methods are used almost exclusively for treating tumor diseases, especially malignant tumors. Radiotherapy and surgery (Chapter 10) are the two most important treatment methods for these serious conditions.

Physical therapy has an exceedingly wide range of application, which is not always well defined: the term is often used to mean rehabilitation of the patient after major operations, taking palliative steps (general measures to alleviate disease or to support treatment) and giving prophylaxis (actions to prevent disease).

RADIOTHERAPY

Radiation therapy is based on two fundamental disciplines, **radiobiology** and **radiophysics**. These make up the theoretical basis for applied radiotherapy.

Radiobiology is the branch of science that deals with the effect of ionizing radiation on cells and tissues. Radiophysics is the branch of science that deals with radiation, especially ionizing radiation.

In radiotherapy, different types of radiation are used. A distinction is drawn between conventional **x-ray therapy**, in which the radiation photon energy is lower than 0.5 MeV, and **super-voltage therapy (megavolt therapy, million-volt therapy)** in which the photon energy is greater than 0.5 MeV. The high-energy radiation can be obtained from **radionuclides**, especially ^{60}Co. It can be generated with **betatrons**, **linear accelerators**, **cyclotrons** and **Van de Graaf generators** as well.

A special form of radiotherapy is **radionuclide therapy**. The nuclides are administered internally by mouth or by intravenous injection and they become concentrated in certain organs—for example, radioiodine is selectively trapped by the thyroid gland during the treatment of cancer or functional disorders of this gland.

Question		*Answer*
13.1	A patient has been operated on for cancer of the breast. At the operation, metastases—daughter tumors—are found in the axilla. The patient is referred to a .... department.	
13.2	An elderly patient has had pain in one shoulder for a fairly long time. The cause is calcification around the joint, and the basic cause of the symptoms cannot be removed. Therefore, an attempt is made to give ultrasonic therapy as a palliative measure. The patient is referred to a department of	radiotherapy
13.3	Radiotherapy is based on two basic sciences, namely, ... in which the effect of the radiation on the cells and tissues is studied, and .... which is the science mainly concerned with ionizing radiation.	physical therapy
13.4	The types of radiation used in radiotherapy are ...., generated with voltages up to 0.5 MeV, and radiation over 0.5 MeV obtained from .... or generated with ...., ..., ... or	radiobiology radiophysics

13.5	A radioactive isotope is injected into a patient, so that it will concentrate at a particular site—for example, in a tumor. This type of treatment is called	conventional x-rays radionuclides betatrons linear accelerators cyclotrons Van de Graaf generators
		radionuclide therapy

Units for radiation and radiation dose

To define quantitative units for the physical effect of ionizing radiation is easy; to define quantitative units for the biological effect of the radiation is considerably more difficult. This is reflected in the many different dose units that are used, the most important of which are the following.

Activity.   The decay of a radionuclide is given by the number of disintegrations per unit time. The old unit is curie, where $1\ Ci = 3.7 \cdot 10^{10}\ s^{-1}$. The SI-unit is **becquerel**, where $1\ Bq = s^{-1}$. Thus, for example, $1\ mCi = 37\ MBq$.

Exposure.   The amount of radiation an object is exposed to is in old units measured in roentgens where $1\ R$ produces ionization of either sign of $2.58 \cdot 10^{-4}$ **coulomb per kilogram** of dry air at STP. In SI-units, the exposure is merely measured in C/kg.
   The exposure unit does not provide a measure of the actual dose—that is, the energy absorbed in a biological tissue or other object. The exposure indicates how much radiation energy is incident on the object and is available for absorption in it. The absorption characteristics of the object for the type of radiation and the dimensions of the object determine the absorbed energy.

Absorbed dose.   The old unit for absorbed dose is the rad = 100 erg per gram of absorbing substance. The SI-unit is **gray**, where $1\ Gy = 1\ J/kg$ (joule per kilogram). The conversion factor is $1\ Gy = 100\ rad$.

Dose equivalence.   The rad unit is not a measure of the biological effect. This is dependent on how the ionizing particles are distributed in the object. For high-energy radiation with a low specific degree of ionization—for example, gamma radiation—the ionizations are randomly distributed throughout the object. In radiation with high specific ionization—for example, alpha-particle radiation—the ions are grouped along relatively few particle paths, and the biological effect will then be different.

Because of this, the unit **rem** (roentgen, equivalent, man) is used to denote the equivalence, *H*, of a particular radiation. 1 rem is the radiation dose that has an effect on man that corresponds to 1 rad of another specified type of radiation, usually 200 kV x-rays.

In matters regarding radiation protection, the dose, D_{rad}, is multiplied by a factor, Q (quality factor), to obtain the dose equivalence in rem:

$$H = D_{rad}Q$$

or in SI units:

$$H = 100 \, D_{Gy}Q$$

In radiotherapy, the factor *RBE* (Relative Biological Effectiveness) is used instead of *Q*. The factor, *RBE*, has values between about 0.8 and 20. The factor not only varies with the radiation type but, for a given type of radiation, it varies somewhat for different tissues. For gamma radiation from ^{60}Co relative to 200 kV x-rays, the *RBE* = 0.8–0.9. For proton radiation and alpha particles the *RBE* lies between 10 and 20.

13.6	The old unit for denoting the disintegration of a radionuclide is .... and the SI-unit	
13.7	Two nuclear engineers locate a radioactive leak with instruments measuring the	Ci (curie) $Bq = s^{-1}$ (becquerel)
13.8	One of them uses a modern instrument giving the exposure in .... (SI unit).	exposure (rate of ionization)
13.9	The other has an old instrument calibrated in	C/kg
13.10	The SI-unit for absorbed dose is	R (roentgen)
13.11	The old unit for absorbed dose is .... which is related to the SI-unit through .... (old) = ... (SI).	Gy (gray)
13.12	The dose unit for the biological effect of ionizing radiation on man is the	rad $1 \, rad = 10^{-2} \, Gy$

13.13	The relation between the dose D expressed in rad and the dose equivalence H in rem is given by the expression	rem
13.14	RBE is the abbreviation for	$H = D \cdot Q$
13.15	RBE varies according to the type of radiation used in radiotherapy and is between about . . . . and	relative biological effectiveness
13.16	The relation between the roentgen and the rem is	0.8 20
		dependent on the object's absorption and the Q or the RBE factor

RADIOBIOLOGY

Ionizing radiation affects living cells. When the radiation is absorbed, a few of the atoms and molecules of the cells are ionized. The ionization leads, either directly or via the formation of free radicals, to chemical reactions in the cells, which are damaged. The chemical and physical mechanisms of this damage are largely unknown.

The great sensitivity of the cells to such ionization is remarkable. A dose of 1,000 rad (10 Gy), which is a small amount of energy—it raises the temperature of 1 ml of water a few thousandths of a degree—and which produces ionization of only 1 molecule out of 10^7, is lethal for practically all vertebrates.

When a number of living cells are irradiated, they are not all affected in the same way, the cell damage being randomly distributed among all the cells. For example, a dose of 50 rad (0.5 Gy) kills only a few eggs of the fruit fly, while 500 rad (5 Gy) kills practically all of them. The surviving cells can be more or less damaged, so that different levels of change occur in the metabolism of the cells and in their structure. The biological effect is apparent only after a latency period, which decreases with the radiation dose. It ranges from a few days to weeks or more; genetic damage does not show up until the next generation.

Cell death after irradiation with the doses used in radiotherapy is probably due to damage to the germ plasma of the cells. Most of the cells survive limited damage in the body, but they die when division occurs. This fact may partially account for the variations in sensitivity to radiation for both normal tissue and tumor tissue, and for the fact that tumor tissues are often more sensitive than the normal tissue from which they originated. Some normal tissues, which are characterized by a comparatively high rate of cell division, have a high radiosensitivity: bone marrow, lymph nodes, gonads (testicles and ovaries), intestinal mucous membranes and skin. The majority of rapidly growing tumors likewise have a high sensitivity to radiation—exceeding that for the above normal tissues. These tumors have a much higher rate of cell division than any of the normal tissues.

A low radiation dose can cause cancer, a high dose kills cancer. This paradoxical finding can be explained by assuming that the radiation damage occurs in the genes of the cells. When healthy tissue receives a moderate dose, moderate damage to the cell genes causes a mutation, with the result that a cancer cell develops and then multiplies. At a high dose, the damage is so great that the cells cannot multiply because of defective genes. An example that supports this theory is experimental leukemia in the mouse. At doses of less than 200–800 rad (2–8 Gy), depending on age, the frequency of leukemia increases with the dose; at higher doses it decreases (Fig. 13.1).

Relative frequency of leukemia

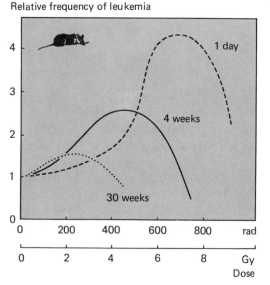

Figure 13.1 Frequency of leukemia in mice of different ages as a function of the dose.

Immunological factors probably play an important part in the body's ability to heal an irradiated tumor. In the rare cases where there is spontaneous healing of a malignant tumor, the immunological defense mechanism may also provide an explanation. The substances in the tumor cells are foreign to the organism and a cell-mediated immunological reaction occurs (page 346). When the body's immunological reaction capacity has been weakened, a tumor can develop and grow from a genetically abnormal cell that has formed in the body. The mechanism in radiotherapy is possibly that the radiation assists the organism's own immunological defense against the tumor—perhaps by damaging a large number of tumor cells so that they cannot divide.

In radiotherapy, radiation damage to tissues around the tumor cannot be avoided. The dose must be adjusted so that the damage to normal tissues does not lead to permanent disability. For this to be possible, careful planning of the dose is required, and this is one of the prime tasks of the radiophysicist (page 624).

13.17	During irradiation with x-rays, gamma rays and particle radiation, damage is caused to living cells because of .... of atoms and molecules.	
13.18	The cause of the cell damage may be that the ionization causes formation of chemically highly reactive	ionization
13.19	During irradiation with a uniformly distributed dose, the damage to all the cells is .... (equal, randomly distributed).	free radicals
13.20	Cell death after irradiation with the doses used in radiotherapy is probably due to damage to the .... of the cells.	randomly distributed
13.21	The most radiosensitive normal tissues are characterized by a high	genes
13.22	Examples of such normal tissues are ...., ..., ..., ... and	rate of cell division
13.23	Because the bone marrow is the most radiosensitive tissue in the body, an early sign of radiation damage is	bone marrow lymph nodes gonads (sex glands) intestinal mucous membrane skin
13.24	At the beginning of the century, when the harmful effects of radiation were unknown, radiologists suffered from changes in the skin on their hands, caused by the radiation dose to which they were exposed, and sometimes .... developed.	blood deficiencies

13.25	Statistical analyses show that American radiologists engaged in work involving exposure to radiation of the whole body were affected by a malignant disease, namely, ... (hint: which tissue is the most radiosensitive?) eight times more often than the normal population. These statistical findings have not been confirmed in an English investigation.	cancer
13.26	These unfortunate consequences do not constitute a reason for giving up radiological work. The risks are well known and there are reliable ways of preventing them, since the spread of, and exposure to, radiation is governed by simple physical laws. (When can the risk of accidents in the community be so well predicted!) A simple and reliable measure is to arrange effective	leukemia (blood cancer)
13.27	A patient with a tumor 5 cm across is given radiotherapy with a dose of 2,000 rad (20 Gy). The tumor consists of 10^8 cells. With the dose given, it is probable that one out of 10^6 cells survives. Nevertheless, the patient survives for more than five years (the patient is then regarded as cured). The remaining 100 cancer cells were probably taken care of by the body's	radiation protection
13.28	The active immunological mechanisms are .... (humoral, cell-mediated).	immunological defense
		cell-mediated (cf. page 346)

Radiosensitivity and cell environment

The radiosensitivity of the cells depends on the environment in which they are located during the time of irradiation. Important factors are the degree of **oxygenation**, and the presence of **radiosensitizers**, which increase the radiosensitivity, and **radioprotective substances**, which prevent cell damage to some extent.

A high degree of oxygenation increases the radiosensitivity. In total hypoxia—the absence of oxygen—the radiation dose required to obtain a given effect is more than twice as great as when the tissue is saturated with oxygen. During radiotherapy, attempts have been made to increase the oxygen tension by performing the treatment in a hyperbaric oxygen atmosphere (page 551). However, it is difficult to increase the radiosensitivity of the whole tumor in this way; in the center of a large tumor vascularization and perfusion are often so poor that this part of the tumor becomes necrotic (dies) and oxygenation in and near the center is then poor.

By supplying radiosensitizers or radioprotective substances, the biological effect of a radiation dose can be modified. A large number of substances have been used to increase the radiosensitivity—for example, certain inorganic salts, a group of compounds known as radiomimetic substances, hormones, chemotherapeutic and cytostatic agents. Cysteine, an amino acid, reduces radiosensitivity.

Radiosensitivity and radiocurability

A high **radiosensitivity**, the sensitivity of a tumor to radiation, is not the same as a high **radiocurability**, the probability of curing the tumor with radiation. Radiosensitivity is often associated with a high degree of malignancy, which means that the tumor spreads and this makes it difficult to cure, even though it can be affected by radiation. Such factors as the tumor's manner of metastasizing (spreading itself), its accessibility for radiotherapy and its size at the time of its discovery crucially affect the results of treatment.

Among the most radiosensitive tumor diseases are leukemia (blood cancer), lymph-node cancer (malignant lymphoma) and some tumors of the skeleton and bone marrow (Ewing's sarcoma, myeloma). It is often not possible to permanently cure these by radiotherapy alone.

Among the moderately radiosensitive tumors are many in the gastrointestinal tract (adenocarcinomas) and cervical cancer in women. Patients with cervical cancer can be treated successfully with radiotherapy alone in 90 percent of the cases.

Among the less radiosensitive tumors are the malignant ones that form from birthmarks (moles forming malignant melanoma), which despite their superficial location cannot be treated by radiotherapy.

13.29	The sensitivity of the cells to a certain radiation dose depends on the environment in which they are located—for example, the degree of . . . . of the tissues—and on the occurrence of two types of substances: . . . . and	
13.30	Malignant lymphomas are extremely radiosensitive. They . . . . (can, cannot) be effectively cured by radiotherapy.	oxygenation radiosensitizers radioprotective substances
13.31	The reason is that they are also highly malignant—in spite of great radiosensitivity they do not have a corresponding level of	cannot

13.32 Besides the radiosensitivity of the tumor, there are several factors that affect the results of treatment. These are the .... for radiotherapy, the .... at the time of discovery and the tumor's manner of spreading itself, that is	radiocurability

accessibility
size
metastasizing

RADIOPHYSICS

Radiotherapy requires careful **treatment planning**, availability of carefully calibrated **radiation sources**, and methods for **dose measurement**. These problems are chiefly of a physical nature, and this has led to the establishment of special radiotherapy departments at hospitals.

Treatment Planning

The purpose of radiotherapy is to deliver a large radiation dose in the tumor and a minimal dose in the surrounding normal tissues, especially the radiosensitive ones. It is important to protect the skin and the mucous membrane of the intestines, for otherwise the radiation can cause nonhealing lesions which lead to a permanent disability. When persons are of fertile age, the gonads (sex glands) must be protected; in most cases this is not a problem because of the age distribution of tumor diseases. In order to achieve the correct therapeutic effect in the individual case, **contour planning** is done as a basis for determining the **physical dose distribution**.

Contour planning

By determining the extent of the tumor and the attenuation of the surrounding tissues, a contour plan can be drawn up for the individual patient. It is important to know whether the surrounding tissues contain air, as in the case of the lungs, and whether the radiation must pass through bone on its path to the tumor. The tissue attenuation must be known in order to determine the tumor dose.

To determine the topography, contour plans of one or more cross-sections of the body are drawn. The most important of these is the cross-section through the center of the tumor, so that the **target volume** can be determined.

As a basis for the contour plans, a plaster cast of the patient's external outline is often made and a number of radiographs taken using reference points on the skin; these consist of radiopaque indicators. In the plans, the boundaries of the tumor are drawn, together with essential anatomic details such as skeletal parts (Fig. 13.2).

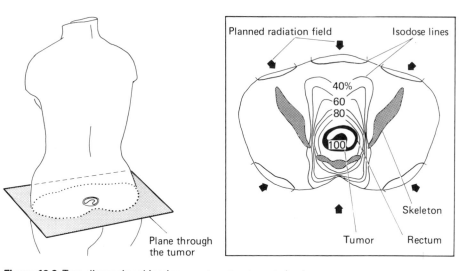

Figure 13.2 Two dimensional isodose contour treatment plan in cobalt treatment of rectal cancer with six radiation fields.

Physical dose distribution

To obtain the optimal effect in each case, a careful choice of the **type of radiation** and the **radiation geometry** is made. The therapy is divided into a number of individual treatments, so-called **fractionation**.

In determining these parameters, the most important factor is the depth of the tumor in the body. The technique is dependent on the depth, and a distinction is made between **brachytherapy** (superficial) and **teletherapy** (deep).

The desired radiation dose in the tumor is important; the dose varies with the type of tumor and usually lies between 4,000 and 8,000 rad (40–80 Gy).

The **type of radiation** is chosen to obtain a suitable depth of penetration. Both **photon** and **particle radiation**, with different energies, can be used.

Photon radiation is gradually attenuated—except in the case of the build-up effect described below—just as the light becomes weaker with increasing depth in the sea; particle radiation has a limited range, just as the shot-putter cannot throw beyond a certain limit.

While photon radiation is usually characterized by half-value thicknesses, particle radiation can be characterized by its maximum range.

In case of superficial tumors, such as skin cancer, low-energy types of radiation are used, which are mainly absorbed by the tumor and which do not penetrate to deeper layers. However, most tumors are located deeper in the body and require higher energies. By this means it is possible to obtain a higher dose at a certain depth than in the skin plane.

Photon radiation is obtained either from conventional x-ray tubes or from gamma-ray emitting nuclides, such as ^{60}Co. A comparison between conventional x-radiation, generated at <250 kV, corresponding to the photon energy maximum at 200–150 keV (cf, Fig. 8.17) and high-energy photon radiation (>500 keV) gives the following differences, which are important in teletherapy:

• High-energy radiation has a lower energy attenuation per gram of tissue and this gives an increased depth of penetration.
• The attenuation at high energies is largely independent of the atomic composition of the tissue (Fig. 13.3). At energies under 100 keV the attenuation is much higher for bone

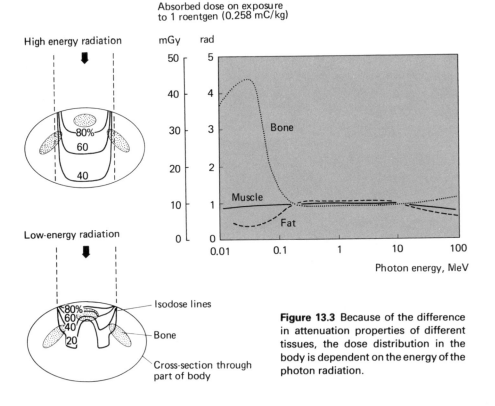

Figure 13.3 Because of the difference in attenuation properties of different tissues, the dose distribution in the body is dependent on the energy of the photon radiation.

than for muscle and fat; the advantage of the higher energy is that the skeletal parts do not cast shadows and that the dose can be calculated more exactly, since no knowledge of the spatial dimensions of the skeleton is required.

- In the case of high-energy radiation, the dose maximum is obtained some distance into the tissues because of a **build-up effect** (Fig. 13.4). This is caused by the generation of

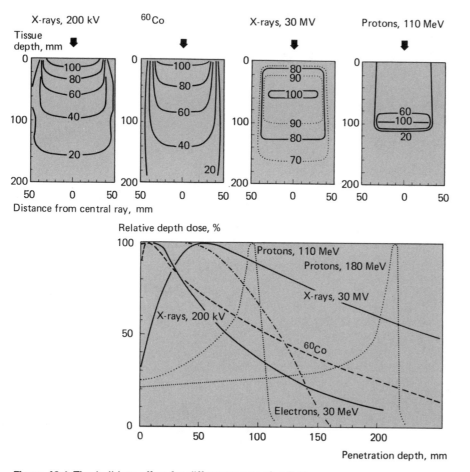

Figure 13.4 The build-up effect for different types of radiation. *Top:* Isodose curves in a homogeneous attenuator (water). *Bottom:* Relative depth dose as a function of depth of penetration.

secondary electrons, which mainly have a forward direction in the beam—that is, coincident with the beam used in the treatment. Secondary electrons have comparatively long ranges, because of the energy of the primary radiation. Compton photons, which are spread forward, also contribute. This build-up effect is important for protecting superficial tissue layers and for obtaining a dose maximum in the tumor mass.

Particle radiation. Because of the limited range of this type of radiation, the dose curves are completely different from those for photon radiation (Fig. 13.4). This means that the surrounding tissues can be better protected with particle radiation. As with photon radiation, there is a build-up effect, but this develops differently for different types of particle radiation because of the different modes of origin. For electrons, the curve is shallow, whereas for proton radiation there is a marked dose maximum—so-called Bragg peak (Fig. 13.4).

Table 13.1 Typical values for radiation from different radiation sources

Radiation source	Type of radiation	Energy MeV	Build-up depth, cm
x-ray tube	photons	0.25	0
^{60}Co teletherapy unit	photons	1.3	0.5
Linear accelerator	photons	4–25	1–3
Betatrons	photons	15–45	3–6
Synchrocyclotron	protons	180	21

Ray geometry. When a contour plan is completed and the type of radiation is chosen, a detailed dose plan is drawn up. Factors to be determined are the required **directions** of the irradiation, the **distance** to the radiation source and the **boundaries of the field**.

It is advantageous to divide the radiation field into a number of directions so that the dose to the skin can be distributed between several sites, while the tumor receives an aggregate dose. An example of treatment divided into six radiation fields is shown in Fig. 13.2. To obtain a wide distribution of the skin dose, the ray source can be rotated around the patient. For a full rotation of 360° around the patient, the center of rotation is the tumor; for a partial rotation the center of the tumor usually does not coincide with the center of rotation. Most ^{60}Co teletherapy units, betatrons and linear accelerators are designed for such **moving field irradiation**.

The field is defined by using appropriate collimators. To compensate for oblique directions of incidence on the body surface—and hence to simplify the calculation of ray geometry—wedge-shaped filters can be inserted between the radiation source and the patient. It is also possible to build up the filter with **bolus** material, which has attenuation properties corresponding to those of soft tissues. The patient's external contours are thus filled out so that a suitable beam geometry is obtained.

The result is a contour treatment plan with **isodose curves** drawn in (Fig. 13.2). The use of a computer can greatly reduce the amount of work required to develop this contour treatment plan.

Fractionation that is, division of the therapy into several irradiation treatments—is performed in order to give the normal tissues time to recover. It is empirically found that tumor tissue does not recover as well as the normal tissues if the total dose is distributed over a number of daily treatments given during a period ranging from a week or so to more than a month.

Dose Measurement

For calibrating radiation sources, measuring doses during radiotherapy and for radiation protection control, different methods of measurement are used. The commonest principle is that of the **ionization chamber**, of which there are many types. The method is simple and reliable. The instrument output is proportional to the therapeutic effect. An ionization chamber can be designed for measuring over wide energy ranges.

For digital recording of the dose, **Geiger-Mueller tubes** or **scintillation detectors** are often used.

Photographic measurement techniques are available for radiation protection control and for rapid determination of the dose distribution in a radiation field. The method has the disadvantage that the sensitivity of the photographic emulsion is dependent on the type of radiation and that the degree of blackening is dependent on the developing process.

When doses within small areas are to be measured, detectors based on the principle of **thermoluminescence** are used. When lithium fluoride is exposed to ionizing radiation, the electrons are raised to an excited state, which persists as long as the material is at room temperature. If the temperature is then increased to a certain level, the electrons leave this state, and energy is liberated in the form of visible light, which is measured.

13.33	The task of the radiophysicist is to prepare .... for each tumor patient, to have calibrated .... available and to be responsible for	
13.34	In treatment planning, a .... plan is first drawn up and then the .... is determined.	treatment planning radiation sources dose measurements
13.35	The purpose of the contour plan is to determine the .... of the tumor and the .... of the surrounding tissue.	contour physical dose distribution
13.36	When calculating the physical dose distribution, the .... is chosen and the .... is determined.	position attenuation

13.37	The choice of radiation source and type is dependent mainly on the . . . . of the tumor in the body.	type of radiation ray geometry
13.38	In superficial tumors, ... -energy radiation is used for so-called . . . .-therapy.	depth
13.39	In deep tumors, where . . . . -therapy is used, the dose can be concentrated in the tumor in two essentially different ways. High energies can be used, which produce, among other things, a . . . . effect and also the treatment can be performed as	low brachy
13.40	The build-up effect results in a higher dose at a certain depth in the body than on the skin; this is due, among other things, to the fact that the primary radiation generates largely coincident . . . . which are responsible for the deeper ionization.	tele build-up moving field irradiation
13.41	By means of moving field irradiation, the dose to the . . . . is dispersed, whereas the dose to the . . . . is concentrated.	secondary electrons
13.42	In radiotherapy, photon radiation is produced with . . . ., ... (radionuclide-charged devices) . . . ., and	normal tissues tumor
13.43	A patient is to receive radiotherapy. A contour plan has been drawn up and the type of radiation has been chosen. The remaining task is to find a suitable . . . ., and for this task, the radiotherapist makes the following determinations relative to the patient: the . . . . of the radiation, the . . . . of the radiation source and the . . . . of the beam.	x-ray tubes ^{60}Co teletherapy units betatrons linear accelerators
13.44	To compensate for oblique angles of incidence on the skin surface, a filter can be placed between the radiation source and patient. The filter is . . . . (shape). It is also possible to build up a filter on the patient from a material having the same attenuation as the soft tissues; this is known as . . . . (name of material).	ray geometry direction distance boundaries
13.45	The device most commonly used in radiophysics for measuring dose is an	wedge-shaped bolus material
		ionization chamber

PHYSICAL THERAPY

Physical therapy is a general term covering a number of different treatment methods. Their purpose is to produce symptomatic, palliative (supporting) or prophylactic effects (page 485).

A number of these methods act by developing heat in the tissues. For a superficial heating effect, the heat sources commonly used are **infrared radiation** from heat lamps or **warm baths**. For deeper effects, high-frequency techniques are used.

Examples of such physical therapy methods are **shortwave diathermy, microwave therapy** and **ultrasonic therapy**. Treatment with **ultraviolet light** differs from these, since it is based on a different mechanism of action: the ultraviolet light acts directly on the cells.

Exercise therapy is also a branch of physical therapy. Just as exercise helps the healthy person to keep in good physical and mental health, it also benefits ill or convalescent patients. For example, after a major operation, breathing exercises are of great importance for avoiding lung complications (pneumonia). Exercise is also important for preventing the development of blood clots in the legs and abdomen after operations. Exercise therapy is an indispensible procedure in modern hospital care; since it does not present any particular technical problems, it will not be considered further here.

Therapeutic effect of heat. The organs are affected by heat in much the same way no matter how it is supplied. When the tissue temperature is increased, so is the cell **metabolism**. This occurs in disease when the temperature is elevated—that is, when fever develops. By means of local heat treatment, the tissue temperature can be increased artificially and hence also its metabolism. This accelerates the process of healing.

When the temperature of the tissues is increased, **hyperemia** develops—that is, an increase in the quantity of blood flowing through the part. The arterioles, the smallest arteries, are dilated and the hydrodynamic impedance is reduced, resulting in an increased blood flow. It is well known that the skin reddens when exposed to heat. The increased blood flow facilitates transport of nutrients to the cells and waste products from them. The increased blood flow is also a way for preventing heat damage to the organism—the heat is conducted away by the blood.

Heat has an **analgesic** effect—that is, it alleviates pain. Pain is due to an oxygen deficiency in the tissues or to an accumulation of pain-eliciting substances: the increased blood flow results in increased oxygenation and facilitates the removal of these substances. The **sedative**, calming, effect of heat may be associated with the analgesic effect.

Depth of penetration in heat therapy. The method of heat treatment is chosen to provide heat at the required depth. Pathological skin conditions can be treated with **infrared radiation** from a heat lamp; this causes the development of heat up to a couple of millimeters deep in the skin, where it produces vasodilation—that is, widening of the vessels. If a deeper effect is required, **high-frequency techniques are used.**

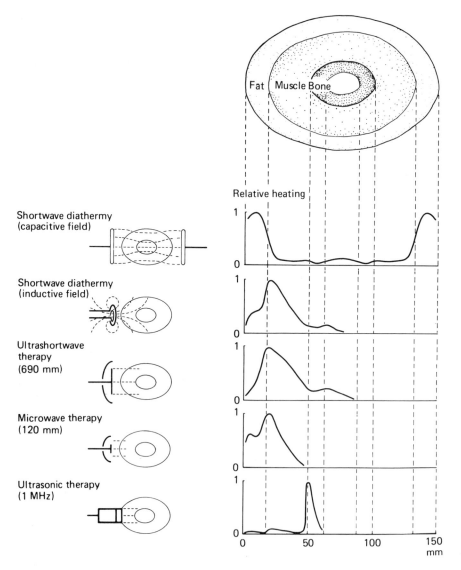

Shortwave diathermy
(capacitive field)

Shortwave diathermy
(inductive field)

Ultrashortwave
therapy
(690 mm)

Microwave therapy
(120 mm)

Ultrasonic therapy
(1 MHz)

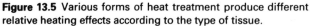

Figure 13.5 Various forms of heat treatment produce different
relative heating effects according to the type of tissue.

The depth of penetration varies for different high-frequency techniques. The heat developed is due to the electrical and ultrasonic losses in the tissues. These losses are different for fat, muscle, blood and bone. For high-frequency currents in the shortwave region (13, 27 or 40 MHz), applied by capacitive fields, the heat development is greatest in the subcutaneous fat layers (Fig. 13.5). This is expected, because the heat development increases with electrical resistivity (and dielectric loss), which is high for fat.

When the patient is placed in an inductive field, the distribution of heat losses differs: the greatest effect is obtained in tissues with a low resistivity—for example, muscle. In this case, the field is short-circuited to a greater extent and the heating effect is due to the generation of circulating currents.

In microwave irradiation using frequencies of 434 MHz and 2,400 MHz, the heat distribution is dependent on the depth of penetration (Fig. 13.5).

With ultrasonic irradiation at about 1 MHz, the maximum heating effect is obtained in the skeletal structures, since the absorption of ultrasound is greatest in bone.

13.46	An elderly patient has pain in his joints due to wear of the cartilage. There is no causal therapy. Therefore, shortwave diathermy is given. In the tissues .... is generated. It produces .... (increased blood flow).	
13.47	Hyperemia produces .... (alleviation of pain) because the increased blood flow improves the .... of the tissues and facilitates the removal of	heat hyperemia
13.48	In order to produce the greatest heat in the subcutaneous fat, ... (method) is used.	analgesia oxygenation pain-eliciting substances
13.49	In order to produce the greatest heat in muscle, as is often desired, one can use .... or	shortwave therapy with a capacitive field
13.50	To produce the greatest heating effect in bone, ... is chosen.	shortwave therapy with an inductive field microwave irradiation
		ultrasonic therapy

REFERENCES

ARENA, V. *Ionizing Radiation and Life.* Saint Louis (C. V. Mosby) 1971. 543 pages.

BARNES, P. and REES, D. *A Concise Textbook of Radiotherapy.* London (Faber & Faber) 1972. 384 pages.

BUSCHKE, F. and PARKER, R. G. *Radiation Therapy in Cancer Management.* New York (Grune & Stratton) 1972. 402 pages.

LICHT, S. *Therapeutic Electricity and Ultraviolet Radiation.* Vol. 4. *Phys. Med. Libr.* New Haven (Licht) 1967. 434 pages.

LICHT, S. *Therapeutic Heat and Cold.* Vol. 2. *Phys. Med. Libr.* New Haven (Licht) 1965. 593 pages.

| chapter 14 | # Hospital Information Systems |

Medical diagnosis and treatment require an involved analysis of gathered information. **Data collection** takes place at many decentralized locations in the hospital, such as the wards, x-ray, clinical chemistry and other laboratories, and from places outside the hospital, such as other clinics where the patient receives treatment. Moreover, the collected information is of a heterogeneous nature: most of it consists of **alphanumeric data**, a considerable portion consists of **analog information**, such as ECG curves and some consists of **image information**, such as radiographs.

The physician uses the collected information in **complex decision-making**. This is based on his evaluation of the collected information—evaluated not only relative to his fund of medical knowledge but also relative to a large number of practical organizational and economic factors associated with the actual medical care situation at the hospital in which the patient is treated.

Other problems are that it must be possible to constantly **up-date** the information, and add to it without limit, and that the information must be kept **confidential** in order to protect the integrity of the patient.

The earlier chapters give examples of the use of computer techniques for solving particular problems in different clinical specialties. But the application of these special data routines is limited. For example, one of the important objectives of processing ECG and EEG data is to obtain **data reduction** so that the diagnostically valuable information can be easily distinguished. This is accomplished by selecting out and rejecting the insignificant data. In clinical chemistry, computer techniques are used for **numerical calculations** of analytical results, for **statistical calculations** (to obtain quality control and error detection) and for a print-out of **patient reports**. In microbiology and hematology, data processing is used more for **administrative control** than for numerical calculation. Most of these medical applications for data processing can be capably handled with computers of modest size.

The integrated processing of the total flow of information in medical care—in a **hospital information system**, with which this chapter deals, is an extremely complex problem. This is because the total volume of information, most of which is collected directly from the patient and which must be accumulated at different times, is considerably greater than that which is analyzed in any of the clinical specialties mentioned above. One of the prime goals of a hospital information system is to replace the conventional medical record with a **computer record**.

Hospital information systems have been tried at many hospitals, but in most cases have proved unworkable or too costly and have been abandoned. Therefore, what follows in this chapter should be considered as an ideal, which may be realized in the coming years as computer costs are reduced and improved systems are developed. Portions of hospital information systems are functioning well in many locations. The integration of an entire system is more difficult.

The object of introducing a hospital information system is to increase the efficiency of medical care. This can be achieved because the **computer record** provides the responsible physician with a **better basis for his decision** in a shorter time and with less effort. The choice of treatment methods can then be made earlier and on a sounder basis and the treatment can be carried out more efficiently. Computer memory provides a better way of **storing** medical care information. Existing diagnostic and therapeutic resources in the hospital can be coordinated with a computerized resource inventory. With the information in computer form, it is possible to perform a continuous **check of the delivery** of medical care. It is possible to follow what treatment is given and where it is given. It is also possible to obtain better **quality control** by subsequently analyzing the results of the treatment, and it is possible to perform scientific evaluations of different diagnostic and therapeutic methods. Linked to some extent with quality control is the importance of the medical record as a **legal** document of what has happened to the patient.

With the **conventional medical record** written manually on a typewriter, many of these processes are difficult to perform. For example, medical records of the conventional type present a great storage problem. Every year the space needs for filing actual hospital records amount to about 2 shelf kilometers per million inhabitants, to which must be added about 1 shelf kilometer of x-rays per million inhabitants. (The growth of other stored documents in government administration amounts to only 0.5 shelf kilometer per million inhabitants per year.) With conventional records, it is virtually impossible to recover the information, and this makes it difficult to improve health care delivery and quality control, since statistical research attempting to evaluate, for example, therapy, becomes impractical. Conventionally stored records often disappear: about 15 percent are not found during the first search and 5 percent are never found.

THE MEDICAL RECORD

Content of the Medical Record

A medical record in the conventional form or designed as a computer record must contain many different kinds of information. The majority consist of alphanumeric data—that is, information that consists of numeric values, text that can be coded with characters or running text that is unsuitable for coding.

Various types of record information can be coded to different degrees. On the average, about 80 percent can be coded, while the remainder must be expressed in readable form for practical reasons. An attempt at complete coding would be doomed to failure and would, moreover, result in such voluminous code lists that they would be unmanageable and also involve a loss of information.

The collection of information presents no essential difficulties, whether done manually or on the computer.

On the other hand, there are many unsolved problems in the analysis of the large volumes of information. The major problems arise in the handling of analog information and image information; in manual handling they are space-consuming and difficult to survey; in computer systems it is very difficult to save these, since they consume large amounts of computer storage.

Identification data   relating to the patient must be reliably inserted to avoid any possible confusion. In Sweden each person has a personal identification number. This is particularly useful for identification in computer systems. In the United States, a number must be assigned to each new patient entering the hospital.

The medical history   is the most important source of information for making the diagnosis (page 105). Extracts from earlier medical records may be included in the medical history.

By using a questionnaire, the medical history can be **structured**: the patient's data are inserted in a standardized questionnaire requiring "yes/no" or multiple choice answers. The structuring enables the information to be easily **coded**—an extremely important concentration of data is obtained and information analysis is thus facilitated. Medical histories can also be acquired directly by the computer. The patient observes a series of questions on a terminal screen and answers by pressing keys on a keyboard. A branching program can assimilate the bulk of the

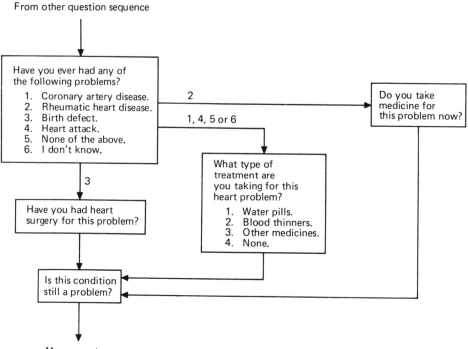

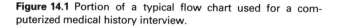

Figure 14.1 Portion of a typical flow chart used for a computerized medical history interview.

required information and present it in summary form to the physician. Figure 14.1 shows a segment of a flow chart for a branching medical history computer program.

Patient's condition.   The **somatic** (physical) condition of the patient is recorded in a definite order on an anatomical basis. The information can be structured and coded to a fairly advanced degree. The physician records any pathological findings, for example, by placing an X in a circle on a questionnaire. For recording the **mental** condition, structured questionnaires can also be used, although a greater amount of free text will probably always be needed for describing a mental pathological condition than a physical one.

Preliminary evaluation.   This is made on the basis of the medical history and the medical record. The data are evaluated and an attempt is made to make one or more alternative tentative diagnoses. These are used as working hypotheses for further investigation of the patient. In manually compiled medical records, the preliminary evaluation is often incompletely reported.

In a computer record, the preliminary evaluation should be more fully reported, since this is of value for laboratories and clinics concerned with the examination of the patient; by appropriate data transmission the preliminary evaluation can be made available for these laboratories and clinics. The preliminary evaluation can be structured so that it can be stored in the computer; however, the report of the preliminary evaluation in this way entails a greater amount of work for the physician. In return, a higher level of efficiency and more rapid routines are obtained.

Daily entries   regarding changes in the patient's condition and changed opinions regarding the preliminary evaluation are inserted in the medical record. Information that may also be inserted as daily entries includes a new goal for investigations, decisions on treatment or observed effects of treatment. It is possible to structure the daily entries for computer storage.

Chemical laboratory data   are chiefly numerical values, which can easily be inserted into and analyzed by computer.

Microbiological laboratory data   can also be computer processed without difficulty. Typical results consist of the name of the type of bacteria observed in a specimen and its resistance properties. The results can also consist of serological titer values (page 355).

Physiological data   at present are difficult to store in unprocessed form in a computer. It is necessary to make an extensive data reduction of analog measurement values, such as ECG, ventilation curves, EEG and EMG before they can be processed and stored. The data reduction involves sampling by analog to digital conversion, and selection of desired parts of the curves. The selection can be performed either manually or in some cases by computer, using special techniques (ECG, page 213, and EEG, page 246).

Radiographic information   cannot be stored with available technology so that it can be used in a hospital information system. The evaluation of radiographs must be performed by physician examination. A statement can be inserted in the computer record in readable or in code form (page 438). Easiest to code are the so-called x-ray signatures that indicate the method, examined organ and the radiological diagnosis.

Statements   by specialists such as ophthalmologists, ear specialists, gynecologists and pathologists (statements mainly relating to biopsy tests, page 116, and autopsies) can be structured and thus coded to facilitate computer analysis.

Operation reports,   summarized descriptions of the procedure for surgical operations and the findings can easily be structured.

Anesthesia records   can easily be structured.

Nursing station data   that are manually entered into the medical record are easy to store in the computer, such as instructions concerning the patient's drugs and other treatment. Other data are usually plotted in graphical form, such as temperature, pulse rate and urine volumes. All of these data must be available as a summary used in the evaluation of the patient at each round.

To present the alphanumeric data is easy. To present plots of graphical data is somewhat more difficult. Such special data presentation systems having the capability of reproducing centrally stored analog and alphanumeric data on cathode ray tube screens are usually reserved for sophisticated intensive care units because of their high cost.

The summary   of the medical record is written after a particular treatment is complete. It may be written at the time of the patient's discharge or subsequently. Important diagnostic findings and treatment are described in an abstract form. The summary may be structured for computer entry. The diagnosis may be coded according to the system recommended by the World Health Organization, WHO.

Purpose of the medical record

The medical record thus contains a large volume of data which is being constantly added to and which therefore must be updated. The medical record must serve as a basis for three medical decisions concerning the patient: **diagnosis**, **choice of treatment** and **prognosis** (Fig. 2.1). It should also serve as a basis for research.

Design of the Medical Record

The information contained in a medical record is stored and presented in different forms. In the conventional manually compiled medical record, the information is written by hand on various forms. In the computer medical record, the information is stored in the usual types of computer storage media—for example, magnetic tape and disc memories. The data presentation takes the form of a print-out of all or selected parts of the stored information. In certain intensive care units, the data are presented on special terminals with cathode ray tube screens.

The conventional medical record

The conventional medical record has many disadvantages, most due to the fact that pages are usually added in chronological sequence. Since the material is inserted in unstructured form, this complicates retrieval. It is true that the data are arranged in repetitive patterns, but because of the daily insertion of new data, the bundle of pages comprising the medical record increases steadily in size and the final result is difficult to survey. It has been mentioned above that a search for information in the stored medical records is practically impossible; most of the accumulated experience in medical care is therefore very difficult to find. A significant part of the personnel time in medical care consists of manual work concerned with entering information in the medical record and transfer of data between different locations in the hospital. Each medical record can be read by only one person at a time.

The conventional medical record also has certain advantages. When it is typewritten, it is typographically more easily read than the computer records. (Most medical records are handwritten.) In addition, the physician can insert his findings without being required to adopt a standardized form of expression, as with a structured recording method. Also, he doesn't have to go to a terminal to record or retrieve data.

The computer record

In the computer record, the desired information can be made available in a convenient way. The stored material can be grouped and sorted according to different principles, depending on its purpose. It can be concentrated so that only the most relevant information is presented each time a decision is to be made. Constant updating is possible and new information goes into the right place. The information can be made available for many users at the hospital simultaneously via multiple printouts or via multiple computer terminals.

The computer record can be easily designed as a **problem oriented medical record, POMR**. This means that it contains a listing of all the patient's problems, not only those for which the patient happened to consult the physician. A "problem" consists of a symptom or sign; for example, fever or a pathological finding discovered during the patient examination, such as a skin eruption or abnormal laboratory result. The problems are listed separately because they are described and followed one at a time. The description of each problem is expanded as new data are acquired, such as new laboratory values and radiological findings.

The problem-oriented record results in better medical care. It is very common for several diseases to occur simultaneously, and there is a risk of overlooking important diagnoses if different symptoms and findings are not separated in this easily traceable manner.

The introduction of the computer to store medical records presents great practical problems. The use of structured information can lead to difficulties if the physician must adapt himself to a rigid system that is the same for all physician–patient situations. In order to avoid loss of important information, free text comments must be permitted at many points in the structured information. This makes special demands on the design of the computer system. The presentation of information in a computer record is not optimal. As printed out by the computer, the medical record may be typographically difficult to read, but this presents no practical problems after a period of training. An important psychological point is that when a conventional medical record system is used, the physician takes the medical history by writing his own notes and by dictating. This makes a much stronger impression on his memory than just reading a completed text. Such disadvantages are compensated for by the fact that a hospital information system reduces the overall work load of the physician. It also enables him to localize problem areas, for example, via self-administered questionnaires, and then use the interview to delve more deeply.

The need for secrecy presents special problems in a hospital information system. Although absolute secrecy is not required—legal precedent provides that in certain cases the content of a medical record can be made available—the records should not be accessible to unauthorized persons. Secrecy requirements place demands on the organizational conditions governing the collection of medical data. An advantage is that it is easy to record who has requested the information.

By means of data processing, the medical records can be compiled more conventionally. The computer can store information, perform a search for it and process it; the computer cannot define problems, create the medical record or make medical decisions.

PLANNING OF MEDICAL CARE

By means of a hospital information system, it is possible to obtain better **planning** of medical care.

A consultation may be conducted in the following way: A patient who wishes to see a physician must first fill in a structured medical history form. This is sent to the hospital, where the information is transferred to computer-readable and coded form, after which computer analysis is performed. If the patient has stated that he is troubled by certain symptoms, these are compiled on a list. With the guidance of this list, certain laboratory tests and special examinations are planned. An administration center schedules the examinations at various laboratories such as x-ray. The appointments are printed out by the computer and sent to the patient in the form of an appointment notice. The patient is then examined at the various laboratories according to the appointments. All the results are continuously recorded in the data bank, which can update, retrieve and print out any desired information. When the patient visits the physician for the first time, he has considerable relevant information on the patient and his illness, for instance, the medical history, laboratory and x-ray results. The physician can then devote more time to the patient. A disadvantage of this scheme is that the tests cannot be as selectively chosen as when the patient sees the physician initially.

COMPUTER DIAGNOSIS

The mental process that leads to a diagnosis is complex. The physician first systematically collects a number of observations relating to the patient. According to his experience, he then assigns these observations to three classes: the ones that are normal, the ones that are abnormal and observations that cannot reliably be assigned to either of these two groups. With the collected and sorted information he makes a mental comparison with the number of known diseases and symptom complexes—altogether the number is considered to be about 35,000. There are again three alternative possibilities. First, there can be complete, or almost complete, agreement with one or more diseases—if this is the case he considers the diagnosis as established. Second, there can be incomplete agreement with one or more different diseases—in this case he performs further examinations to determine the diagnosis. (This is an extremely common situation in the investigation of patients where the diagnosis is not immediately clear.) Third, the physician can find himself in the situation where there is no agreement at all between his findings and known diseases. Then, either the observations are incorrect, his fund of experience is incomplete or he cannot remember the disease. It is seldom a question of a new disease.

Attempts have been made to use computers to perform the extremely sophisticated information analysis required by the diagnostic procedure. These attempts have had only a very limited success. It is possible to perform computer diagnoses within narrowly limited disease groups—for example, congenital heart failure or blood diseases—with a diagnostic reliability that is as good as that for the medical specialist who programmed the computer. However, this requires that the computer be fed with the results of all the examinations required for the diagnosis. The choice of these rests entirely with the physician.

A direct and complete computer diagnosis of each case would require a very large number of examinations on each patient; this would not be acceptable from an economic, practical or ethical aspect. It must be borne in mind that many diagnostic procedures incur some risk, and it is not in the patient's interest to perform them unless they are necessary.

Computer assisted diagnosis is therefore designed as a dialog between the physician and the computer. The initial findings are fed to the computer, which suggests certain possible diagnoses. These require new examinations to clarify the situation. The computer can be programmed so that the most urgent examinations receive priority. It is also possible to make an optimal choice of further examinations to minimize the total costs of medical care, including the costs of the examinations, the room charges, the physician's charges and the patient's loss of work time.

The use of computers in diagnostic work will probably be limited to the above-described logic functions, while completely automated diagnosis using the methods of examination known today will never be realizable in practice.

REFERENCES

BEKEY, G. A. and SCHWARTZ, M. D. (Eds.). *Hospital Information Systems.* New York (Marcel Dekker) 1972. 402 pages.

COLLEN, M. F. *Hospital Computer Systems.* New York (Wiley) 1974. 768 pages.

THE EDITORS. HIS—Physician Friend or Foe? *Computers and Medicine.* Vol. 3, July/August 1974.

GALL, J. E. The Application of the MIS-1 System at El Camino Hospital. *Advances in Automated Analysis.* Vol. 5, 1972. Pp. 87–90.

SIMMONS, D. A. *Medical and Hospital Control Systems; the Critical Difference.* Boston (Little, Brown) 1972. 739 pages.

Appendix

Internationally adopted SI units

Category	Quantity	Unit Name	Unit Symbol	Expressed in other SI units	Conversion
Space	length	meter	m	—	1 in = 0.0254 m
					1 foot = 0.305 m
					1 yard = 0.914 m
					1 Å = 100 pm
	area	square meter	m^2·	—	1 in^2 = 6.45 cm^2
					1 ft^2 = 9.29 dm^2
					1 yd^2 = 0.836 m^2
	volume	cubic meter	m^3	—	1 in^3 = 16.39 cm^3
					1 ft^3 = 28.3 dm^3
					1 yd^3 = 0.765 m^3
	angle	radian	rad	—	1 rad = 57.3°
		degree	°	—	1° = $\pi/180$ rad
	solid angle	steradian	sr	—	

Internationally adopted SI units (continued)

Category	Quantity	Unit Name	Unit Symbol	Expressed in other SI units	Conversion
Time, space-time	time	second	s	—	
		minute	min	60 s	
		hour	h		3600 s
	frequency	hertz	Hz	s^{-1}	$1\ Hz = 1\ s^{-1}$
	velocity	meter per second	m/s	—	1 km/h = 0.278 m/s
					1 mile/h = 1.609 km/h
					= 0.477 m/s
					1 ft/s = 0.305 m/s
	acceleration	meter per second squared	m/s^2	—	
Mass and force	mass	kilogram	kg	—	1 pound (lb) = 0.454 kg
					1 ounce (oz) = 28.4 g
	density	kilogram per cubic meter	kg/m^3	—	$1\ lb/in^3 = 27.8\ g/cm^3$
					$1\ lb/ft^3 = 16.02\ kg/m^3$
	force	newton	N	$kg \cdot m/s^2$	1 kilopound (kp) = 9.81 N
					1 pound-force (lbf) = 4.45 N
	moment of force	newton meter	Nm	$kg\ m^2/s^2$	
	pressure	pascal	Pa	N/m^2	$1\ kp/cm^2 = 98.1\ kPa$
					1 bar = 100 kPa
					1 torr = 133.3 Pa
					1 mm Hg = 133.3 Pa
					1 atm = 760 torr = 101.3 kPa
					1 atm = 98.1 kPa
	amount of substance	mol	mol	—	
Energy, power	energy, work	joule	J	Nm, Ws	1 kcal = 4.19 kJ
					1 kWh = 3.6 MJ
					1 BTU = 1055 J
					1 hph = 2.70 MJ
	power	watt	W	J/s	1 kpm/s = 9.81 W
					1 kcal/s = 4.19 kW
					1 kcal/h = 1.163 W
					1 hp = 745 W
					1 hp (metric) = 735 W

Internationally adopted SI units (continued)

Category	Quantity	Unit Name	Unit Symbol	Expressed in other SI units	Conversion
Electricity and magnetism	electric current	ampere	A	—	
	electric charge	coulomb	C	As	
	electric potential	volt	V	W/A	
	conductance	siemens	S	A/V	
	resistance	ohm	Ω	V/A	
	capacitance	farad	F	C/V	
	inductance	henry	H	Wb/A	
	magnetic flux	weber	Wb	Vs	
	magnetic flux density	tesla	T	Wb/m^2	
Optical radiation	luminous intensity	candela	cd	—	
	luminance	candela per square meter	cd/m^2	—	
	luminous flux	lumen	lm	$cd \cdot sr$	
	illumination	lux	lx	lm/m^2	
Ionizing radiation	activity	becquerel	Bq	s^{-1}	1 Ci (curie) $= 3.7 \cdot 10^{10}$ Bq
	exposure	coulomb per kilogram	C/kg		1 R (roentgen) $= 2.58 \cdot 10^{-4}$ C/kg
	absorbed dose	gray	Gy	J/kg	1 rad $= 10$ mGy

Index

Abdomen:
anatomy, 35
physical examination, 110
by palpation, 122
Abdominal cavity, tumor, diagnosis of, 118
Abduction, *terminology,* 41
ABO system, blood groups, 363
Abortion:
definition, 592
induced, 592
terminology, 592
uterine infection, example (Q 1.160), 32
Abscess, 30
abdominal, treatment of, example (Q 10.72), 532
surgical treatment, 531
Absorbance, 304
Absorbed dose:
SI unit, 647
units, 617
Absorption disorders (*see* Malabsorption)
Absorption photometry, 302

Acceleration, *SI unit,* 646
Accommodation, 97
Acetylcholine, transmitter substance, 21
Acetylsalicylic acid, effect (Q 9.39), 494
Achlorhydria, 299
Acid-base balance, and intensive care, 574
Acid-base disturbances, cause of, 574
Acid-fast bacteria, 325
Acidosis, 157-59, 574-77
metabolic, 157
and potassium ions, 273
respiratory, 157
Acid phosphatases and prostate carcinoma, 284
Acoustic impedance:
ear, 100
and ultrasonic imaging, 463
Acoustic meatus, *anatomy,* 99
Acoustic pathways, 81
Acoustic resonators, in speech formation, 57
Acromegaly, example (Q 9.6), 481

Action potential(s):
of heart muscle fibers, 189
from motor units, 254
in nervous system, 231
of skeletal muscles, 231, 253, 256
Active immunization, 349
Activity:
decay of radionuclide, 617
SI unit, 647
-acusia, 100
Adams-Stokes attacks, 196
pacemaker treatment, 219
Adaptation:
of eye, 97
of sensory organs, 96
Addiction, 494
Addison's disease, and sodium ions, 272
Adduction, *terminology,* 41
Adenocarcinoma:
radiosensitivity of, 623
terminology, 33
Adenosine diphosphate, 19
Adenosine triphosphate, 19
Adipose tissue, 17

ADP, 19
Adrenal cortex, 75
Adrenal glands, 75
Adrenal medulla, 75
Adrenergic nerves, 21
Adrenocortical hyperfunction:
  and potassium ions, 273
  and sodium ions, 272
Adrenocortical hypofunction:
  and potassium ions, 273
  and sodium ions, 272
Aerobic bacteria, 325
Aerobic process, in muscles, 19
Afferent fibers, 49
Afferent pathways:
  definition, 77
  spinal, 84
Agar, 330
Agglutination:
  of antigens, 347
  of microorganisms, 355
Agranulocytosis, due to drug
  hypersensitivity, 493
Air:
  acoustic impedance, 464
  as contrast medium, 382
  density, 464
  double-contrast, 393
  velocity of sound, 464
Air embolus, 29
  example (Q 1.150), 30
Airway(s):
  obstruction, intensive care, 540
  partial pressures in, 153
  tumor, diagnosis of, 118
Airway resistance, 150
  measurement, 151
Alanine-amino-transferase, 284
Alarm signal, in intensive care
  monitoring, 586
ALAT, 284
Albumin:
  in blood plasma, 279
  and colloid osmotic pressure, 280
  labeled, 184
Albuminuria, 296
Alcohol:
  disinfection by, 338
  overdose of, example (Q 3.62), 159
Alcoholism, chronic, cause of death
  in, example (Q 1.134), 28
ALG, in transplantation, 526
-algia, 9
Alkalosis, 157-59, 574-77
  metabolic, 157
  respiratory, 157
Allergic diseases, 350
  terminology, 480
Allergic reactions, and bleeding, 291
Allergy, 351
  terminology, 480
Allograft, 372
  transplantation of, 526
"All-or-nothing-law," 20
Alphanumeric data, 635
Alpha-particle, and dose equivalence,
  617
Alpha wave(s), 236
  synchronization with light pulses,
  240

Alveolar ventilation, 145
  determination, 154
Alveoli:
  anatomy, 56
  partial pressures in, 153
Amino acids, 277
  analysis, 312
  intravenous nutrition, 570
Amniotic fluid, 596
Amniotic sac, 596
  rupturing during delivery, 601
Amplifier(s):
  current limited, 207
  differential (*illus.*), 205
  for electrocardiography, 204-9
  neurophysiological, 261
    input impedances of, 261
A(n)-, 5
Anabolism, 284
Anaerobe culture technique, 330
Anaerobic bacteria, 325
Anaerobic infections, hyperbaric oxygen treatment, 553
Anaerobic process, in muscles, 19
Analgesia, in heat therapy, 631
Analgesia inhaler, 603
Analgesia stage, 511
Analog information, 635
Analyses, blood gas, 154
Analytical methods:
  automated, in clinical chemistry,
    312-18
  chemical, 302-18
  chromatography, 310-12
  electrochemical, 307-10
  optical, 302-7
  quantitative radiological, 439
  radioimmunological, 356
  using radionuclides, 318-20
Anaphylactic shock, 351, 558
  in blood transfusion, 362
Anastomosis, *terminology,* 530
Anatomy, *terminology,* 35
Anemia:
  cause of, 286
  example (Q 5.43), 290
  fetal, 365
  sign of radiation damage, 400
  symptoms, 286
  terminology, 29
  treatment blood transfusion, 360
Anesthesia, 505-18
  in Cesarean section, 607
  control by electroencephalogram,
    244
  in delivery, 603
  depth of, 509
  gaseous agents, 508
  general, and electroencephalogram,
    244
  risks in, 517
  stages of, 511
Anesthesia machines, 513-17
Anesthesia records, and hospital information systems, 640
Anesthesiology, *terminology,* 500
Angina pectoris, 107
Angiocardiography, 391
Angiography, 390
  of central nervous system, 398

-angioma, 33
Angle, *SI unit,* 645
Angle of scapula, 111
Animal starch, 60, 275
Ankle, *anatomy,* 36
Antebrachium, *anatomy,* 36
Anterior, *terminology,* 37
Anterior axillary line, *terminolog*
  110
Anti-, 5
Antiadrenergic substances (Q 9.3
  492
Antibacterial, *terminology,* 5
Antibiotic, 332
Antibiotics, treatment with, 495
Antibody, antibodies, 346-57
  to blood group antigen, 362
  definition, 346
  fluorescing, 358
  formation of, 346
  naturally occurring, 362
Anticoagulant therapy, in myocard
  infarction, 561
Antigen(s), 346-57
  definition, 346
  on red cells, 362
  transplantation, 374
Antilymphocytic globulin,
  transplantation, 526
Antimetabolites, in transplantatic
  526
Antisepsis, in surgery, 502
Antispasmodic, *terminology,* 5
Antitoxin, *terminology* (Q 1.21), 7
Anuria, *terminology* (Q 1.19), 7
Anus, *anatomy,* 53
Aorta (*illus.*), 60
  anatomy, 59
  aortic arch,
    baroreceptors in, 93
    chemoreceptors in, 90
  blood flow in (*illus.*), 173
  blood flow velocity in, 172
  pressure curves in, 173
  pulse waves in (*illus.*), 173
Aortic insufficiency, blood pressure
  (Q 2.98), 136
Aortic stenosis, x-ray examinatio
  390
Aortic valve(s), 128
  defects, catheterization of, 164
  insufficiency, murmur, 131
  stenosis, murmur, 131
Apex of lungs, *anatomy,* 56
Appendicitis:
  and body posture, 115
  example (Q 2.69), 123
Appendicitis abscess, 531
Appendix, *anatomy,* 53
Aqueous humor, *anatomy,* 97
Arachnoid, 82
Area, *SI unit,* 645
Arm:
  anatomy, 36
  bone of, *anatomy,* 44
Aromatic acids, analysis of, 312
Arrhythmia, 194-98
  cardioversion of, 218
  pacemaker treatment, 219-27
  (*see also* Heart arrhythmia)

rrhythmia detectors, 586
rteri-, 62
rterial walls, elasticity of, 172
rteriography, 391
 and thermography, 457
rterioles:
 anatomy, 59
 pressure drop in, 65
rteriosclerosis, 498
 and peripheral circulation, 186
 and serum cholesterol, 276
rteriovenous shunt, in hemodialysis,
 579
rteritis, *terminology,* 62
rtery, arteries:
 anatomy, 59, 60
 aorta (*illus.*), 60
 axillary (*illus.*), 60
 brachial (*illus.*), 60
 carotid (*illus.*), 60
 collateral, 186
 embolism, 186
 femoral (*illus.*), 60
 iliac (*illus.*), 60
 popliteal (*illus.*), 60
 radial (*illus.*), 60
 renal (*illus.*), 60
 ulnar (*illus.*), 60
 x-ray examination of, 391
rtifacts:
 in electroencephalography, 249
 in intensive monitoring, 582
rtificial hearts, 569
rtificial ventilation, 145, 540
 in cardiac arrest, 554
 and intrathoracic pressure, 546
 manual aids, 542
 manual methods for, 541
SAT, 284
-scan, ultrasonic, 464
scending colon, *anatomy,* 53
citic fluid, culture medium, 330
parate-amino-transferase, 284
phyxia:
 in anesthesia, 512
 during pregnancy and delivery, 604
 piration, risk in anesthesia, 509
 sisted breathing, 545
 sisted circulation, 562, 568-70
 apparatus for, 568
 thma, (Q 1.257), 58
 and air flow resistance, 150
 attack of, example (Q 11.6), 543
 cause of, 351
 FEV value, 150
 intensive care, 540
 ystole, 196
 and potassium ions, 273
 electasis, x-ray examination of, 387
 hlete's foot, example (Q 6.26), 328
 P, 19
 rial fibrillation, 196
 rial flutter, 196
 rial septal defect, 177
 illus.), 178
 rial septum, puncture during
  catheterization, 164
 rial systole, 128
 rioventricular node, 195

Atrophy:
 of muscles, 48, 252
 terminology, 9
Attenuation coefficient, ultrasonic,
 473
Aura, 241
Auscultation, 127-32
 of heart, 128
 of lungs, 127
AutoAnalyzer:
 for blood typing, 368
 for chemical analysis, 313
Autoclaving, 336
Autograft, 372
 transplantation of, 526
Autoimmune diseases, 352
 systemic, 353
Autoimmunity, 352
Automatic analysis:
 by continuous flow, 313
 with discrete samples, 314
Automation:
 in analytical chemistry, 312-18
 blood pressure measurement,
  583-85
 blood typing, 368
 drug administration, 588
 in microbiological diagnosis, 357
Autonomic nervous system, 87
 and blood pressure regulation, 93
 control of heart rate by, 160
 and light adaptation of eye, 97
Autoradiography, 450
AV block, 195
AV node, 195
Axon, 20

Bacteremia, 30
Bacteria, 324
 acid-fast, 325
 aerobes, 325
 anaerobes, 325
 bacilli, 324
 classification of, 331
 cocci, 324
 colonies, 330
 culture technique, 330
 facultative, 325
 gram negative, 325
 gram positive, 325
 growth curves, 334
 spirilla, 324
 spirochete, 324
 staining properties of, 324
Bacterial resistance, determination,
 332
Bacteriological diagnosis, automated,
 357
Balance, sense of, 100
Barbituate drugs, in delivery, 603
Barbiturates, for intravenous
 anesthesia, 508
Barium, as contrast medium, 382
Barium sulphate:
 as contrast medium, 393
 double-contrast, 393
Barium titanate:
 acoustic impedance, 464

 density, 464
 velocity of sound, 464
Baroreceptors, 93
Basal ganglia, 77
Base excess, 575
Base of lungs, *anatomy,* 56
Basophilic granulocytes (*illus.*), 23
Batteries, for pacemakers, 220
BCG vaccination, 349
becquerel, 647
Benign tumor, 32
Betatrons, 616
Beta waves, 237
Bi-, 5
Bicarbonate ions:
 in blood serum, 273
 concentration in blood, 157
Bicycle ergometer, 227
Bifocal lens, *terminology,* 5
Bilateral, *terminology,* 37
Bile, 52
 function of, 299
Bile duct(s):
 anatomy, 52
 common, *anatomy,* 52
 concretions in, 30
Bile pigment, 277
Biliary stasis, and jaundice (Q 1.251),
 55
Biliary tract diseases, and composition
 of urine, 295
Bilirubin, 277
Biliverdin, 277
Biological effect, of ionizing radia-
 tion, units for, 617
Biopsy, instruments for, 116
Bipolar technique, in electroencephalography, 235
Birth:
 after, *terminology,* 592,
 before, *terminology,* 592
 first four weeks after, *terminology,*
  592
 period of, *terminology,* 592
 (*see also* Delivery)
Birthweight, and stage of maturity,
 592
Blank value, photometry, 303
Bleeding:
 and anemia, 286
 postoperative, example (Q
  10.63-10.64), 529
 in surgery, 524
 from uterus, 593
Bleeding diseases, 291-93
Bleeding time, 291
Blood:
 analysis of, 270-93
 carbon dioxide tension in, 154
 clotting of, 291-93
 coagulation, 291-93
 differential count, 289
 electrolytes in, 272-75
 in feces, 299
 fetal circulation, ultrasonic
  monitoring of, 612
 functions of, 271
 glucose concentration, 275
 hemoglobin, normal values, 286

hemolysis, 288
infectious agent specimen technique, 329
infusion of, 370
oxygen tension in, 153
pH, 157-59
regulatory function of, 271
shelf-life of, 370
storage of, 370
sugar, threshold value, in kidneys, 294
total volume of, 184
and transplantation, 359-76
Blood cancer, 289
radiosensitivity of, 623
Blood capillaries, epithelial tissue of, 15
Blood cell counter, automatic, 287
Blood cells, 23
and bone marrow, 286
examination of, 285
function of, 285
red, 286-88
white, 288
function of, 289
Blood circulation:
monitoring in intensive care, 583
and shock, 557
Blood diseases, 285-91
mortality, 484
Blood donor, 369
Blood flow:
determination, 174-83
by Fick principle, 175
by indicator dilution method, 175
by indirect methods, 175
electromagnetic measurement of, 181
flow profile determination, 183
instantaneous measurement of, 181
measurement of, during catheterization, 161
peripheral, determination of, 186
ultrasonic measuring methods, 182
velocity in aorta, 172
Blood gas(es), 153-57
analyses of, 154
in intensive care monitoring, 583
sampling during catheterization, 161
Blood group(s), 362
definition, 361
and heredity, 361
percentage distribution (Q 7.24–7.27), 366-67
Blood-group serology, 361
Blood picture, sign of radiation damage, 400
Blood plasma, 271-85
proteins in, 279-82
Blood platelets (*see* Thrombocytes)
Blood pressure(s), 66
arterial, monitoring in intensive care, 583
automatic measurement, in intensive care, 583-85
automatic regulation by controlled dosage of drug, 588
differences in extremities, 135

dynamic measurement of, 171
mean, in circulatory system (*illus.*), 65
measurement of, 170-74
during catheterization, 161
in physical diagnosis, 133
normal values, 135
reference point for, 170
regulation of, 92
static measurement of, 170
Blood pumps, 567
Blood serum, 271-85
low-molecular weight organic substances in, 275-79
nitrogen-containing substances in, 277
opalescent, 276
Blood transfusion, 369-72
general requirements for, 364
and hepatitis B, 342
in shock, 559
unit for (*illus.*), 371
Blood type, 361
Blood typing, 367
automated, 368
manual, 367
Blood vessels, disorders of, 291
Blood volume, and colloid osmotic pressure, 280
Blood withdrawal, 369
Blunt dissection, 519
Body:
heat loss, 455
parts of, 35
Body fluids, 26
Body height, correlation to body surface, 388
Body plethysmograph, 148, 151
Body posture and physical diagnosis, 114
Body surface, calculation of, 388
Body temperature, 94, 136
Body water, 26
measurement of, 185
Body weight, correlation to body surface, 388
Bolus, in radiotherapy, 628
Bone:
cancellous, 42
compact, 42
acoustic impedance, 464
density, 464
velocity of sound, 464
infection, x-ray diagnosis of, 383
intercellular substance, 17
spongy, 42
tissue, 17
trabecular, 42
transplantation of, 526
ultrasonic imaging of, 467
Bone-marrow:
damage, and bleeding, 291
due to drug hypersensitivity, 493
puncture, 286
radiosensitivity of, 620
red, 42
tumors, radiosensitivity of, 623
yellow, 42
Bone mineral, 17

assay of, 440, 444, 445
Bone tumors, x-ray diagnosis of, 383
Brachial artery, *anatomy,* 60
Brachium, *anatomy,* 36
Brachytherapy, 625
Bradycardia, 122
Bragg peak, use in radiotherapy, 628
Brain:
angiography of vessels, 390
bleeding, ultrasonic diagnosis o 467
and Rh immunization, 365
ventricles, x-ray examination o 398
ventricular system of, 448
Brain death, 245
Brain membranes, 82
Brain stem, 82
Brain tumors:
diagnosis of, 139 (*see also* Tum and Tomography, co puterized axial)
and electrical activity, 243
and epilepsy, 241
ultrasonic diagnosis of 467
Brain waves:
amplitude of, 233
frequency of, 236-37
types, 236-40
Breastbone, *anatomy,* 44
Breasts:
anatomy, 73
tumors of, and thermography, 45
Breathing exercise, 631
Breathing rate, 145
monitoring in intensive care, 583
Breech presentation, 601
Bronchi:
anatomy, 56
x-ray examination of, 387
Bronchial carcinoma, x-ray exami tion of, 387
Bronchial hygiene, in intensive ca 540
Bronchial sound, 127
Bronchiectasis, after whooping cou example (Q 9.44), 496
Brochioles, *anatomy,* 56
Bronchitis, *terminology,* 57
Bronch(o)-, 57
Bronchography, 387
Bronchopneumonia, 57
Bronchoscope, 118
Bronchospasm, (Q 1.257), 58
Brow presentation, 601
B-scan, linear, ultrasonic, 464
Bubble oxygenators, 566
Bucky grids, x-ray technique, 409
Buffer base, 575
Build-up effect, in radiothera 627-28
Bullet wound in abdomen, example 6.8), 323
Bundle block, 196
Bundle of His, 195
Burns:
hyperbaric oxygen treatment of, hyperkalemia, example (Q 5. 274

intensive care of, 539
intravenous nutrition in, 571
treatment of fluid balance in, (Q 11.86), 574

Caffeine, pharmacological effect, 491
Calcium, analysis of, 305, 307
Calcium ions:
in blood, control of, 74
in blood serum, 273
and clotting of blood, 292
Cancellous bone, 42
Cancer:
gastrointestinal tract, treatment of, 532
mammary, treatment of, 532
ovarian, treatment of, 532
(see also Tumor)
Capacitance, SI unit, 647
Capacitive field, depth of penetration in physical therapy, 633
Capillaries:
and bleeding, 291
bleeding in surgery, 525
Carbohydrates:
in blood serum, 275
breakdown of, 299
intravenous nutrition, 570
Carbon dioxide:
contrast medium, 382
double-contrast, 393
Carbon dioxide tension:
in blood, 154
determination of, 155
Carbon monoxide:
as indicator, 185
poisoning, hyperbaric oxygen treatment of, 553
Carbonic acid, in blood, 157
carcinoma, 33
Cardiac arrest:
first aid, 554
treatment of, 554
Cardiac arrhythmia, in myocardial infarction, 560
Cardiac catheterization, 161-67
leakage current during, 165
during physical work, 227
risks in, 164
Cardiac defibrillation, 217
Cardiac orifice, anatomy, 51
Cardiac output, 160
determination of, 175, 187
and intrathoracic pressure, 546
and pulse rate, 228
thermodilution method, 177
Cardi(o)-, 61-62
Cardiogenic shock, 557
Cardiologist, terminology, 61
Cardiology:
terminology, 480
and ultrasonic diagnosis, 469
Cardiopulmonary physiology, 142-228
Cardioscope, 118, 586
Cardiospasm, terminology, 62
Cardioversion, 218
Care, types of, 481

Carotid arteries:
baroreceptors in, 93
chemoreceptors in, 90
internal, impairment of circulation, 457
Carotid sinus, 93
Carpus, anatomy, 36
Cartilage, 17, 44
articular, 45
prosthesis, 528
CAT, 447
Catabolism, 284
Catgut, for suturing, 523
Catheter(s):
compliance of, 171
dynamic properties of, 171
Catheter-transducers, pressure, resonant frequency and damping factor of, 171
Caudal, terminology, 38
Causal treatment, 485
Cecum, anatomy, 53
Cell(s), 12
blood, 23
body, 12
cilia, 13
death after irradiation, 619
glial, 20
irritability of, 13
membrane, 12
permeability of, and calcium ions, 273
metabolism of, 13
and heat therapy, 631
motility of, 13
mutation after irradiation, 620
nerve, 20
nutrition of, 61
physiology, terminology, 35
proteins, 283
reproduction, 13
respiration, 142
sensitivity to ionizing radiation, 619
size of, 12
Cell-mediated immunity, 346
and autoimmunity, 352
and transplantation, 373
Cellular tests, in tissue typing, 374
Central nervous system, 79-83
electroencephalography, 232-51
intensive care of diseases, 538
x-ray examination by computerized axial tomography, 398, 448-49
Central venous pressure, 558
monitoring in intensive care, 583, 585
tumors, and protein in cerebrospinal fluid, 301
x-ray examination of, 398
Centrifuge analyzers, 315
Cephalic presentation, 601
Cerebell-, 78
Cerebellar, terminology, 78
Cerebellum, 82
Cerebral, terminology, 78
Cerebral aneurysm, example (Q 9.17), 484
Cerebral angiography, 391
(illus.), 390

Cerebral cortex, 79
and membrane potential of neurons, 233
Cerebral death, 141
Cerebral hemorrhage, and muscular paralysis, 251
Cerebral meningitis, example (Q 5.49), 292
Cerebr(o)-, 78
Cerebromalacia, (Q 1.336), 79
Cerebrospinal, terminology, 78
Cerebrospinal fluid, 82, 301
composition of, 301
formation of, 301
Cerebrum, anatomy, 79
Cervical cancer, radiosensitivity of, 623
Cervical vertebrae, anatomy, 44
Cervix, widening during delivery, 599
Cesarean section, 607
Chemical analysis, methods, 302-18
Chemical corrosion, and electrosurgery, 521
Chemical disinfection, 338
Chemical laboratory data, and hospital information systems, 639
Chemical sterilization, 337
Chemoreceptors, 90
Chemotherapeutic agent, 332
and radiosensitivity, 623
Chemotherapeutic drugs, treatment with, 495
Chest organs, surgical diseases of, terminology, 500
Cheyne-Stokes breathing, (Q 2.47), 115
Chickenpox:
incubation time, 326
infectious agent in, 326
Child:
definition, 592
gestation periods, 592
immature, definition, 592
mature, 592
premature, definition, 592
terminology, 592
Children, diseases of, terminology, 480
Children's diseases, and antibodies, 347
Chloramine, disinfection, 338
Chloride ions:
in blood serum, 273
and electrolyte balance, 573
treatment with, 576
Chloroform, 508
Chol-, 54
Cholangiography:
example, 536
intravenous, 395
operative, 395
Cholangitis, terminology, 54
Cholecyst-, 52, 54
Cholecystectomy, example, 536
Cholecystitis, 534 (Q 1.246), 55
and peritonitis, (Q 1.252), 55
Cholecystography, 395
Choledochotomy, example, 536

Cholelithiasis, 30
  example of surgical treatment,
    533-37
Cholesterol, in blood serum, 276
Cholinergic nerves, 21
Chorionic gonadotropin, 595
Choroid, *anatomy,* 97
Chromatin granules, 12
Chromatography, 310-12
Chromosomes, 12
Chronic care, 482
Chronic infections, and anemia, 286
Cilia, 13
Circulation, 160-227
  during anesthesia, 510
  assisted, 562, 568-70
  extracorporeal, 562-68
  fetal, ultrasonic monitoring of, 612
  and intensive care, 554-62
  of interstitial fluid, 281
  peripheral, 186-88
Circulatory diseases, treatment of, 497
Circulatory disorders, 28
  and thermography, 457
Circulatory failure, 554-62
  intensive care of, 554-62
  in myocardial infarction, 561
Circulatory organ diseases and mor-
    tality, 484
Circulatory organs, x-ray examination
    of, 388
Circulatory system, 58-67
Cisternal puncture, in diagnostic
    radiology, 398
Clark electrode, 154
  (*illus.*), 155
Clavicle, *anatomy,* 44
Clearance, 297
  definition, 297
Clinical chemistry, 267-320
  reliability in, 317
Clinical death, 140
Clinical microbiology, 321-43
Clinical neurophysiology, 230-65
Clotting time:
  determination of, 292
  and surgery, 525
⁶⁰Co:
  radiation source, for sterilization,
    337
  in radiotherapy, 626
Coagulation, 291
Cocci, 324
Coccyx, *anatomy,* 44
Cochlea, *anatomy,* 99
Coding, of medical records, 637
Coefficient of reflection, ultrasonic,
    464
Coitus, and pregnancy, 594
Col-, 54
Coliform bacteria, growth curve, 334
Colitis:
  terminology, 54
  ulcerative (Q 1.250), 55
Collagen fibers, 17
Collagenoses, 353
Collar bone, *anatomy,* 44
Collimators:
  for rectilinear scanning, 450

x-ray technique, 408
Colloid osmotic pressure, 280
  and fluid balance, 572
  and serum albumin, 280
Colon:
  anatomy, 53
  endoscopy in ulcerative colitis (Q
    2.62), 121
  excretory function of, 67
  position of (*illus.*), 112
  tumor (Q 1.171), 34
  diagnosis of, 118
  x-ray examination of (*illus.*), 393
Colonies, of bacteria, 330
Color changes, and physical
    diagnosis, 115
Color sensitivity, eye, 97
Colostomy, *terminology,* 54
Combustion products, excretion of,
    67
Compact bone, 42
Compartment volume, determination
    of, 184
Compatibility, immunological, 374
Complement fixation, serological
    diagnosis, 355
Compliance, 151
  of catheters, 171
  definition, 152
  determination of, 152
  of ventricular walls, 160
Compound B-scan, ultrasonic, 466
Compression loss, in ventilator, 549
Computer, average response, for
    evoked potentials, 265
Computer analysis:
  in electrocardiography, 214
  in electroencephalography, 246-49
Computer classification, in electrocar-
    diography, 215
Computer diagnosis, 643
Computer record, 636
Computerized axial tomography,
    447-49
  of central nervous system, 398,
    448-49
Conception, 594
Concretions, 30
Conductance, *SI unit,* 647
Conduction velocity:
  in motor nerves, 256-58
  in nerve fibers, 258
Cones, *anatomy,* 97
Congenital deformities, mortality, 484
Congestive heart failure, 497
Connective tissue, 17
  diseases of, and mortality, 484
Consciousness, level of:
  and electroencephalogram, 244
  in intensive care monitoring, 587
Contact dermatitis, cause of, 351
Continuous suture, 523
Contourograph, 586
Contour planning, in radiotherapy,
    624
Contraceptive pills, toxic effect of, (Q
    9.43), 494
Contrast, in x-ray imaging, 380
Contrast discrimination, of eye, 433

Contrast enhancement of x-ray image
    420
Contrast medium, 382
  excretion by kidneys, 396
  negative, 382
  positive, 382
Controlled breathing, 545
Contusion, *terminology,* 34
Convolution process, in computerized
    tomography, 448
Corium, *anatomy,* 72
Cornea:
  anatomy, 97
  transplantation of, 526
Corneal reflex, 138
Coronal plane, 37
Coronary angiography, 391
Coronary arteries, *anatomy,* 61
Coronary arteriosclerosis, 498
Coronary care unit, 561
Coronary insufficiency, 498
  electrocardiogram in, 200, (Q
    3.169-3.170) 201
  (*illus.*), 199
Coronary vessels, x-ray examination
    of, 391
Corpus callosum, *anatomy,* 79
Corpuscular hemoglobin, 288
Corpuscular volume, 288
Correlation analysis, in elec-
    troencephalography, 246
Corrosive gases, and alveolar diffu-
    sion, 145
Cortical layer, of brain, 77
Cortico-, 76
Corticoids, 75
  terminology, 76
Corticotropic, *terminology,* 76
Costae, *anatomy,* 44
Costal arch, 111
Cotton swab, 329
Cowpox, 349
Coxsackie virus, 327
CPK, 284
Cranial, *terminology,* 38
Cranial nerves, 83
Cranium, *anatomy,* 35
Creatine, 277
Creatine phosphokinase, 284
Creatinine, 277
Creatinine clearance, 297
Crosscorrelation analysis, in elec-
    troencephalography, 247
Crossmatching, 370
Crus, *anatomy,* 36
Cryotechnique, 521
Culture media, for infectious agent
    330-32
Culture technique:
  anaerobe, 330
  for bacteria, 331
  microbiological, 329-35
  reinoculation, 330
  using animals, 333
  for viruses, 334
Curare, 517
Cushing's syndrome, and sodiu
    ions, 272
Cutan-, 73

Cutis, *anatomy,* 72
Cutting, *terminology,* 530
CVP, 558
Cyanide poisoning, and cell respiration, 143, (Q 3.19) 146
Cyanosis, 28
  and diffusion resistance, 145
Cyclopropane, 508
Cyclotrons, 616
Cysteine, and radiosensitivity of tissues, 623
Cystic duct, *anatomy,* 52
Cystitis:
  example (Q 1.291), 69
  terminology, 68
Cyst(o)-, 68
Cystography, 396
Cystolithiasis, *terminology,* 68
Cystoscope, 118
Cystoscopy, anesthesia for (Q 10.22), 507
Cyt(o)-, 13
Cytology, *terminology,* 13, 35
Cytoplasm, 12
Cytostatic agents, and radiosensitivity of tissues, 623

Dacron, prosthesis material, 528
Daily entries, and hospital information systems, 639
Damped percussion note, 125
Dark and light adaptation, 98
Data collection, in hospital information systems, 635
Data presentation, in intensive care monitoring, 587
Data processing:
  in clinical chemistry, 315
  in clinical microbiology, 358
  in diagnostic radiology, 434
  of electrocardiogram in myocardial infarction, 561
  in electrocardiography, 213
  in fetal electrocardiography, 610
  in hospital information systems, 635-44
  in intensive care, 582-89
  of medical records, 637-42
Data reduction:
  in electrocardiography, 213
  in electroencephalography, 246, 249
  in hospital information systems, 636
  in intensive care monitoring, 586
Data storage:
  in electrocardiography, 212
  in hospital information systems, 636
  in intensive care monitoring, 587
Data tomogram, 448
Daughter tumor, 33
Day-care, 482
Death, clinical, 140
Decantation tee, 368
Decision-making, and data processing, 635
Deep, *terminology,* 39
Deep sensibility, 49
Deep sleep, 244
Defense mechanisms:
  nonspecific, 343
  specific, 344
Defibrillation, 217-20
  external, 217
  internal, 217
  in myocardial infarction, 561
  synchronized, 218
Defibrillators, types of, 218
Degeneration, of tissues, 27
Dehydration:
  and creatinine in blood serum, 277
  and fluid balance, 592
  and Hb value, 286
  and sodium ions, 272
  treatment of, 573
Delirium stage, in anesthesia, 512
Delivery, 599-610
  Cesarean section, 607
  date of, 597
  example, (Q 12.21–12.30) 602-3
  first stage, 599
  forceps, 608
  instrumental extraction, 608
  second stage, 601
  simultaneous monitoring of heart rate and intrauterine pressure, 613
  third stage, 602
  vacuum extraction, 608
Delta waves, 237
Demand pacemaker, 222
Dendrites, 20
Denervation, 251
Density, *SI unit,* 646
Density, of x-ray film, 414
Depolarization, of heart muscle fibers, 189
Depth of field, in radiography, 378
Derma-, 73
Dermatitis:
  cause of, 351
  terminology, 73
Dermatology, *terminology,* 480
Dermatomycosis, *terminology,* 73
Dermatophytoses, infectious agent in, 326
Dermis, *anatomy,* 72
Descending colon, *anatomy,* 53
Dexter, *terminology,* 37
Di-, 5
Diabetes mellitus, 75
  acidosis in, example (Q 3.61), 159
  and blood glucose, 275
  coma:
    automatic treatment of, 589
    example (Q 11.89–11.90), 576
  example (Q 1.129), 26
  and glucosuria, 294
  smell of acetone, example (Q 2.66), 121
Diagnosis:
  bacteriological, 329
  with chemical tests, 270-302
  with computer, 643
  neurological, 230
  radiological, 377-478
  serological, 355
  with thermography, 457
Dialysis:
  and fluid balance, 578
  and hepatitis B, 342
  and intensive care, 577-82
Diaphragm:
  anatomy, 35
  observation of movements, 379
  position of (*illus.*), 112
Diarrhea:
  and sodium ions, 272
  treatment of dehydration, example (Q 11.84-11.85), 573, 574
Diastole, 66, 128
Diastolic pressure, 66
Dichotomy, *terminology,* 5
Diencephalon, 82
Diet, and arteriosclerosis, 498
Diethyl ether, 508
Differential amplifier:
  (*illus.*), 205
  neurophysiological, 261
Differential count, 289
Differential diagnosis, 102
Diffusion:
  alveolar, 142, 145
  in dialysis, 578
Digestion, 299
Digestive organs:
  diseases of, 484
  x-ray examination of, 393
Digestive system, 51
  diseases of, *terminology,* 480
Digitalis, 497
  in myocardial infarction, 561
Digits, *anatomy,* 36
Diptheria, infectious agent in, 324
Diplococci, 324
Disc, intervertebral, *anatomy,* 44
Disc herniation (Q 1.359–1.360), 85, 86
  location of, 84
Diseases:
  allergic, 350
  autoimmune, 352
  general terminology of, 10
  immunological, 350
  infections, 323
Diseases of the elderly, *terminology,* 480
Disinfection, 338-40
  definition, 335
Dislocation, *terminology,* 34
Distal, *terminology,* 37
Distribution, skew, of normal values, 269
Dodging, of x-ray image, 420
Doppler, frequency shift, 183
Doppler principle, for measuring flow, 182
Doppler ultrasonic method, in fetal monitoring, 611-12
Dorsal, *terminology,* 37
Dorsal roots, 83
Dorsiflexion, *terminology,* 40
Dose, accumulated, for radiological personnel, 401
Dose, of ionizing radiation:
  in diagnostic radiology, 400-401, 412
  and image information, 421-27
  and image intensification, 411-12
  maximum permissible, 401
  in radionuclide organ visualization, 449
  units, 617

Dose equivalence, 617
Dose measurement, in radiotherapy, 629
Double blind tests, 486
Double-contrast, 393
Drainage, of abscess, 531
Dressing techniques, 529
Driven right leg ground, 205-7
Drowning, example (Q 5.44–5.45), 290
Drug(s):
  addiction, 494
  administration of, 488
  analysis of, 312
  automatic administration of, 588
  effects of, 490-93
  and hypersensitivity, 351
  interaction of, 491
  metabolism of, 491
  resistance, 332, 495
  side effects of, and bleeding, 291
  slow release of, 489
  substitution therapy, 491
  toxic effect of, 493
Dry-heat sterilization, 336
Du Bois formula, 388
Ductus arteriosus, 177, (illus.) 178
Ductus deferens, anatomy, 69
Duodenal ulcer (Q 1.249), 55
  example (Q 5.79), 301
Duodenum:
  anatomy, 52
  endocrine function of, 75
Dura mater, 83
Dys-, 5
Dysfunction, terminology, 5
Dyspepsia, terminology, 5

Ear:
  anatomy, 99
  inflammation of (see Otitis)
Ear, nose and throat, diseases of, terminology, 500
Ear drum, perforation, diagnosis of, 118
ECG (see Electrocardiography)
Echo encephalography, 468
Echo virus, 327
Echocardiography, 469
Eclampsia, 605
Edema, 28
  and colloid osmotic pressure, 281
  and fluid balance, 572
  and Hb value, 286
  pulmonary, 28
  and sodium ions, 272
  in toxemia of pregnancy, 605
EEG (see Electroencephalography and Electroencephalogram)
Efferent fibers, 49
Efferent pathways:
  definition, 77
  spinal, 84
Elastic fibers, 17
Electric charge, SI unit, 647
Electric current, SI unit, 647
Electric potential, SI unit, 647
Electric shock, and ventricular fibrillation, 217

Electrocardiogram:
  analysis of curves, 198-202
  AV-block, 200
  bundle block, 200, (Q 3.172) 202 (illus.), 199
  in coronary insufficiency, 200, (Q 3.169–3.170) 201 (illus.), 199
  in intensive care monitoring, 585
  interpretation of, 200 (illus.), 199
  in myocardial infarction, 200, (Q 3.171) 202 (illus.), 199
  observation in myocardial infarction, 561
Electrocardiography, 188-217
  amplifiers, 204-9
    current limited, 207
    and grounding of patient, 205
    interference from power lines, 205
    time constant, 204
  bipolar limb leads, 189
  calibration signal, 207
  computer analysis in, 214
    value of, 215
  computer interpretation of, 214
  corrected orthogonal leads, 192
  data reduction, 213
  display type, 210
  electrodes, 203
  Frank lead system, 192
  interference from muscle potentials, 207
  lead systems, 189-94
  measurement considerations, 202-09
  monitoring during catheterization, 164
  multivariate classification technique, 215
  during physical work, 227
  precordial leads, 192
  presentation systems, 210
  recording techniques, 209
  standard leads, 189
  storage, 212
  telemetry, 212
  transmission techniques, 209
  unipolar chest leads, 192
  unipolar limb leads, 191
  vectorcardiography, 210
Electrocorticography, 242
Electrodes:
  in electrocardiography, 203
  in electrosurgery, 520
  impedance, measurements of, 203
  in neurophysiology, 260
  for pacemakers, 225, 226
  polarization of, 203, 261
Electroencephalogram, 232
  alpha waves, 236
  beta waves, 237
  and brain death, 245
  and brain tumors, 243
  and cerebral hemorrhage, 243
  clinical use of, 241
  and deep sleep, 244
  delta waves, 237

diagnosis of epilepsy, 241
frequency of waves, 236-37
and level of consciousness, 244
provocation:
  by hyperventilation, 240
  by light pulses, 240
  by sleep, 240
and REM sleep, 244
and sleep (illus.), 237
spikes and waves, 237
synchronization of cortex cells, 233 238
theta waves, 237
wave types, 236
Electroencephalography:
  analysis of transients, 249
  automatic signal analysis, 246
  bipolar recording technique, 235
  computer analysis, 246
  correlation analysis, 246
  cross correlation analysis, 247
  data reduction, 246
  display systems for, 250
  electrodes:
    contact impedance of, 235
    placement on scalp, 234
  Fourier analysis, 246
  frequency analysis in, 248
  parameter estimation, 246
  recording techniques, 234
  stationary processes, analysis of 246
  spectral density determination, 246
  unipolar recording technique, 235
  variance analysis, 248
Electrolyte balance, 272
  and intensive care, 573
Electrolytes:
  in blood, 272-75
  in blood serum, normal value (table), 274
Electromagnetic measurement of blood flow, 181
Electromyography, 253-56
  discharge frequency, 254
  fibrillations, 255
  and muscle denervation, 255
  potentials, 254
Electroneurography, 258-59
Electrophoresis, 308
  free, 309
  gel, 309
  immuno-, 309
  paper, 309
  separation of serum proteins, 280
  zone, 308
Electrophoretic mobility, 309
Electroshock treatment, 241
Electrosurgery, 520
  damage from, 521
  examples (Q 10.48–10.50), 522-2
  in hemostasis, 525
  risk of explosion in anesthesi 518
Embolus, 29, (Q 1.148) 30
  abdominal operation, example (1.269), 63
  arterial, thermography diagnosis of 457
  in myocardial infarction, 561

mia, 24
mission photometry, 304-7
nanthem, 115
ncephal-, 77
ncephalitis:
  infectious agent in, 327
  terminology, 77
ncephalography, 398
ncephalon, *anatomy,* 79
nd(o)-, 5
ndocarditis, infectious agent in, 326
ndocrine diseases, mortality in, 484
ndocrine glands, 16
  anatomy, 74
ndocrine system, 74
  regulatory function of, 88
ndocrinology, *terminology,* 480
ndogenous, *terminology,* 5
ndometritis, (Q 1.300), 72
ndometrium:
  anatomy, 71
  and menstrual cycle, 593
ndoscope, 116
ndoscopy, 116
  anesthesia for, 505
ndotracheal tube, 510
nema:
  for administration of drugs, 489
  contrast medium, 393
nergy, *SI unit,* 646
nergy metabolism, 284
nterovirus, 327
nzyme(s):
  in cells, 13
  gastrointestinal, 299
  measure of activity, 284
  for specific analysis:
    by polarography, 308
    by potentiometry, 307
  stomach secretion, 51
nzyme diagnosis, 284
nzyme pattern, 284
osinophilic granulocytes:
  function of, 289, 347
  (*illus.*), 23
pidemic parotitis, and sterility, (Q
    1.296), 71
pidemiology, *terminology,* 480
pidermis, *anatomy,* 72
pididymis, *anatomy,* 69
pididymitis, and sterility, (Q 1.297),
    71
pilastrium, 110
pilepsy:
  aura, 241
  in brain tumors, 243
  and electroencephalogram, 241
  focal, 241, 242
  grand mal, 241
  jacksonian attacks, 242
  petit mal, 241
pileptic attacks, provocation by
    photostimulation, 240
pinephrine:
  and blood pressure regulation, 93
  secretion by adrenal medulla, 75
piphyseal line, 43
ithelial cells, in urine, 296
ithelial tissue(s), 15

Erysipelas:
  incubation time, 326
  infectious agent in, 326
Erythrocyte sedimentation rate, 288
Erythrocytes, 23, 286-88
  hemolysis, 288
Esophagoscope, 118
Esophagus:
  anatomy, 51, 57
  bleeding from veins, diagnosis, 118
  diagnosis of tumor, 118
ESR, 288
-esthesia, 9
Estrogen, 75
Ether, anesthesia, example (Q 10.36),
    513
Ethylene oxide sterilization, 337
Eustachian tube, *anatomy,* 99
Evan's blue, 184
Evoked potentials, 265
Evoked response, 265
Ewing's sarcoma, radiosensitivity of,
    623
Exanthem, 115
Exchange transfusion, 365
Excision, *terminology,* 530
Excitatory postsynaptic potential, 232
Excretion, of waste products, 293
Excretory organs, x-ray examination
    of, 396
Excretory system, kidneys, 67
Exercise electrocardiogram, 200, (Q
    3.170), 201
Exercise tests, 227
Exercise therapy, 631
Exhaustion shock, 558
Exocrine glands, 16
Exophthalmos, 114
Expiration, 56
  in ventilator treatment, 546
Expiratory reserve volume, 147
Exposure:
  amount of radiation, units, 617
  SI unit, 647
Extension, *terminology,* 40
External, *terminology,* 38
External rotation, of fetus, 607
Extinction, 304
Extinction coefficient, 304
Extirpation, *terminology,* 530
Extra-, 5
Extracellular fluid, 26
  and fluid balance, 572
Extracellular ions:
  calcium, 273
  sodium, 272
Extracorporeal circulation, 562-68
  total duration of, 564
Extracorporeal dialysis, 578
Extradural hematoma, example (Q
    8.183), 471
Extraperitoneal, *terminology,* 5
Extrasystole(s), 196
  atrial, 196
  automatic detection of, 561
  during catheterization, 164
  nodal, 196
  ventricular, 196

Extrauterine pregnancy, 594
Extremities, work capacity and cir-
    culation, 186
Exudate, 30
Eye, 97
  anesthesia for, 505
  cataract, ultrasonic diagnosis of,
    469
  contrast discrimination and
    diagnostic radiology, 411, 433
  diseases of, *terminology,* 500
  fixation nystagmus, 433
  perceivable image contrast, 425
  perceivable image elements, 425
  perception of contrast and image
    noise, 423
  pressure in, 133
  retinal detachment, ultrasonic
    diagnosis of, 469
  and spatial illumination gradient
    (*illus.*), 433
  tumor, diagnosis of, 118
Eye damage, and autoimmunity, 353
Eye movements, in anesthesia, 511

Fabric, prosthesis material, 528
Face, *anatomy,* 35
Face presentation, 601
Fallopian tube:
  anatomy, 70
  inflammation of, and sterility, (Q
    1.299), 71
  and pregnancy, 593
Fascia, transplantation of, 526
Fast Fourier Transform, application
    in electroencephalography, 246
Fat:
  acoustic impedance, 464
  breakdown of, 299
  density, 464
  embolus, 29
    example (Q 1.149), 30
  in feces, 300
  intravenous nutrition, 570
  transport of, in blood, 276
  velocity of sound, 464
Fatty tissues, and x-ray image con-
    trast, 381
Febrile, 95
Feces, 299-301
  blood in, 299
  fat in, 300
  infectious agent specimen techni-
    que, 329
f-ECG, 610
Feedback, and muscular contraction,
    49
Femoral artery, *anatomy, 61*
Femoral neck:
  anatomy, 45
  fracture, example (Q 2.46), 114
    (*illus.*), 384
Femur:
  anatomy, 36, 45
  fracture, 383
    (*illus.*), 384

657

Fertilization, 594
  probability of, 594
Fetal membranes, 596
Fetus:
  anatomy, 71
  anemia, 365
  asphyxia, 604
    example (Q 12.34–12.35), 606
  development of, 596
  electrocardiography, 610
  fetal sounds, 598
    irregularity of, 605
  heartbeats, 598
  heart rate and asphyxia, 605
  intrauterine death, 604
    in toxemia of pregnancy, 605
  leading part in delivery, 601
  movements of, 595, 598
  passage through pelvis (*illus.*), 600
  passive immunization of, 349
  phonocardiography, 611
  position of, 601
  pulse rate determination, ultrasonic
    method for, 183
  Rh positive, 364
  simultaneous monitoring of heart
    rate and intrauterine pressure,
    613
  size of, 597-98
  x-ray examination of, 610
FEV, 150
Fever:
  due to drug hypersensitivity, 493
  and ketone bodies, 277
Fiber optics, in endoscopes, 117, 119
Fibrillations, 255
Fibrin, 292
Fibrinogen, 292
Fibroma, *terminology,* 33
Fibrosis, 27
Fibrous tissue, 17
Fibula, *anatomy,* 45
Fick principle, 175
Field block anesthesia, 506
Film oxygenators, 566
Film(s), in diagnostic radiology, 413
Filtration, of blood plasma, in
    kidneys, 293
Fingers, *anatomy,* 36
Flame photometry, 304
Fleas, vector of infection, 325
Flexion, *terminology,* 40
Floors, conducting, in operating
    rooms, 518
Flowmeters, for oxygen and gaseous
    anesthetics, 513
Flow resistance, 150
Fluid balance, 27, (Q 1.133), 27
  and dialysis, 578
  and intensive care, 572
Fluid compartments:
  of the body, 26
  determination of, 184
Fluid(s):
  body, 26
  extracellular, 26
  interstitial, 26
  intracellular, 26
Fluorography, 415

Fluorometry, 305
Fluoroscopy, 378
  imaging techniques in, 410
  integration time in, 421
  and transmission of information,
    423
Focus, in cerebral cortex, 241
Food, and arteriosclerosis, 498
Food poisoning, infectious agent in,
    326
Foot, *anatomy,* 36
Footling presentation, 601
Force, *SI unit,* 646
Forced expiratory volume, 150
Forceps technique, 608
Foreign bodies:
  gastrointestinal, x-ray examination
    of, 395
  observation of, 379
Foreskin, *anatomy,* 69
Fossae, 110
Fovea centralis, *anatomy,* 97
Fractionation, in radiotherapy, 629
Fracture(s):
  reduction of:
    anesthesia and muscle relaxation,
      505
    during fluoroscopy, 379
  terminology, 34
  x-ray examination of, 383
Frank lead system, 192
FRC, 147
Frequency, *SI unit,* 646
Frequency analysis:
  in electroencephalography, 248
  of heart sounds, 167
Frequency filtering, in fetal elec-
    trocardiography, 610
Frontal lobe(s):
  anatomy, 79
  function of. 79-81
Frontal plane, 37
Functional residual capacity, 147
Fungi, 324

⁶⁷Ga, visualization of organs with, 449
Gall bladder:
  anatomy, 52
  removal of, 536
  x-ray examination of, 395
    (*illus.*), 394
Gallstone(s), 30
  and cholecystitis (Q 1.246), 55
  example of surgical treatment,
    533-37
  operation, vitamin K prophylaxis,
    example (Q 9.33), 492
  preoperative treatment, example (Q
    5.51), 293
  x-ray examination of, 395
    (*illus.*), 394
Gamma, of x-ray film, 415
Gamma cameras, 452
Gamma globulins:
  and passive immunization, 349
  preparation of, 349
  synthesis of, 280
Ganglia, sympathetic, 88

Ganglion, 77
Gangrene, 27
Gas chromatography, 310
Gas gangrene, 27
  hyperbaric oxygen treatment of, 5?
Gas sterilization, 337
Gastr-, 51
Gastric juice, 299-302
  bactericidal action of, 344
Gastric ulcer (Q 1.248), 55
  and body posture in physic
    diagnosis, 115
  diagnosis of, 118
  example (Q 7.5), 361
  operation, anesthesia for, examp
    (Q 10.42), 517
Gastric washings, infectious age
    specimen technique, 329
Gastritis:
  acute (Q 3.59), 159
  diagnosis of, 118
  and hyposecretion, 299
  terminology, 54
Gastr(o)-, 54
Gastroenteritis, *terminology,* 54
Gastroenterology, *terminology,* 480
Gastrointestinal tract, x-ray examin
    tion of, 393
Gastroscope, 118
Gastroscopy, and photography, 453
Gaussian curve, 268
Geiger-Mueller tube, 629
Gelfoam, in hemostasis, 525
-gen, 9
General anesthesia, 505, 508-18
  example, in gallstone operation, 5?
General condition of patient, descri
    tion, 109
General symptoms, 105
Genes, 12
-genesis, 9
Genesis, 10
Geometric enlargement, in radi
    graphy, 378
Geriatric care, 482
Geriatrics, *terminology,* 480
German measles:
  incubation time, 326
  infectious agent in, 326
Glands:
  anatomy, 74
  endocrine, 16
  exocrine, 16
  radiosensitivity of, 400
Glandular epithelium, 16
Glans, *anatomy,* 69
Glass electrode:
  internal resistance of, 158
  for pH measurement, 158
Gli-, 22
Glial cells, 20
Glioma, 33
  terminology, 22
Gliosarcoma, *terminology,* 22
Globulins, in blood plasma, 279
Glomerulonephritis, example (
    5.69), 298
Glomerulus, glomeruli, 293
  measurement of function, 297

Glucose:
  analysis of, 308
  in blood serum, 275
Glutamic-oxalacetic transaminase, 284
Glutamic-pyruvic transaminase, 284
Glutaric aldehyde sterilization, 337
Glycogen, 60, 275
Gonadotropin, 595
Gonads:
  endocrine function of, 75
  radiosensitivity of, 620
Gonorrhea:
  diagnosis of, 329
  incubation time, 326
  infectious agent in, 324
Gout:
  and composition of urine, 295
  example (Q 5.68), 298
Grand mal, 241
Granulocytes, 24
  normal values, 288-89
  phagocytic function of, 343
Gravida:
  definition, 592
  terminology, 592
gray, 647
  definition, 617
Gray matter, 77
Grids, x-ray technique, 408
Grounding:
  and interference, 262
  of patient, 205-7
Ground loop, 262
Growth curves, bacteria, 334
Gynecology:
  terminology, 500
  and ultrasonic diagnosis, 469

Halothane, 508
Hand, *anatomy,* 36
Hay fever, cause of, 351
Hb value, 286
Headache, in toxemia of pregnancy, 605
Headache tablets, toxic effect of (Q 9.42), 494
Hearing, sense of, 99
  reflex control of, 99
Hearing center, *anatomy,* 81
Heart:
  action potentials, 189
  anatomy, 57, 58
  angiography of, 390
  artificial, 569
  asystole, 196
    in myocardial infarction, 560
  atria, *anatomy,* 59
  auscultation of, 128
  AV node, 195
  and calcium ions, 273
  cardiac output, 150
  catheterization of, 161
  compression, external, in cardiac arrest, 555
  conduction system, 195
  congenital deformations, x-ray examination of, 389

congenital malformations of, 177
  (*illus.*), 178
congestion, 497
coronary arteriosclerosis, 498
coronary vessels, x-ray examination of, 391
defibrillation, 217-20
determination of cardiac output, 175-81, 187
electric field vector, 189
electrocardiogram, 188-217
intensive care monitoring of, 585
murmur, 131
muscle, 18
myocardial infarction, 560
organic defect, diagnosis of, 161
pacing centers in, 194
physical examination of, 110
position of (*illus.*), 112
and potassium ions, 273
pressure in, 129
pulsations, observation of, 379
sinus node, 194
stroke volume, 160
transplantation of, 526
ventricles, *anatomy,* 59
vulnerable period, 217, 218
work output of, 66
x-ray examination of, 386, 388
(*see also* Electrocardiography *and* Electrocardiogram)
Heart arrhythmias, 194-98
  cardioversion of, 218
  extrasystoles, 196
    automatic detection of, 561
    example (Q 3.161–3.162), 198
  fibrillation, 196
    and calcium ions, 273
  flutter, 196
  pacemaker treatment, 219-27
  preventive treatment, 561
  prognostic significance of, 560
  treatment of, 497
  ventricular extrasystoles in myocardial infarction, 560
  ventricular fibrillation, 196
    in hypothermia, 564
    in myocardial infarction, 560
Heart block, 195 (*see also* Heart arrhythmias)
Heart diseases:
  diagnosis during work, 227
  terminology, 480
Heart failure, treatment of, 497
Heart-lung bypass, 562
Heart-lung machines, 563
Heart rate:
  control of, 160
  during exercise, 227
  limitation of, 228
  maximum, 228
  monitoring in intensive care, 586
Heart rhythm, 194-98
  disturbances of, 194-98
Heart sounds:
  analysis of, 167
  time relation of, 168
Heart valve(s), 128
  diseases, treatment of, 497
  location of sound (*illus.*), 131

prosthesis, 528
  operation, 562
  sounds, 130
Heart volume:
  correlation to blood volume, 388
  correlation to body surface, 388
  x-ray determination, 388
    (*illus.*), 389
Heat, therapeutic effect of, 631
Heat emission, and fever (Q 2.101), 138
Heat generation, 94
  and fever (Q 2.100), 138
Heat loss, 94
Heat sterilization, 336
Heat therapy:
  analgesic effect of, 631
  depth of penetration, 631
  high-frequency techniques in, 632-33
  hyperemia in, 631
  sedative effect of, 631
Heel effect, x-ray tube, 441
Hemangioma, *terminology,* 24, 33
Hemato-, 24
Hematocrit value:
  determination of, 287
  normal range, 287
Hematogenous, *terminology,* 9
Hematology, 271, 285-91
Hematoma, 29
Hematuria, 296
Heme group, 277
Hemi-, 5
Hemianopia, *terminology,* 5, 9
Hemiparesis, *terminology,* 5
Hemiplegia, *terminology,* 9
Hemispheres, *anatomy,* 79
Hem(o)-, 24
Hemodialysis, 579
  apparatus, control circuits, 580
Hemodynamics, 64, 160-88
Hemoglobin:
  amount of, in erythrocytes, 286
  in blood, normal values, 286
  breakdown of, 277
  oxygen saturation of, 153
  total amount of, 185
Hemolysins, 288
Hemolysis, 288
  and antigens, 347
  and artificial hearts, 569
  and blood pumps, 567
  and duration of extracorporeal circulation, 564
  in heart-lung machine, 563
  in oxygenators, 566
Hemolytic anemia, 288
  cause of, 353
Hemolytic states, and bilirubin in blood serum, 278
Hemolytic streptococcal infections in family, example (Q 6.27), 328
Hemolytic streptococci:
  cause of valvular heart disease, 497
  and glomerulonephritis, example (Q 5.69), 298
Hemophilia, 292
Hemorrhage, 29
  capillary, due to drug hypersensitivity, 493

in central nervous system, x-ray examination of, 398
cerebral, 29
treatment by blood transfusion, 360
Hemorrhagic shock, 557
Hemorrhoids, (Q 1.124), 25
diagnosis of, 118
Hemostasis, 291
compression of wound, 529
during operations, 524
Hemostat, 525
Hemothorax, percussion of, 126
Henderson-Hasselbalch equation, 157
and acid-base disturbances, 575
Hepat-, 52
Hepatic artery, *anatomy,* 60
Hepatic coma, due to drug hypersensitivity, 493
Hepatic duct, *anatomy,* 52
Hepatic vein, *anatomy,* 60
Hepatitis (Q 1.251), 55
disinfection, 338
enzyme diagnosis, 284
terminology, 31
viruses, 327
Hepatitis A:
antibody against, 349
incubation time, 326
Hepatitis B:
and blood transfusion, 370
example (Q 6.24), 328
and hospital infections, 342
incubation time, 326
Heredity, 105
and arteriosclerosis, 498
Hexachlorophene, disinfection, 338
High-frequency physical therapy, depth of penetration, 633
High-frequency techniques, in heat therapy, 632-33
Hip joint prosthesis, 528
Histology, *terminology,* 35
HL-A system, 374
Homeostasis, 88
Horizontal plane, 37
Hormonal disorders, and composition of urine, 295
Hormonal disturbances, x-ray diagnosis of, 383
Hormones, 74-77
analysis of, 305, 356
and radiosensitivity of tissues, 623
Hospital hygiene, 340-43
Hospital infections, 342
Hospital information systems, 635-44
Human lymphocyte antigens, 374
Humerus, *anatomy,* 44
Humoral immunity, 346
Hydrochloric acid, 51
in stomach, 299
Hydrodynamic impedance, 64
Hydrogen ions, 24-hour production of, 574
Hydronephrosis, *terminology,* 67
Hydrostatic pressure, in vessels, 281
Hydrothorax, percussion of, 126
Hydroxyapatite, 17
as ion exchanger, 42
in skeleton, 273
Hyper-, 5

Hyperbaric oxygen atmosphere in radiotherapy, 622
Hyperbaric oxygen treatment, 551
Hyperbaric oxygenation, and tissue storage, 375
Hyperemia, 28
in heat therapy, 631
Hyperesthesia, *terminology,* 9
Hyperglycemia (Q 1.128), 26
Hyperinsulinism, and blood glucose, 275
Hyperkalemia, 273
Hyperopia, *terminology,* 5, 9
Hyperparathyroidism:
and blood serum calcium and phosphate, 273
and kidney stones, 273
Hypersecretion, 299
Hypersensitive reactions:
calcium therapy (Q 5.17), 275
delayed, 351
immediate, 351
Hypersensitivity, to drugs, 493
and bleeding, 291
and leukopenia, 289
Hypertension, 66
example (Q 2.95), 135
symptoms (Q 1.286), 66
in toxemia of pregnancy, 605
Hyperthyroidism, 74, 114
diagnosis by radionuclides, 318
example (Q 1.316), 76
example (Q 5.119), 320
Hypertonia:
blood vessels in eye, example (Q 2.60), 120
operation on narrow kidney artery, example (Q 10.56), 527
and renal failure, example (Q 5.71), 298
Hypertrophy:
of muscle, 48
terminology, 5, 9
Hyperventilation:
and acid-base disturbance, 575
alkalosis due to, example (Q 3.60), 159
provocation of brain waves by, 240
Hypervolemia, and fluid balance, 573
Hyp(o)-, 6
Hypoacusia, *terminology,* 100
Hypoesthesia, *terminology,* 9
Hypoglycemia, example (Q 1.129), 26
Hypokalemia, 273
Hypoparathyroidism:
and blood serum calcium and phosphate, 273
example (Q 5.18), 275
Hypophysis, 74
Hyposecretion, 299
Hypostatic spots, 141
Hypotension, 66
symptoms (Q 1.285), 66
Hypothalamus, 74, 82
and body temperature, 94
Hypothermia, 564
and tissue storage, 375
terminology, 6
Hypothyroidism, 74, 114
and autoimmunity, 353

diagnosis by radionuclides, 318
Hypotonic solutions, and hemolysis 288
Hypotrophy, *terminology,* 6
Hypovolemic shock, 557
example (Q 11.46), 559
and fluid balance, 572
Hypoxia:
intrauterine, 604
terminology, 6
Hypoxic metabolic acidosis, 558

¹³¹I, visualization of organs with, 449
Iatrogenic damage, 486
Iatrogenic disease, 486
Identification data, and hospital information systems, 637
Ileocecal valve, *anatomy,* 53
Ileum, *anatomy,* 52
Iliac crest, 111
Iliac fossa, 110
Iliac spine, anterior superior, 111
Illumination:
for endoscopy, 117
SI unit, 647
Image converter, infrared, 460
Image distortion, ultrasonic, 473
Image information, 635
Image intensifier, x-ray, 411
Image reconstruction, in computerized tomography, 448
Imaging:
with thermography, 454-63
ultrasonic, 463-77
with x-rays, 377-437
Immature child, *terminology,* 592
Immobilization treatment, 532
Immune reaction, suppression of, 526
Immunity:
cell-mediated, 346
and transplantation, 372
Immunization, 348
active, 349
passive, 348
Immunoelectrophoresis, 309
Immunological compatibility, 359
Immunological diseases, 350
Immunological factors, in radiotherapy, 620
example (Q 13.27), 622
Immunology, 343-58
in transplantation, 526
Impedance plethysmography, 187
in automatic blood pressure measurement, 585
in intensive care monitoring, 583
Impetigo, infectious agent in, 326
Implantation:
of pacemaker, 225
of prosthesis, 527
Incision, *terminology,* 530
Incisional surgical methods, 519
Incus, *anatomy,* 99
Indicator dilution method, 148
for compartment volume determinations, 184
for flow determinations, 175
Inductance, *SI unit,* 647

660

ductive field, depth of penetration in physical therapy, 633
fant, *definition,* 592
farct, 29
farction (Q 1.262), 63
myocardial, 560
fection(s):
of clean surgical wounds, 342
definition, 30
and gamma globulins (Q 5.31), 282
in hospitals, 342
and intensive care, 538
lowered resistance to, 289
nonspecific defense mechanism, 343
prevention by immobilization, example (Q 10.65), 529
routes of, 341
sources of, 340
specific defense mechanism, 344
spread of, 340
surgical treatment of, 531
susceptibility of object, 341
fectious agent(s):
attenuated, 349
carrier of, 340
culture media, 330-32
killed, 349
specimen-taking, 329
fectious diseases:
diagnosis of, 329
mortality for, 484
(table), 495
terminology, 480
treatment of, 495
ferior, *terminology,* 38
ferior vena cava, *anatomy,* 59
filtration anesthesia, 506
flammation:
signs of, 30
and thermography, 458
fluenza, mortality for, 495
formation:
amount of, and x-ray dose, 401
coding of medical records, 637
collection in hospital information systems, 637
content, x-ray image, 380, 416
total volume in hospital information systems, 636
transmission through axon, 20
formation loss:
in diagnostic radiology, 411
in fluoroscopy, 412
in x-ray imaging, 413
fraclavicular fossa, 110
frared radiation:
in heat therapy, 631
in physical therapy, 631
fusion, intravenous, 570
halation anesthesia, 508
methods for, 513
hibition, pharmacological effect, 491
hibitory postsynaptic potential, 232
juries and accidents, mortality, 484
-patient care, 482
Sb detector, for thermography, 461
sect sting, and hypersensitivity, 351
spection, in physical diagnosis, 114
spiration, 56

Inspiratory reserve volume, 146
Instrumental extraction, of fetus, 608
Insufficiency, 130
Insufflation, in ventilator treatment, 546
Insulin, 75
automatic administration of, 589
Intellectual functions, center of, 79
Intensifying screen, x-ray, 413
Intensive care, 482, 538-90
in respiratory failure, 540-54
technical aspects of, 582-89
Intensive care monitoring:
arrhythmia detectors, 586
cardioscopes, 586
and level of consciousness, 587
parameters in, 582
and temperature measurement, 587
Intensive observation, 539
Intensive treatment, 539
Inter-, 6
Interaction, of drugs, 491
Intercellular, *terminology,* 6
Intercellular substance, 17
Intercostal, *terminology,* 6
Intercostal spaces, 110
Interference:
by capacitive coupling, 261
in electrocardiography amplifiers, 205
by incorrect grounding, 262
by inductive coupling, 262
in neurophysiological amplifiers, 261
Interferon, 344
Intermittent, *terminology,* 6
Internal, *terminology,* 38
Internal environment, and intensive care, 570-82
Internal medical diseases, examples of treatment, 494
Internal medicine, 479-99
specialties of, 479-81
Internal rotation, of fetus, 607
Interrupted suture, 523
Interstitial, *terminology,* 6
Interstitial fluid, 26
circulation of, 281
and fluid balance, 572
Interstitial space, 61
Interstitial tissue space, and colloid osmotic pressure, 281
Intervertebral, *terminology,* 6
Intervertebral discs, *anatomy,* 44
Intestinal juice, 299-301
Intestinal mucosa, spatial frequency content of, 420
Intestinal mucous membranes, radiosensitivity of, 620
Intestines:
communication between, terminology, 530
disorders of, 299
excretion of drugs by, 491
radiosensitivity of mucous membrane, 624
Intra-, 6
Intra-arterial, *terminology,* 6
Intracellular, *terminology,* 6
Intracellular fluid, 26
and fluid balance, 572

Intracellular ions, potassium, 272
Intracorporeal dialysis, 578
Intracranial, *terminology,* 6
Intracranial pressure, 132
Intracutaneous, *terminology,* 73
Intramuscular, *terminology,* 6
Intramuscular administration of drugs, 489
Intrathoracic pressure, in ventilator treatment, 546
Intrauterine, *terminology,* 6
Intrauterine fetal death, 604
Intravascular, *terminology,* 6
Intravenous administration of drugs, 489
Intravenous anesthesia, 508
Intravenous drip, in intensive care, 570
Intubation, 510
in intensive care, 540
Iodine, as contrast medium, 382
Ion exchanger, bone as, 42
Ionization chamber dose measurement, 629
Ionizing radiation:
accumulated dose, 401
biological effect of, 400
and bleeding, 291
cumulative effect of, 400
diagnostic use of, 377
dose in diagnostic radiology, 400-401, 412
dose and image information, 421-27
dose in radionuclide organ visualization, 449
effect on living cells, 619
lethal power of, 400
maximum permissible dose, 401
sterilization by, 337
SI units, 647
units, 617
Iris, *anatomy,* 97
Iron lung, 545
Irreversible shock, 558
Irritability of cells, 13
Ischemia, 29
Islets of Langerhans, 75
Iso-, *terminology,* 362
Isoagglutinins, 362
Isodose curves, in radiotherapy, 628
Isogenic graft, 372
Isografts, transplantation of, 526
Isometric contraction, 48
Isotonic contraction, 48
Iterative process, in computerized tomography, 448
-itis, 31

Jacksonian attacks, 242
Jaundice:
and biliary stasis (Q 1.251), 55
and bilirubin in blood serum, 278
Jejunum, *anatomy,* 52
Joint(s), friction in, 45

Katal, 284
Ketone bodies, in blood serum, 277
Kidney(s):
anatomy, 67

diseases of, *terminology,* 480
excretion of drugs, 491
functions of, 293
   determination by radionuclides, 319
   x-ray determination of, 396
inflammation of,
   and anemia, 286
   example (Q 5.69), 298
   and hematuria, 296
   and proteinuria, 296
   (*see also* Nephritis)
parenchyma, 11
position of (*illus*), 112
renal circulation, disturbed, 578
renal damage:
   chronic, dialysis treatment, example (Q 11.94), 581
   determination of, 277
   due to drug hypersensitivity, 493
   partial, 578
   and potassium ions, 273
   and sodium ions, 372
renal failure:
   acidosis in, 577
   acute, 578
   chronic, 578
   and composition of blood plasma, 296
   dialysis, 577
   treatment of, 577
renal pelvis, x-ray examination of, 396
   (*illus.*), 397
transplantation of, 526 (Q 10.58) 527
urea in blood serum, 277
x-ray examination of, 396
Kidney stones, 30
   and body posture in physical diagnosis, 115
   x-ray examination of, 396
Kidney tumors, x-ray examination of, 396
Knee cap, *anatomy,* 45
Kolff kidney, 580
Kyphoses, 44

Labeled compound, 449
Labor, contractions of uterus, 599
Laboratory automation:
   in clinical chemistry, 312-18
   in microbiology, 357
Labyrinth, *anatomy,* 99
Lactic dehydrogenase, 284
Lambert-Beer's law, 303, 381
Laminagraphy, 427
Laparoscope, 118
Laryngitis, *terminology,* 57
Laryng(o)-, 57
Laryngoscope, 118
Laryngospasm, *terminology,* 57
Larynx:
   anatomy, 56
   tumors, diagnosis of, 118
Lasers, use in surgery, 521
Latency period, of biological effect after irradiation, 619
Lateral, *terminology,* 37
Laughing gas, 508

LDH, 284
Leakage current, in catheter, during catheterization, 165
Left atrium, *anatomy,* 59
Left ventricle, *anatomy,* 59
Left ventricular failure, 497
Left-right shunt (*illus.*), 178
Leg, *anatomy,* 36
Leg ulcers, hyperbaric oxygen treatment of, 553
Length, *SI unit,* 645
Lens, *anatomy,* 97
Leprosy:
   incubation time, 326
   infectious agent in, 324, 326
Lethality, 10, 483
Leukemia, 289
   example (Q 5.48), 291
   in mouse after irradiation, 620
   radiosensitivity of, 623
Leukocytes, 24
   immature forms of, 289
Leukocytosis, example (Q 5.47), 290
Leukopenia, 289
Lice, vector of infection, 325
Lidocaine, in myocardial infarction, 561
Ligaments, 44
Ligature, 524
Light sensitivity, 97
Linear accelerators, 616
Lines, for indicating position, 110
Lipase, 299
Lipemia, *terminology,* 17
Lipidosis, 27
Lipids, *terminology,* 17, 33
Lip(o)-, 17
Lipoma, *terminology,* 17, 33
Lipoproteins, 276
Liquid chromatography, 310
Liquid jet recorder, 210
Liquid sterilization, 337
Liquid tissue, 23
Liquid-liquid oxygenators, 566
-lith, 31
Lithiasis, 31
Lithium, analysis of, 305
Lithium fluoride, thermoluminescent effect, 629
Live birth, *definition,* 592
Liver:
   anatomy, 52
   damage,
      in cholelithiasis, 534
      enzyme diagnosis of, 284
   detoxification of drugs, 491
   disorders due to drug hypersensitivity, 493
   heat production in, 457
   inflammation of (*see* Hepatitis)
   parenchyma, 11
   position of (*illus.*), 112
   and RES, 343
   rhythm, example (Q 5.21), 279
   transplantation of, 526
   visualization with radionuclides, 449
Lobar pneumonia, 57
Lobotomy, 80
Local anesthesia, 505

Local pain, 107
Locomotive system, 42-51
Longitudinal presentation, 601
Lordoses, 44
Lowenstein-Jensen agar, 333
Lumbar puncture, 301
   in diagnostic radiology, 398
   in spinal anesthesia, 506
Lumbar vertebrae, *anatomy,* 44
Luminance, *SI unit,* 647
Luminous flux, *SI unit,* 647
Luminous intensity, *SI unit,* 647
Lung(s):
   airway resistance, 150
   anatomy, 56
   auscultation of, 127
   compliance, 151
   determination of volumes, 148
   diffusion, 142
   embolism (Q 3.18), 146
   excretory function of, 67
   function tests of, 146-59
   intensive care of diseases, 538
   interstitial fibrosis (Q 3.16), 146
   lobes of, 57
   parenchyma, 11
   partial pressures in, 153
   physical examination of, 110
   position of (*illus.*), 112
   rupture in ventilator treatment, 54
   transplantation of, 526
   ventilation of, 142
   x-ray examination of, 386
Lung capacity, total, 147
Lung tumors, x-ray examination 387
Lupus erythematosus, cause, 353
Lymph(-), 24, 62
   anatomy, 61
Lymphadenitis:
   example (Q 1.130) 26, (Q 2.73),
   terminology, 24
Lymphangioma, *terminology,* 24, 3
Lymphangitis:
   example (Q 1.130), 26
   terminology, 24, 62
Lymph(atic) capillaries:
   anatomy, 61
   terminology, 24
Lymph ducts, *anatomy,* 61
Lymph nodes:
   anatomy, 61
   cancer, radiosensitivity of, 623
   metastases, example (Q 2.74), 124
   palpation of, 109, 122
   radiosensitivity of, 620
   and RES, 343
Lymphocytes, 24
   and cell-mediated immunity, 346
   function of, 289
   normal value, 289
   and tissue typing, 374
Lymphosarcoma, *terminology,* 33
Lysis, of antigen cell, 347
Lysozyme, 344

Mach effect, 434
Macr(o)-, 6
Macrocyte, *terminology,* 6

acroscopic, *terminology,* 6
agnetic flux, *SI unit,* 647
agnetic flux density, *SI unit,* 647
alabsorption, 300
and anemia, 286
alaria:
example (Q 6.25), 328
incubation time, 326
infectious agent in, 324
temperature curve in (*illus.*), 136
aldigestion, 300
alignancy, degree and radiosensitivity, 623
alignant lymphoma, radiosensitivity of, 623
alignant tumor, 32
alingering, 114
alleus, *anatomy,* 99
ammae, *anatomy,* 73
ammillary line, *terminology,* 110
anometers for static blood pressure measurements, 170
anus, *anatomy,* 36
As, 402
ass, *SI unit,* 646
ass attenuation coefficient, and x-ray image contrast, 381
astectomy, 533
aterials:
carcinogenic, 528
choice for prosthesis, 528
attress suture, 523
ature child, *terminology,* 592
aximum voluntary ventilation, 148
ayo stand, 503
easles:
antibody against, 349
diagnosis of (Q 2.48), 115
immunity, 349
incubation time, 326
infectious agent in, 326
temperature curve in (*illus.*), 137
-ECG, 610
edial, *terminology,* 37
edian line, *terminology,* 110
edian plane, 37
ediastinoscope, 118
ediastinum, *anatomy,* 57
edical care:
and planning of hospital information systems, 642
quality control of, 636
specialties of, 479-81
types of, 481
edical checkups, 482
edical history, 105
and hospital information systems, 637
structured, 637
edical record, 102
comparison between conventional and computer record, 636
content and hospital information systems, 637-40
design of:
computer record, 641
conventional record, 641
and hospital information systems, 637-42

as legal document, 636
problem oriented, 641
storage of, 636
summary and hospital information systems, 640
Medical terminology, 1-100
Medicine, definition, 479
Medulla oblongata, 82
circulatory center in, 93
respiratory center in, 90
Mega-, 6
Megacolon, *terminology,* 6
Megavolt therapy, 616
Melanoma, radiosensitivity of, 623
Membrane oxygenators, 566
Membrane potentials, in neurons, 232
Membranes, in hemodialyzers, 580
Meninges, 82
Meningitis:
bacterial, mortality for, 495
epidemic cerebral, incubation time, 326
example (Q 5.84), 302
infectious agent in, 324
and protein in cerebrospinal fluid, 301
viral, infectious agent in, 327
Menstrual cycle, 593
Menstruation:
absence of, 594
and anemia, 286
Mental state, and inspection of patient, 114
Mesentery, *anatomy,* 53
Metabolic acidosis, 157
base excess in, 575
in cardiac arrest, 556
and combustion of fat, 277
example (Q 3.61), 159, (Q 11.89-11.90), 576
hypoxic, in shock, 557
standard bicarbonate value in, 575
treatment of, 575
ventilation of carbon dioxide in, 575
Metabolic alkalosis, 157
base excess in, 575
example (Q 3.59), 159, (Q 11.93), 577
standard bicarbonate value in, 575
treatment of, 576
Metabolic apparatus, 51-69
Metabolism, 283
and blood pH, 157
and body temperature, 94
rate of, 74
in hypothermia, 564
Metacarpus, *anatomy,* 36
Metastases of tumors, 33
lung, x-ray examination of, 387
visualization with radionuclides, 449
Metatarsus, *anatomy,* 36
Methoxyflurane, 508
Micro-, 6
Microbiological diagnosis, technical aspects, 357
Microbiological laboratory data, and hospital information systems, 639

Microcyte, *terminology,* 6
Microelectrodes, in neurophysiology, 261
Microorganisms:
defense mechanisms against, 343
nonpathogenic, 323
pathogenic, 323
protection against, in surgery, 529
some pathogenic (*table*), 326
Microscopic anatomy, *terminology,* 35
Microscopic examination:
of blood cells, 285
of cerebrospinal fluid, 301
of urine, 296
of white blood cells, 288-89
Microtia, *terminology,* (Q 1.30), 8
Microwave irradiation, depth of penetration in physical therapy, 633
Microwave therapy, 631
Micturition, 67
Midaxillary line, *terminology,* 110
Midbrain, 82
Midclavicular line, *terminology,* 110
Midline echo, 467-68
Milliequivalent, 274
Million-volt therapy, 616
Mingograph, 210
Minute ventilation, 145
Miscarriage, *definition,* 592
Mites, vector of infection, 325
Mitral valve(s), 128
defect, catheterization of, 164
insufficiency and murmur, 131
stenosis:
example (Q 8.186), 471
and murmur, 131
ultrasonic diagnosis of, 469
x-ray examination of, 389
Mixed lymphocyte culture, 374
^{99}Mo, visualization of organs with, 449
Modulation transfer function, in diagnostic radiology, 418
mol, 646
Moment of force, *SI unit,* 646
Monocytes, 24
phagocytic function of, 343
Morbidity, 10, 483
Morphine:
in myocardial infarction, 561
pharmacological effect of, 491
in premedication, 509
Mortality, 10, 483
maternal in placenta previa, 605
in myocardial infarction, 561
for some infectious diseases (*table*), 495
Motility of cells, 13
Motor center, in cerebral cortex, 81
Motor nerve, 48
Motor pathways:
definition, 77
spinal, 84
Motor unit, 48
action potentials from, 254
Mouth:
anatomy, 51
inspection of, 109

Mouth-to-mouth method, 541
Moving field irradiation, 628
Mucosa, spatial frequency content of, 420
Mucous membranes, radiosensitivity of, 400
Mucus, stomach secretion, 51
Multigravida, 592
Multipara, 592
Multiple sclerosis:
  and muscular paralysis, 251
  reflexes in, example (Q 2.106), 140
Mumps:
  antibody against, 349
  and sterility (Q 1.296), 71
Murmur(s), 131
  presystolic (Q 2.89), 132
Muscle(s):
  acoustic impedance, 464
  antagonists (*illus.*), 48
  atrophy of, 48, 252
  contraction:
    and calcium ions, 273
    energy, 19
    and fatigue, 19
    and potassium ions, 272
  coordination of, 82
  denervated, 251
  and electromyography, 255
  density, 464
  in digestive apparatus, 53
  efficiency of, 48
  electromyography, 253-56
  hypertrophy, 48
  paralysis of, 251
  paresis of, 48, 251
  potentials from 254
  ultrasonic imaging, 467
  velocity of sound, 464
Muscle fibers, 18, 48
  action potentials, 189
Muscle relaxation, in anesthesia, 505
Muscle spindles, 49
Muscular contraction, 48
  regulation of, 48
Muscular system, 47
Muscular tissue(s), 18
  heart, 18
  smooth, 18
  striated, 18
Mutation, after irradiation, 620
MVV, 148
Myalgia, *terminology,* 9
Myasthenia gravis:
  cause, 353
  and creatine in blood serum, 277
  and muscular weakness, 252, 255
Mycology, 322
Mycoses, 324
Myelography, 398
Myeloma, radiosensitivity of, 623
My(o)-, 19
Myocardial infarction, 498, 560
  asystole in, 560
  electrocardiogram in, 200, (Q 3.171), 202
    (*illus.*), 199
  enzyme diagnosis of, 284
  mortality, 560

observation of, 561
treatment of, 560-61
ventricular extrasystoles in, 560
ventricular fibrillation in, 560
Myocarditis, *terminology,* 62
Myocardium, *terminology,* 62
Myoglobin, *terminology,* 19
Myoma, *terminology,* 19
Myopathy, *terminology,* 9
Myopia, *terminology,* (Q 1.42), 10
Myotonia, 252
Myxedema, 74, 114

Narcotics:
  addiction, 494
  overdose of, example (Q 3.62), 159
Natal, *terminology,* 592
Neck, *anatomy,* 35
Necrosis, 27
Needle electrodes, neurophysiological, 260, 261
Negative contrast, 282
Neonatal, *terminology,* 592
Neoplasm, 32
Nephritis, 578
  and anemia, 286
  example (Q 1.290), 69
  terminology, 31, 67
Nephr(o)-, 67
Nephroangiography, 391
Nephrogenic, *terminology,* 67
Nephrolithiasis, 30
Nephrology, *terminology,* 480
Nephron, 293
Nephrosis, *terminology,* 67
Nerve(s):
  adrenergic, 21
  cholinergic, 21
  conduction velocity in, 256-58
  cranial, 83
    (*illus*), 84
  electroneurography, 258-59
  femoral (*illus.*), 84
  median (*illus.*), 84
  peripheral, lesion in, 251
  peroneal (*illus.*), 84
  phrenic (*illus.*), 84
  propagation of impulse, 20
  radial (*illus.*), 84
  rejoining of, 525
  saphenous (*illus.*), 84
  sciatic (*illus.*), 84
  spinal (*illus.*), 84
  synapse, 21
  tibial (*illus.*), 84
  tiss̮ṿo, 20
  transmitter substances, 21
  ulnar (*illus.*), 84
Nerve block anesthesia, 506
Nerve cell(s), 20
  conduction:
    and calcium ions, 273
    and potassium ions, 272
    (*see also* Neuron)
Nerve fibers, 20
  afferent, 49
  conduction velocity, 20
  efferent, 49

and muscular contraction, 48
pulse frequency modulation in, 20
Nervous system, 77
  autonomic, 87
  central, 79-83
  diseases of,
    mortality, 484
    terminology, 480
  peripheral, 83-88
  regulatory function of, 88
  surgical diseases of, terminolog 500
  x-ray examination of, 398
Nervous tissue:
  acoustic impedance, 464
  density, 464
  velocity of sound, 464
Nettle rash, cause of, 351
Neuralgia, *terminology,* 9
Neuritis, *terminology,* 22
Neur(o), 22
Neurogenic, *terminology,* 9
Neurogenic shock, 558
  example (Q 11.49–11.52), 559-60
Neurology:
  definition, 230
  terminology, 480
  and ultrasonic diagnosis, 467
Neuron(s), 20
  membrane potential in, 232
  polarization of, 232
  synchronization by subcortic centers, 233, 238
Neuropathy, *terminology,* 9
Neurophysiology, 230-65
  amplifiers for, 261
  electrodes, 260
  impedance of electrodes, 260, 261
  measurement techniques, 260-66
  recording techniques, 265
Neurosurgery, *terminology,* 500
Neurotoxins, *terminology,* 22
Neurotransmitters, 21
Neutrophilic granulocytes (*illus.*), 23
Neutrophilic leukocytes, function c 289
Newborn, mortality in diseases, 484
newton, 646
newton meter, 646
Niche, stomach (*illus.*), 392
Nitrogen-containing substances, blood serum, 277
Nitroglycerine, treatment arteriosclerosis, 498
Nitrous oxide, 508
Nitrous oxide anesthesia, in deliver 603
Nonrebreathing system, 514
Noradrenalin, 21
Norepinephrine:
  and blood pressure regulation, 93
  secretion by adrenal medulla, 75
  transmitter substance, 21
Normal distribution, 268
Normal range, 269
Normal values:
  and diagnosis, 268
  of electrolytes in blood seru (*table*), 274

of low-molecular weight substances in blood serum (*table*), 276

in medical examinations (Q 5.5–5.6), 270

Nose, anesthesia for, 505

Nosocomial infections, 340, 342-43

Nucleic acids, 12

Nucleus, 12

  group of neurons, 77

Nullipara, 592

Numerical calculations, in hospital information systems, 636

Nursing station data, and hospital information systems, 640

Nutrients:

  in blood serum, 275

  and intensive care, 570

Nylon, for suturing, 523

Nystagmus, fixation, and contrast discrimination, 433

Objective signs, 105

Obstetrics, 591-614

  care, 591

    complications, 604

  diagnosis, technical aspects of, 610

  surgical techniques in, 607

  terminology, 500, 591, 592

  and ultrasonic diagnosis, 469

Obstructive, *terminology*, 186

Occipital lobe, *anatomy*, 79

Occlusion, *terminology*, 186

Occlusive disease, 498

Olfactory organ, 97

oma, 33

Oophor-, 71

Oophortis, *terminology*, 71, (Q 1.301), 72

Operating suite, 502

Operation(s):

  abdominal:

    anesthesia for, 507

      and muscle relaxation, 505

  example of, 533-37

  for hemorrhoids, anesthesia for, (Q 10.24), 507

  gynecological, anesthesia for, 507

  preparatory measures, 534

  radical, 533

  urological, anesthesia for, 507

Operation reports, and hospital information systems, 640

Ophthalm(o)-, 98

Ophthalmology:

  terminology, 500

  and ultrasonic diagnosis, 468

Ophthalmoscope, 118

-opia, 9, 98

-opsia, 9, 98

Optic nerve, 83, 97

Optical receptors, 97

Optics, infrared, 461

Oral airway, 510

Orchi-, 71

Orchitis:

  and sterility (Q 1.296), 71

  terminology, 71

Organ(s), 11

  determination of function by radionuclides, 318

  reattachment of detached, 526

  visualization by radionuclides, 449

  x-ray examination of, 383-98

Organ-specific autoimmune diseases, 353

Orthogonal lead system, 192

Orthopedics, *terminology*, 500

Os, ossa, 44

Oscillometry, 186

  in automatic blood pressure measurement, 585

-osis, 28

Osmosis, in dialysis, 578

Osmotic pressure, and hemolysis, 288

Osteitis, x-ray diagnosis of, 383

Oste(o)-, 17

Osteogenetic, *terminology*, 17

Osteogenic, *terminology*, 17

Osteology, *terminology*, 17

Osteomyelitis, infections agent in, 326

Osteoporosis:

  and malabsorption, 300

  terminology, 17

Osteosarcoma, *terminology*, 33

Otitis, *terminology*, 31

Ot(o)-, 100

Otolaryngology, *terminology*, 500

Otosclerosis (Q 1.397), 100

Otoscope, 118

Out-patient care, 482

Oval window, *anatomy*, 99

Ovaries:

  anatomy, 70

  and pregnancy, 593

  radiosensitivity of, 620

Overdose stage, in anesthesia, 512

Overweight, and arteriosclerosis, 498

Oviduct, *anatomy*, 70

Ovulation, 594

  extra, 594

  and pregnancy, 594

Ovum:

  survival time of, 594

  transport of fertilized, 594

Oxygen:

  content in blood, 153

  as contrast medium, 382

  physically dissolved in plasma, 154, 551

  tension in blood, 153

  transport, and hyperbaric treatment, 551

  treatment with, 497

  uptake, 153

Oxygenation, degree and radiosensitivity of tissues, 622

Oxygenators, 565-67

Oxygen deficit, in muscles, 19

Oxygen tension, determination of, 154

Oxygen uptake, during exercise, 228

Oxytocin, 599

P wave, 198

Pacemaker(s), 219-27

  and airport security metal detectors, 223

  atrial synchronization of, 222

  batteries, 220

  with constant frequency, 221

  demand type, 222

  and diathermy, 223

  electrodes, 225, 226

  energy requirements, 219

  implantation of, 225

  manually adjustable, 221

  risk of ventricular fibrillation, 220, 222

  sensitivity to external interference, 223

  types of, 221

  ventricular inhibited, 222

  ventricular synchronized, 222

  therapy, 219-27

PAH (*see* Para-aminohippuric acid)

Pain:

  local, 107

  location of, 106

  migration in kidney stones (*illus.*), 108

  organs sensitive to, 107

  referred, 107

  sign of inflammation, 30

  site of:

    in angina pectoris (*illus.*), 107

    in gallstones (*illus.*), 108

  as symptom of disease, 106

Pain sensors, skin, 96

Palliative treatment, 485

Palma manus, 40

Palmar flexion, *terminology*, 40

Palpation, 122

Pancreas:

  anatomy, 52

  endocrine function of, 75

  position of (*illus.*), 112

Pancreatic tumor, and jaundice, example (Q 5.67), 298

Pancreatitis:

  and gallstones (Q 1.247), 55

  risk in cholelithiasis, 534

Para-, 6

  definition, 592

  terminology, 592

Para-aminohippuric acid, for renal clearance determinations, 175

Paralysis, 251

  of radial nerve, example (Q 4.97), 258

Paraplegia, *terminology*, 9

Parasite, *terminology*, 6

Parasternal line, *terminology*, 110

Parasympathetic system, 88

  and blood pressure regulation, 93

Parathyroid glands, 74

  and blood serum calcium and phosphate, 273

Paratyphoid fever:

  incubation time, 326

  infectious agent in, 326

  terminology, 6

  vaccination against, 349

Parenchyma, 11

Parenteral administration of drugs, 489

Paresis, 48, 251

Paresthesia, *terminology,* 9
Parietal lobe, *anatomy,* 79
Parkinson's disease, example (Q 9.7), 481
Partial rebreathing systems, 516
Particle radiation, in radiotherapy, 628
Parturition, 599-610
pascal, 646
Passive immunization, 348
Patella, *anatomy,* 45
Patellar reflex, 139
-path, 9
Path(o)-, 6
Pathogenic, *terminology,* 6
Pathognomonic symptoms, 105
Pathological *terminology,* 27-35
Pathology, *terminology,* 6
Pathophysiology, *terminology,* 35 (Q 1.32), 8
-pathy, 9
Pediatrics, *terminology,* 480
Pelvis, *anatomy,* 35, 45
Penicillin, 495
Penicillinase, 495
Penis, *anatomy,* 69
Pepsin, 51, 299
Peptic ulcer:
  and anemia, 286
  and bleeding, 299
Per-, 6
Percussion, 124
Percutaneous, *terminology,* 73
Percutaneous technique, 162
Perforation, *terminology,* 6, 34
Perfusion, and tissue storage, 375
Peri-, 6
Periarthritis, *terminology,* (Q 1.34), 8
Pericarditis:
  terminology, 62
  ultrasonic diagnosis, 469
Pericardium, *terminology,* 6, 62
Perinatal, *terminology,* 592
Perioral, *terminology,* 6
Periosteum, 43
Peritoneal dialysis, 580
  apparatus, 580
Peritoneal membrane, as dialysis membrane, 580
Peritoneum, *anatomy,* 53
Peritonitis, rupture of gallbladder (Q 1.252), 55-56
Peripheral arteries, circulation in, 186
Peripheral circulation, 186-88
Peripheral nerve(s):
  anatomy, 77
  and muscles, 251-260
Peripheral nervous system, 83-88
Peristaltic movements, 53
  observation of, 379
Permeable, *terminology,* 6
Permeation anesthesia, 505
Pernicious anemia, 286
  and achlorhydria, 299
  cause, 353
Peroral, *terminology,* 6
Peroral administration of drugs, 488
Per rectum, *terminology,* 6
Pes, *anatomy,* 36

Petit mal, 241
Petri dish, 330
pH:
  in blood, 157
  measurement of, 158
Phagocytosis, 343
Pharmaceutical preparations, 479
Pharmacological effects, 491
Pharmacology, 488
Pharmacotherapy, 488
Pharynx, *anatomy,* 56
Phenol, disinfection by, 338
Phenylketonuria, 312
Phlebectasia, *terminology,* 62
Phlebitis, *terminology,* 62
Phleb(o)-, 62
Phlebography, 391
Phonocardiography, 167-70
Phosphate ions, in blood, 273
Photofluorography, 415
Photography, 453
Photon radiation:
  attenuation of, 625
  half-value thickness, 625
  high energy, in radiotherapy, 626
  in radiotherapy, 626
Photospot filming, 415
Physical activity, and arteriosclerosis, 498
Physical diagnosis, 102-41
Physical dose distribution, 625
Physical examination, 109-40
Physical exercise, catheterization during, 161
Physical therapy, 631-33
Physical work capacity, 227-28
Physiological data, and hospital information systems, 639
Physiology, *terminology,* 35
Pia mater, 82
PID regulator for automatic drug administration, 588
Pimple, 531
Pituitary, 74
Placebo, 486
Placenta:
  anatomy, 71
  detachment in delivery, 602
  endocrine function of, 76
  and fetal development, 596
  insufficiency of, 604
  location by thermography, 458
  ultrasonic determination of position, 469
Placentia previa, 605
Planes, for indicating position, 37
Planigraphy, 427
Plantar flexion, *terminology,* 41
Plasma, 23, 271
  clotting time of, 292
  separation of, 369
  transfusion of, 360
  transfusion in shock, 559
  volume of, 184
Plasma protein(s), 279-82
  concentrate, 369
Plasma volume, and fluid balance, 572
Plaster dressing, 529

Plastic operation, *terminology,* 530
Plastic surgery, *terminology,* 500
Platelet concentrate, 369
Platelet factor, 291
Platelets:
  separation of, 369
  transfusion of, 360
-plegia, 9
Plethysmography:
  for airway resistance determinatio (*illus.*), 151
  for blood flow determination, 186
  impedance, 187
  for lung volume determinatio (*illus.*), 148
  venous occlusion, 186
Pleur-, 57
Pleura, *anatomy,* 57
Pleural cavity:
  anatomy, 57
  percussion of, 126
  tumor, diagnosis of, 118
Pleural exudate, *terminology,* 57
Pleural puncture, *terminology,* 57
Pleurisy, *terminology,* 57
Pneumo-, 57
Pneumography, 398
Pneumonia:
  infectious agent in, 324, 326
  mortality for, 495
  temperature curve in (*illus.*), 137
  terminology, 57
  viral, infectious agent in, 326
  x-ray examination, 387
Pneumotachograph, 150
Pneumotachometer, 150
Pneumothorax, (Q 1.261), 58
  percussion of, 126
  x-ray examination of, 387
Poisoning, and intensive care, 538
Polarization, of electrodes, 261
Polarography, 307
  for oxygen tension determination 154
Poliomyelitis:
  carriers of, 340
  and creatine in blood serum, 277
  infectious agent in, 327
  and muscular paralysis, 251
  vaccination against, 349
  virus, 327
Poly-, 7
Polyarthritis, *terminology,* 7
Polycythemia, 286
  example (Q 5.42), 290
Polyethylene, gas permeability of, 566
Polyneuritis, reflexes in, example (Q 2.107), 140
Polyp, of colon (*illus.*), 394
Polysaccharide(s):
  as antigen, 346
  terminology, 7
POMR, 641
Pons, 82
Portal circulation, *anatomy,* 60
Portal vein, *anatomy,* 60
Portio vaginalis, *anatomy,* 71
Positive contrast, 282
Posterior, *terminology,* 37

osterior axillary line, *terminology,*
110
ostnatal, *terminology,* 592
ostsynaptic potentials, 232
otassium, analysis of, 305, 307
otassium ions:
and acid-base balance, 573
in blood, 272
and electrolyte balance, 573
and heart fibrillation, 273
otentials, evoked, 265
otentiometry, 307
ower, *SI-unit,* 646
-R interval, 200
ecipitation, of antigens, 347, 355
efixes, *terminology,* 5
egnancy, pregnancies, 593-99
diagnosis of, 594
by fetal electrocardiography, 610
by ultrasonic method, 611
duration of, 597
extrauterine, 594
hormone, 595
intermittent bleeding during, 605
medication during, 493
number of, *terminology,* 592
signs of, 594
tests, 595
and thermography, 458
toxemia of, 605
ultrasonic method for monitoring,
183
egnancy periods, 592
emature child, *terminology,* 592
emedication, 508
example, 534
enatal, *terminology,* 592
epuce, *anatomy,* 69
eservation of tissues, 375
essure:
direct measurement in physical
diagnosis, 133
intracranial, 132
measurement in physical diagnosis,
132-136
SI unit, 646
essure necrosis, and electrosurgery,
521, (Q 10.48) 522
essure receptors, skin, 96
etransfusion testing, 370
eventive treatment, 485
imary tumor, 33
imigravida, 592
imipara, 592
octoscope, 118
ogesterone, 75
ognosis, in cholelithiasis, 534
ogression of disease, 10
ogressive muscular dystrophy, 252
and creatine in blood serum, 277
onation, *terminology,* 41
ophylactic treatment, 485
ostat-, 71
ostate gland, *anatomy,* 69
ostatic hypertrophy, treatment of,
example (Q 9.23–9.26), 487
ostatitis, *terminology,* 71 (Q 1.298)
71
ostatomegaly, *terminology,* 71

Prosthesis:
implantation of, 527
materials for, 528
Protein(s):
absorption in intestines, 277
analysis by electrophoresis, 308
as antigen, 346
in blood serum (*table*), 280
breakdown of, 299
Protein error, in absorption
photometry, 304
Proteinuria, 296
in toxemia of pregnancy, 605
Proteus, and hospital infections, 342
Prothrombin, 291
Prothrombin activity, 292
Prothrombin time, 292
Proximal, *terminology,* 37
Pseudomonas, and hospital infec-
tions, 342
Psittacosis, infectious agent in, 326
Psychiatry, *definition,* 230
Psychic blindness, 81
Psychic shock, 558
Psychopathy, *terminology,* 9
Psychosomatic, 10
Psychosomatic diseases, therapy of,
486
Psychotherapy, 486
Pulmonary artery:
anatomy, 59
pressure in, 164
Pulmonary circulation, *anatomy,* 58
Pulmonary edema, 28
and diffusion, 145
in left ventricular failure, 497
ventilator treatment of, 548
Pulmonary embolus after abdominal
operation, example (Q1.270), 63
Pulmonary valve(s), 128
insufficiency, murmur, 131
stenosis, murmur, 131
Pulse:
absence of, sign of cardiac arrest,
554
pressure, 122
rate, 122
in hypovolemic shock, 558
during physical work, 227
rhythm, 122
type, 122
waves:
in arterial system, 172
reflection of, 173
Pulse frequency modulation in nerves,
20
Pupil:
anatomy, 97
dilated, sign of cardiac arrest, 554
Pupil size, in anesthesia, 511
Pupillary reflex, 138
Purkinje fibers, 195
Pus, 30
infectious agent specimen technique, 329
PVC, 196
Pyelitis:
example (Q 1.291), 69

terminology, 67
Pyel(o)-, 67
Pyelography:
intravenous, 396
retrograde, 396
Pyelonephritis:
infectious agent in, 324, 326
terminology, 67
Pyemia, 30
Pyloric orifice, *anatomy,* 52
Pyramidal tract, 80

QRS complex, 198
width of, 200
Quadriplegia, *terminology,* 9
Quality control of medical care, 636
Quanta, types of in diagnostic
radiology, 422-23
Quantitative radiological
measurements, 439-48
Quartz:
acoustic impedance, 464
density, 464
velocity of sound, 464

Rabies, infectious agent in, 327
rad, *definition,* 617
Radial artery, *anatomy,* 60
Radial deviation, *terminology,* 41
Radial nerve, paralysis of, example (Q
4.97), 258
Radiation, and latency time, 400
Radiation damage, signs of, 400
Radiation detection, in thermography,
460
Radiation sources, for x-ray spectrophotometry, 443
Radiation sterilization, 337
Radical operation, 533
Radiobiology, 619
terminology, 616
Radiocurability, 623
Radiograph, 378
depth of field of, 378
distortion of, 378
geometric enlargement of, 378
information content of, 416
as a shadow picture, 378
(*see also* X-ray image)
Radiographic information, and
hospital information systems,
639
Radiography:
and fluoroscopy, 378
integration time in, 421
Radioimmunological assay, 356
Radiology:
definition, 377
diagnostic, 377-478
Radiomimetic substances and
radiosensitivity, 623
Radionuclide therapy, 616
Radionuclides:
in radiotherapy, 616
visualization of organs with,
318-20, 449
Radiopacity, 382

Radiophysics, 624-30
  terminology, 616
Radioprotective substances, 622
Radiosensitivity, 623
  and cell environment, 622
  of x-ray object, 400
Radiosensitizers, 622
Radiotherapy, 615-34
  contour planning, 624
  dose measurement, 629
  and immunological reaction capacity, 620
  moving field irradiation, 628
  physical dose distribution, 625
  ray geometry, 628
  type of radiation, 625
Radius, *anatomy,* 44
Raynaud's disease, 457
RBE, 618
Reabsorption, in kidneys, 293
Reactor accident, example (Q 5.50), 292
Rebreathing system, 514
Receptors:
  baro-, 93
  chemo-, 90
  for muscle control, 49
  optical, 97
  pressure, 96
  taste, 97
  touch, 96
  warm and cold, 96
Recorder, liquid jet, 210
Recording techniques:
  in electrocardiography, 209
  in electroencephalography, 234
  in neurophysiology, 265
Rectal administration of drugs, 489
Rectal anesthesia, 508
Rectal temperature, 94
Rectilinear scanning, 450
Rectum:
  anatomy, 53
  palpation of, 110
  tumor, diagnosis of, 118
Red blood cells, 286-88
  diameter, 288
  frozen, 370
  hemolysis, 288
  life span of, 364
  number of, 287
  separation of, 369
  transfusion of, 360
  volume of, 184
Reddening, sign of inflammation, 30
Reductions, 500
Referred pain, 107
Reflexes, 77, 88
  absent, 139
  blink, in anesthesia, 511
  conditioned, 89
  corneal, 89, 138
  deep tendon, 138
  inborn, 89
  increased, 139
  monosynaptic, 89
  patellar, 89, 139
  in physical diagnosis, 138
  polysynaptic, 89

  pupillary, 89, 138
  sneezing, 89
  tendon jerk, 89
Regeneration, of tissues, 27
Regional anesthesia, 505
  in delivery, 603
Regression of disease, 10
Regulatory function(s):
  and blood, 271
  blood pressure, 92
  of body and intensive care, 570
  body temperature, 94
  compound, 90
  endocrine, 74
  failure in neurogenic shock, 558
  fluid and electrolyte balance, 293
  nervous, 77
  of parathyroid gland and calcium and phosphate ions, 273
  reflexes, 88
  ventilation, 90
Regulatory systems, 74
Regurgitation, cardiac, 128
Reinoculation, 330
Rejection, immunological, 526
Relative Biological Effectiveness, 618
rem, *definition,* 618
REM sleep, 244
Ren-, 67
Renal:
  terminology, 67
  (*see also* Kidneys)
Renal and urinary tract diseases, mortality, 484
Renal artery, *anatomy,* 67
Renal clearance, 175
Renal function, 293 (*see also* Kidneys)
Renal pelvis, *anatomy,* 67
Renograms, 319
Replacement transfusion, 360
Repolarization, of heart muscle fibers, 189
Reproduction of cells, 13
Reproductive system, 69
RES, 343
Resection, *terminology,* 530
Residual volume, 146
Resistance:
  bacterial, 332, 495
  due to insufficient antibiotic treatment, example (Q 9.46), 496
  SI unit, 647
Resolution, in ultrasonic imaging, 472
Resorption, impaired intestinal, 299
Respiration, 145-59
  and acid-base balance, 575
  during anesthesia, 509
  in anesthesia, 511
  and blood pH, 157
  and intensive care, 540-54
  monitoring in intensive care, 583
  purpose of, 142
  ventilatory volumes, 146
Respiratory acidosis, 157
  example (Q 3.62) 159, (Q 11.88) 576
  ventilator treatment, 546
Respiratory alkalosis, 157
  example (Q 3.60) 159, (Q 11.91) 577
  oxygenators, 566

  in ventilator treatment, 546
Respiratory arrest, sign of cardiac rest, 554
Respiratory center, 90
  narcotic effect on, example 3.62), 159
  paralyzation of, and intensive ca 540
Respiratory failure:
  and acid-base disturbance, 575
  intensive care of, 540
Respiratory movements, paradoxic example (Q 11.11), 544
Respiratory organs:
  mortality in diseases, 484
  x-ray examination of, 386
Respiratory system, 56
Respiratory work, 150-53
  elimination in ventilator treatme 546
Resuscitation:
  in myocardial infarction, 561
  of traffic accident victims, exam (Q 11.11–11.14), 544-45
Reticuloendothelial system, 343
  and synthesis of gamma globuli 280
Retina:
  anatomy, 97
  contrast discrimination of, 433
Retinal detachment:
  diagnosis of, 118
  operation, 521
Retro-, 7
Retrograde, *terminology,* 7
Retrograde catheterization, 164
Retrograde filling, of contr medium, 396
Retroperitoneal, *terminology,* 7
Retrosternal, *terminology,* 7
Rh immunization:
  during pregnancy, 364
Rh system, 364
Rheography, 187
Rheumatic diseases, *terminology,* 4
Rheumatic fever:
  and heart murmurs, example 2.90), 132
  laboratory finding in, example 5.3), 270
  and valvular heart disease, 497
Rheumatoid arthritis:
  cause of, 353
  and decalcification (*illus.*), 386
Rheumatology, *terminology,* 480
Rhodopsin, 98
Ribs, *anatomy,* 44
Ricksettsia, 325
Right atrium, *anatomy,* 59
Right bypass, 562
Right catheterization, 164
Right-left shunt (*illus.*), 178
Right ventricle, *anatomy,* 59
Right ventricular failure, 497
Rigor mortis, 141
Risk(s):
  in anesthesia, 517
  assessment of, in diagno radiology, 401

associated with cholecystectomy, 534
in blood transfusion, 370
in cardiac catheterization, 164
of confusion, in anesthesia, 518
of explosion, in anesthesia, 518
grounding of patient, 206
    example (Q 3.185), 208
in hyperbaric oxygen treatment, 552
of infection in peritoneal dialysis, 580
in instrumental extraction of fetus, 609
in intrauterine pressure recordings, 613
lung rupture in ventilator treatment, 547
myocardial damage during defibrillation, 218
pacemaker and ventricular fibrillation, 220, 222
in parenteral injection, 490
postoperative complications, 509
in radiological work (Q 13.25–13.26), 622
tissue damage from electrosurgery, 521
    examples (Q 10.48, 10.49, 10.50), 522-23
    through unreliable chemical analysis, 317
Rocky Mountain spotted fever, infectious agent in, 325
Rods, *anatomy*, 97
roentgens, *definition*, 617
Roller blood pump, 567
Rotation:
    in obstetrics, 607
    terminology, 41
Rouleaux, 288
Rupture, *terminology*, 34

Sacrum, *anatomy*, 44
Sagittal plane, 37
Saliva, bactericidal action of, 344
Salmonella bacteria, 324
Salping-, 71
Salpingitis:
    and sterility, (Q 1.299), 71-72
    terminology, 72
Salpingography, *terminology*, 71
Salt error, in absorption photometry, 304
-sarcoma, 33
Scalpel, 519
Scapula, *anatomy*, 44
Scapular line, *terminology*, 110
Scarlet fever:
    carriers of, 340
    incubation time, 326
Scattered radiation, 399
Scintillation detector dose measurement, 629
Scissors, use in surgery, 519
Sclera, *anatomy*, 97
Sclerosis, 27
Scoliosis, 44
-scope, 9

Scopolamine in premedication, 509
Screening, 482
    microbiological diagnosis, 358
Scrotum, *anatomy*, 69
Secondary sex characteristics, 76
Secondary tumor, 33
Secretion, in kidneys, 293
Section radiography, 427
Sedative effect, in heat therapy, 631
Seldinger's method, 162
Semicircular canals, *anatomy*, 100
Seminal vesicles, *anatomy*, 69
Sensitization, allergic, 351
Sensory center, in cerebral cortex, 81
Sensory epithelium, 16
Sensory organs, 96-100
Sensory pathways:
    definition, 77
    spinal, 84
Sepsis, 30
Septal defects, 177, (*illus.*), 178
Serological diagnosis, 355
Serological reactions, use of, 354
Serological tests, in tissue typing, 374
Serology, 354-57
Serous fluid, 28
Serum, 271
Severinghaus electrode (*illus.*), 155
Sex glands, radiosensitivity, 400
Sexual drive, 593
    regulation of, 75-76
Sexual intercourse, and pregnancy, 594
SGOT, 284
SGPT, 284
Sheep blood cells, sensitized, 595
Shin bone, *anatomy*, 45
Shingles, infectious agent in, 326
Shock, 557-60
    anaphylactic, 351, 558
    blood transfusion treatment, example (Q 7.4), 360
    cardiogenic, 557
    exhaustion, 558
    hemorrhagic, 557
    hypovolemic, 557
    irreversible, 558
    neurogenic, 558
    and potassium ions, 273
    prevention of, 558
        in anesthesia, 505
    psychic, 558
    supervision of, 558
    surgical, 558
    toxic, 558
    treatment of, 558
        by blood transfusion, 360
        treatment of acidosis in, 575
    types of, 557
Shortwave diathermy, in physical therapy, 631
Shoulder blade, *anatomy*, 44
Sigmoid colon, *anatomy*, 53
Sigmoidoscope, 118
Signal analysis:
    automatic:
        in electrocardiography, 214
        in electroencephalography, 246
Signal recording, for electrocardiography computer analysis, 214

Signs, of disease, 105
Silastic, prosthesis material, 528
Silicon rubber:
    gas permeability of, 566
    prosthesis material, 528
Silk, for suturing, 523
Simulation, of symptoms, 114
Sinister, *terminology*, 37
Sinus node, 194
SI units, internationally adopted, 645
Skeletal system, 42
Skeleton:
    amount of calcium in, 273
    anatomy, 44
    hereditary disorders, x-ray diagnosis of, 383
    hydroxyapatite in, 273
    tumors, radiosensitivity of, 623
    x-ray examination of, 383
    and x-ray image contrast, 381
Skin:
    anatomy, 72
    conductivity of, 203
    contact impedance of, 203
    epithelial tissue, 15
    function of, 72-73
    infrared photography of, 460
    radiosensitivity of, 400, 620, 624
    sensory system in, 96
    somatic sensory system, 96
    transplantation of, 526
Skin and its diseases, *terminology*, 480
Skin eruption(s):
    cause of, in children, example (Q 9.40), 494
    due to drug hypersensitivity, 493
Skin temperature, measured by thermography, 456
Skull, *anatomy*, 35
Sleep:
    and electroencephalogram (*illus.*), 237
    provocation of brain waves, 240
Sleep difficulties, and liver rhythm, example (Q 5.21), 279
Sleep physiology, and electroencephalogram, 244
Sleeping pills:
    overdose of, example (Q 3.62), 159
    poisoning, example (Q 11.91), 577
Smallpox:
    incubation time, 326
    infectious agent in, 326
    vaccination against, 349
Smell:
    of acetone in physical diagnosis (Q 2.66–2.67), 121-22
    in physical diagnosis, 121
Smoking, and arteriosclerosis, 498
Smooth muscle, 18
Sodium, analysis of, 305
Sodium bicarbonate, shock treatment with, 575
Sodium chloride, and fluid balance, 572
Sodium ions:
    in blood serum, 272
    and electrolyte balance, 573
Sodium lactate, shock treatment with, 575

Soft tissues:
  ultrasonic imaging of, 467
  and x-ray image contrast, 381
Solid angle, *SI unit,* 645
Somatic, 10
Somatic care, 479
Somatic sensory system, 73, 96
Somatize, 486
Spatial frequency, and electronic subtraction, 430
Spatial frequency content, of x-ray objects, 420
Specific symptoms, 105
Specimen-taking technique, infectious agent, 329
Spectral distribution of heat radiation from body, 455
Speech formation, 57
Sperm, 69
  survival time of, 594
  transport of, 594
Spikes and waves, 237
Spinal-, 78
Spinal anesthesia, 506
  terminology, 78
Spinal canal, x-ray examination of, 398
Spinal cord:
  anatomy, 82
  (*illus.*), 84
Spinal puncture, *terminology,* 46
Spine:
  anatomy, 44
  terminology, 46
Spine of scapula, 111
Spirochete, 324
Spirometer (*illus.*), 147
Spirometry:
  dynamic, 150
  static, 147
Spleen:
  position of (*illus.*), 112
  and RES, 343
  rupture of, examples (Q 2.45), 114, (Q 2.70) 123
Spongy bone, 42
Spontaneous abortion, 592
Spores, of bacteria, 335
Spore tests, sterilization, 336
Sputum, infectious agent specimen technique, 329
S-T depression and work capacity, 227
S-T interval, 198
Staining properties of bacteria, 324
Stainless steel, for suturing, 523
Standard bicarbonate, 575
Standard deviation, *definition,* 268
Stapes, *anatomy,* 99
Staphylococci, 324
  and hospital infections, 342
Starvation:
  and ketone bodies, 277
  and smell of acetone, example (Q 2.67), 122
Stasis, 28
Statistical calculations, in hospital information systems, 636
Steatorrhea, 300
  example (Q 5.81–5.82), 301
Stefan-Boltzmann's law, 455
Stenosis, 130

Sterile area, of operating suites, 502
Sterility, caused by infection (Q 1.296–1.300), 71-72
Sterilization, 336-38
  definition, 335
Sternal, *terminology,* 46
Sternal line, *terminology,* 110
Sternal puncture, *terminology,* 46
Sternum, *anatomy,* 44
Steroids:
  analysis of, 312
  in blood serum, 276
Stethoscope, 127
  electronic, 127
  frequency response of, 127, (*illus.*), 128
Still birth, *definition,* 592
Stimulation, pharmacological effect, 491
Stimuli, and coordination of reflexes, 77
Stomach:
  anatomy, 51
  bleeding, photography of, 454
  disorders, 299
  endocrine function of, 75
  hydrochloric acid production in, 299
  and pernicious anemia, 353
  position of (*illus.*), 112
  tumor:
    diagnosis of, 118
    example (Q 2.58), 120
Stomach cancer, and hyposecretion, 299
Stomach ulcer, x-ray examination of (*illus.*), 392
-stomy, 530
Stooping position, 541
Stratigraphy, 427
Streptococci, 324
Streptomycin, 495
Stress, and arteriosclerosis, 498
Striae, 595
Striated muscle, 18
Stroke volume, 160
Sub-, 7
Subacute, *terminology,* 7
Subclinical, *terminology,* 7
Subcortical centers, and synchronization of neurons, 233, 238
Subcutaneous, *terminology,* 73
Subcutaneous administration of drugs, 489
Subcutaneous tissue, *anatomy,* 72
Subdural hematoma, example (Q 8.184), 471
Subfebrile, 95
Subjective symptoms, 105
Sublingual administration of drugs, 489
Substance, amount of, *SI unit,* 646
Substitution therapy, 485, 491
Substrate competition:
  example (Q 9.36), 492
  pharmacological effect, 491
Subtraction:
  electronic, of x-ray images, 419
  photographic technique, 428
Suffixes, *terminology,* 9

Suggestion therapy, 486
Suicide, attempted:
  example (Q 10.33), 512
  intensive care of, 538
  sleeping pills, dialysis treatment of example (Q 11.95), 581
Super-voltage therapy, 616
Superficial, *terminology,* 39
Superior, *terminology,* 38
Superior vena cava, *anatomy,* 59
Supination, *terminology,* 41
Suppository, 489
Supraclavicular fossa, 110
Supraren-, 76
Suprarenal, *terminology,* 67, 76
Suprarenal glands, 75
Surface active components, disinfection by, 338
Surface anatomy, 110
Surface anesthesia, 505
Surface electrodes, neurophysiological, 260
Surfactant, 592
Surgery, 500-537
  electrosurgery, 520
  general, 500
  intensive care after, 539
  operating suite, 502
  planning of operation schedule, 50
  reconstructive, *terminology,* 500
  sponges, radiopaque marking of 535
  techniques, 518-30
  treatment principles, 501-30
    endocrine, 533
  working routines, 503
Surgical anesthesia, stage of, 512
Surgical diathermy, 520
Surgical diseases, examples of treatment, 530
Surgical nurse, working routine, 503
Surgical shock, 558
Surgicel, in hemostasis, 525
Suturing, 523
Sweat, bactericidal action of, 344
Sweat glands, excretory function of 67, 73
Swelling, sign of inflammation, 30
Symbiosis, between animals and bacteria, 323
Sympathetic ganglia, 88
Sympathetic ophthalmia, 353
Sympathetic system, 88
  and blood pressure regulation, 93
Symptomatic treatment, 485
Symptoms, 105
  simulation of, 114
Synapse, 21
Synaptic potentials, in nervous system, 231
Synthetic materials, for suturing, 523
Syphilis:
  and heart murmur, example (2.91), 132
  infectious agent in, 324
  light and pupillary reflexes (2.105), 140
  serological diagnosis, 355
  treatment of (Q 9.45), 496
Systemic circulation, *anatomy,* 58

Systole, 66, 128
Systolic pressure, 66

T wave, 198
Tachycardia, 122
Target volume, in radiotherapy, 624
Tarsus, *anatomy,* 36
Taste receptors, 97
⁹⁹ᵐTc, visualization of organs with, 449
Teflon, prosthesis material, 528
Telemetry, of electrocardiogram, 212
Teletherapy, 625
Temperature:
    measurement of, 136
    monitoring in intensive care, 587
    oral, 136
    rectal, 136
    regulation of, 94
    underarm, 136
Temporal lobe, *anatomy,* 79
Tendon sheath, treatment of infec-
    tion, example (Q 10.73), 532
Teratogenic effects, 493
Terminology:
    of diseases, general, 10
    of general anatomy, 35-42
    general medical, 2-35
    indicating location, 37
    movement of extremities, 40
    of organs, 35-100
    pathological, 27
    prefixes, 5
    suffixes, 9
    of tissues, 11-27
Testicles:
    anatomy, 69
    radiosensitivity, 620
Testo-, 71
Testosterone, 75
    terminology, 71
Tetanus:
    agent in, 325
    incubation time, 326
    and parathyroid glands, 74
    vaccination against, 349
Tetanus infection, 325
Tetracycline, 495
Thalamus, 82
THAM, shock treatment with, 575
Therapy:
    acid-base balance disorders, 574
    artificial ventilation, 540
    contrasexual, of tumors, 533
    dialysis, 577-82
    of electrolyte balance disorders, 573
    exchange transfusion, 365
    of fluid balance disorders, 572
    forms of, 485
    general principles, 485-94
    heat, 631-33
    hyperbaric oxygen, 551
    intensive care, 538-90
    internal medicine, 479-99
    nutrition in intensive care, 570
    obstetric care, 591-614
    physical, 631-33
    surgery, 500-37
    ventilator, 545

Thermistor, use in breathing rate
    monitoring, 583
Thermodilution method, 177
Thermography, 454-63
    image presentation in, 462
    medical applications of, 457
    physical basis of, 455
    radiation detection in, 460
Thermoluminescence dose measure-
    ment, 629
Theta waves, 237
Thigh, *anatomy,* 36
Thigh bone, *anatomy,* 45
Thirst, and salty food (Q 5.15), 274
Thoracic duct, *anatomy,* 61
Thoracic surgery, *terminology,* 500
Thoracic vertebrae, *anatomy,* 44
Thoracoscope, 118
Thorax, *anatomy,* 35
Throat:
    anesthesia for, 505
    infection:
        and glomerulonephritis, example
            (Q 5.69), 298
        infectious agent in, 324
        infectious agent specimen from, 329
Thrombin, 291
Thrombocytes, 24
    disorders of, 291
    reduced number of, 291
Thrombocytopenia, 291
    cause of, 353
    example (Q 5.50), 292
Thrombosis, venous, and temperature
    curve, example (Q 2.103), 138
Thrombus, 29, (Q 1.147) 29
Thymus, and antibodies, 346
Thyro-, 76
Thyrogenic, *terminology,* 76
Thyroid gland, 74
    determination of function, 318
    palpation of, 109
    visualization with radionuclides, 449
Thyroid hormones, 74
Thyroidectomy, *terminology,* 76
Thyroiditis, chronic, 353
Thyrotoxicosis, 114
Thyrotropic, *terminology,* 76
Thyroxin, 74
Tibia, *anatomy,* 45
Ticks, vector of infection, 325
Tidal volume, 145, 146
Time, *SI unit,* 646
Tissue(s), 11
    adipose, 17
    breakdown and composition of
        urine, 295
    connective, 17
    degeneration of, 27
    epithelial, 15
    fetal, radiosensitivity of, 400
    fibrous, 17
    glial, 20
    imaging of structures, 464
    inflammation of, 30
    inflammatory reaction by sutures,
        523
    liquid, 23
    muscular, 18

nerve, 20
    radiosensitivity of, 400, 619
    regeneration of, 27
    soft, and x-ray image contrast, 381
    storage, 375
    terminology, 11-27
    transfer of, *terminology,* 530
    types of, 15-26
    typing of, 374
Tissue compartments, determination
    of, 184
Tissue damage:
    and enzyme diagnosis, 284
    from incorrect electrosurgery, 521
        examples (Q 10.48, 10.49, 10.50),
        522-23
Tissue fluid, 61
Titration, serological, 355
To-and-fro system, 514
Toes, *anatomy,* 36
Tomography:
    computer-assisted, 449
    computerized axial, 447
    computerized transverse, 449
    x-ray, 427
    -tomy, 530
Topical anesthesia, 505
Topographical anatomy, *terminology,*
    35
Total block, 196
Touch receptors, skin, 96
Toxemia, 30
    of pregnancy, 605
        example (Q 12.36–12.37), 606
        treatment of, 605
Toxi-, 7
Toxic effects, of drugs, 493
Toxic goiter, 114
Toxic shock, 558
Toxicity, *terminology,* 7
Toxicology, *terminology,* 7
Toxicosis, *terminology,* 7
Toxin(s):
    and bleeding, 291
    and hemolysis, 288
    inactivated, 349
    precipitation of, 347
    terminology, 7
Toxo-, 7
Toxoid, 349
Toxoplasmosis, infectious agent in,
    324
Trabecular bone, 42
Trachea:
    anatomy, 56, 57
    tumor, diagnosis of, 118
Tracheotomy:
    in intensive care, 540
    ventilator treatment, 545
Traffic accident, example (Q
    11.11–11.14), 544-45
Transducer(s):
    for blood pressure measurement,
        171
    pressure,
        compliance of, 171
        types of, 172
Transfusion reaction, hemolytic, 362,
    370
Transmitter substances, 21

Transplantation, 372-76
  antigens, 374
  and blood groups, 374
  and hepatitis B, 342
  immunology, 526
  techniques, 525
  terminology, 530
Transseptal catheterization, 164
Transverse colon, *anatomy,* 53
Transverse plane, 37
Transverse presentation, 601
Trauma, *terminology,* 34
Traumatology, *terminology,* 34
Travenol kidney, 580
Treatment, forms of, 485
Treatment planning, in radiotherapy, 624
Treatment principles, 485-94
Tricuspid valve, 128
  insufficiency, murmur in, 131
  stenosis, murmur in, 131
Triglycerides, in blood serum, 276
Tris, shock treatment with, 575
Tris-hydroxymethyl-amino methane, shock treatment with, 575
-trophy, 9
Trypsin, 299
Tubercle bacilli, and hospital infections, 342
Tuberculin reaction, 351
Tuberculosis:
  cultivation of infectious agent, 333-34
  incubation time, 326
  infectious agent in, 324
  intestinal, route of infection, 325
  mortality for, 495
  vaccination against, 349
Tubule, 293
Tumor(s):
  and anemia, 286
  benign, 32
  brain:
    diagnosis of, 139
    and electrical activity, 243
    ultrasonic diagnosis of, 467
  in central nervous system, x-ray examination of, 398
  choice of radiation in radiotherapy of, 625
  colon (Q 1.171), 34
  diseases, 32
    investigation and treatment of, example (Q 9.9–9.16), 483
    mortality, 484
    surgical treatment of, 532
  dose in radiotherapy, 624
  expansive growth, 32
  gastrointestinal, x-ray examination of, 395
  immunology, 354
  implantation, 32
  infiltrative growth, 32
  intestinal, example (Q 5.65–5.77), 300
  lung, x-ray examination of, 387
  malignant, 32
    spontaneous healing of, 620
  metastases, 33
  primary, 33

radiocurability of, 623
radiosensitivity of, 619, 623
resistance to, 354
secondary, 33
sensitivity to radiation, 32
spread of, 32
and thermography, 458
vaccine, 354
visualization with radionuclides, 449
Two-corridor system, in operating suite, 503
2-D reconstruction, 449
Tympanic membrane, 99
  infection, diagnosis of, 118
Tympanitic percussion note, 125
Typhus:
  infectious agent in, 325
  vaccination against, 349

Ulcer:
  gastrointestinal, x-ray examination of, 395
  terminology, (Q 1.248), 55
Ulcerative colitis:
  cause of, 353
  example (Q 2.62), 121
Ulna, *anatomy,* 44
Ulnar, artery, *anatomy,* 60
Ulnar deviation, terminology, 41
Ultrafiltration, in dialysis, 578
Ultrasonic diagnosis:
  in fetal monitoring, 611
  medical applications, 467-71
  of placenta previa, 605
  technical aspects of, 472
Ultrasonic Doppler, in automatic blood pressure measurement, 585
Ultrasonic flowmeters, 182
Ultrasonic imaging, 463-77
  A-scan, 464
  compound B-scan, 466
  distortion, 475
  linear B-scan, 464
  physical principles, 463
  resolution, 472
Ultrasonic irradiation, depth of penetration in physical therapy, 633
Ultrasonic therapy, 631
Ultrasonic tomogram, 465
Ultrasound, attenuation in tissues, 473
Umbilical cord, 596
  complications during pregnancy and delivery, 604
  prolapse of, 605
Umbilical plane, 37
Unconsciousness, sign of cardiac arrest, 554
Unipolar technique:
  in electrocardiography, 191
  in electroencephalography, 235
Universal donor (*illus.*), 364
Universal recipient (*illus.*), 364
Unsterile area, of operating suites, 502
Urea, 277
  analysis of, 307

Urease, 307
Uremia, 577
  due to drug hypersensitivity, 493
  terminology, 24, 67
Uretero-, 67
Ureters:
  anatomy, 67
  x-ray examination of (*illus.*), 397
Urethra:
  anatomy, 67, 69
  anesthesia for, 505
  infectious agent specimen from, 32
  x-ray examination, 396
Urethritis, *terminology,* 68
Urethr(o)-, 68
Urethrocystography, 396
Uric acid, and gout, 295
Urinary bladder:
  anatomy, 67
  anesthesia for, 505
  tumor, diagnosis of, 118
  x-ray examination of, 396 (*illus.*), 397
Urinary obstruction, x-ray examination of, 396
Urinary organs, diseases of *terminology,* 500
Urinary tract:
  and hospital infections, 342
  infections, peroral treatment of, 48
  stones, diagnosis of, 118
  x-ray examination of, 396
Urine, 293-98
  composition of, 295
  infectious agent specimen technique, 329
  poisoning of the blood *terminology,* 67
  port-colored, 534
  sediment analysis of, 296
Ur(o)-, 68
Urobilin, 278
Urobilinogen, 277
Urographic examination (*illus.*), 397
Urography, 396
Urology, *terminology,* 500
Uterine cervix, *anatomy,* 71
Uterus:
  anatomy, 70
  contractions during delivery, 599
  growth of in pregnancy, 593
  intrauterine pressure, monitoring during delivery, 613
  and pregnancy, 593
  ultrasonic imaging of pregnant, 46

Vaccination, 349
Vaccine, against tumor, 354
Vacuum extraction, of fetus, 608
Vagina, *anatomy,* 71
Vagus nerve, 83
  and blood pressure regulation, 93
Valve system:
  of heart, 128
    defects, x-ray examination of, 389
Van de Graaf generators, 616
Vaporizer, for liquid anesthetics. 51

aricose veins, gastrointestinal, x-ray examination of, 395
ascular damage, due to drug hypersensitivity, 493
ascularization, *terminology,* 62
as(o)-, 62
asoconstriction, 93
 terminology, 62
asodilation, 93
 terminology, 62
asodilators, in arteriosclerosis, 498
asomotor, *terminology,* 62
asomotor centers, failure in neurogenic shock, 558
ectorcardiography, 210
 loops, 211
 redundancy in, 212
ein(s):
 anatomy, 60
 axillary (*illus.*), 60
 brachial (*illus.*), 60
 femoral (*illus.*), 60
 great saphenous (*illus.*), 60
 iliac (*illus.*), 60
 inferior vena cava (*illus.*), 60
 jugular (*illus.*), 60
 left subclavian, *anatomy,* 61
 popliteal (*illus.*), 60
 portal (*illus.*), 60
 radial (*illus.*), 60
 right subclavian, *anatomy,* 61
 subclavian, *anatomy,* 61
 superficial, infrared photography of, 454
 superior vena cava (*illus.*), 60
 ulnar (*illus.*), 60
 vena cava, *anatomy,* 59
 x-ray examination of, 391
\elocity, *SI unit,* 646
\elocity of sound (*table*), 464
\ena cava, *anatomy,* 59
\enereal diseases, *terminology,* 480
\enerology, *terminology,* 480
\en(o)-, 62
\enous blood, mixed, sampling of, 164
\enous occlusion plethysmography, 186
\enous thrombosis, abdominal operation, example (Q 1.269), 63
\ntilation, 142, 145
 adequate in ventilator treatment, 545
 alveolar, 145
 determination of, 154
 artificial, 145, 540
 control of, 90
 controlled, in anesthesia, 513
 monitoring in intensive care, 583
 in operating rooms, 502
 spontaneous, in anesthesia, 513
 work required, 150
\ntilators, 545
 compression loss in, 549
 flow-limited, 546
 pressure-limited, 546
 servo-controlled, 548
 volume-limited, 547
\ntilatory volumes, 146
\ntral, *terminology,* 37

Ventral roots, 83
Ventricles, brain, 82
Ventricular diastole, 128
Ventricular fibrillation, 196
 cause, 217
 by electric current, 207
 in hypothermia, 564
Ventricular septal defect, 177 (*illus.*), 178
Ventricular systole, 128
Ventriculography, 398
Vertebra, *anatomy,* 44
Vertebral column, *anatomy,* 44
Vertex presentation, 601
Vesicular breathing, 127
Vesicular sound, 127
Vessels:
 communication between, *terminology,* 530
 prosthesis, 528
 sewing in transplantation, 525
Vestibulocochlear nerve, 83
Virology, 322
Viruses, 325-29
 classification of, 325, 334
 culture technique, 334
 exanthem, 326
 inhibition of synthesis of, 344
 neurotropic, 326
 respiratory, 326
 size of, 325
Viscera:
 anatomy, 35
 position of:
  relation to skeleton (*illus.*), 112
  relation to surface anatomy, 111
Visual acuity, 98
Visual center, *anatomy,* 81
Visual pathways, 81
Visual sense, 97
Visualization of organs by radionuclides, 318
Vital capacity, 147
Vitallium, 528
Vitamins, analysis of, 305
Vitamin B_{12} deficiency, 286, 353
Vitamin C deficiency, and bleeding, 291
Vitamin D deficiency, x-ray diagnosis of, 383
Vitamin K, and clotting time, 292
Vitreous humor, *anatomy,* 97
Vocal cords, *anatomy,* 57
Volume, *SI unit,* 645
Vomiting:
 alkalosis due to, example (Q 3.59), 159
 and intravenous nutrition, 571
Vulnerable period, heart, 217-18

Warm and cold receptors, skin, 96
Warm baths, in physical therapy, 631
Warmth, sign of inflammation, 30
Wassermann reaction, 355
Water:
 body, total amount of, 185
 circulation of, 26
 excretion of, 67
Water balance, and sodium ions, 272

Wedging, during catheterization, 164
White blood cells, 288
 function of, 289
 microscopic examination of, 289
White substance, 77
Whole blood, 360
Whooping cough:
 antibody against, 349
 in infant (Q 9.44), 496
 mortality for, 495
Widal's reaction, 355
Wien's displacement law, 455
Word deafness, 81
Work, *SI unit,* 646
Work capacity:
 of extremities, and circulation, 186
 physical, 227-28
Wound, *terminology,* 34
Wounds:
 infected:
  immobilization of, 529
  infectious agent in, 324
 treatment of, anesthesia for, 506
W.R., 355
Wrist, *anatomy,* 36

X-ray radiation, in radiotherapy, 626
X-ray collimators, 408
X-ray diagnosis, 377-449
X-ray examination:
 of children, and exposure time, 399
 of organs, 383-98
X-ray film, 413
 contrast, 414
 densitometry, 439
 density, 414
 exposure latitude, 431
 gamma value, 415
 number of developable grains, 413-14
X-ray fluorescent screens, and transmission of information, 423
X-ray fluoroscopic screens, efficiency of, 411
X-ray generators, 402-10
X-ray grids, 408
X-ray intensifying screens, 413
X-ray image:
 computerized tomography, 447
 contrast, 416
  and choice of tube voltage, 380
  definition, 425
  and modulation transfer function, 418
 contrast resolution and noise, 423
 demands:
  on resolution, 399
  on short exposure time, 399
 detection, 410-15
 dodging, 430
 dose and information, 400, 421-27
 electronic subtraction, 429
 and exposure time, 399
 information and number of quanta, 421-27
 information content, 380, 416
 information selection, 427
 integration time, 421
 intentional unsharpness, 428

673

methods for recording, 413
movement unsharpness, 419
noise content, 421
noise level, 423
number of quanta in forming, 422-23
perceivable contrast, 425
primary dodging, 431
and pulsation of organs, 399
resolution, 416, 418
    and quantum noise, 425
secondary dodging, 431
size of image elements, 425
spatial intensity gradient, 434
subtraction, 428
tomography, 427
types of quanta in forming, 422-23
unsharpness, 416
unwanted spatial frequency, 430
X-ray image intensifier(s), 411
    and modulation transfer function, 419

number of photons absorbed, 423
and transmission of information, 423
X-ray investigation:
    and field size, 408
    scattered radiation, and image contrast, 408
    skin dose, 405
X-ray modulation transfer function, 418
X-ray object(s):
    composition and spectrophotometry, 443
    elementary composition of, 399
    physical properties of, 399
    radiosensitivity of, 400
    spatial frequency content of, 420
X-ray photofluorography, 415
X-ray photospot filming, 415
X-ray screens, types of, 414
X-ray spectrophotometry, 442-47
X-ray techniques, 399-416

X-ray television system, 411
    and modulation transfer function, 419
X-ray therapy, 616
X-ray tubes, 402
    bremsstrahlung, 405
    characteristic radiation, 407
    energy distribution, 405-7
    focal spot, 402
    focus and modulation transfer function, 418
    generation efficiency, 403
    heel effect, 441
    inherent filtration of, 403
    line focus, 404
    load, 403
    output of, 402
        and type of rectification, 404
    thermal focus, 404
X-ray videotape system, 415
Xylocaine, in myocardial infarction, 561